Management of Chronic Kidney Disease

Mustafa Arici
Editor

Management of Chronic Kidney Disease

A Clinician's Guide

Springer

Editor
Mustafa Arici, MD
Department of Nephrology
Faculty of Medicine
Hacettepe University
Ankara
Turkey

ISBN 978-3-662-52294-3 ISBN 978-3-642-54637-2 (eBook)
DOI 10.1007/978-3-642-54637-2
Springer Heidelberg New York Dordrecht London

Printed on acid-free paper

Springer is part of Springer Science+Business Media (www.springer.com)

To my admirable wife Esra, and my lovely daughters Ayse and Zeynep, for their love, support, time and patience, but above all, for them being "all my reasons" for life

To my parents and brothers, for their continuous love, encouragement and wisdom

Preface

> To study the phenomena of disease without books is to sail an uncharted sea, while to study books without patients is not to go to sea at all.
>
> William Osler

I am very pleased to offer the first edition of *Management of Chronic Kidney Disease: A Clinician's Guide*. Actually, there are many textbooks devoted to general nephrology or books that are particularly focused on dialysis or renal transplantation. However, there is a real deficiency of books devoted particularly to the care of chronic kidney disease (CKD) patients. This book attempts to fulfill this gap by providing a comprehensive, guideline-based, practice-oriented management plan for physicians who continuously take care of adult CKD patients.

Chronic kidney disease is now a significant public health problem worldwide. CKD globally affects almost 10 % of general population. Incidence and prevalence of CKD figures are still rising especially in developing countries. The rise in CKD figures are fuelled by aging of the populations and growing problems of obesity, diabetes, high blood pressure and cardiovascular diseases. Today, the number of CKD patients from stage 1 to 5 not on dialysis exceeds the number of patients with end-stage renal disease (ESRD) by a factor of 50–100. Practicing nephrologists come across much more CKD patients than dialysis or renal transplantation cases. CKD management is, therefore, a major item in the agenda of nephrology practice, and its pressure will increase more in the following years. Physicians in the other disciplines will also see more CKD patients in their daily practice due to increasing prevalence of CKD. This book covers adult CKD patients, starting from "at risk" for CKD to CKD stage 5 not on renal replacement therapies. The book's major target audience is nephrologists and residents/fellows and attending physicians in nephrology. The book, however, may also serve as a multidisciplinary resource for many doctors, including family physicians, internists, endocrinologists, cardiologists, and geriatrists, who frequently encounter many CKD patients at earlier stages.

The book is intended to cover the whole journey of a CKD patient as:

- Defining and diagnosing CKD
- Assessing and controlling risk factors of CKD
- Stopping/slowing progression in CKD
- Assessing and managing complications of CKD
- Caring for CKD patients under special conditions
- Caring for CKD patients just before initiating renal replacement therapies

In the book, diagnostic and therapeutic approaches were presented according to latest staging system of CKD, from earlier to late stages. The book have some novel chapters such as "Quality of Life in CKD", "Pain Management in CKD", "CKD in Intensive Care Unit", "CKD and Cancer", "CKD Management Programs and Patient Education" and "Conservative/Palliative Treatment and End-of-Life Care in CKD". These chapters aim to complement some neglected but substantial steps in CKD care. In this book, many special chapters were written by non-nephrologists but specialists of that particular field like radiologists, cardiologists, neurologists, surgeons, obstetricians, dermatologists, psychiatrists, etc. As CKD care needs a multidisciplinary action, this book intends to increase communication between different disciplines while looking after the same CKD patient.

All chapters start and end with boxes titled as "Before You Start: Facts You Need to Know" and "Before You Finish: Practice Pearls for the Clinician". Most chapters have also "What the Guidelines Say You Should Do?" and "Relevant Guidelines" boxes for easy access to guidelines and guideline recommendations. These boxes will suffice to distill "practical practice pearls" from the bulky volumes of guidelines and other sources of information with a "5-min attention" of busy clinicians. Each chapter has a very selective list of references restricted to 15–20 in maximum. I encourage all who use this book to send their suggestions and comments both for the content and the design of the book.

The book is intended for a global coverage of CKD problem. The contributing authors are world-known experts in their fields and act as executive members of many national and international associations in nephrology. Most authors have participated in writing guidelines on CKD.

This book will not be possible were it not for so many people. Firstly, I have been fortunate that many distinguished authors, colleagues and friends have kindly accepted to contribute to this book. I would like to take this opportunity to thank them all very warmly. They have generously spent their most valuable hours to produce high-quality and up-to-date chapters. They were very considerate and rigorous during the review processes. Secondly, I would like to express my sincere gratitude to Portia Levasseur, the Developmental Editor for the book. Without her excellent support and enthusiasm, it will be impossible to hold this book in your hands. Last but not least, I thank all the staff of Springer, but particularly Sandra Lesny who gave me the opportunity to edit this book.

I also would like to acknowledge my mentors, colleagues, my residents/fellows and my students in Hacettepe University. I have learned many things from them and they helped me to be who I am. My major inspiration in nephrology practice is seeing the joy in the faces of patients when their CKD progression were slowed down or halted completely. It is a privilege for me to care for them and they have been the powerful source of my motivation, dynamism and knowledge.

Increasing the awareness of CKD, mounting the chances for early recognition and definition of CKD and managing better for preventing or delaying/halting progression of CKD and its complications were major aims of this book. If the readers will apply at least some of those to their clinical practice, the editor and the authors will feel rewarded for their efforts.

Ankara, Turkey Mustafa Arici

Contents

Contributors

Marcin Adamczak, MD, PhD Department of Nephrology, Endocrinology and Metabolic Diseases, Medical University of Silesia, Katowice, Poland

Rajiv Agarwal, MD, FASN, FAHA, FASH Department of Medicine, Indiana University School of Medicine, Indianapolis, IN, USA

Mustafa Arici, MD Department of Nephrology, Faculty of Medicine, Hacettepe University, Ankara, Turkey

Zülfikar Arlier, MD Neurology Department, Baskent University Medical Faculty, Adana Teaching and Research Hospital, Adana, Turkey

Ria Arnold, BS Department of Neurological Sciences, Prince of Wales Hospital, Sydney, NSW, Australia

Sean M. Bagshaw, MD, MSc, FRCPC Department of Critical Care Medicine, Faculty of Medicine and Dentistry, University of Alberta, Clinical Sciences Building, Edmonton, AB, Canada

Guido Bellinghieri, MD Department Clinical and Experimental Medicine, University of Messina, Messina, Italy

Edwina A. Brown, DM (Oxon), FRCP Imperial College Kidney and Transplant Centre, Hammersmith Hospital, London, UK

Jorge B. Cannata-Andía, MD, PhD Bone and Mineral Research Unit, Hospital Universitario Central de Asturias, Instituto Reina Sofía de Investigación (REDinREN-ISCIII), Oviedo, Asturias, Spain

Natalia Carrillo-López, PhD Bone and Mineral Research Unit, Hospital Universitario Central de Asturias, Instituto Reina Sofía de Investigación (REDinREN-ISCIII), Postdoctoral Fellow Hospital Universitario Central de Asturias, Oviedo, Asturias, Spain

Devasmita Choudhury, MD Department of Medicine, University of Virginia, Salem VA Medical Center, Salem, VA, USA

Kai Ming Chow, MBChB, FRCP Division of Nephrology, Department of Medicine and Therapeutics, Prince of Wales Hospital, Chinese University of Hong Kong, Hong Kong, China

Ricardo Correa-Rotter, MD Department of Nephrology and Mineral Metabolism, Instituto Nacional de Ciencias Médicas y Nutrición Salvador Zubirán, Mexico City, DF, Mexico

John M. Davison, MD, FRCPE, FRCOG Institute of Cellular Medicine, Royal Victoria Infirmary and Newcastle University, Newcastle upon Tyne, Tyne and Wear, UK

Sara N. Davison, MD, MSc Department of Medicine and Dentistry, University of Alberta Hospital, Edmonton, AB, Canada

Rosa Maria De Santo Italian Institute for Philosophical Studies, Naples, Italy

Garabed Eknoyan, MD Department of Medicine, Baylor College of Medicine, Houston, TX, USA

Andrew Ferguson, MB, BCh, BAO, Med, FRCA, FFICM Department of Anaesthetics, Craigavon Area Hospital, Portadown, Co. Armagh, UK

Pedro Fidalgo, MD Division of Critical Care Medicine, Faculty of Medicine and Dentistry, University of Alberta, Clinical Sciences Building, Edmonton, AB, Canada

Semih Giray, MD Neurology Department, Baskent University Medical FacultyAdana Teaching and Research Hospital, Adana, Turkey

Coral Graham, MSc School of Nursing and Midwifery, De Montfort University, Leicester, UK

Kevin Harris, MD, MB, BS, FRCP John Walls Renal Unit, Leicester General Hospital, University Hospitals of Leicester, Leicester, UK

S. Susan Hedayati, MD, MHSc Division of Nephrology, Department of Internal Medicine, University of Texas Southwestern Medical Center and Veterans Affairs North Texas Health Care System, Dallas, TX, USA

Jean L. Holley, MD Department of Internal Medicine and Nephrology, University of Illinois, Urbana-Champaign and Carle Physician Group, Urbana, IL, USA

Joshua S. Hundert, MD Renal Division, Department of Medicine, Brigham and Women's Hospital, Boston, MA, USA

T. Alp Ikizler, MD Division of Nephrology, Department of Medicine, Vanderbilt University School of Medicine, Nashville, TN, USA

Michel Jadoul, MD Department of Nephrology, Cliniques Universitaires Saint-Luc, Université catholique de Louvain, Brussels, Belgium

Nishank Jain, MD, MPH Division of Nephrology, Department of Internal Medicine, University of Texas Southwestern Medical, Dallas, TX, USA

Vivekanand Jha, MD, DM, FRCP Department of Nephrology, Postgraduate Institute of Medical Education and Research, Chandigarh, India

Jan T. Kielstein, MD Department of Nephrology and Hypertension, Hannover Medical School, Hannover, Germany

Jeffrey A. Kraut, MD Division of Nephrology, VHAGLA Healthcare System, Los Angeles, CA, USA

UCLA Membrane Biology Laboratory, David Geffen UCLA School of Medicine, Los Angeles, CA, USA

Arun V. Krishnan, MBBS, PhD, FRACP Department of Neurology, Prince of Wales Hospital, Sydney, NSW, Australia

Vivek Kumar, MBBS, MD, DM Department of Nephrology, Postgraduate Institute of Medical Education and Research, Chandigarh, India

Vincent Launay-Vacher, PharmD Service ICAR – Department of Nephrology, Pitié-Salpetrière University Hospital, Paris, France

Jenna Lester, BA Department of Dermatology, Warren Alpert Medical School of Brown University, Providence, RI, USA

Moshe Levi, MD Department of Internal Medicine/Division of Renal Diseases and Hypertension, University of Colorado Denver AMC, Aurora, CO, USA

Philip Kam-tao Li, MD, FRCP, FACP Department of Medicine and Therapeutics, Princes of Wales Hospital, Chinese University of Hong Kong, Hong Kong, China

Peter Marckmann, MD, DMSc Department of Nephrology, Roskilde Hospital, Roskilde, Denmark

Peter A. McCullough, MD, MPH Department of Cardiovascular Medicine, Baylor Heart and Vascular Institute, Baylor University Medical Center, Baylor Jack and Jane Hamilton Heart and Vascular Hospital, Dallas, TX, USA

The Heart Hospital, Plano

Rachael L. Morton, MScMed(Clin Epi)(Hons), PhD Sydney School of Public Health, University of Sydney, Sydney, NSW, Australia

Nuffield Department of Population Health, Health Economics Research Centre, University of Oxford, Headington, Oxfordshire, UK

Mohammad Nasser, MD Department of Internal Medicine, Providence Hospitals and Medical Centers, Southfield, MI, USA

Yousef W. Nielsen, MD, PhD Department of Diagnostic Radiology, Copenhagen University Hospital, Herlev, Denmark

Kosaku Nitta, MD, PhD Department of Medicine, Kidney Center, Tokyo Women's Medical University, Shinjuku-ku, Tokyo, Japan

Sharidan K. Parr, MD Division of Nephrology and Hypertension, Department of Medicine, Vanderbilt University Medical Center, Nashville, TN, USA

Rajeev Raghavan, BS, MD Department of Medicine, Department of Medicine, Baylor College of Medicine, Houston, TX, USA

Juan C. Ramírez-Sandoval, MD Department of Nephrology and Mineral Metabolism, Instituto Nacional de Ciencias Médicas y Nutrición Salvador Zubirán, Mexico City, DF, Mexico

Stephanie Riggen, MD Department of Medicine, Indiana University School of Medicine, Indianapolis, IN, USA

Leslie Robinson-Bostom, MD Division of Dermatopathology, Warren Alpert Medical School of Brown University, Providence, RI, USA

Department of Dermatology, Rhode Island Hospital, Providence, RI, USA

Minerva Rodríguez-García, MD, PhD Department of Nephrology, Hospital Universitario Central de Asturias REDinREN, Oviedo, Spain

Domenico Santoro, MD Department Clinical and Experimental Medicine, University of Messina, Messina, Italy

Ersilia Satta, MD Department Clinical and Experimental Medicine, University of Messina, Messina, Italy

Rebecca J. Schmidt, DO Department of Medicine, Nephrology Section, West Virginia University School of Medicine, Morgantown, WV, USA

Susan Sharman, DiPHE, BA John Walls Renal Unit – Renal Community Team, Leicester General Hospital, Leicester, UK

Edward D. Siew, MD, MSCI Division of Nephrology and Hypertension, Department of Medicine, Vanderbilt University Medical Center, Nashville, TN, USA

Ajay K. Singh, MBBS, MBA Renal Division, Brigham and Women's Hospital, Boston, MA, USA

Merlin C. Thomas, MBChB, PhD, FRACP Department of Biochemistry of Diabetes Complications, Baker IDI Heart and Diabetes Institute, Melbourne, VIC, Australia

Henrik S. Thomsen, MD, DMSc Department of Diagnostic Radiology, Copenhagen University Hospital, Herlev, Denmark

Faculty of Medical and Health Sciences, University of Copenhagen, Copenhagen, Denmark

José-Vicente Torregrosa, MD Department of Nephrology and Renal Transplant, Hospital Clinic REDinREN, University of Barcelona, Barcelona, Spain

Richard M. Treger, MD Division of Nephrology, Department of Internal Medicine, VHAGLA Healthcare System, Los Angeles, CA, USA

David Geffen School of Medicine, UCLA, Los Angeles, CA, USA

Meryem Tuncel Kara, MD Department of Internal Medicine, University of Connecticut School of Medicine/John Dempsey Hospital, Internal Medicine/Calhoun Cardiology Center, University of Connecticut Health Center, Farmington, CT, USA

Angela C. Webster, MBBS MM (Clin Epid) PhD Sydney School of Public Health, University of Sydney, Sydney, NSW, Australia

Centre for Transplant and Renal Research, Westmead Hospital, Sydney, NSW, Australia

Caroline West, MBChB, MRCP, FCARCSI Department of Anaethetics, Craigavon Area Hospital, Portadown, Co.Armagh, UK

Andrzej Więcek, MD, PhD, FRCP (Edin), FERA Department of Nephrology, Endocrinology and Metabolic Diseases, Medical University of Silesia, Katowice, Poland

Sarah Winfield, MBBS, MRCOG Department of Obstetrics and Gynaecology, Leeds Teaching Hospitals NHS Trust, Leeds General Infirmary, Leeds, West Yorkshire, UK

Rahmi Yilmaz, MD Department of Nephrology, Hacettepe University Hospital, Medical Faculty of Hacettepe University, Ankara, Turkey

Part I

Chronic Kidney Disease: Basics and Clinical Assessment

What Is Chronic Kidney Disease?

1

Rajeev Raghavan and Garabed Eknoyan

Before You Start: Facts You Need to Know

- Chronic kidney disease (CKD) is defined as having abnormalities of kidney structure or function for at least 3 months with implications for the health of the individual.
- CKD is classified based on cause (C), GFR category (G; G1 to G5), and albuminuria (A; A1 to A3).
- CKD is common (1 in 10 adults, 500 million persons worldwide), harmful, treatable, and a major public health problem worldwide.
- CKD is easily diagnosed from urinalysis and the estimated GFR (eGFR) calculated from serum creatinine.
- There is a strong graded and consistent relationship between the severity of the two hallmarks of CKD: reduced eGFR and increased albuminuria.
- CKD is more common in the elderly, males, and individuals of African or Latino descent.
- Detection of CKD is best accomplished with serial measurements of blood pressure, serum creatinine, and urinalysis in select populations at a higher risk of disease.

1.1 Introduction

Diseases of the kidney have afflicted humans from time immemorial. Medical interest in the detection and treatment of kidney disease can be traced to antiquity, but all past efforts have been fragmentary and almost entirely focused on its symptomatic manifestations as a change in urine color (hematuria) and flow (obstruction) or pain due to stones or obstruction. It is only in the past decade that the actual burden of kidney disease has been documented and identified as a global public health problem [1, 2].

The traditional lineage of detecting and defining kidney disease is traced to Richard Bright (1789–1858), who in 1827 described the autopsy findings of the kidneys in 24 albuminuric, dropsical patients who had died of kidney failure. Bright considered his disease an inflammatrory lesion (nephritis) that was rather rare as reflected in his statement that "Inflammation of one or both kidneys, as a primary idiopathic disease, is

R. Raghavan, BS, MD (✉)
Division of Nephrology, Department of Medicine,
Baylor College of Medicine,
1709 Dryden ST, Ste 900, Houston, TX 77030, USA
e-mail: rajeevr@bcm.edu

G. Eknoyan, MD
Department of Medicine, Baylor College of Medicine,
One Baylor Plaza, Houston, TX 77030, USA
e-mail: geknoyan@bcm.edu

M. Arici (ed.), *Management of Chronic Kidney Disease*,
DOI 10.1007/978-3-642-54637-2_1, © Springer-Verlag Berlin Heidelberg 2014

less frequently met than most other forms of phlegmasiae." In his textbook on the practice of medicine published in 1839, he devotes most of the discussion of nephritis to calculous or obstructive diseases rather than the rare disease he had identified. In the century that followed, the acute and chronic forms of Bright's disease were defined, their diagnosis from urinalysis was refined, and their microscopic renal lesions were described; but its therapy remained symptomatic and outcome fatal much as it had been in 1827 when Bright described his eponymous disease. It was the conceptual and technical advances in medicine during and after the Second World War that were to change it all, most notably that of the introduction of the artificial kidney that was to transform the fatal disease of Bright into a treatable one, a milestone achievement that catapulted the growth of nephrology in the closing decades of the past century [1].

Ironically, it was the treatment of Bright's end-stage renal disease (ESRD) with dialysis that focused attention on the broader and more serious issue of chronic kidney disease (CKD). Dialysis started as an exploratory effort to sustain the life of acute renal failure patients in the years that followed the Second World War; it evolved in the 1970s into a lifesaving therapy for patients whose CKD had progressed to kidney failure necessitating renal replacement therapy (RRT) with dialysis. For most of the years thereafter, the problem of kidney disease came to be viewed in the context of ESRD, which affects about 0.1 % of the population. As administrative data from national dialysis registries accrued in the 1980s, it became evident that the care of patients with ESRD should have been started well before they presented for dialysis having sustained already the ravaging consequences of progressive loss of kidney function. It was this concern that at the turn of the century prompted the first efforts at the definition, classification, and evaluation of CKD [1, 2].

1.2 Definition of CKD

In 2002, the Kidney Disease Outcomes Quality Initiative (KDOQI) developed guidelines for a working definition of CKD, independent of the cause of the disease, based on the presence of either kidney damage (proteinuria, abnormal kidney biopsy, or imaging studies) or a glomerular filtration rate (GFR) of less than 60 ml/min/1.73 m^2 for more than 3 months [3]. The guidelines also proposed a classification of CKD based on severity determined by the level of kidney function calculated from the serum creatinine and expressed as the estimated GFR (eGFR). They proposed the classification of CKD into 5 stages: with stages 1 and 2 as covert disease requiring the presence of kidney damage (proteinuria, abnormal urinalysis, biopsy, or imaging studies) and stages 3, 4, and 5 as overt diseases (i.e., when the eGFR was less than 60 ml/min/1.73 m^2) with eGFR of 30–59, 29–15, and <15 ml/min/1.73 m^2, respectively. The conceptual model of CKD used in proposing this classification is shown in Fig. 1.1. The five stages of CKD classification do not appear in this cartoon. Rather, stages 1 and 2 are grouped together and implicitly represented in the ellipse-labeled "injury" and flagged for albuminuria and stages 3 and 4 in the ellipse-labeled "decreased GFR" and flagged <60 ml/min/1.73 m^2. These guidelines were a major step forward in the evolution of our understanding of kidney disease as they provided a uniform definition of CKD that replaced the inchoate, ambiguous, and descriptive terms that had been used theretofore such as pre-end-stage renal disease, pre-dialysis, renal insufficiency, azotemia, uremia, and chronic renal failure. The proposed common terminology of CKD and its standardized classification provided new tools whereby kidney disease could be explored and the results compared across different studies, regions, and countries.

Methodological issues associated with the initial definition of CKD were addressed in the following years and to some extent resolved. Serum creatinine measurements have now been standardized, the equation to calculate eGFR refined, and many clinical laboratories have integrated the reporting of eGFR in their laboratory results. Recently, the cystatin C level has been added to that of creatinine and integrated in the formula used to calculate the eGFR. This new CKD-EPI equation based on serum creatinine alone is more reliable in predicting the morbidity and mortality

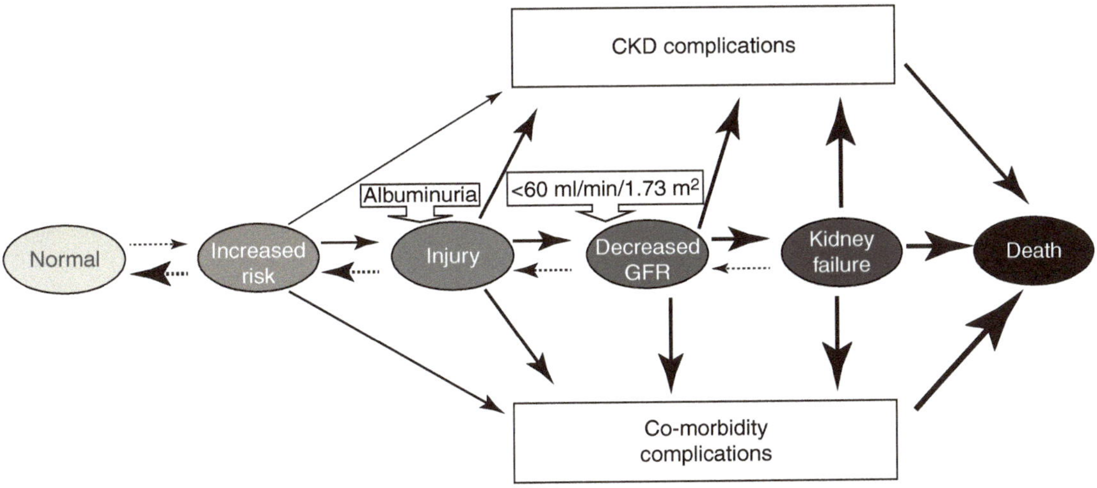

Fig. 1.1 A conceptual model of the course, complications, and outcomes of chronic kidney disease. The ellipses represent the progressive stages and consequences of progressive chronic kidney disease (*CKD*). The first two ellipses are antecedent stages representing cohorts at increased risk of developing CKD. The next two ellipses are flagged for the two hallmarks used in the definition and staging of CKD: albuminuria (stages 1 and 2) and a glomerular filtration rate of <60 ml/min/1.73 m^2 (stages 3 and 4). The gradually increasing thickness of the *arrows* connecting the ellipses reflects the increasing risk of progressing from one stage to the next stage of CKD as the disease progresses. The *dotted arrows* connecting the ellipses indicate the potential for improvement from one stage to its preceding stage due to treatment or variable natural history of the primary kidney disease. The rectangle at the top indicates the complications of CKD (anemia, mineral and bone disorders, hypertension, hyperparathyroidism). The rectangle at the bottom indicates the risk multiplier effect of CKD of coexistent comorbidities, principally that of cardiovascular disease. The gradually increasing thickness of the *arrows* connecting the ellipses to the upper and lower rectangle represents the increased risk of the complications as the CKD progresses from one stage to the next

outcomes of CKD [4] and is further improved when the serum cystatin level is incorporated in the equation [5]. The standardization and reporting of urinary albumin measurements are under active investigation but remain to be refined.

In defining CKD as kidney damage for at least 3 months, the guidelines also set the stage for the identification of another form of kidney disease, the potentially reversible form of acute kidney injury (AKI) of less than 3 months duration that is now the subject of its own guideline. A discussion of AKI is beyond the scope of this chapter, but familiarity with its guideline is essential for the care of CKD patients who are the subjects most susceptible to AKI and sustain its poorest outcomes of morbidity, mortality, the additional loss of residual kidney function, and accelerated progression to ESRD [6].

Importantly, based on available evidence then, the KDOQI guidelines documented the increased number of systemic complications (anemia, hypertension, mineral and bone disorders), morbidity, and mortality associated with declining eGFR and described the greater risk of death of CKD patients from cardiovascular disease than from their progression to kidney failure and ESRD [3, 4]. During the decade that followed the issue of these guidelines, epidemiologic data has validated, refined, and provided convincing evidence that CKD is common, harmful, treatable, and a major public health problem worldwide [7, 8]. CKD is definitely much more common than had been appreciated theretofore. The prevalence of CKD is over 10 % of the general population and increases in high-risk populations (diabetic, hypertensive, obese, elderly), some ethnic groups (Latin Americans, African Americans, Pima Indians), and those with predisposing genetic composition. Importantly, there is now persuasive evidence that the presence and severity of CKD adversely affects the outcome of not only cardiovascular disease but also other prevalent diseases such as that of diabetes, hypertension, and obesity [9]. The reciprocity of these major chronic diseases is shown in Fig. 1.2, in which the overall interaction of chronic diseases

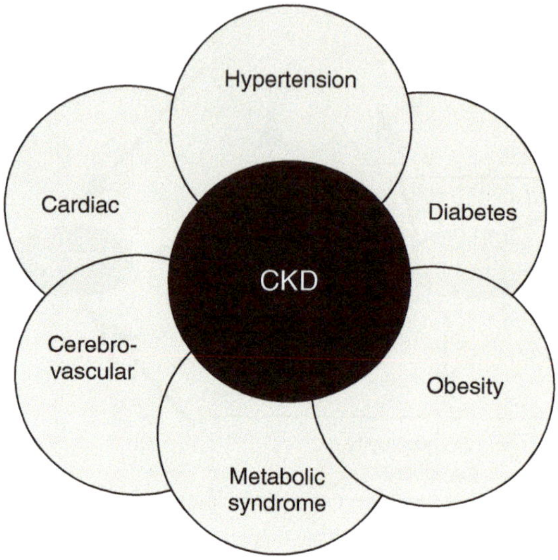

Fig. 1.2 The cluster of comorbidities associated with and aggravated by chronic kidney disease (*CKD*). Where there is clinical intersection of the circle representing a given comorbidity with that of CKD, the presence of CKD emerges as a risk multiplier of the outcome of that disease, and conversely the severity and course of CKD are aggravated by that of the disorder with which it overlaps. In areas where there is overlap of more than one circle, the risks are further magnified

can be viewed as an overlap phenomenon whereby the presence of CKD emerges as a risk multiplier of the morbidity and mortality of the other major chronic diseases. The risk of each disease increases in the areas of their overlap with CKD, and the magnitude of this detrimental effect is related to the severity of CKD [9, 10]. Thus, both detection of CKD in these conditions and evaluation of the severity of CKD are essential to appropriately estimate its impact on outcomes.

1.3 Staging of CKD

By any criteria, the paradigm shift created by the 2002 KDOQI guidelines for the definition and the classification of CKD is a milestone in the evolution of nephrology, but was not without its limitations. Despite the effort that went into developing the evidence base of the proposed classification, a major limiting factor was the quality and quantity of evidence then available. Fortunately, one of the most fruitful derivatives of that initial step forward has been the stimulus it provided for new research and hence the subsequent incremental accrual of new evidence for their support as well as their refinement. Apart from information on the epidemiology and outcomes of CKD, the new evidence revealed a strong, graded, and consistent relationship between the severity of the two hallmarks of CKD: reduced eGFR and increased albuminuria [10]. As a result, the Kidney Disease Improving Global Outcomes (KDIGO) released a new guideline for the staging of CKD that integrates albuminuria as a determinant of severity of the disease. The new guideline refines the definition of CKD as abnormalities of kidney structure or function, present for >3 months, with implications for health of the individual, and classifies CKD based on cause (C), GFR (G), and albuminuria (A) category (CGA) [11]. The classification of CKD by the level of eGFR and albuminuria (the GA of **CGA**) and their impact on prognosis is shown in Fig. 1.3. That of the cause (C) is based on the presence and absence of systemic diseases and the location of the disease within the kidney (glomerulus, tubule, vasculature, cystic, or genetic). The principal systemic diseases that overlap with CKD and are affected by and in turn affect the severity of CKD are shown in Fig. 1.2.

The importance of considering the cause (the C of **CGA**) of CKD, now part of the new definition, is highlighted in the conceptual model of CKD shown in Fig. 1.1. The dotted arrows in the figure reflect the potential for reversibility at each stage of CKD. This improvement may be part of the natural course of the cause of some diseases but is also and to a greater extent the result of detection and proper treatment of individual cases. Thus, a patient with malignant hypertension who presents in ESRD requiring dialysis can recover sufficient kidney function after control of the blood pressure to cease requiring maintenance dialysis and revert to a stage 3 or 4 CKD patient. Similarly, a patient with congestive cardiomyopathy, who requires dialysis at presentation in

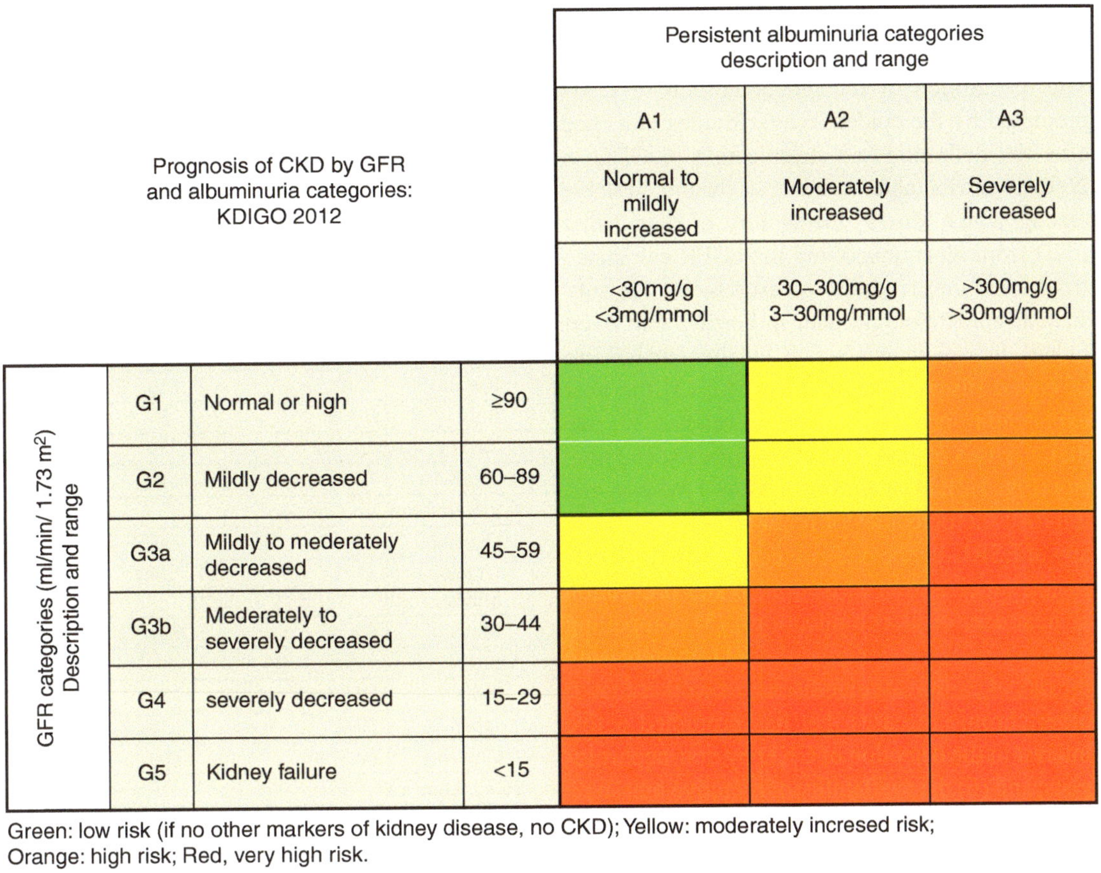

Fig. 1.3 Staging and prognosis of chronic kidney disease (CKD) by glomerular filtration rate and albuminuria (Reproduced with permission from Kidney Disease: Improving Global Outcomes (KDIGO) [11])

ESRD, can recover sufficient kidney function following treatment of the heart failure to perfuse the kidneys well enough to move to an earlier stage of CKD. The same argument can be made for all CKD patients whose kidney function is aggravated by poor management of the comorbid conditions with which it overlaps (Fig. 1.2). By the same token, improvement of kidney function with regression to an earlier stage can be achieved by the proper therapy (steroids, immunosuppression) of the cause of the kidney disease in selected cases (lupus nephritis, IgA nephropathy, etc.) or the reduction of the magnitude of their albuminuria with angiotensin-converting enzyme inhibitors (ACEIs) and antihypertensive agents. In those whose CKD continues to progress, their outcomes can be improved by preventing the complications of continued loss of kidney function (anemia, mineral and bone disorders) to forestall the otherwise serious systemic ravages of CKD. This underscores the vital importance of detecting kidney disease in its earliest stages before the onset of serious and irreversible complications.

Whereas albuminuria is used in the grading of CKD, the evaluation of the individual patient with CKD should include all abnormalities detected on urinalysis that are usually equally important in diagnosis and affect CKD outcomes, especially that of hematuria. As with its predecessor, the new 2012 KDIGO staging is not an end but a beginning for the accrual of new information that could further refine the definition and grading of CKD in future iterations of the guideline.

1.4 Epidemiology of CKD

The recognition of the global burden of CKD prompted by the epidemiologic studies launched after the definition and stratification of CKD in 2002 is attributable to several factors, notable among which are (1) the facility of diagnosing CKD from albuminuria and the eGFR calculated from a serum creatinine measurement; (2) substantial epidemiologic data indicating that overt kidney disease (stages 3–5) is the tip of an iceberg of covert disease (stages 1 and 2); (3) the near exponential increase in the prevalence of two major causes of kidney disease, diabetes, and obesity (Fig. 1.2); (4) attempts to control the cost and improve the outcomes of renal replacement therapy of ESRD by the early detection of overt CKD for the amelioration of its course and prevention or treatment of its complications; (5) compelling evidence of the major role of CKD in increasing the risk of cardiovascular disease as well as that of other chronic diseases that has prompted active interest in the detection of CKD by non-nephrologists; and (6) the availability of effective measures to prevent the progression of CKD, reduce its complications, and ameliorate its outcomes (Fig. 1.1). While these factors render control of CKD an achievable goal of healthcare planning in the developed world, the problems they delineate in the developing world are challenging and remain to be adequately addressed.

Aggregate estimates suggest that CKD affects as many as 1 in 10 adults (10 %) or over 500 million people worldwide [8]. However, concrete data regarding the true incidence and prevalence of CKD is hampered by the paucity of proper record keeping and national renal registries, particularly in poorer countries (Table 1.1). In 2010, approximately 13.1 % of US adults age 20 or older, or 70,000 per million persons, had CKD – defined as an estimated GFR less than 60 ml/min/1.73 m^2 or a urine albumin-to-creatinine ratio (ACR) of ≥30 mg/g [12]. Because of the high mortality from cardiovascular disease in patients with CKD, for every patient who progresses to end-stage renal disease (ESRD), there are more than 200 with overt chronic kidney disease (stage 3 or 4) and almost 5,000 with covert disease (stage 1 or 2) who succumb to cardiovascular disease without ever progressing to ESRD [8, 11, 12]. Those who progress to ESRD present a challenge of their own. Nearly two million people in the world have ESRD and receive maintenance dialysis [3, 8]. The average worldwide incidence of ESRD is estimated at 150 per million persons [8]. In the United States, this number is 350 per million persons. Both the incidence and prevalence of ESRD are higher in developed countries, driven largely by healthcare agenda for its treatment (availability of dialysis and transplantation) [12]. Hence, it is not surprising that most of the world's dialysis patients are located in high-income countries, with 52 % of the patients residing in just four countries: the United States, Japan, Brazil, and Germany, which

Table 1.1 Prevalence of CKD and ESRD in different parts of the world

	Prevalence of CKD (percentage per adult population)	Prevalence rate of ESRD (number of adults per million)
Global estimates	10 %	400
Europe		
United Kingdom	9 %	659
Germany	5.4 %	1,020
Spain	5.1 %	991
Russia	N/A	130
Italy	6.4 %	755
Turkey	15.7 %	756
Australia	11 %	778
North America		
Canada	9.5 %	1,007
United States	13 %	1,641
Mexico	8.1 %	929
Asia		
India	N/A	15
Japan	10 %	1,956
China	10.8 %	150
South America		
Brazil	N/A	520
Africa		
Nigeria	1.6–12 %	N/A

All reported data was collected and published between 2005 and 2012. The definition of CKD includes persons with estimated glomerular filtration rate (eGFR <60 ml/min/1.73 m^2) or albuminuria. Prevalence rate of ESRD is defined as the number of persons sustained on dialysis

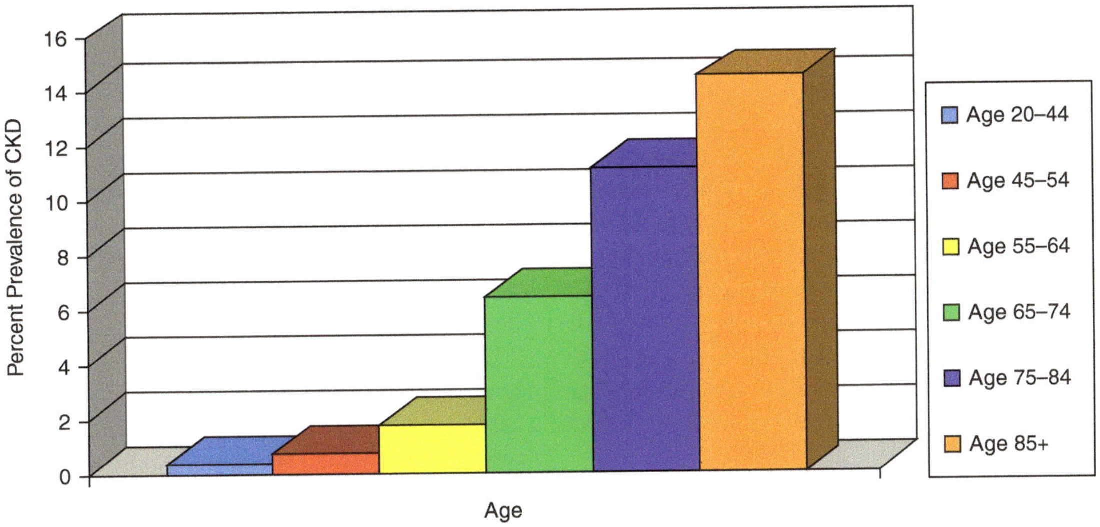

Fig. 1.4 Age as a determinant of the prevalence of chronic kidney disease. Almost 15 % of the US population aged 85 years or older have CKD (Data from the 2012 US Renal Database Report [12])

collectively represent only 12 % of the world population. Because RRT is costly and simply unaffordable for many low-income countries, the emphasis must be on preventing CKD by detecting it in its early stages, then slowing its progression with therapeutic agents and lifestyle changes, and preventing its complications by appropriate measures. Governments must play an active role in implementing programs that utilize cost-effective methods (urinalysis, blood pressure) to detect covert CKD in high-risk populations (Fig. 1.2). The proper implementation of the KDIGO 2012 CKD guidelines requires a certain basic infrastructure, which remains lacking in some countries. Such infrastructure includes that of the uniform standardization of creatinine and proteinuria assays and implementation of eGFR reporting. National health agencies must take the initiative to close these gaps.

Data from the National Health and Nutrition Examination Survey (NHANES) indicate that the prevalence of CKD is rising, particularly in stage 3, probably due to the increased prevalence of obesity and diabetes (Fig. 1.2). Between one-quarter to one-third of diabetics will develop diabetic nephropathy, which is the leading cause of CKD [7]. It is estimated that the number of people worldwide diagnosed with diabetes will rise from 171 million in 2000 to 366 million in 2030, resulting in additional millions of new cases of CKD. A change to a more "Western" diet and the rising rates of obesity along with genetic predisposition are all considered as potential etiologies that account for the rising incidence of ESRD in regions with a high prevalence of diabetes, obesity, and hypertension [13]. Yet another contributing factor to the rise in CKD is the increase in cases of AKI. In the past two decades, there has been an increase in the incidence of dialysis-requiring AKI of >7 % per year. Two principal reasons for this are (1) procedures using nephrotoxic agents such as contrast dye and (2) survival from severe sepsis, a major risk factor for AKI. Furthermore, all patients with an AKI hospitalization (regardless of whether there is underlying CKD) have a risk of either ESRD (5 %) or death (25 %) in the year following their hospitalization [12].

The onset and progression of CKD depend on the occurrence of both modifiable (obesity, smoking, poorly controlled hypertension or diabetes, diet) and non-modifiable (age, gender, race, genetics) risk factors. Figure 1.4 shows the distribution of CKD by cohorts of increasing age. Older age is a well-established risk factor for CKD, but there has been ongoing debate as to whether the age-related GFR decline is "normal" or pathological. The age-related decline in GFR, which affects up to 40 % of people aged over 65 years, could lead to overestimating the actual burden of CKD because many of these elderly people have impaired but stable kidney function [7]. However, the elderly with stable but reduced residual renal function are at increased risk of drug toxicity and of detrimentally affecting coexisting chronic diseases (Fig. 1.2). Actually, a reduced eGFR in the elderly is often a predictor of reduced "overall" health due to comorbid conditions (hypertension, heart disease, stroke). Thus, with increasing age, especially in patients above 75 years, the likelihood of death outweighs the risk of developing ESRD even when the eGFR is severely reduced (below 29 ml/min/1.73 m^2) [8, 14].

The data comparing the prevalence of CKD in men and women is not straightforward and remains a topic of some controversy. Feminine hormones have been proposed to favorably alter the onset, course, and progression of chronic kidney disease, through alterations in the renin–angiotensin system, reduction in mesangial collagen synthesis, modification of collagen degradation, and upregulation of nitric oxide synthesis [15]. The USRDS database indicates that women have a 22 % lower risk of being diagnosed with CKD ($p<0.001$) and a lower incident rate of ESRD, but the definite worldwide effect of gender in CKD remains to be determined [12, 14, 15].

CKD has a higher incidence among African Americans and Latin Americans in the United States than among their Caucasian counterparts. Even among patients of African descent, the incidence of CKD is lower in Africa and Europe than in the United States, highlighting the importance of modifiable lifestyle risk factors in the development of CKD. Another non-modifiable risk factor in the pathogenesis of CKD is genetics. Even after adjusting for known genetic causes of CKD (such as polycystic disease or Alport's syndrome), family members of dialysis patients tend to have a higher prevalence of CKD [8].

1.5 Etiology of CKD

A detailed inventory of the etiologies of CKD is beyond the scope of this chapter. In the United States, the vast majority of CKD cases (up to 80 %) are secondary to diabetes or hypertension (Fig. 1.2). These systemic diseases and their contribution to CKD are increasing worldwide. The WHO estimates that approximately one billion individuals are now classified as overweight or obese [14]. Apart from its association with diabetes and hypertension, obesity is linked to earlier onset and faster progression of CKD in general and of the glomerulonephritides in particular [2]. The importance of weight control in all CKD obese patients cannot be overemphasized.

Disparities in the cause of CKD are affected by racial, geographic, and economic factors (Table 1.1). In developing countries, chronic glomerulonephritis (GN) and interstitial nephritis are a more frequent cause of CKD, in many cases reflecting kidney disease secondary to a bacterial, viral, and parasitic infection [13]. The incriminated infectious agents include tuberculosis (200 million affected worldwide), streptococcal infections, hepatitis C virus (170 million), human immunodeficiency virus (40 million), and schistosomiasis (200 million), depending on the region. IgA nephropathy is common in Southeast Asia and the Pacific region (accounting for up to 35–45 % of glomerulonephritides) [13]. Focal segmental glomerulosclerosis (FSGS) is another common cause of CKD in developing countries such as India, possibly as a consequence of the low nephron mass associated with low birth weight. Finally, the magnitude of environmental pollution's contribution on CKD remains debatable: an association has been documented only for occupational exposure to lead, cadmium, and mercury.

1.6 Detection

CKD is potentially a progressive disease with the definite likelihood of ongoing loss of kidney function even after the initial injury is no longer present. Patients with CKD are often asymptomatic until they reach the more advanced stages (sometimes stage 3, but more often stage 4). Hence, it seems intuitive that earlier detection will facilitate timely treatment, disease awareness, and promote the necessary lifestyle and medication changes to retard the progression of CKD and prevent its complications. Three diagnostic tests employed to detect latent CKD

Table 1.2 Select international guidelines in screening specific adult populations for CKD

Organization	Population	Screening test
American Diabetes Association (ADA) http://care.diabetesjournals.org/content/36/Supplement_1/S4.full.pdf+html	Adults with diabetes	Serum creatinine and urinalysis for albumin (microalbuminuria)
Joint National Committee (JNC): 7th edition http://www.nhlbi.nih.gov/guidelines/hypertension/jnc7full.pdf	Adults with hypertension	Serum creatinine and urinalysis for albumin
Japanese Society of Nephrology http://www.jsn.or.jp/en/guideline/pdf/guideline2009.pdf	Adults with diabetes	Serum creatinine (with eGFR) and urinary albumin–creatinine ratio (ACR) in a spot urine sample
National Institute for Health and Clinical Excellence (NICE) http://www.nice.org.uk/nicemedia/live/12069/42116/42116.pdf	Adults with diabetes, hypertension, cardiovascular disease, structural renal tract disease, renal calculi, prostatic hypertrophy, multisystem diseases with potential kidney involvement (e.g., lupus), family history of hereditary kidney disease or stage 5 CKD	Offer CKD testing with urinary albumin–creatinine ratio (ACR) and/or serum creatinine (with eGFR)
	Adults prescribed nephrotoxic drugs or receiving long-term systemic nonsteroidal anti-inflammatory drug (NSAID) treatment	Serum creatinine (with eGFR)
	Obese individuals	No specific screening recommended
Canadian Society of Nephrology http://www.cmaj.ca/content/suppl/2008/11/17/179.11.1154.DC1/guide-hemm-1-at.pdf	Adults at high risk of kidney disease: diabetes, hypertension, vascular disease, autoimmune disease, estimated glomerular filtration rate <60 ml/min/1.73 m^2, or edema	Urinary protein–creatinine ratio or albumin–creatinine ratio (ACR)
Kidney Disease: Improving Global Outcomes (KDIGO) http://www.kdigo.org/clinical_practice_guidelines/pdf/CKD/KDIGO_2012_CKD_GL.pdf	Adults with CKD	Estimated GFR (eGFR) and urinalysis for albumin
United States Preventative Task Force (USPTF) www.uspreventiveservicestaskforce.org/	Asymptomatic adults	No specific screening recommended
National Kidney Foundation (NKF) www.kidney.org/	Adults at "increased risk" of CKD (not specified)	Monitoring of blood pressure, serum creatinine (with eGFR) and urinary albumin–creatinine ratio (ACR)

are the dipstick urinalysis for albuminuria, serum creatinine (to calculate eGFR), and blood pressure. Although relatively cheap, these have not proven cost-effective when applied to the screening of the general population. In the last decade, several countries now mandate reporting of the estimated GFR along with serum creatinine value, in persons aged 18 and older, but whether this will translate into the anticipated improved outcomes for patients with CKD is under investigation but remains to be documented. Targeting specific susceptible subpopulations, for example, patients with diabetes, hypertension, obesity, or cardiovascular disease, is a more economical approach to screening to detect CKD. Recommendations regarding which "high-risk" group should be screened vary between national and international organizations (Table 1.2).

Efforts at diligent detection and early identification are just a beginning; unfortunately there is frequently failure to achieve therapeutic targets, due to lack of awareness of available clinical practice guidelines or their ineffective implementation. Planned programs at detection must incorporate the next important step of proper follow-up and therapy.

Treatment of CKD will be addressed in separate chapters. However, the six general interventions targeted in slowing the progression of CKD include dietary modification, weight loss, blood pressure control, reducing the amount of proteinuria, optimizing glycemic control, controlling lipids, and avoiding smoking.

Although the worldwide epidemic of obesity and diabetes extend to children, screening for kidney disease in this population is also controversial. The most commonly used and cost-effective screening tool in children is urinalysis for blood and albumin. Two challenges facing mass screening campaigns are (1) determining the right population (such as children's age or country of origin) to screen and (2) assuring the accuracy of random urinalysis. Detection of proteinuria is most accurate with the first morning void; hence, all persons who screen positive on a random sample should have a confirmatory urinalysis done on a first-void morning specimen shortly thereafter.

The goals of implementing a school screening program for children are listed in Table 1.3 [16]. Mass urinary screening programs were initially implemented in France and have been routine practice in Asian countries such as Japan, Taiwan, and Korea for decades. Perhaps due to the high prevalence of IgA nephropathy, childhood screenings in Japan have been reported as "successful" [15]. In 2002, 246,000 elementary and 115,000 junior high school Japanese children were screened. Proteinuria was detected in 0.11 % and confirmed on repeat urinalysis in 0.05 % of the elementary school children; the results of junior high school screens were 0.6 and 0.32 %, respectively. The number of Japanese adolescents who develop ESRD has decreased between 1984 and 2002 suggesting that screening children has the potential to reduce the incidence of ESRD. However, there seems to be a movement away from mass screening in North America and Europe due to issues of its cost-effectiveness. For example, the American Academy of Pediatrics (AAP) does not recommend urinalyses during childhood to screen for kidney disease.

Given this data, all children with risk factors for CKD, including those who are obese, are hypertensive, or have relocated from areas of the world with a high endemic burden of CKD, should have a screening urinalysis and if abnormal should be followed by a repeat first morning urinalysis.

Table 1.3 Goals of a school screening program to detect CKD

1. Program should be based on relatively simple tests that have been documented to provide reproducible results
2. Tests should have a high level of sensitivity (to avoid missing cases of CKD) and preferably associated with high specificity (to reduce number of false positives)
3. Infrastructure of screening program should be set up in such a way to identify abnormal results and schedule confirmatory tests in a short period of time
4. Close communication with the parents of children with abnormal results should be maintained throughout all stages of the screening program
5. Appropriate consultation with a pediatric nephrologist should be expedited for all children who have persistently abnormal results
6. Cost-effectiveness of the program should be confirmed periodically in order to maintain enthusiasm for the program

Source: Reproduced with permission from the American Society of Nephrology [16]

Before You Finish: Practice Pearls for the Clinician

- CKD is a major public health problem that is common, harmful, and treatable.
- Detection of CKD is best accomplished with serial measurements of blood pressure, serum creatinine, and urinalysis in select populations at a higher risk of disease (Table 1.2)
- CKD staging combines albuminuria (A) and cause (C), with GFR (G), to improve prognostication (Fig. 1.3).
- The two principal hallmarks of CKD that affect its outcomes are levels of reduced eGFR and increased albuminuria.
- Because of the epidemic of obesity and diabetes, the incidence of CKD is increasing, particularly for persons with overt stage 3 disease (eGFR 30–59 ml/min/1.73 m^2) (Fig. 1.2).
- Six general interventions to slow the progression of CKD include dietary modification, weight loss, blood pressure control, reducing the amount of proteinuria, optimizing glycemic control, controlling lipids, and avoiding smoking.

References

1. Eknoyan G. The early modern kidney. Nephrology in and about the nineteenth century (part 1). Semin Dial. 2013;26:73–84.
2. Eknoyan G, Lameire N, Barsoum R, Eckhardt KU, Levin A, Levin N, et al. The burden of kidney disease: improving global outcomes. Kidney Int. 2004;66:1310–4.
3. National Kidney Foundation. KDOQI clinical practice guidelines for chronic kidney disease: evaluation, classification, and stratification. Am J Kidney Dis. 2002;39(Suppl 1):S1–S266.
4. Matsushita K, Mahmood BK, Woodward M, Emberson JR, Jafar TH, Jee SH, et al. Comparison of risk prediction using CKD-EPI equation and the MDRD study equation for estimated glomerular filtration rate. JAMA. 2012;307:1941–51.
5. Inker LA, Schmid CH, Tighiouart MS, Eckfeldt JH, Feldman HI, Greene T, et al. Estimating glomerular filtration rate from serum creatinine and cystatin C. New Engl J Med. 2012;367:20–9.
6. KDIGO clinical practice guideline for acute kidney injury. Kidney Int Suppl. 2012;2:1–138
7. Coresh J, Selwin E, Stevens LA, Manzi J, Kusek J, Eggers P, et al. Prevalence of chronic kidney disease in the United States. JAMA. 2007;298:2038–47.
8. Couser WG, Remuzzi G, Mundi S, Tonelli M. The contribution of chronic kidney disease to the global burden of noncommunicable diseases. Kidney Int. 2011;80:1258–70.
9. Fried LF, Katz R, Sarnak MJ, Schlipak MG, Chaves PHM, Jenny NS, et al. Kidney function as a predictor of noncardiovascular mortality. J Am Soc Nephrol. 2005;16:3728–35.
10. Van der Velde M, Matsushita K, Coresh J, et al. Lower estimated glomerular filtration rate and higher albuminuria are associated with all-cause mortality. A collaborative meta-analysis of high risk population cohorts. Kidney Int. 2011;79:1341–52.
11. KDIGO 2012 clinical practice guideline for the evaluation and management of chronic kidney disease. Kidney Int Suppl. 2013;3:1–150.
12. US Renal Data System. USRDS 2012 annual data report: atlas of chronic kidney disease and end-stage renal disease in the United States. Bethesda: National Institutes of Health, National Institute of Diabetes and Digestive and Kidney Diseases; 2012.
13. Barsoum RS. Chronic kidney disease in the developing world. N Engl J Med. 2006;354:997–9.
14. WHO. Preventing chronic diseases: a vital investment. WHO global report. World Health Organization. 2005. http://www.who.int/chp/chronic_disease_report/full report.pdf. Accessed 6 Feb 2013.
15. Seligera SL, Davis C, Stehman-Breen C. Gender and the progression of renal disease. Curr Opin Nephrol Hypertens. 2001;10:219–25.
16. Hogg RJ. Screening for CKD in children: a global controversy. Clin J Am Soc Nephrol. 2009;4:509–15.

Clinical Assessment of a Patient with Chronic Kidney Disease

2

Mustafa Arici

Before You Start: Facts You Need to Know

- A focused history and physical examination is essential in the assessment of patients with chronic kidney disease (CKD).
- A CKD patient's history should differentiate CKD from acute kidney disease, define duration and chronicity, find a causative or contributory disease, and assess complications and comorbidities.
- Physical examination should cover all systems but has a special emphasis on blood pressure and orthostatic changes, volume assessment, and cardiovascular examination.
- Serum creatinine and estimation of glomerular filtration rate (GFR) with an equation using serum creatinine should be done as a part of initial assessment in all CKD patients.
- A complete urinalysis and measurement of albumin in the urine should be carried out in all CKD patients.

2.1 History and Physical Examination of a Chronic Kidney Disease Patient

Chronic kidney disease (CKD) is usually a silent condition. Signs and symptoms, if present, are generally nonspecific (Box 2.1) and unlike several other chronic diseases (such as congestive heart failure, chronic obstructive lung disease), they did not reveal a clue for diagnosis or severity of the condition. Typical symptoms and signs of uremia (Box 2.2) appear almost never in early stages (Stage 1 to 3A/B, even Stage 4) and develop too late *only in some patients* in the course of CKD. Still, all newly diagnosed CKD patients, patients with an acute worsening in their kidney function, and CKD patients on regular follow-up should have *a*

Box 2.1. Symptoms and Signs of Early Stages of CKD

Weakness
Decreased appetite
Nausea
Changes in urination (nocturia, polyuria, frequency)
Blood in urine or dark-colored urine
Foamy or bubbly urine
Loin pain
Edema
Elevated blood pressure
Pale skin

M. Arici, MD
Department of Nephrology, Faculty of Medicine, Hacettepe University, Ankara 06100, Turkey
e-mail: marici@hacettepe.edu.tr

M. Arici (ed.), *Management of Chronic Kidney Disease*,
DOI 10.1007/978-3-642-54637-2_2, © Springer-Verlag Berlin Heidelberg 2014

Box 2.2. Symptoms and Signs of Late (Uremic) Stages of CKD

General (*lassitude, fatigue, elevated blood pressure, signs of volume overload, decreased mental acuity, intractable hiccups, uremic fetor*)

Skin (*sallow appearance, uremic frost, pruritic excoriations*)

Pulmonary (*dyspnea, pleural effusion, pulmonary edema, uremic lung*)

Cardiovascular (*pericardial friction rub, congestive heart failure*)

Gastrointestinal (*anorexia, nausea, vomiting, weight loss, stomatitis, unpleasant taste in the mouth*)

Neuromuscular (*muscular twitches, peripheral sensory and motor neuropathies, muscle cramps, restless legs, sleep disorders, hyperreflexia, seizures, encephalopathy, coma*)

Endocrine-metabolic (*decreased libido, amenorrhea, impotence*)

Hematologic (*anemia, bleeding diathesis*)

focused history and physical examination. This will be the key to perceive *real* "implications of health" associated with decreased kidney function in CKD.

In a newly diagnosed CKD patient, the history should be focused *to differentiate an acute kidney injury/disease from CKD* and get clues for duration and chronicity of kidney dysfunction. Any previous kidney function tests, urine findings, and imaging studies should be obtained and reviewed. If CKD diagnosis is confirmed, history should be focused *to find an underlying cause*. Patients should be questioned for any sign or symptom of an underlying (causative or contributory) disease(s) for CKD. All medications (including current and prior medications, over-the-counter and non-prescription medications) should be carefully reviewed and documented. Any previous surgical intervention, especially genitourinary interventions, should be reviewed. A detailed family history should be obtained to exclude presence of a familial, hereditary kidney disorder (Box 2.3).

Box 2.3. Clues to the Underlying (Causative or Contributory) Disease in a CKD Patient

Previous lab tests, imaging, or biopsy findings (*provide definite evidence for CKD if they show previously decreased GFR and/or presence of kidney damage, presence of bilateral small kidneys*)

System review:

- Cardiovascular (*history of myocardial infarction, coronary intervention, and heart failure provide evidence for cardiorenal connection and impaired renal perfusion*)
- Immunologic/Infectious (*provide evidence for autoimmune or infectious causes of CKD*)
- Gastrointestinal (*history of hepatitis, cirrhosis*)
- Genitourinary (*frequent urinary tract infection, recurrent kidney stones, and urinary symptoms related to bladder neck obstruction provide evidence for pyelonephritis, obstruction, and stones*)

Past medical history (*history of long-standing hypertension or diabetes, glomerulonephritis in early childhood, renal complications during pregnancy, any previous acute kidney injury episode, any previous urologic intervention*)

Family history (*anyone with CKD diagnosis among first-degree relatives*)

Medication history (*frequent use of NSAIDs or pain killers, long-term exposure to nephrotoxic antibiotics, frequent exposure to radiocontrast agents, chemotherapeutic use, etc.*)

Source: Reprinted from KDOQI clinical practice guidelines for chronic kidney disease: evaluation, classification, and stratification [1], Copyright 2002, with permission from Elsevier. Available from: http://www.kidney.org/professionals/KDOQI/guidelines_ckd/toc.htm

In each visit, the *stage of CKD and presence of any comorbidity and complications* related to loss of kidney function and *cardiovascular status* should be evaluated. All body systems should be thoroughly reviewed as CKD may have various manifestations in any of them. Patients should be specifically questioned for dermatological, pulmonary, cardiovascular, cerebrovascular, peripheral vascular, gastrointestinal, genitourinary, musculoskeletal, and neurological symptoms. *Potential risk factors for sudden deterioration and progression* of CKD, along with *a careful review of medications*, should be sought in each visit.

Physical examination of a CKD patient includes a few specific points beyond general rules. Patient's general health, nutritional status, appetite, and weight changes should be determined in each visit. Blood pressure and pulse should be assessed both in upright and supine positions for determining orthostatic changes. Hypertensive or diabetic changes in the eye should be examined by fundoscopy. Patients should be examined for signs of hypovolemia or volume overload. Skin should be evaluated for finding an underlying disease and signs of CKD (anemia, pruritus, sallow appearance). A careful evaluation of the cardiovascular system is important. The abdomen should be palpated for large kidneys and bladder distention. Abdominal bruits should be noted for potential renovascular disease. Costovertebral tenderness may be a sign of infection and/or stone disease in kidneys. In men, rectal examination is required for determining prostatic enlargement. Neurological evaluation should be focused on signs of neuropathy and muscular problems. Examination for any sign of a systemic disease causing or contributing to CKD should be carefully sought. Findings consistent with uremia should be determined and followed in each visit (Box 2.4).

Box 2.4. What the Guidelines Say You Should Do: History and Physical Examination

- Review past history and any previous measurement for GFR or markers of kidney damage to determine the duration of kidney disease.
- Evaluate the clinical context, including personal and family history, social and environmental factors, medications, physical examination, laboratory measures, imaging, and pathologic diagnosis to determine the causes of kidney disease.

Source: Data from KDIGO 2012 clinical practice guideline for the evaluation and management of chronic kidney disease [2]

2.2 Estimating or Measuring Glomerular Filtration Rate in CKD

Glomerular filtration rate (GFR) is usually accepted as the best index of kidney function. Persistently decreased GFR (<60 ml/min/1.73 m^2) is a hallmark for CKD, even in the absence of any marker for kidney damage. GFR usually correlates well with the prognosis and complications of CKD like anemia, mineral-bone disorders, and cardiovascular disease. GFR should be determined for confirming diagnosis, staging the disease, estimating the prognosis and making decisions about treatment in all CKD patients. GFR level may also be used to decide appropriate timing to start renal replacement therapies. GFR should be regularly monitored in CKD patients according to the stage and severity of CKD. There is however no consensus on the monitoring frequency of GFR in various stages (Table 2.1).

GFR is traditionally measured as renal clearance of an "ideal" filtration marker, such as inulin from plasma. This measured GFR is considered *the gold standard* but is not practical for daily clinical use due to complexity of the measurement procedure. Estimating GFR based on a filtration marker (usually serum creatinine) is now widely accepted as an initial test. Several GFR prediction equations that use serum creatinine or some other filtration markers along with certain patient characteristics (like age, gender, and race) are giving precise estimates of GFR in various clinical settings [3].

1. *Serum creatinine, Creatinine clearance, and GFR estimating equations*: These are the most

Table 2.1 How often should GFR be monitored in CKD?

Stage	Testing frequency (once in every)[a]
Stage 1 and 2	6–12 months
Stage 3A	4–6 months
Stage 3B	3–4 months
Stage 4	2–3 months
Stage 5	1 month

Source: Adapted by permission from Macmillan Publishers Ltd: Kidney Disease: Improving Global Outcomes (KDIGO) CKD Work Group [2] and National Institute for Health and Clinical Excellence (NICE) [4]. Available from: http://www.kdigo.org/clinical_practice_guidelines/CKD.php

[a]Testing frequency may change according to progression rate and albuminuria level in each stage. All CKD patients have GFR measurement during any intercurrent illness, any operation, any hospitalization, and any radiocontrast administration

common methods used for assessing kidney function in clinical practice.

- *Serum creatinine measurement* is a very convenient, cheap, and readily available technique. It is, therefore, the most commonly used parameter to evaluate kidney function in routine clinical practice. Serum creatinine (SCr) levels are largely determined by the balance between its generation and excretion by the kidneys. Creatinine generation is affected by muscle mass and dietary meat intake. Age, gender, and racial differences in creatinine generation depend to changes in muscle mass. In a CKD patient, reduced protein intake, malnutrition, and muscle wasting may reduce creatinine generation. These factors may blunt the rise of serum creatinine in spite of a decrease in GFR levels, especially in late stages of CKD.

  Creatinine is freely filtered through the glomerulus and is also secreted by the proximal tubules (5–10 % of the excreted creatinine). Tubular secretion of creatinine increases with decreasing kidney function. Another problem is the increased extrarenal elimination of creatinine with decreasing kidney function. Both factors lead to underestimation of kidney function by using only serum creatinine levels. In early stages of CKD, serum creatinine usually stays in normal limits despite large reductions (~30–40 %) in real GFR due to increased tubular secretion and extrarenal elimination of creatinine [5].

  Serum creatinine is commonly measured by alkaline picrate (Jaffé method), enzymatic, or high-performance liquid chromatography (HPLC) methods. These different methods of measuring serum creatinine are recently standardized to the isotope dilution mass spectrometry (IDMS). Standardized measurements usually yield 5 % lower values for serum creatinine concentrations. The alkaline picrate method is subject to interference by various serum constituents and drugs. The differences in assays and inter- and intra-laboratory variability may also affect the accuracy of serum creatinine measurements [6].

  All these factors (differences in creatinine generation, tubular secretion, extrarenal elimination, and variations in assay methods) may affect diagnostic sensitivity and correct interpretation of serum creatinine. *Serum creatinine alone is not anymore accepted as an adequate marker of kidney function.*

- *Creatinine clearance (Ccre) measurement* is a frequently used clinical method for measuring GFR. Its calculation depends on 24-h urine collection. This is a cumbersome procedure, especially in elderly. An incomplete or prolonged collection of urine alters the accuracy of the results. If creatinine generation is stable and there is no extrarenal elimination of creatinine, a complete collection may be determined by calculating total excretion of creatinine in the urine as follows:

$$\begin{aligned}&\text{Urine creatinine} \times \text{urine volume}\\&= 20-25\ \text{mg/kg/day for men},\\&\ 10-15\ \text{mg/kg/day for women}\end{aligned}$$

  Calculation of creatinine clearance assumes that all of the filtered creatinine (equal to the product of the GFR and the serum creatinine concentration (SCr)) is equal to all of the excreted creatinine (equal to product of the urine creatinine concentration (UCr) and the urine flow rate) and ignores the tubular secretion of creatinine. In this condition, the formula is as follows:

$$Ccre = [UCr \times V] / SCr, \text{ where Ucr (Urine creatinine) is mg/ml, V (urine volume) is ml and SCr (Serum creatinine) is mg/dl. If the finding is divided to 1,440 (24h} \times \text{60 min), creatinine clearance is expressed as ml/min.}$$

Creatinine clearance formula overestimates true GFR by approximately 10–20 % because of disregarding tubular secretion. As already mentioned, tubular secretion of creatinine increases with decreasing kidney function causing higher overestimations in late stages of CKD.

- The *reciprocal serum creatinine concentration (1/SCr) curve* is used to follow changes in the kidney function of patients with CKD. It assumes that GFR is inversely proportional to the serum creatinine. If creatinine generation, extrarenal elimination, and tubular secretion remain stable, a plot of 1/SCr against time will be linear with a constant decrease in GFR. Due to several caveats, this method is not popular anymore for following progression among CKD patients.
- *GFR estimating equations based on serum creatinine* were developed in order to eliminate several limitations of serum creatinine use. These equations were derived from different studies and populations and usually combine serum creatinine levels with other determinants of GFR like age, gender, and race and body size. The most common equations used are the Cockcroft-Gault, the Modification of Diet in Renal Disease (MDRD) Study, and the Chronic Kidney Disease Epidemiology Collaboration (CKD-EPI) equations.
- The *Cockroft-Gault equation* is the oldest (developed in 1973) but simplest equation for everyday clinical use. It has been derived using data from 249 men with a creatinine clearance ranging from approximately 30–130 ml/min [7].

$$Ccre(ml/min) = \{[(140 - age) \times \text{body weight}] / (72 \times Scr)\} \times (0.85 \text{ if female}), \text{ where age is expressed in years, weight in kilograms, and serum creatinine (Scr) in milligrams per deciliter.}$$

This equation was derived when standardized creatinine assays were not in use. In labs where standardized creatinine assays were used, this equation will cause an overestimation (10–40 %) of actual GFR. This equation has not been adjusted for body surface area. It is less accurate in obese patients (overestimate), in patients with normal or mildly decreased GFR (underestimates), and in the elderly (underestimates) [6, 8].

- The *MDRD Study equation* was developed in 1999 by using data from 1628 CKD patients (primarily white subjects, with nondiabetic kidney disease) with a GFR range between 5 and 90 ml/min/1.73 m^2. The equation was re-derived in 2006 for use with the standardized serum creatinine assays [9, 10].

$$GFR\ (ml/min/1.73\ m^2) = 186.3 \times Scr^{-1.154} \times age^{-0.203} \times (0.742 \text{ if female}) \times (1.210 \text{ if African American}),$$
where Scr is expressed in mg/dl and age is expressed in years.

$$GFR\ (ml/min/1.73\ m^2) = 175 \times Scr^{-1.154} \times age^{-0.203} \times (0.742 \text{ if female}) \times (1.210 \text{ if African American}),$$
where a standardized Scr (mg/dl) measurement is done.

MDRD equation is the most widely used formula in recent years. Many laboratories automatically report MDRD equation GFR estimate along with serum creatinine measurements. This equation is more accurate in estimating GFR than 24-h urine creatinine clearance and Cockroft-Gault formula. It is also more accurate in patients with lower GFR levels (<60 ml/min/1.73 m2). Its accuracy differs in various ethnic groups. It is less accurate in obese patients and in patients with normal or mildly decreased GFR.

- *The CKD-EPI equation* has been derived in 2009 from a large study population that included patients with or without kidney disease with a wide range of GFR. When compared with MDRD, CKD-EPI has found to be more accurate in people especially with higher GFR levels (>60 ml/min/1.73 m^2) [11].

$$\text{GFR (ml/min/1.73 m}^2) = 141 \times \min(\text{SCr}/\kappa, 1)^{\alpha} \times \max(\text{SCr}/\kappa, 1)^{-1.209} \times 0.993^{\text{Age}} \times (1.018 \text{ if female}) \times (1.159 \text{ if African American}),$$

where SCr is serum creatinine (in mg/dl), κ is 0.7 for females and 0.9 for males, α is –0.329 for females and –0.411 for males, min indicates the minimum of SCr/κ or 1, and max indicates the maximum of SCr/κ or 1

Female

<0.7 mg/dl	$\text{GFR} = 144 \times (\text{Scr}/0.7)^{-0.329}$	
>0.7 mg/dl	$\text{GFR} = 144 \times (\text{Scr}/0.7)^{-1.209}$	× (0.993)Age × 1.157 [if black]

Male

<0.9 mg/dl	$\text{GFR} = 141 \times (\text{Scr}/0.9)^{-0.411}$
>0.9 7mg/dl	$\text{GFR} = 141 \times (\text{Scr}/0.9)^{-1.209}$

The CKD-EPI equation has been found to result in lower prevalence estimate of CKD across a broad range of populations and categorized mortality and ESRD risk better than MDRD. Given the data on the improved performance, especially in general population at higher levels of GFR, *"KDIGO 2012 clinical practice guideline for the evaluation and management of chronic kidney disease" recommends to use CKD-EPI equation for GFR estimation.*

All GFR equations have some imprecision and do not provide an accurate estimate of GFR due to several limitations. Some of the limitations are related to the serum creatinine itself (Box 2.5) and some are linked to the populations and studies that the equations have been derived. All GFR equations should be used in stable settings where serum creatinine has no rapid alterations (i.e., not used in acute kidney injury/disease). They are not recommended for use in patients under the age of 18, in patients with extremes in body size or muscle mass, in patients with severe alterations in dietary intake (vegetarians, using creatine supplements), in very elderly (>85 years), or in pregnant patients.

2. *Blood urea and Urea clearance*: Urea is the most well-known nitrogenous waste and it was used as one of the first indicators to measure GFR. It is also measured as an indicator of uremic burden and uremic symptoms in late stages of CKD. Although blood urea nitrogen (BUN) has an inverse relationship with GFR, it is not an ideal filtration marker. Urea production is variable and is largely dependent on protein intake. BUN concentration increases as its production increases with high protein intake, tissue breakdown, trauma, hemorrhage, or glucocorticoid use. In contrast, BUN concentration decreases when its production decreases with low protein intake or in liver disease.

Urea is freely filtered from the glomerulus, but 40–50 % is reabsorbed in the tubules. Urea reabsorption increases substantially in states of decreased renal perfusion (volume depletion, congestive heart failure, diuretic use). In all these conditions, BUN levels will increase out of proportion to a decrease in GFR and

Box 2.5. Sources of Error by Using Serum Creatinine in GFR Estimation

Non-steady state (*e.g., acute kidney injury*)

Variable creatinine generation (*e.g., race, extremes of muscle mass, extremes of body size, high protein diet, creatinine supplements, muscle wasting*)

Variable tubular secretion (*e.g., decrease by trimethoprim, cimetidine, fenofibrate*)

Variable extrarenal elimination (*e.g., decrease by inhibition of gut creatininase by antibiotics, increase by large volume losses*)

Higher GFR (*e.g., higher measurement errors in patients with higher GFR*)

Interference with assay (*e.g., spectral interferences from bilirubin and some drugs or chemical interferences from glucose, ketones, bilirubin, and some drugs*)

Source: Adapted by permission from Macmillan Publishers Ltd: Kidney Disease: Improving Global Outcomes (KDIGO) CKD Work Group [2]. Copyright 2013. Available from: http://www.nature.com/kisup/index.html

will result in an increased ratio of BUN to SCre. Increased BUN-to-SCre ratio is suggestive of a prerenal state and may indicate an acute deterioration in a CKD patient.

Urea clearance is not a reliable indicator of GFR also due to variable tubular reabsorption rates of urea. GFR may be underestimated almost as half as the real level by urea clearance. *The only clinical setting where urea clearance use has been advocated is the late stages of CKD for deciding appropriate timing of dialysis* [12]. As urea clearance underestimates and creatinine clearance overestimates GFR, it is recommended that the average of these two clearances (*GFR* = (*creatinine clearance* + *urea clearance*)/*2*) is preferred for estimating GFR in advanced CKD. The use of this formula is also compromised by problems related to proper urine collection.

3. *Serum cystatin C and GFR equations*: Limitations inherent to the use of serum creatinine are the major drive for seeking alternative filtration markers in the serum. Among them, cystatin C is considered to be a potential alternative to serum creatinine for estimating GFR. Cystatin C is a low molecular weight (13-kDa) cysteine protease inhibitor that is produced by all nucleated cells. It is freely filtered by the renal glomerulus. It is reabsorbed and completely catabolized by tubular cells. In contrast to creatinine, cystatin C does not undergo any tubular secretion. The generation of cystatin C was believed to be less variable and affected less by age and sex. Later epidemiological studies, however, have suggested that cystatin C generation rate and serum levels have been influenced by age, sex, cell turnover rate, steroid use, body mass index, inflammation, and diabetes. Studies have also shown that there is an extrarenal elimination of cystatin C at low levels of GFR. Serum cystatin C measurements are not standardized yet and still evolving. Studies have shown that cystatin C measurements also have higher intra-individual variation than serum creatinine.

Several studies have shown that cystatin C concentrations may correlate more closely with GFR than serum creatinine. Similarly, GFR estimates based on cystatin C may be more powerful predictors of clinical outcomes than creatinine-based eGFR. These findings have been the strongest for mortality and CVD events, and the prognostic advantage of cystatin C is most apparent among individuals with GFR >45 ml/min/1.73 m^2. Recently, a single equation combining both serum creatinine and cystatin C has been found to be more accurate in determining GFR [13]. The role of cystatin C measurements or use of cystatin C-based equations in CKD care has yet to be determined. "KDIGO 2012 clinical practice guideline for the evaluation and management of chronic kidney disease" has recommended to measure cystatin C to confirm CKD in adults if eGFR based on serum creatinine was between 45 and 59 ml/min/1.73 m^2 without any markers of kidney damage. KDIGO recommends to use either cystatin C-based eGFR equation or cystatin C and creatinine-based eGFR equations in confirming the presence of CKD. The use of cystatin C equations has also several limitations (Boxes 2.6 and 2.7).

Box 2.6. Sources of Error by Using Serum Cystatin in GFR Estimation

Non-steady state (e.g., *acute kidney injury*)

Variable cystatin generation (e.g., *race, thyroid function disorders, corticosteroid use, diabetes, obesity*)

Variable extrarenal elimination (e.g., *increase by severe decrease in GFR*)

Higher GFR (e.g., *higher measurement errors in patients with higher GFR*)

Interference with assay (e.g., *heterophilic antibodies*)

Source: Adapted by permission from Macmillan Publishers Ltd: Kidney Disease: Improving Global Outcomes (KDIGO) CKD Work Group [2]. Copyright 2013. Available from: http://www.nature.com/kisup/index.html

Box 2.7. What the Guidelines Say You Should Do: Glomerular Filtration Rate

- Use serum creatinine and a GFR estimating equation for initial assessment.
- Use a GFR estimating equation to derive GFR from serum creatinine (eGFRcreat) rather than relying on the serum creatinine concentration alone.
- Understand clinical settings in which eGFRcreat is less accurate.
- Clinical laboratories should report eGFRcreat in adults using the 2009 CKD-EPI creatinine equation.
- Clinical laboratories that measure cystatin C should report eGFRcys and eGFRcreat-cys in adults using the 2012 CKD-EPI cystatin C and 2012 CKD-EPI creatinine-cystatin C equations.

Source: Data from KDIGO 2012 clinical practice guideline for the evaluation and management of chronic kidney disease [2]

CKD-EPI Cystatin C equation:

$$\text{GFR (ml/min/1.73 m}^2) = 133 \times \min(\text{SCysC}/0.8, 1)^{-0.499} \times \max(\text{SCysC}/0.8, 1)^{-1.328} \times 0.996\text{Age} \; [\times 0.932 \text{ if female}],$$

where SCysC is serum cystatin C (in mg/l), min indicates the minimum of SCysC/0.8 or 1, and max indicates the maximum of SCysC/0.8 or 1.

CKD-EPI Creatinine-Cystatin C equation:

$$\text{GFR (ml/min/1.73 m}^2) = 135 \times \min(\text{SCr}/\kappa, 1)^{\alpha} \times \max(\text{SCr}/\kappa, 1)^{-0.601} \times \min(\text{SCysC}/0.8, 1)^{-0.375} \times \max(\text{SCysC}/0.8, 1)^{-0.711} \times 0.995^{\text{Age}} \; [\times 0.969 \text{ if female}] \; [\times 1.08 \text{ if black}],$$

where SCr is serum creatinine (in mg/dl), SCysC is serum cystatin C (in mg/l), κ is 0.7 for females and 0.9 for males, α is –0.248 for females and –0.207 for males, min(SCr/κ, 1) indicates the minimum of SCr/κ or 1,and max(SCr/κ, 1) indicates the maximum of SCr/κ or 1; min(SCysC/0.8, 1) indicates the minimum of SCysC/0.8 or 1 and max(SCysC/0.8, 1) indicates the maximum of SCysC/0.8 or 1.

All these equations may be reached in various websites as electronic calculators, such as http://touchcalc.com/bis2.html or http://www.hdcn.com/calcf/gfr2.htm.

4. *Measuring GFR with exogenous markers*: In clinical settings where GFR estimates from serum creatinine or creatinine-based GFR estimating equations cannot be performed (such as pregnancy, acute kidney disease, etc.) or when there is a need for a more precise determination (such as for living donor assessment) of GFR, clearance measurements should be performed with several filtration markers (inulin, iothalamate, iohexol, DTPA,

or EDTA) [14]. Measuring GFR with the use of these markers is complex, expensive, and difficult to do in clinical practice. The measurement of GFR with these markers has also some limitations and rarely used in clinical practice for CKD care except research settings. In a CKD patient, a measured GFR may only be required if the patient is chronically ill with severe reduction in muscle mass, if there will be a prolonged exposure to nephrotoxic drugs, or if there is a discrepancy between severely reduced eGFR and symptoms of uremia before deciding to start renal replacement therapy.

5. *Novel biomarkers*: There is still ongoing research for finding one or more potential, alternative markers for estimating GFR. In this sense, several low molecular weight molecules such as beta-trace protein (BTP), beta(2)-microglobulin (B2M), and symmetric dimethyl arginine have been investigated. BTP and B2M have been found to be more accurate than serum creatinine in some studies. It is yet to be determined whether one or several of them have a role in CKD patients alone or in combination with creatinine or cystatin C.

2.3 Urinalysis and Albuminuria in CKD

Urinalysis and assessment of albuminuria are very informative, noninvasive tests for both screening and diagnosing CKD. Albuminuria is also an important measure for defining severity of kidney dysfunction, estimating prognosis of CKD-related outcomes, and associated cardiovascular risk. The presence of albuminuria and its severity also guides treatment alternatives in CKD.

1. *Urinalysis*: A complete urinalysis should be carried out in the first examination of all CKD patients. Along with a targeted history and physical examination, urinalysis provides important information for differential diagnosis of acute and chronic kidney disease. Urinalysis may also provide clues for underlying etiologies of chronic kidney disease. There is, however, no evidence-based information whether urinalysis is required in each follow-up visit of a CKD patient.

   A detailed discussion of the diagnostic uses of urinalysis or specific tests of urine (metabolic diseases, urine electrolytes, etc.) is beyond the scope of this chapter and may be found in other sources. Here, only essential features of urinalysis for the care of CKD patients will be covered.

   An accurate urine analysis should start with a proper collection of a urine sample. First-void (early) morning urine is usually preferred as formed elements will more likely be seen in concentrated urine with a low pH. The sample should be analyzed within 2–4 h from collection.

   A complete urinalysis consists of three components, as physical (gross) examination, chemical (dipstick) analysis, and microscopic evaluation of the urinary sediment. In routine clinical practice, most of the physical and chemical parameters are examined by a dipstick. A dipstick provides a semiquantitative examination of several urinary characteristics by a series of tests embedded on a reagent strip. Among physical parameters, color (usually normal in CKD), turbidity (usually normal in CKD), and specific gravity (usually a fixed, isosthenuric urine is produced in CKD, i.e., specific gravity is 1010) are assessed. In chemical analysis, urine dipstick assesses pH (low or normal in CKD), glucose (usually normal in CKD), ketones (usually normal in CKD), bilirubin and urobilinogen (usually normal in CKD), nitrite and leukocyte esterase (usually normal in CKD), blood, and protein. *The dipstick test for blood* detects peroxidase activity of erythrocytes. The dipstick test is commonly considered to be sensitive for detection of microscopic hematuria. False-negative results are unusual, i.e., a negative dipstick for blood excludes hematuria. However, myoglobin and hemoglobin also will catalyze this reaction, so a positive test result may indicate hematuria, myoglobinuria (from rhabdomyolysis), or hemoglobinuria (from intravascular hemolysis). When it is positive, visualization of intact erythrocytes on microscopic examination of the urinary sediment should be done for confirmation of hematuria. Hematuria may be observed in patients with CKD due to various underlying causes. *The dipstick test for protein* is most sensitive to albumin and may not detect low concentrations of globulins, tubular proteins, and Bence Jones proteins. The dipstick measurement of urine protein allows only an approximate quantification of urine albumin, expressed on a scale from negative trace to 1(+) to 4(+). Dipstick tests for trace amounts of protein yield positive results at concentrations of 5–10 mg/dl—lower than the threshold for clinically significant proteinuria. Dipstick protein may miss moderately increased albuminuria levels in the range of 30–300 mg/day (formerly called microalbuminuria) in most cases. A result of 1+ corresponds to approximately 30 mg of protein per dl and is considered positive; 2+ corresponds to 100 mg/dl, 3+ to 300 mg/dl, and 4+ to 1,000 mg/dl. In addition, dipstick protein measurement is dependent on the concentration of the urine specimen, where concentrated urine may give false-positive and dilute urine may give false-negative results. Thus, it is important to quantify the amount of proteinuria detected on urine dipstick analysis with other methods. Protein can be quantified in random samples, in timed or untimed overnight samples, or in 24-h collections. Although 24-h urine protein amount represents the gold standard method, problems related with 24-h collection (over or under collection) are a major source of error. It is also a cumbersome procedure for many patients. Still, adequately collected 24-h urine protein concentrations are accepted as the most accurate way to monitor proteinuria under active treatment (such as active immunosuppressive use). A complete collection may be determined by the amount of expected 24-h urine creatinine excretion (see above). *Protein-creatinine ratio (PCR)* in a random urine sample is accepted as an alternative to 24-h urine collection. PCR may correct problems arising from variability of urine volume and concentration. It is easy to obtain and showed a strong correlation with 24-h urine collection. However, when urine protein levels are greater than 1 g/l, spot protein-creatinine correlation with 24-h urine may not be accurate. Thus, spot protein-creatinine level may act as a simple screening for proteinuria, i.e., if it is negative, there is no need for a 24-h urine collection.

In cases where presence of non-albumin proteins (such as gamma globulins, Bence Jones proteins) is suspected, other precipitation methods like sulfosalicylic acid test should be used. Trichloroacetic acid can be used in place of sulfosalicylic acid to increase the sensitivity to gamma globulins.

Microscopic examination of urine sediment should be done in all patients with CKD and in patients with high risk for CKD. In the urine sediment, cellular elements (red blood cells, white blood cells), casts, and crystals should be thoroughly examined. Some findings in the urine sediment may help to diagnose some underlying causes of CKD. There is, however, no characteristic finding in the urinary sediment of a CKD patient, except broad casts which are typically associated with advanced stages of CKD.

2. *Albuminuria*: Albumin is the predominant protein in major proteinuric diseases causing CKD. Albumin measurement in urine has greater sensitivity and improved precision for the detection of low levels of proteinuria compared to protein measurements. It is therefore accepted as a more sensitive method for screening/diagnosing not only diabetic but also nondiabetic CKD. Most of the recent studies also showed strong evidence linking increased albuminuria and outcomes of CKD.

   Urinary concentrations of albumin <150 mg/l are below the detection limit of the "dipstick" tests used in routine urinalysis. Albumin in the urine may be detected by radioimmunoassay, immunoturbidimetric technique, and nephelometry, ELISA, or HPLC. Reagent strip methods were also developed for urine albumin screening but have increased false-positive or false-negative ratios.

   Twenty-four-hour urine collection is also the gold standard for the detection of high albuminuria (formerly, microalbuminuria).

Box 2.8. Sources of Error When Using ACR for Albuminuria

Transient, false elevations in albuminuria (e.g., *menstrual blood contamination, urinary tract infection, fever, exercise, orthostatic, severe uncontrolled hyperglycemia, or hypertension*)

Variability due to sample storage (*e.g., degradation of albumin before analysis*)

Variability in creatinine excretion (*e.g., lower in children, women, or elderly, higher in black, lower due to decreased muscle mass, variability due to non-steady state*)

Interference with assay (*e.g., samples with very high albumin levels may falsely be reported as low or normal due to antigen excess effect in some assays*)

Source: Adapted by permission from Macmillan Publishers Ltd: Kidney Disease: Improving Global Outcomes (KDIGO) CKD Work Group [2]. Copyright 2013. Available from: http://www.nature.com/kisup/index.html

Albuminuria screening however may be done with spot early morning urine collections, timed urine collections, or as a ratio of albumin to creatinine in the urine (ACR). The ACR is the preferred method as it does not require timed collections, it correlates with the 24-h urine values over a large range of proteinuria, it is cheap to perform, and repeat values can be easily obtained to be certain that high albuminuria, if present, is persistent. A value of 30–300 mg/g of creatinine (or, using standard (SI) units, 3.4–34 mg/mmol of creatinine) suggests that albumin excretion is between 30 and 300 mg/day and therefore that high albuminuria is probably present. A false reading for ACR may occur after vigorous exercise, in the presence of fever, urinary infection, congestive heart failure, acute severe elevations of blood pressure or blood sugar, or menstruation. There are some other sources of error in the assessment of ACR (Box 2.8) [15].

Box 2.9. What the Guidelines Say You Should Do: Albuminuria

- Use the following measurements for initial testing of proteinuria (in descending order of preference, in all cases an early morning urine sample is preferred):
  1. Urine albumin-to-creatinine ratio (ACR)
  2. Urine protein-to-creatinine ratio (PCR)
  3. Reagent strip urinalysis for total protein with automated reading
  4. Reagent strip urinalysis for total protein with manual reading
- Confirm reagent strip-positive albuminuria and proteinuria by quantitative laboratory measurement and express as a ratio to creatinine wherever possible
- Confirm ACR >30 mg/g (>3 mg/mmol) on a random untimed urine with a subsequent early morning urine sample
- Measure albumin excretion rate or total protein excretion rate in a timed urine sample for a more accurate estimate

Source: Data from KDIGO 2012 clinical practice guideline for the evaluation and management of chronic kidney disease [2]

Most national and international guidelines (including KDIGO 2012 clinical practice guideline for the evaluation and management of chronic kidney disease) recommend ACR measurement with an early morning urine sample over other methods. Albuminuria assessment is recommended to be done at least annually in CKD patients. The frequency of assessment of albuminuria may depend on clinical situation, i.e., rate of progression or monitoring the effect of anti-albuminuric treatment (Boxes 2.9 and 2.10).

2.4 Other Lab Tests in CKD

CKD patients may need further tests as a part of their general assessment or for finding any other marker of kidney damage like renal tubular

Box 2.10. Relevant Guidelines

1. *KDIGO Guideline*:
   Kidney Disease: Improving Global Outcomes (KDIGO) CKD Work Group. KDIGO 2012 clinical practice guideline for the evaluation and management of chronic kidney disease. Kidney Int Suppl. 2013;3:1–150.
   http://www.kdigo.org/clinical_practice_guidelines/CKD.php
2. *CARI Guideline*:
   Diagnosis, classification and staging of chronic kidney disease. July 2012
   http://www.cari.org.au/CKD_early_CKD/Diag_Classification_Staging_ECKD.pdf
3. *The Renal Association Guideline*
   Detection, monitoring and care of patients with CKD. Final Version (28 February 2011).
   http://www.renal.org/Clinical/GuidelinesSection/Detection-Monitoring-and-Care-of-Patients-with-CKD.aspx
4. *Japanese Society of Nephrology Guideline*
   Evidence-based Practice Guideline for the Treatment of CKD. Clin Exp Nephrol. 2009;13:533–66.
   http://www.jsn.or.jp/en/guideline/pdf/guideline2009.pdf
5. *National Institute for Health and Clinical Excellence (NICE) Guideline*
   Chronic Kidney Disease. National clinical guideline for early identification and management in adults in primary and secondary care. 2008, Royal College of Physicians.
   http://www.nice.org.uk/nicemedia/live/12069/42116/42116.pdf
6. *Canadian Society of Nephrology Guideline*:
   Guidelines for the management of chronic kidney disease. CMAJ. 2008;179(11):1154–62.
   http://www.cmaj.ca/content/suppl/2008/11/17/179.11.1154.DC1
7. *NKF KDOQI Guideline*:
   KDOQI Clinical practice guidelines for chronic kidney disease: evaluation, classification, and stratification. Am J Kid Dis. 2002;39(2 Suppl 1):S11–266.
   http://www.kidney.org/professionals/KDOQI/guidelines_ckd/toc.htm

disorders or for assessment of the complications of CKD (such as anemia, mineral-bone disorders, malnutrition, neuropathy, cardiovascular tests). These tests will not be covered in detail here. It is however important to note that some tests need a cautious interpretation especially in patients who are in the late stages (Stages 4 or 5) of CKD. Among those tests, there are serum ALT, AST, amylase, lipase concentrations, troponins, and BNP/NT-proBNP levels which may have diagnostic and/or therapeutic importance. With a decrease in GFR, there is a trend of false alterations in these tests: Liver transaminases tend to decrease to very low levels, pancreatic amylase and lipase, troponins, and BNP/NT-proBNP levels tend to increase above cutoff concentrations. All these alterations should be interpreted carefully, and "real" implications of test results should be assessed within the clinical context of the patient.

Before You Finish: Practice Pearls for the Clinician

- In each visit, a CKD patient should be assessed for general well-being, for progression and any factor for acute deterioration of CKD, for presence of any complications or comorbidity, and for cardiovascular health.
- Patients who are in late stages of the disease should be assessed for the presence of any uremic symptom, and the need for renal replacement therapy should be evaluated.
- Blood pressure, orthostatic changes, volume, and cardiac status should be checked in all visits.
- CKD patients should have an assessment of eGFR and albuminuria as a part of their initial assessment. eGFR and albuminuria should be rechecked at least annually in all CKD patients.
- eGFR should be calculated by 2009 CKD-EPI equation derived from serum creatinine. Patients who are in the late stages, who have a higher risk for progression, who have any intercurrent illness/medication use/operation, and who have changes in treatment may have frequent eGFR assessments.
- Keep in mind the limitations of eGFR or ACR measurements mostly caused by creatinine measurements.
- The use of direct methods to measure GFR should be considered in clinical situations in which estimation equations are known to be suboptimal.
- Albuminuria should be assessed by albumin-creatinine ratio measured from an early morning urine sample. Patients who have severely increased albuminuria or patients who are under antiproteinuric treatment may have frequent albuminuria assessments.

References

1. KDOQI clinical practice guidelines for chronic kidney disease: evaluation, classification, and stratification, 2002. Am J Kidney Dis. 2002;39(2 Suppl 1):S11–266. http://www.kidney.org/professionals/KDOQI/guidelines_ckd/toc.htm.
2. Kidney Disease: Improving Global Outcomes (KDIGO) CKD Work Group. KDIGO 2012 clinical practice guideline for the evaluation and management of chronic kidney disease. Kidney Int Suppl. 2013;3:1–150. http://www.kdigo.org/clinical_practice_guidelines/CKD.php.
3. Stevens LA, Coresh J, Greene T, Levey AS. Assessing kidney function-measured and estimated glomerular filtration rate. N Engl J Med. 2006;354:2473–83.
4. National Institute for Health and Clinical Excellence (NICE). Chronic kidney disease. National clinical guideline for early identification and management in adults in primary and secondary care [internet]. London: Royal College of Physicians; 2008. http://www.nice.org.uk/nicemedia/live/12069/42116/42116.pdf. Cited 6 Mar 2013.
5. Levey AS, Perrone RD, Madias NE. Serum creatinine and renal function. Annu Rev Med. 1988;39:465–90.
6. Myers GL, Miller WG, Coresh J, Fleming J, Greenberg N, Greene T, National Kidney Disease Education Program Laboratory Working Group, et al. Recommendations for improving serum creatinine measurement: a report from the Laboratory Working Group of the National Kidney Disease Education Program. Clin Chem. 2006;52:5–18.
7. Cockcroft DW, Gault MH. Prediction of creatinine clearance from serum creatinine. Nephron. 1976;16:31–41.
8. Creatinine Standardization Recommendations [Internet]. Bethesda: National Kidney Disease Education Program. http://www.nkdep.nih.gov/lab-evaluation/gfr/creatinine-standardization/recommendations.shtml#pharmacists. Updated 1 Mar 2012; cited 3 Mar 2013.
9. Levey AS, Bosch JP, Lewis JB, Greene T, Rogesr N, Roth D. A more accurate method to estimate glomerular filtration rate from serum creatinine: a new prediction equation. Modification of Diet in Renal Disease Study Group. Ann Intern Med. 1999;130:461–70.
10. Levey AS, Coresh J, Greene T, Stevens LA, Zhang YL, Hendriksen S, et al. Using standardized serum creatinine values in the modification of diet in renal disease study equation for estimating glomerular filtration rate. Ann Intern Med. 2006;145:247–54.
11. Levey AS, Stevens LA, Schmid CH, Zhang YL, Castro 3rd AF, Feldman HI, et al. Using standardized

serum creatinine values in the modification of diet in renal disease study equation for estimating glomerular filtration rate. Ann Intern Med. 2009;150:604–12.
12. Tattersall J, Dekker F, Heimbürger O, Jager KJ, Lameire N, Lindley E, ERBP Advisory Board, et al. When to start dialysis: updated guidance following publication of the Initiating Dialysis Early and Late (IDEAL) study. Nephrol Dial Transplant. 2011;26(7):2082–6.
13. Inker LA, Schmid CH, Tighiouart H, Eckfeldt JH, Feldman HI, Greene T, et al. Estimating glomerular filtration rate from serum creatinine and cystatin C. N Engl J Med. 2012;367:20–9.
14. Stevens LA, Levey AS. Measured GFR as a confirmatory test for estimated GFR. J Am Soc Nephrol. 2009;20:2305–13.
15. Miller WG, Bruns DE, Hortin GL, Sandberg S, Aakre KM, McQueen MJ, National Kidney Disease Education Program–IFCC Working Group on Standardization of Albumin in Urine, et al. Current Issues in Measurement and Reporting of Urinary Albumin Excretion. Clin Chem. 2009;55:24–38.

Imaging in Chronic Kidney Disease

3

Yousef W. Nielsen, Peter Marckmann, and Henrik S. Thomsen

Before You Start: Facts You Need to Know

- Intravascular contrast media cannot be used for imaging of kidneys, ureters and urinary bladder in advanced renal failure (GFR <30 ml/min/1.73 m^2) due to poor imaging quality.
- Chronic kidney disease patients may experience serious adverse reactions to both gadolinium- and iodine-based contrast agents, namely, nephrogenic systemic fibrosis and contrast nephropathy – complications correlated with increased morbidity and mortality.
- Awareness of these issues is of utmost importance.
- Appropriate precautions to avoid these adverse reactions should be taken; all departments should have guidelines for the handling of patients at risk.

3.1 Diagnostic Imaging in CKD

The patients with chronic kidney disease can undergo exactly the same imaging examinations as patients with normal kidney function with one important exception, namely, when glomerular function is part of the examination as it is in renography, intravenous urography, CT urography, and magnetic resonance imaging urography where excretion of the contrast agent is an integrated part of the examination.

In most cases, the process towards end-stage renal disease is long. Diabetic nephropathy rarely occurs before the patient has had diabetes mellitus for 10 years. Multiple cysts can be seen in patients with adult dominant polycystic kidney from their early twenties, whereas end-stage renal disease typically first occurs in their fifties. Thus, the major work for radiology/nuclear medicine in patients with chronic kidney disease is not imaging of the kidneys themselves, but the complications to chronic kidney disease, e.g., vascular problems (arteriography, venography), cardiac incompensation (chest X-ray), infections, and cerebral diseases. In any case, the patient should always be referred

Y.W. Nielsen, MD, PhD
Department of Diagnostic Radiology, Copenhagen University Hospital, Herlev Ringvej 75, Herlev DK-2730, Denmark
e-mail: ywnielsen@gmail.com

P. Marckmann, MD, DMSc
Department of Nephrology, Roskilde Hospital, Kogevej 7-13, Roskilde, DK-4000, Denmark
e-mail: peter.marckmann@dadlnet.dk

H.S. Thomsen, MD, DMSc (✉)
Department of Diagnostic Radiology, Copenhagen University Hospital, Herlev Ringvej 75, Herlev DK-2730, Denmark

Faculty of Medical and Health Sciences, University of Copenhagen, Copenhagen, Denmark
e-mail: henrik.thomsen@regionh.dk

M. Arici (ed.), *Management of Chronic Kidney Disease*,
DOI 10.1007/978-3-642-54637-2_3, © Springer-Verlag Berlin Heidelberg 2014

to the most optimal imaging to verify or rule out a suspected lesion. When there is reduced glomerular filtration rate or it is absent, other ways to visualize the lumen of the pelvis, ureter, and bladder tract than the usual imaging method, e.g., CT urography, should be performed. One has to inject the contrast medium directly into the ureter/pelvis and/or bladder using a catheter. When the contrast medium has been injected, CT or plain films should be done. Alternatively, MR hydrography using the water in the urinary tract should be performed. There may be instances where MRI and CT are equal with regard to diagnostic workup; in those cases, MRI should be chosen for patients with chronic kidney disease so that radiation is avoided.

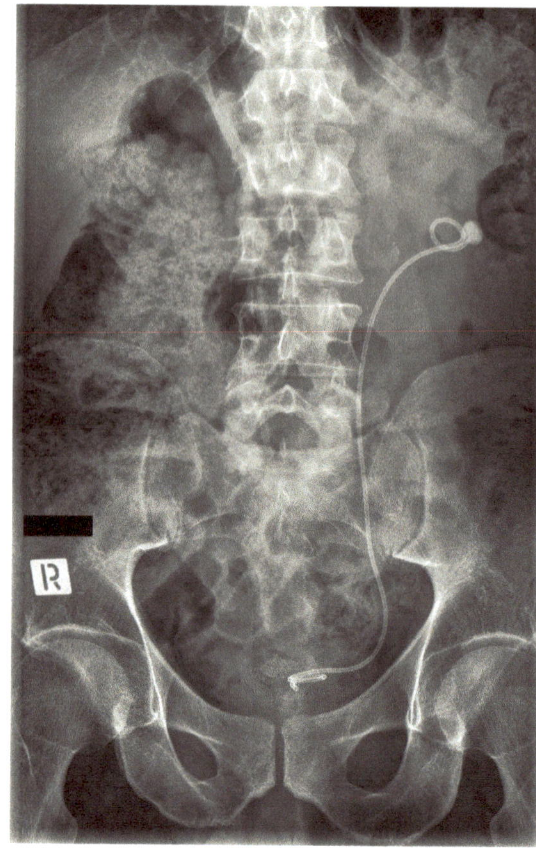

Fig. 3.1 A plain film of the urinary tract showing a left-sided double J-stent

3.2 Radiological Investigations

3.2.1 Conventional Radiography

A plain film of the urinary tract gives information about the calcifications within and outside the urinary tract as well as various medical devices, e.g., nephrostomy tube, double J-stent, and artificial sphincter (Fig. 3.1). As in other patients chest X-ray is used to evaluate heart size, pulmonary congestion, pneumonic infiltrations, pneumothorax, location of catheters, and fluid in the pleural space (Fig. 3.2). It is frequently used in patients with severely reduced kidney function or on dialysis as they develop chest problems easier (e.g., incompensation, inflammations) than patients with normal kidney function.

Intravenous urography or pyelography has no role in patients with reduced kidney function or on dialysis as the kidneys cannot filter enough contrast agents per time unit to enhance the lumen of the urinary tract for imaging. Visualization of the urinary tract (lumen) is possible using conventional imaging methods like direct pyelography where the contrast medium is injected through a catheter inserted percutaneously (nephrostomy) or via a catheter placed in the ureter during cystoscopy. These examinations are called antegrade pyelography and retrograde pyelography, respectively (Fig. 3.3). They are rarely used today as most information can be obtained by magnetic resonance imaging and CT scanning.

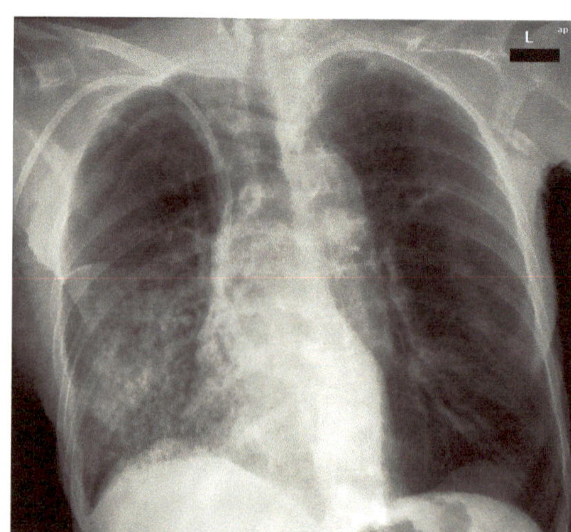

Fig. 3.2 Chest X-ray. Right-sided pneumonia in a CKD patient

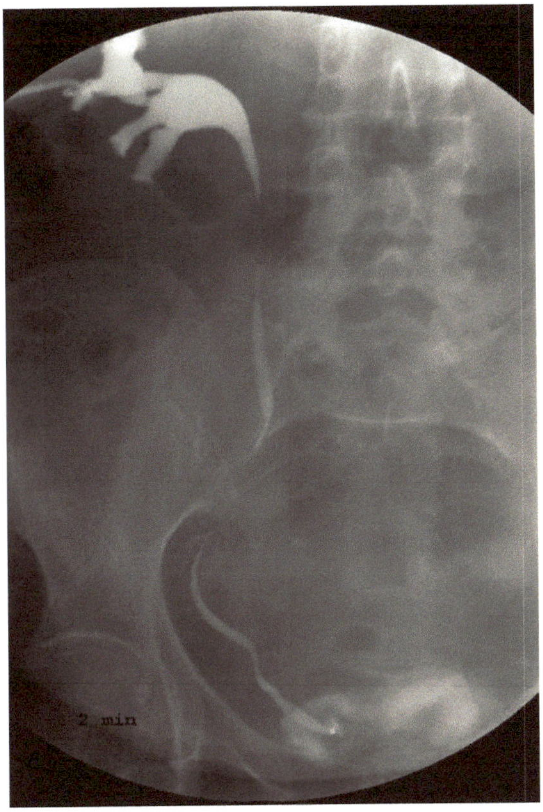

Fig. 3.3 Normal antegrade pyelography. Note the nephrostomy tube

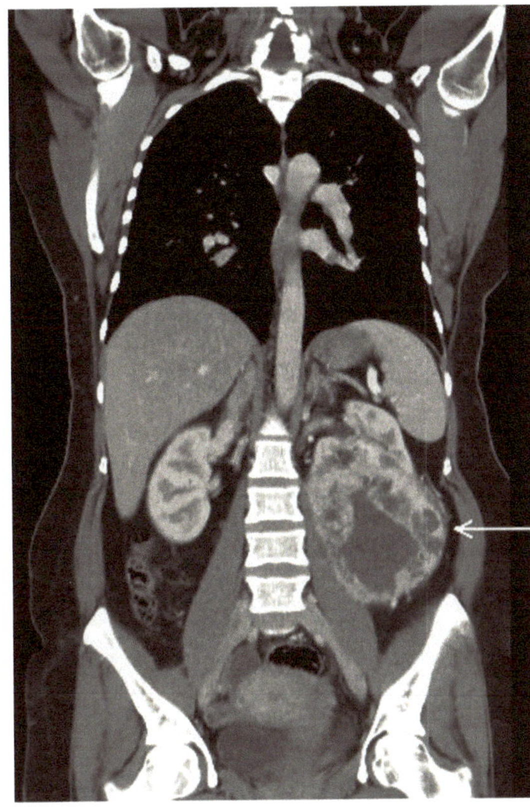

Fig. 3.4 Contrast-enhanced CT showing a large left-sided renal cell carcinoma with central necrosis (*arrow*)

However, direct pyelography does not include intravascular injection and the patient has no risk of contrast nephropathy. Regarding radiation during CT and/or conventional radiography, patients with CKD are subject to the same risks as patients with normal kidney function. The risk of developing a cancer due to radiation exposure decreases with age. Those at highest risk are children. In such patients, the use of CT and radiography should always be considered carefully, and it should be discussed whether the same diagnostic information can be obtained without radiation. In older patients, the risk/benefit ratio is different. In many instances, the benefit outweighs the risk.

3.2.2 CT Imaging

CT imaging can be performed with or without administration of intravenous iodine-based contrast media (CM). Unenhanced CT imaging can be performed in CKD patients without special precautionary measures, whereas contrast-enhanced studies may result in contrast nephropathy (see Sect. 3.7.1). Due to the risk of contrast nephropathy, the role of enhanced CT imaging in CKD patients is limited.

Unenhanced CT may show obstruction, tumors, cysts, or calculi. In some cases, both the level and degree of urinary tract obstruction can be clearly visualized by this method. For patients with low kidney function, however, the hydrostatic pressure in glomeruli and tubuli may not generate enough pressure to enlarge the pelvic cavity in the presence of obstruction. Thus, a normal-sized pelvic cavity does not exclude obstruction in patients with poor kidney function. Some renal tumors can be detected with unenhanced CT; however, detection of small renal cell carcinomas requires contrast media administration (Fig. 3.4). Presence of a normal

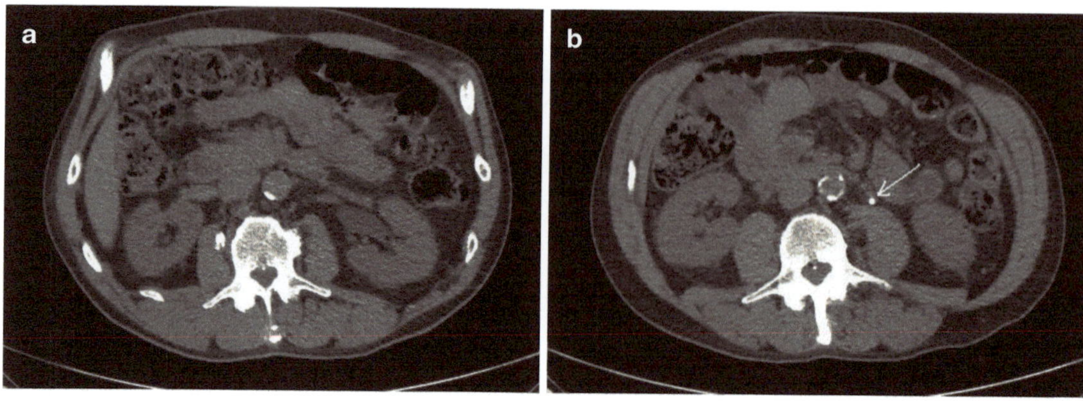

Fig. 3.5 Unenhanced CT showing left-sided hydronephrosis (**a**). The cause was a 6 mm calculus (*arrow*) in left proximal ureter (**b**)

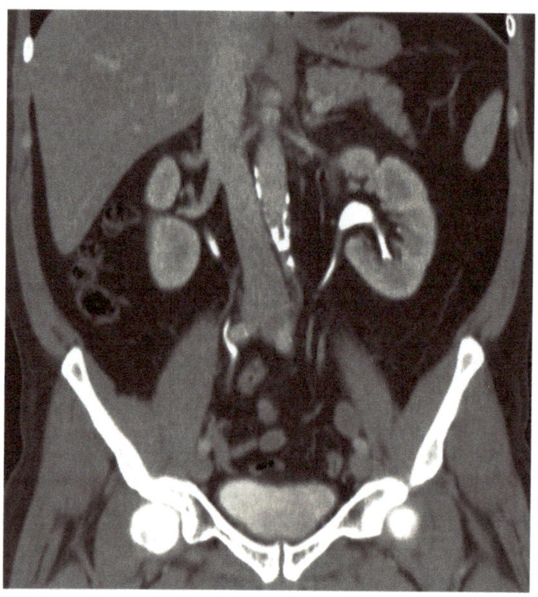

Fig. 3.6 CT urography. After intravenous contrast administration, there is enhancement of renal parenchyma as well as contrast in the urinary tract

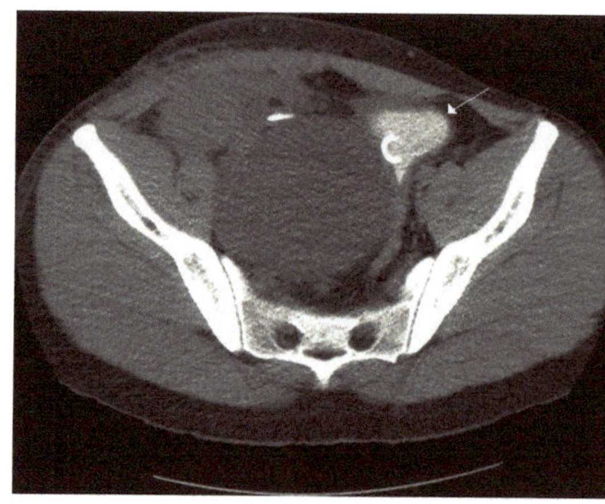

Fig. 3.7 Posttransplant complication. A large lymphocele is present in the pelvis. The bladder (*arrow*) is compressed and displaced by the lymphocele

contoured kidney does not exclude malignancy in renal parenchyma. It may be very difficult to detect small tumors in the upper urinary tract without the use of contrast medium; this also applies to patients with acquired cystic disease. Presence of fat within renal lesions is suggestive of angiomyolipoma, but again small amounts of fat may be found in renal cell carcinomas. Unenhanced CT is the best imaging method for detection of urinary tract calculi (Fig. 3.5a, b).

Contrast-enhanced CT performed as CT urography is the method of choice to detect renal as well as urothelial carcinomas outside the bladder (Fig. 3.6). The strength of CT urography is the excellent enhancement of renal parenchyma combined with contrast filling in the collecting system and ureters. The major drawback in CKD patients is that the method requires glomerular filtration of the contrast medium. Thus, it is not possible to perform CT urography when GFR is reduced.

Other indications for contrast-enhanced CT in CKD patients are by large related to vascular diseases. CT angiography performed in modern multislice CT scanners is suitable for detection of renal artery stenosis, as well as peripheral and coronary artery disease (see Sect. 3.5).

In renal transplant patients, CT may be used in problem solving of posttransplant complications (fluid collections or hematomas) (Fig. 3.7).

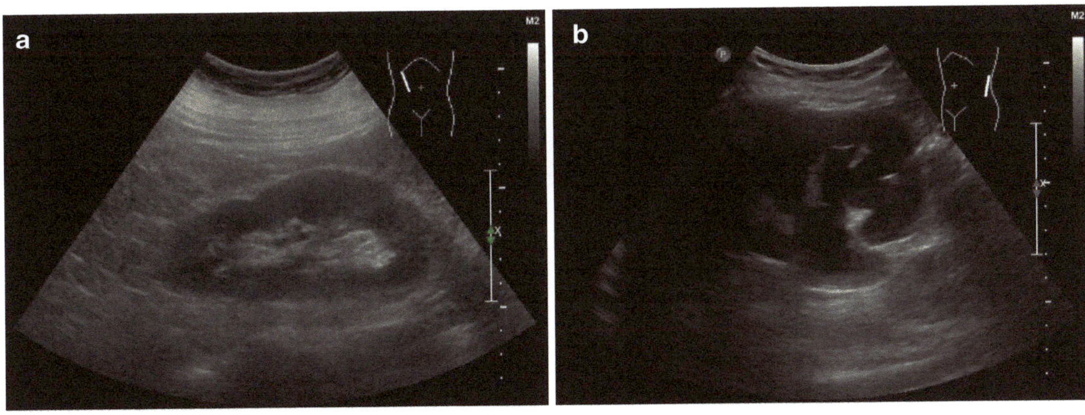

Fig. 3.8 Ultrasound showing a normal kidney (**a**), and a kidney with hydronephrosis (**b**)

The key point in each CKD patient is whether or not the diagnostic question can be answered with unenhanced or enhanced CT. If unenhanced CT fails in answering the question and enhanced CT is ruled out because of the risk of contrast nephropathy, other imaging studies (MRI or ultrasound) should be performed. However, this does not apply to all parts of the body, e.g., the lungs in workup of a lung cancer.

One should remember that in anuric patients (no water excretion at all), iodine-based contrast media can be administered without any risk of contrast nephropathy.

3.3 Ultrasound

Ultrasonography is frequently used in patients with reduced kidney function. It can give information about the size of the kidney and presence of hydronephrosis (Fig. 3.8a, b). However, absence of hydronephrosis does not exclude obstruction. Doppler can provide information about vascularization of the kidney. Resistive index (RI) determined by Doppler in CKD patients is considered as a marker of kidney function, histological damage, and renal prognosis. RI >0.65–0.70 is associated with severe interstitial fibrosis and arteriosclerosis and kidney function decline, acute tubular necrosis and more. RI may also be used to screen for renal artery stenosis (Box 3.1). Patients with CKD should be referred to renal ultrasound if they have (1) progressive CKD (eGFR decline more than 5 ml/min/1.73 m^2 within 1 year or more than 10 ml/min/1.73 m^2 within 5 years), (2) have visible or persistent invisible hematuria, (3) have symptoms of urinary tract obstruction, (4) have a family history of polycystic kidney disease and are aged over 20 years, (5) have CKD stage 4 or 5, or (6) are considered by a nephrologist to require a renal biopsy.

Box 3.1. Resistive Index (RI)

RI: Measures the degree of intrarenal arterial impedance

RI definition: [peak systolic velocity – end diastolic velocity]/peak systolic velocity

RI is best measured in the kidneys interlobar arteries

Normal values:

$RI_{interlobar}$ 0.54 ± 0.20

RI_{hilum} 0.65 ± 0.17

RI >0.7 is discriminative between normal and pathological resistance to flow.

Elevated RI may be seen with following conditions:

Nephrocalcinosis

Arterial hypertension

Renal artery stenosis

Tubular-interstitial kidney disease

Graft-rejection

3.3.1 Renal Artery Stenosis (RAS)

Difference in RI >0.05–0.07 between the two kidneys is suggestive of RAS.

RI may be used as a prognostic marker in RAS.

- Renal artery stenting does not improve symptoms and kidney function when RI >0.8 [Radermacher et al. N Eng J Med. 2001;344:410–7].
- Renal artery stenting improves renal function in 29 % of patients when RI >0.8 [Garcia-Criado et al. J Ultrasound Med. 2006;24:1641–7]. However, recent research have questioned this value [Cooper et al. N Engl J Med 2014;370:13-22].

3.4 MR Imaging

MRI can be used to image the urinary tract in CKD patients. Similar to CT, MRI can be used to evaluate structural abnormalities like tumors, cysts, and obstruction. However, compared with CT, MRI is relatively insensitive for detecting urinary tract calculi, so an unenhanced CT may be complementary to the MRI. Other disadvantages of MRI include long imaging times, susceptibility of motion artifacts, and lower spatial resolution than CT and radiography. Considerable advantages of MRI are excellent soft-tissue visualization and no use of ionizing radiation.

Typical MR techniques used for imaging urinary tracts are MR hydrography and excretory MR urography. For the remaining parts of the body, the same examinations for patients with normal kidney function are done in patients with CKD; the only issue is whether it should be enhanced or not as gadolinium-based contrast media may only be used with caution in patients with a glomerular filtration rate below 30 ml/min/1.73 m^2. The technical foundation of MRI is complicated and in-depth description of MR hydrography and excretory MR urography falls beyond the scope of this book. The basic principles of the imaging methods are presented.

In MR hydrography, the so-called T2-weighted imaging sequences (that renders water/urine bright) are used to produce MR urograms. The method was the earliest means of urinary tract MRI. MR hydrography does not rely on excretion of contrast media and is therefore useful for visualizing the collecting system of an obstructed,

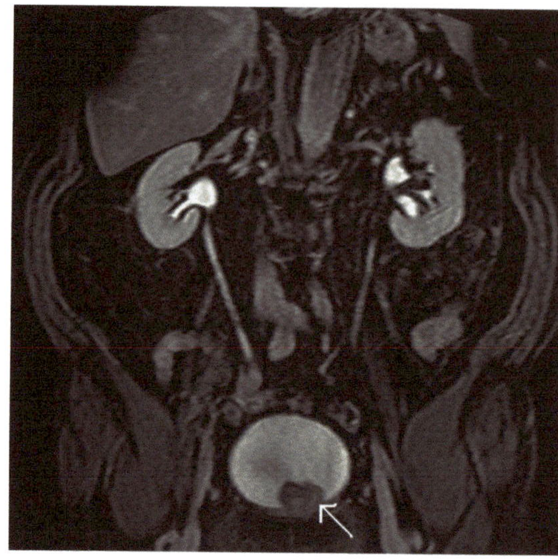

Fig. 3.9 Excretory MR urography. There is contrast enhancement in renal parenchyma as well as contrast material in the ureters and bladder. Note the tumor in the bladder (*arrow*)

poorly excreting kidney. MR hydrography can be performed in CKD patients to evaluate if any obstruction is present, but it is dependent on whether the kidney can generate a pressure that enlarges the pelvic cavity. If one is suspicious of an obstructed normal-sized pelvic cavity, the only way to solve the issue is to catheterize the pelvic cavity and see whether kidney function improves. In patients with normal renal function, renography can often answer the question.

Excretory MR urography is similar to CT urography. A contrast medium is injected intravenously followed by imaging in the renal excretory phase. In excretory MR urography, gadolinium-based MR contrast agents are used, just as iodine-based contrast media are used in CT urography. However, pharmacokinetic profiles of the contrast agents are similar, with the agents being eliminated by renal filtration. T1-weighted images are used to produce bright MR urograms (Fig. 3.9). The reason for this is that the paramagnetic effects of gadolinium shorten T1 relaxation times in adjacent tissue. A common problem in excretory MR urography is that gadolinium becomes concentrated in the urine. This leads to inhomogeneity in the magnetic field and signal loss on the MR urogram. In order to reduce this problem, a lower dose of gadolinium contrast agent should be used for excretory MR urography as compared to other contrast-enhanced MR procedures (typical 0.05 mmol/kg body weight in MR urography vs. standard MR dose of 0.1 mmol/kg).

Furthermore, image quality of excretory MR urography can be improved by administration of low-dose diuretics (5–10 mg furosemide in adults). The diuretic administration improves image quality as urine flow is enhanced and the contrast material is diluted and distributed more uniformly throughout the urinary tract. The role of excretory MR urography in CKD patients is limited, as the kidney(s) cannot filtrate enough contrast medium per minute in order to obtain an adequate visualization of renal pelvis, ureter, and bladder. For all other enhanced studies of the body, the most stable agents should be used, since the less stable gadolinium-based contrast agents are linked to development of nephrogenic systemic fibrosis (NSF) in patients with renal failure (see Sect. 3.7.2). Administration of diuretics is also ineffective for anuric patients.

3.5 Angiography

In patients with severe hypertension, it may be relevant to perform angiography to rule out renal artery stenosis. It can be performed as conventional X-ray-based angiography with direct arterial puncture or as CT or MR angiography (CTA, MRA). Today, most diagnostic studies of renal arteries are performed as CTA or MRA (Fig. 3.10). The sensitivity and specificity of both CTA and MRA for detection of renal artery stenosis are close to that of conventional X-ray angiography (the gold standard method). Both CTA and MRA utilize contrast media injection and fast imaging techniques ensuring acquisition during the arterial transit phase, i.e., the arterial first-pass phase that follows intravenous injection of contrast media. However, recent developments in MRA have made it possible to visualize the vascular system without the use of contrast media.

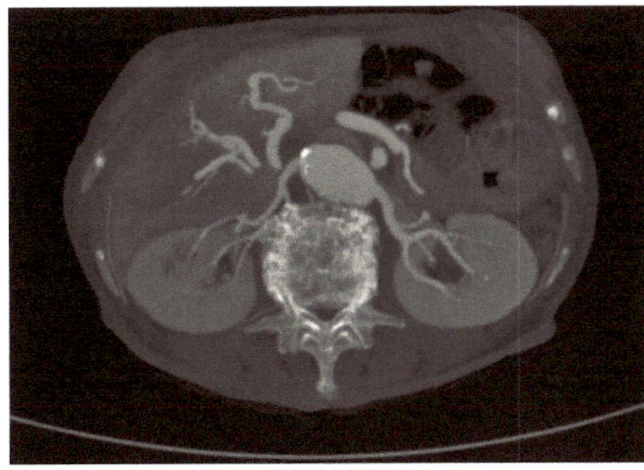

Fig. 3.10 Normal renal CT angiography

Conventional X-ray angiography, typically performed via femoral artery, is rarely applied for diagnostic studies after the introduction of CTA and MRA. However, conventional angiography combined with interventional procedures (percutaneous transluminal angioplasty – PTA) is applicable for treatment of renal artery stenosis. Doppler ultrasound suffers from high interobserver variation, but it may be useful in highly experienced hands.

CTA or MRA of iliac arteries may be relevant in pre-transplant CKD patients to rule out significant stenosis of the vessels that are going to be connected to the transplant kidney and in patients with symptoms and signs of vascular disease.

3.6 Nuclear Scanning

Nuclear medicine also has an important role in patients with reduced renal function. Primarily, it is used for determination of the glomerular filtration rate. Although it can be calculated from scintigraphic data, the method using blood sampling at various times after the injection is used in most cases. For the examination, both ^{51}Cr-EDTA and ^{99m}Tc-DTPA can be used as they are exclusively excreted through glomerular filtration [1]. They provide better determination of kidney function than estimated glomerular filtration rate based on serum creatinine measurements and are easier to perform than the optimal, but cumbersome inulin clearance.

The scintigraphic examinations include renography and renal scintigraphy. For renography, ^{99m}Tc-DTPA and ^{99m}Tc-MAG_3 can be used. Renography provides information about perfusion, excretion, and split function. Excretion data, however, cannot be obtained in patients with severely reduced kidney function and furosemide (diuresis renography) has no effect. DTPA is purely excreted by glomerular filtration, whereas MAG_3 is secreted via tubular cells, with increasingly poor kidney function. ^{99m}Tc DMSA is taken up by the tubular cells. It provides information about the size and contours of the kidney(s). Split function can also be determined and it has a long image window. Today, ^{99m}Tc-MAG_3 is the most frequently used isotope for renal scintigraphy and renography.

Nuclear imaging includes injection of isotopes. Thus, the whole body is subject to radiation and not only the part of the body that is subject to imaging as it is regarding radiography, including CT scanning. Furthermore, the reduced kidney function causes it taking longer time before the isotopes leave the body than in patients with normal renal function.

3.7 Serious Adverse Events

3.7.1 Contrast Nephropathy in CKD

Contrast nephropathy is defined as a condition in which a decrease in kidney function occurs within 3 days of intravascular administration of contrast media [2]. Thus, it is a diagnosis of exclusion, but there are other causes of a decrease in kidney function that could be present, e.g., cholesterol emboli. Initially, it was diagnosed when anuria occurred, but today measurement of serum creatinine 48–72 h after contrast medium is the way to the diagnosis. An increase in serum creatinine levels from preinjection measurement of 0.3 mg/dl (26 μmol/l), 0.5 mg/dl (44 μmol/l), 1.0 mg/ml (88 μmol/l), 25 %, 50 %, or 100 % has been used as a sign of contrast nephropathy. The optimal cutoff level is still debated, but luckily most authors use 0.5 mg/dl (44 μmol/l) and/or 25 % allowing for comparison of various studies. Furthermore, fluctuations in levels of serum creatinine are naturally occurring, probably more in inpatients than outpatients. In most patients, kidney function returns to preinjection levels within 7 days, but a few may develop anuria. Of clinical concern is the fact that patients who develop temporary decrease in kidney function after exposure to iodine-based contrast media have an increased morbidity and mortality within 2 years at least. Contrast nephropathy is almost only seen after administration of iodine-based contrast media for radiography including CT scanning. There is no difference in nephrotoxic potential between various nonionic agents (monomers and dimer), whereas the old ionic agents from the 1950s are more nephrotoxic than more recent nonionic agents (Table 3.1).

Despite many years of research, there is no agreement about the pathophysiology. It is believed that it is a combination of direct toxicity (chemotoxicity) on tubular cells and increased vascular resistance due to a change in the balance between vasoconstrictors and vasodilators in kidney vasculature.

Table 3.1 Classification of iodine-based contrast media

Group	Contrast agents	Nephrotoxic potential
Ionic monomers	Amidotrizoate (Cystografin) Iothalamate (Conray) Ioxithalamate (Telebrix)	High
Ionic dimers	Ioxaglate (Hexabrix)	High
Nonionic monomers	Iohexol (Omnipaque) Iopentol (Imagopaque) Ioxilan (Oxilan) Iomeprol (Iomeron) Ioversol (Optiray) Iopromide (Ultravist) Iobitridol (Xenetix) Iopamidol (Isovue)	Low
Nonionic dimer	Iodixanol (Visipaque)	Low

When contrast nephropathy has occurred, only symptomatic treatment is possible. Therefore, prevention plays a major role. The first issue is to identify patients at risk. Patients with normal kidney function are not at risk, and thus, our primary goal is to find patients with reduced kidney function. This can be done by measuring serum creatinine and calculate estimated glomerular filtration rate within 7 days before the examination and select the patients with reduced kidney function through a questionnaire. When a patient with reduced kidney function has been identified, one should decide whether the requested examination should be performed or another type of examination, e.g., magnetic resonance imaging, is possible. If it is decided that enhanced radiography including CT is the way to go, one should use the smallest amount of a nonionic agent necessary for a diagnostic result and organize volume expansion with either normal saline or sodium bicarbonate. A suitable protocol is intravenous normal saline 1.0–1.5 ml/kg/h for at least 6 h before and after contrast medium. An alternative protocol is intravenous sodium bicarbonate 3 ml/kg/h for 1 h before contrast medium and 1 ml/kg/h for 6 h after contrast medium [3].

However, volume expansion is not 100 % preventive but several studies have shown that it reduces the incidence. Pharmacologic prophylaxis with kidney vasodilators, receptor antagonists of endogenous vasoactive mediators, or cytoprotective drugs including N-acetylcysteine has not yet been shown to offer consistent protection against contrast nephropathy. Hemodialysis immediately after administration has no preventive effect of the development of contrast nephropathy. As a matter of fact, it may bring a patient with poor kidney function into permanent dialysis at an earlier time. [4, 5].

Contrast nephropathy is very rarely seen after administration of gadolinium-based contrast media used for magnetic resonance imaging, and it has not been reported after contrast media administration for ultrasound.

Key points of the current guidelines on contrast nephropathy are summarized in Boxes 3.2 and 3.3.

3.7.2 Nephrogenic Systemic Fibrosis

Nephrogenic systemic fibrosis is a serious adverse event to some gadolinium-based contrast media [7]. Fibrosis may develop in most parts of the body. It may vary from being a little plaque to being almost generalized. The lower extremities are almost always involved, whereas the head is spared. The first signs may come within the first 24 h after injection, but generally occur within the first 3 months. It has been seen even years after the last injection. The patient develops pain, pruritus, swelling, and erythema in the lower extremities followed by thickened skin and subcutaneous tissues, woody texture, and browny plaques. The diagnosis requires visual inspection of the skin as well as a deep biopsy from the skin. Based on dermatologic and dermatopathologic findings, it is concluded whether it is nephrogenic systemic fibrosis or another skin lesion. It is not an easy diagnosis. Demonstration of gadolinium in the skin may be indicative of nephrogenic systemic fibrosis, but in itself it is not an evidence of the adverse event. Whether hemodialysis immediately after imaging examination reduces the risk of developing nephrogenic systemic fibrosis is unknown. It requires about 12 h of effective hemodialysis to get most of the contrast medium out of the body. For continuous ambulatory peritoneal dialysis (CAPD), it takes weeks to remove the agent.

For more than 30 years, it has been known that the heavy metals belonging to the lanthanide group in the periodic table could cause changes in the skin. Lanthanides are not naturally occurring in the human body and they are extremely toxic. Around 0.1 mmol/kg of gadolinium chloride is enough to kill a human being. At the same time researchers found that one of the lanthanides – gadolinium – was excellent for magnetic resonance imaging due to its high relaxativity compared to other ions under similar conditions. In order to detoxify, it was necessary to chelate gadolinium as well as the relativity increased significantly. Two principally different chelates were used: (1) the linear chelate DTPA known for years

Box 3.2. What the Guidelines Say You Should Do

Key points of current ESUR guidelines on contrast nephropathy [3]:

- Identify the patient at risk of contrast nephropathy at time of the referral.
- The risk of contrast nephropathy is lower with intravenous than intra-arterial iodinated contrast media.
- eGFR of 45 ml/min/1.73 m^2 is considered contrast nephropathy risk threshold for intravenous contrast medium and 60 ml/min/1.73 m^2 for intra-arterial injection.
- Hydration with either saline or sodium bicarbonate reduces contrast nephropathy incidence and should be used in patients at risk.
- Patients with eGFR ≥45 ml/min/1.73 m^2 receiving contrast medium intravenously can continue metformin normally.

Key points of most recent KDIGO guidelines for CKD care [6]:

- It is recommend that all people with GFR <60 ml/min/1.73 m^2 (GFR categories G3a-G5) undergoing elective investigation involving the intravascular administration of iodine-based contrast media should be managed according to the KDIGO Clinical Practice Guideline for AKI including:
  - Avoidance of high osmolar agents (1B)
  - Use of lowest possible radiocontrast dose (Not Graded)
  - Withdrawal of potentially nephrotoxic agents before and after the procedure (1C)
  - Adequate hydration with saline before, during, and after the procedure (1A)
  - Measurement of GFR 48–96 h after the procedure (1C)

Key points of current ESUR guidelines on nephrogenic systemic fibrosis (NSF) [3]:

- Patients with GFR below 30 ml/min/1.73 m^2 have increased risk of developing NSF.
- Low stability gadolinium contrast media show the strongest association with NSF.
- Following the guidelines regarding gadolinium-based contrast agents minimizes the risk of NSF.
- Use only intermediate or low-risk agents.
  - These agents should be used with CAUTION in patients with CKD 4 and 5 (GFR <30 ml/min).
  - There should be at least 7 days between two injections.
  - Pregnant women: Can be used to give essential diagnostic information.
  - Lactating women: The patient should discuss with the doctor whether the breast milk should be discarded in 24 h after contrast medium.

Key points of most recent KDIGO guidelines for CKD care [6]:

- It is recommended not to use gadolinium-containing contrast media in people with GFR <15 ml/min/1.73 m^2 (GFR category G5) unless there is no alternative appropriate test (1B).
- It is suggested that people with a GFR <30 ml/min/1.73 m^2 (GFR categories G4-G5) who require gadolinium-based contrast media are preferentially offered a macrocyclic chelate preparation (2B).

from nuclear medicine where it was used together with ^{99m}Tc and (2) the cyclic chelate DOTA which cages around the ion. Both chelates became available in an ionic and nonionic version. In order to lower the osmolality which had been shown to be a major step forward in patient safety and comfort regarding iodine-based contrast media, two amid groups replaced two carboxyl groups in the linear chelates. Amid groups hold the gadolinium less strongly than carboxyl groups do, and they introduce weak binding points for the gadolinium on plain chelate. Thus, they increase the risk of transmetallation with one of the free ions in the body, e.g., Zn^{++}. When liberated from the chelate, gadolinium binds to phosphate and calcium, so free gadolinium is not circulating around in the plasma. Instead, it may be found in skin, liver, lymph nodes, and bone. The longer the less stabile gadolinium-based contrast media are in the blood, the more gadolinium can be liberated from

Box 3.3. Relevant Guidelines

1. European Society of Urogenital Radiology (ESUR) Guidelines:
   - Stacul F, van der Molen AJ, Reimer P, Webb JAWW, Thomsen HS, Morcos SK, et al. Contrast Media Safety Committee of the European Society of Urogenital Radiology. Contrast nephropathy: updated ESUR Contrast Media Safety Committee guidelines. Eur Radiol. 2011;21:2527–41 [2].
   - Thomsen HS, Morcos SK, Almén T, Bellin MF, Bertolotto M, Bongartz G, et al. Nephrogenic systemic fibrosis and gadolinium based contrast media: updated ESUR Contrast Medium Safety Committee guidelines. Eur Radiol. 2013;23:307–18 [7].
   - ESUR.org [internet]. Vienna: European Society of Urogenital Radiology; 2013. Available from www.esur.org. Cited 26 Mar 2013[3].
2. KDIGO Guidelines:
   - The ad hoc working group of ERBP: Fliser D, Laville M, Covic A, Fouque D, Vanholder R, Juillard L, et al. A European Renal Best Practice (ERBP) position statement on the Kidney Disease Improving Global Outcomes (KDIGO) Clinical practice guidelines on acute kidney injury: Part 1: definitions, conservative management, and contrast-induced nephropathy. Nephrol Dial Transplant. 2012;27:4263–72 [5].
   - Kidney Disease: Improving Global Outcomes (KDIGO) CKD Work Group. KDIGO 2012 clinical practice guidelines for the evaluation and management of chronic kidney disease. Kidney Int. 2013;(Suppl 3):1–150 [6].

the chelate through transmetallation. More than 98 % of the injected extracellular agent is out of the body within 24 h in patients with normal kidney function, whereas it may take weeks for patients with severely reduced kidney function.

Very quickly after the link between exposure to less stable gadolinium-based contrast agents (agents based on nonionic linear chelates) and development of nephrogenic systemic fibrosis was discovered, three factors were found to be present in patients who got the disease/adverse event: (1) nonionic linear chelates had been used in most patients developing the disease, (2) that the patient should have advanced renal insufficiency (GFR <30 ml/min/1.73 m^2 in large majority of cases), and (3) a third – but unknown – factor must be present as not all patients with poor kidney function or on dialysis develop nephrogenic systemic fibrosis after exposure to a nonionic linear chelate agent [8]. In some patients, only 0.1 mmol/kg (standard dose for magnetic resonance imaging) is needed before nephrogenic systemic fibrosis develops, whereas in other patients much higher doses, eventually given for a long period (lifetime dose), are required for the development of the disease. The good thing is that the adverse event has been almost erased after the use of less stable agents was stopped and switched to more stable agents (the cyclic ones). Today, the authorities have contraindicated the use of the least stable agents in patients with reduced kidney function or on dialysis (Table 3.2). The long-term consequences of using less stable agents in patients with normal or moderately reduced kidney function are still unknown. There are patients with reduced kidney function who develops nephrogenic systemic fibrosis years after the last exposure to a gadolinium-based contrast agent. Long-term consequences may also be other adverse reactions than nephrogenic systemic fibrosis.

The fear of nephrogenic systemic fibrosis should not lead to inadequate imaging in patients with symptoms of a disease. One should never deny a patient a clinically well-indicated enhanced magnetic resonance imaging examination with the smallest amount of contrast medium necessary for a diagnostic result [3]. Sadly, many radiologists still deny giving patients with eGFR below 30 or even 60 ml/min/1.73 m^2 gadolinium-based contrast medium despite clinical symptoms and signs of disease and no diagnostic solution based on the unenhanced scan.

Key points of the current guidelines on contrast nephropathy are summarized in Boxes 3.1 and 3.2.

Table 3.2 Classification of MRI contrast agents

Contrast agent	Chemical stability	Molecular structure
Gadodiamide (Omniscan)	Low	Nonionic linear
Gadopentetate dimeglumine (Magnevist)	Medium	Ionic linear
Gadoversetamide (Optimark)	Low	Nonionic linear
Gadobenate dimeglumine (Multihance)	Medium	Ionic linear
Gadofosveset trisodium (Ablavar)	Medium	Ionic linear
Gadoxetate disodium (Primovist, Eovist)	Medium	Ionic linear
Gadobutrol (Gadovist, Gadavist)	High	Nonionic macrocyclic
Gadoterate meglumine (Dotarem)	High	Ionic macrocyclic
Gadoteridol (ProHance)	High	Nonionic macrocyclic

Before You Finish: Practice Pearls for the Clinician

- In patients with chronic kidney disease, contrast nephropathy and nephrogenic systemic fibrosis are serious adverse reactions to contrast agents.
- Contrast nephropathy is seen after all available iodine-based contrast agents to the same extent, whereas nephrogenic systemic fibrosis is only seen after some gadolinium-based agents.
- One should not deny a patient with obvious symptoms and signs of a disease an enhanced examination if the unenhanced study was inadequate from a diagnostic point of view. This applies to all parts of the body.

References

1. Blaufox MD, Aurell M, Bubeck B, Fommei E, Piepsz A, Russell C, et al. Report of the radionuclides in Nephrourology Committee on renal clearance. J Nucl Med. 1996;37:883–90.
2. Stacul F, van der Molen AJ, Reimer P, Webb JAWW, Thomsen HS, Morcos SK, et al. Contrast Media Safety Committee of the European Society of Urogenital Radiology. Contrast induced nephropathy: updated ESUR Contrast Media Safety Committee guidelines. Eur Radiol. 2011;21:2527–41.
3. ESUR. www.esur.org [internet]. Vienna: European Society of Urogenital Radiology; 2013. Available from www.esur.org. Cited 26 Mar 2013.
4. Morcos SK, Thomsen HS. Urogenital imaging. A problem-oriented approach. West Sussex: Wiley-Blackwell; 2009.
5. The ad-hoc working group of ERBP, Fliser D, Laville M, Covic A, Fouque D, Vanholder R, Juillard L, et al. A European Renal Best Practice (ERBP) position statement on the Kidney Disease Improving Global Outcomes (KDIGO) clinical practice guidelines on acute kidney injury: Part 1: definitions, conservative management and contrast-induced nephropathy. Nephrol Dial Transplant. 2012;27:4263–72.
6. Kidney Disease: Improving Global Outcomes (KDIGO) CKD Work Group. KDIGO 2012 Clinical Practice Guideline for the Evaluation and Management of Chronic Kidney Disease. Kidney Int. 2013;(Suppl 3):1–150.
7. Thomsen HS, Morcos SK, Almén T, Bellin MF, Bertolotto M, Bongartz G, et al. Nephrogenic systemic fibrosis and gadolinium based contrast media: updated ESUR Contrast Medium Safety Committee guidelines. Eur Radiol. 2013;23:307–18.
8. Thomsen HS, Webb JAW, editors. Contrast media. Safety issues and ESUR guidelines. 3rd ed. Heidelberg: Springer; 2014.

Part II

Chronic Kidney Disease Risk Factors: Assessment and Management

4 Diabetes and Chronic Kidney Disease

Meryem Tuncel Kara, Moshe Levi, and Devasmita Choudhury

Before You Start: Facts You Need to Know

- Diabetic nephropathy remains the most common cause for CKD in those with type 1, type 2, and other secondary forms of diabetes mellitus.
- Lifetime risk of developing nephropathy is similar for type 1 and type 2 diabetes.
- Predisposing factors for diabetic kidney disease include positive family history; race, particularly if African American, Hispanic, or Pima Indian; obesity; poor blood glucose control; and poor blood pressure control.
- Urinary albumin excretion is a clinical hallmark for the presence of diabetic nephropathy.
- Expansion of mesangium, glomerular basement membrane thickening, and glomerular sclerosis are the major histologic changes of diabetic nephropathy.

M.T. Kara, MD
Department of Internal Medicine, University of Connecticut School of Medicine/John Dempsey Hospital, Internal Medicine/Calhoun Cardiology Center, University of Connecticut Health Center, 263 Farmington Avenue, Farmington, CT 06030, USA
e-mail: tuncelkara@uchc.edu

M. Levi, MD
Division of Renal Diseases and Hypertension/Department of Internal Medicine, University of Colorado Denver AMC, 12700 East 19th Avenue, Research 2, Room 7002, C281, Aurora, CO 80045, USA
e-mail: moshe.levi@ucdenver.edu

D. Choudhury, MD (✉)
Department of Medicine, University of Virginia, Salem VA Medical Center, 1970 Roanoke Blvd., Salem, VA 24153, USA
e-mail: devasmita.dev@va.gov

4.1 Epidemiology

Worldwide prevalence of diabetes is expected to increase from an estimated 285 million in 2010 to approximately 439 million by 2030 for ages between 20 and 79 years with estimated health expenditures approximated at 561 billion dollars. Diabetic kidney disease is the leading cause of end-stage renal disease (ESRD) in developed countries with 20–30 % of those with diabetes expected to develop chronic kidney disease (CKD). While the development and progression of diabetic kidney disease has been most studied in those with type 1 DM, clinical and pathologic progression and changes appear to be similar for those with type 2 DM. *Factors predisposing* to the development of nephropathy include a *positive family history* of diabetic kidney disease and

M. Arici (ed.), *Management of Chronic Kidney Disease*,
DOI 10.1007/978-3-642-54637-2_4, © Springer-Verlag Berlin Heidelberg 2014

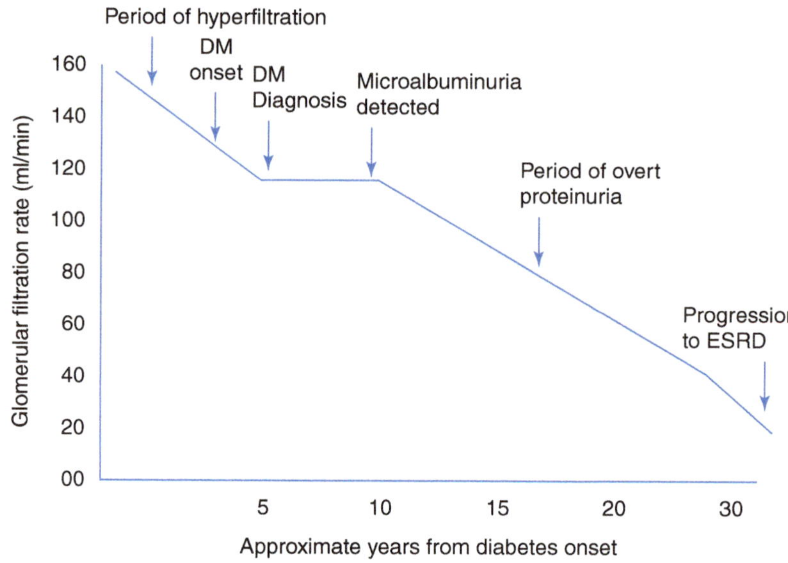

Fig. 4.1 Proposed clinical progression of diabetic kidney disease

ethnicity with particular high prevalence seen in those of African American origin and Hispanic origin and in Pima Indians. In addition, obese individuals seem to be more predisposed to the development of diabetic kidney disease as well as those that have or develop high blood pressure and/or have poor control of their diabetes. Of the modifiable risk factors, smoking and the use of oral contraceptives are noted to have added risk for the development of diabetic nephropathy. Diabetic nephropathy (DN) is clinically characterized by hyperfiltration early on with subsequent occurrence of microalbuminuria, progression to macroalbuminuria over the course of 10–20 years, and then progression to ESRD (Fig. 4.1).

4.2 Clinical Presentation of Diabetic Kidney Disease

Kidney disease develops in approximately 30 % of patients with either type 1 DM or type 2 DM. Diabetic nephropathy is generally a *pathologic diagnosis of diabetic kidney disease* in diabetic patients who have undergone renal biopsy. Diabetic kidney disease is more generally used for the presumed *clinical diagnosis* given to patients with long-standing diabetes with proteinuria in the presence of other diabetic microvascular complications, particularly diabetic retinopathy. Patients with this clinical diagnosis generally undergo clinical evaluation to rule out other secondary glomerular or renal pathology. In patients with long-standing diabetes and CKD without proteinuria or other evidence of microvascular complications such as retinopathy, the presumption of diabetic kidney disease is less certain, and renal biopsy may need to be considered particularly if progression of CKD is rapid (Box 4.1).

Mogensen best characterized the *presentation and progression of diabetic nephropathy* into *5 stages* (Table 4.1): (1) *hyperfiltration* (increased renal plasma flow and increased glomerular filtration) with renal hypertrophy, (2) *normoalbuminuria with pathologic changes* of basement membrane thickening and mesangial expansion, (3) microalbuminuria with early hypertension, (4) *overt urine protein excretion*, and (5) advanced kidney failure with *end-stage renal disease*.

Glomerular hyperfiltration may be noted early in patients with DM and in some patients preceding the diagnosis of diabetes [1]. Several factors can lead to hyperfiltration in the diabetic patient including renal vasodilation induced by elevated blood glucose levels and glycosylated proteins, insulin-like growth factor, atrial natriuretic peptide, as well as increased proximal tubular NaCl reabsorption. Blood glucose control and

Box 4.1. Criteria for Renal Biopsy in Patients with Diabetes and Kidney Disease to Rule Out Other Glomerular Pathologies

1. Rapid deterioration of renal function
2. Diabetes duration <10 years
3. No evidence of microalbuminuria or gross proteinuria despite long-standing diabetes
4. No evidence of other microvascular complications such as retinopathy in the presence of diabetes
5. Signs and symptoms of other systemic diseases
6. Sudden onset or rapidly increasing levels of proteinuria or nephrotic syndrome
7. Active urine sediment

Source: Recommendations based on authors' clinical practice. See also NKF Clinical Practice Guidelines [21]

Table 4.1 Clinical stages of presentation and progression of diabetic kidney disease

Stage 1	Hyperfiltration with renal hypertrophy	Increased renal plasma flow and increased glomerular filtration
Stage 2	Normoalbuminuria	Pathologic changes of basement membrane thickening and mesangial expansion
Stage 3	Microalbuminuria (30–300 mg albumin/g creatinine)	Early hypertension
Stage 4	Overt proteinuria >300 mg albumin/g creatinine	Increased urine protein excretion
Stage 5	Advanced kidney failure	Progression to end-stage renal disease

blood pressure control are noted to decrease hyperfiltration.

Microalbuminuria *defined* as urine albumin excretion of 20–200 ug/min (or 30–299 mg/24 h or 30–300 mg albumin/g creatinine in a random urine sample) hallmarks the early onset of diabetic kidney disease with overt proteinuria noted within 10 years of persistent microalbuminuria. Though regression to normoalbuminuria can be seen in some patients with good metabolic control, progression to macroalbuminuria frequently occurs with intermittent and gradual increase of urine protein. Persistent and increasing overt proteinuria over 5–10 years frequently results in gradual loss of renal function, fluid retention and edema, and eventual need for renal replacement therapy. Urine sediment is often bland for patients with diabetic kidney disease; however, microhematuria may also occur. An active urine sediment with dysmorphic red cells, red or white cell casts, or persistent significant hematuria should be investigated to rule out other glomerular or genitourinary pathologies. In addition, glomerulopathy other than diabetic nephropathy should also be entertained in patients that have onset of diabetes less than 10 years or have no evidence of other microvascular disease, microalbuminuria, or proteinuria or in those with diabetes who appear to have a rapid deterioration in their kidney function.

Screening for microalbuminuria should be at least yearly from the time of diabetes diagnosis with a positive result confirmed for persistence of proteinuria over the next 3–6 months. Microvascular disease including retinopathy and neuropathy is often evident in those with both type 1 and type 2 diabetes even prior to the diagnosis of diabetic nephropathy. These findings are less reliable in those with type 2 DM with 60–70 % presenting with concurrent microvascular disease. Therefore, careful screening and follow-up for microvascular disease in patients with diabetes is also important (Box 4.2).

Box 4.2. What the Guidelines Say You Should Do: Screening Recommendations for Diabetic Kidney Disease

1. Urine albumin creatinine ratio (ACR) in spot urine, serum creatinine with calculated estimated GFR at 5 years after type 1 DM diagnosis, or at diagnosis of type 2 DM, then yearly.
2. Follow up confirmation of microalbuminuria and proteinuria within 3–6 months if noted on initial screening.

Source: Data from KDOQI [21]

4.3 Pathologic Manifestations and Proposed Mechanisms of Diabetic Nephropathy

Changes in *renal histology* associated with diabetes can usually be seen within 3–5 years of diabetes onset, although glomerular and tubular basement membrane thickening has been noted as early as 1.5–2.5 years after the onset of type 1 DM. Glomerular basement membrane thickening with proteinuria may also precede the clinical diagnosis of diabetes in some patients. Changes in glomerular hemodynamics may not necessarily parallel these early changes in histology. Glomerular filtration rate by inulin clearance and effective renal plasma flow by para-aminohippurate clearance did not change significantly when compared to renal biopsy changes at 1 year and 6 years in type 1 DM patients with mean diabetes duration of 10 years at initial biopsy. Further changes in the mesangium with matrix expansion may be seen within 5–7 years of diabetes onset although interstitial expansion occurs [2] and progresses in a variable manner over 15–20 years in both type 1 and type 2 DM. These *changes* have been recently *classified* by expert renal pathologists and summarized as presented in Table 4.2. Figures 4.2, 4.3, and 4.4 represent classic pathologic changes in diabetic nephropathy.

Increased blood glucose affects various pathways leading to podocyte injury and cell apoptosis. Hyperglycemia is associated with oxidative stress-induced production of reactive oxygen species, proinflammatory transcription of nuclear factors, increased flux of polyol and hexosamine pathways with increased protein kinase C, transforming growth factor-β, renin-angiotensin-aldosterone, and advanced glycation end products. These effects result in extracellular matrix protein deposition in the glomerulus and tubulointerstitium. Laboratory studies have also noted *abnormal insulin signaling as contributing to changes in podocyte structure and function*. Both mitogen-activated protein kinase (MAPK) and phosphoinositide-3 kinase (PI3K) pathways work via the insulin receptor to remodel the actin cytoskeleton of podocytes with abnormal signaling leading to altered actin dynamics and podocytopathy. The concept of *metabolic memory* has also been suggested to *play a role* in the continued *pathogen-*

Table 4.2 Classification of diabetic glomerular changes

Class 1	Glomerular basement membrane thickening	Isolated glomerular basement membrane thickening and only mild, nonspecific changes by light microscopy that do not meet the criteria of classes II through IV
Class II	Mesangial expansion, mild (IIa) or severe (IIb)	Glomeruli classified as having mild (<25 %) or severe (>25 %) mesangial expansion but without nodular sclerosis (Kimmelstiel-Wilson lesions) or global glomerulosclerosis in more than 50 % of glomeruli
Class III	Nodular sclerosis (Kimmelstiel-Wilson lesions)	At least one glomerulus with nodular sclerosis but does not meet criteria for class IV
Class IV	Advanced diabetic glomerulosclerosis	Lesions from class I–III plus >50 % glomeruli with global glomerulosclerosis

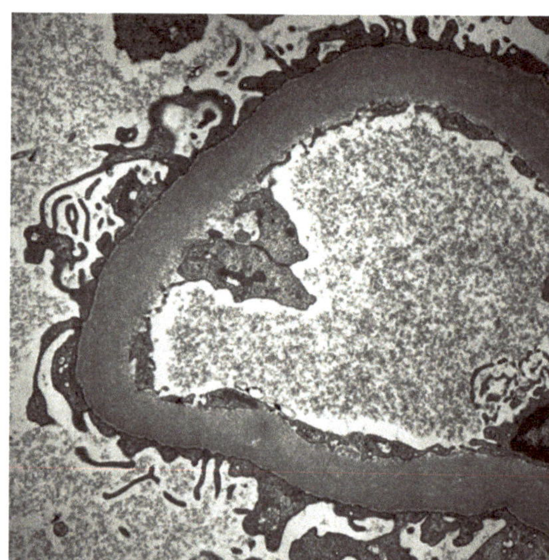

Fig. 4.2 Electron microscopy of thickened glomerular basement membrane in diabetic nephropathy (Courtesy of Irfan Warraich, MD)

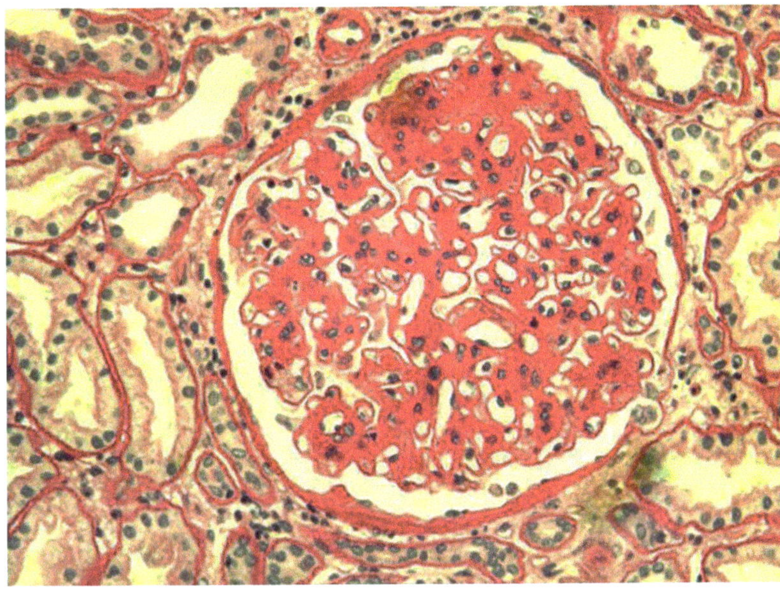

Fig. 4.3 Mesangial expansion and thickened basement membrane in diabetic nephropathy on light microscopy with PAS staining (Courtesy of Irfan Warraich, MD)

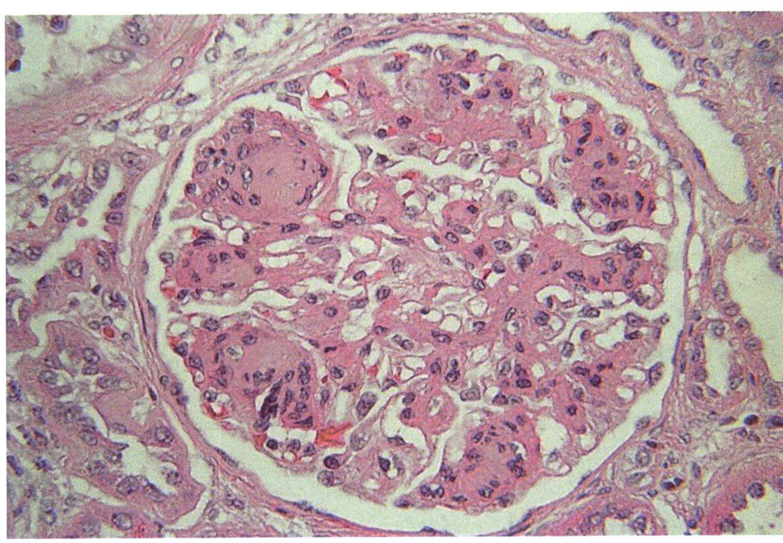

Fig. 4.4 Classic changes of diabetic Kimmelstiel-Wilson nodules in addition to mesangial expansion and basement membrane thickening on light microscopy with H&E stain (Courtesy of Irfan Warraich, MD)

esis of diabetic nephropathy despite achievement of blood glucose control. Epigenetic mechanisms such as hyperglycemia-mediated post-transcriptional histone acetylation, deacetylation, methylation, demethylation, phosphorylation, ubiquitination, and activation of microRNAs may serve as metabolic memory that leads to gene regulation when transient hyperglycemia occurs despite good blood glucose control. These important biologic associations are important for further understanding of pathologic changes in diabetic nephropathy with hopes of treatment that can prevent these irreversible processes.

4.4 Prevention and Treatment of Diabetic Nephropathy

A multi-targeted approach in *treating the risk factors leading to diabetic kidney disease* as well as avoidance of nephrotoxins that can affect

Table 4.3 Medications associated with poor glycemic control

Medication or class of medication	Mechanism of poor glycemic control
Steroid agents	Weight gain, increased hepatic glucose production, decreasing peripheral insulin sensitivity
Calcineurin inhibitors Tacrolimus > cyclosporine	Impaired insulin secretion, possible islet cell damage
Sirolimus	Decreased insulin sensitivity and insulin content and decreasing islet cell mass
Antidepressants (Doxepin, imipramine, mirtazapine, phenelzine, tranylcypromine)	Weight gain
Antipsychotics (Fluphenazine, haloperidol, paliperadone, perphenazine < quetiapine, risperidone, thioridazine < clozapine, olanzapine)	Weight gain (clozapine and olanzapine dysregulate insulin and carbohydrate metabolism)
Mood stabilizers (Carbamazepine < gabapentin < lithium, valproate)	Weight gain

renal function appears to be best for those with diabetes. Treatment in the progression of DN should start with *strict control of hyperglycemia* (glycosylated hemoglobin A1C <7.0 %), *normalizing elevated blood pressure*, and avoidance of hyperfiltration [3, 4]. With dyslipidemia adding to microvascular damage and progression of DN, *lipid lowering* becomes an important part of the treatment. An *LDL goal of <100 mg/dl* (<70 mg/dl for those at high risk) is advocated in DM patients [5]. Since tobacco users are at increased risk of micro- and macrovascular complications, *smoking cessation* must also be advocated early on in patients with DM. Careful use and follow-up are necessary with various medications associated with poor glycemic control including steroids, calcineurin inhibitors, sirolimus, as well as several antipsychotic agents, particularly in those with diabetes or predisposed to diabetes (Table 4.3). Similarly the presence of hepatitis C virus (HCV) infection is associated with insulin resistance, decreased glucose uptake, glycogenesis, as well as pancreatic β cell toxicity. In addition, poor glycemic control often results with various bacterial infections. Therefore, treatment of acute and chronic infections in those with underlying diabetes can improve glycemic control. *Weight control* becomes important as increased weight and obesity are associated with an increase in protein excretion in patients with diabetes. Furthermore, vigilance in *avoiding or minimizing exposure* of patients with diabetic kidney disease or high risk for diabetic kidney disease *to common nephrotoxins* including intravenous radiocontrast agents, nonsteroidal anti-inflammatory drugs, aminoglycoside antibiotics, or herbal and/or oral supplements of unclear sources should be practiced.

4.4.1 Glycemic Control

Hyperglycemia exacerbates microvascular complications of retinopathy, nephropathy, and neuropathy in DM; therefore, *strict glycemic control* to reach near-normal blood glucose levels *delays development and progression of diabetic nephropathy* [4, 6]. The Diabetes Control and Complications Trial (DCCT), a prospective study of 1441 type 1 DM patients randomly assigned to either intensive or conventional therapy, demonstrated that intensive therapy targeted at maintaining near-normal blood glucose levels markedly reduced the risks of development or progression of microvascular complications over an average of 6.5 years' follow-up period [6]. In a smaller study of Japanese individuals, intensive blood glucose control using insulin in type 2 DM patients with target fasting blood glucose of 110 mg/dl, hemoglobin A1C 6.5 %, and 2 h postprandial blood glucose of 180 mg/dl also confirmed delay in the progression of diabetic retinopathy, nephropathy, and neuropathy in patients with type 2 DM [8]. Reversal of established DN lesions with more than 5 years of normoglycemia with pancreas transplantation further underscores the importance of glycemic control [9].

However, *glycemic targets should be individualized* for each *patient and weighed against the increased risk for hypoglycemia*. Microvascular benefits of intensive glycemic control (target HbA1c of <6.0 %) need also be considered in light of a greater risk for cardiovascular mortality as well as overall mortality in addition to increased risk for weight gain and high risk for hypoglycemia. Cautious monitoring of hemoglobin A1C is essential with a glycosylated hemoglobin A1C value of ≤7.0 % appropriate for most patients; however, glycemic targets are generally higher for children (given hypoglycemia unawareness), adolescents, and older patients (given life expectancy) (Box 4.3).

Exogenous insulin agents are usually necessary to achieve optimal glycemic control for type 1 DM. Lispro, aspart, and glulisine are fast-acting insulin analogs and quickly absorbed. A short duration of action makes these agents useful for blood glucose control during a meal compared to regular insulins. Glargine and detemir are long-acting analogs to mimic basal insulin release with lower peak action in order to decrease the number of hypoglycemic events [10].

Pancreas or islet transplantation provides excellent glycemic control and freedom from insulin use, making these treatments attractive. Insulin independence at 1 year is approximately 80 % with either treatment. However, the morbidity of major surgery for pancreas transplantation, with requirements for long-term immunosuppression with either pancreas or islet transplantation, is an important factor that needs to be considered with these treatment options [11]. Adult stem cells that can induce islet and beta cell function are under current investigation and may provide other treatment options for glycemic control in the prevention of diabetic nephropathy in patients with type 1 DM [12].

A number of *oral agents* are available for patients with type 2 diabetes for blood glucose control prior to using insulin therapy. The use and choice of oral agents should be made on the basis of patient tolerability as well as renal clearance. Oral hypoglycemic classes of *insulin sensitizers* biguanides and thiazolidinediones (TZDs) directly improve insulin action. The biguanide metformin is often not used in patients with decreased GFR given the risk for lactic acidosis. US Food and Drug Administration (US FDA) recommends avoidance in patients with serum creatinine over 1.4 mg/dl for women and 1.5 mg/dl for men, whereas the British National Formulary and Japanese Society of Nephrology recommends avoidance in diabetic patients with renal clearance less than 30 ml/min. TZDs act by stimulating the nuclear hormone receptor PPARγ to decrease insulin resistance with favorable effects of decreasing urinary albumin excretion [13]. However lower doses of TZDs are recommended when used for patients with serum creatinine >2.0 mg/dl and not recommended for use in those with concurrent New York Heart Association class III or IV heart failure as these agents lead to increased fluid retention. In addition, TZDs have potential for hepatotoxicity, decreasing bone density with increased risk for fracture, particularly in women.

Of the *oral insulin secretagogues*, first-generation sulfonylureas are not recommended for use in patients with CKD beyond stage 2 given an increased risk of hypoglycemia. Of the second-generation sulfonylureas, glipizide and gliclazide require no dose adjustment in patients with reduced renal clearance. Of the glinides, dose adjustment is usually not necessary; however, initiation with lower doses of repaglinide is suggested with cautious monitoring given reported cases of hypoglycemia in those with impaired kidney function. Oral dipeptidyl peptidase IV (DPP-IV) inhibitors (sitagliptin and saxagliptin) may be used at reduced doses with renal clearances less than 50 ml/min.

Box 4.3. What the Guidelines Say You Should Do: Recommendations of Diabetes Care in CKD

1. HbA1c at or near 7 % is currently recommended for those with diabetes to prevent microvascular complications.
2. Avoid strict HbA1C <7 for those with risk for hypoglycemia.
3. HbA1c targets above 7 % are acceptable for those with repeated hypoglycemic events or decreased life expectations.

Source: Data from KDOQI [21] and American Diabetes Association [22]

Of the *non-oral insulin secretagogues*, glucagon-like peptide 1 (GLP1) agonists exenatide and liraglutide have increased risk of hypoglycemia when used with insulin, and their use is not recommended in patients with renal clearances <30 ml/min. Of other non-oral agents, amylin analog pramlintide should also be avoided in those with renal clearances <20 ml/min. Any specific effects of these agents on diabetic nephropathy are yet to be determined.

Other oral agents that decrease blood glucose by decreasing intestinal carbohydrate and fat absorption are alpha-glucosidase inhibitors. Alpha-glucosidase inhibitors acarbose and miglitol are not recommended for use in patients with serum creatinine >2.0 mg/dl (177 mmol/l) (Table 4.4).

Another potential target to control blood glucose is selective inhibition of the proximal renal tubule glucose transporter, SGLT2. Found primarily in the S1 segment of the proximal renal tubule, these inhibitors lead to glucosuria and may have beneficial effects on glucose regulation in individuals with type 2 diabetes [14]. Canagliflozin has recently been approved for use in the USA, while dapagliflozin is available outside of the

Table 4.4 Dose adjustment for insulin and oral medications for diabetes and CKD

Medication class and agents	CKD stages 3, 4, and 5 (not on dialysis)
Insulin	
Glargine, detemir, neutral protamine Hagedorn (NPH), Regular, aspart, lispro, Glulisine	Adjust dose based on patient response
First-generation sulfonylureas	
Acetohexamide	Avoid use
Chlorpropamide	Decrease dose 50 % for GFR between 50 and 80 ml/min/1.73 m²
Tolazamide, tolbutamide	Avoid use for GFR <50 ml/min/1.73 m² Avoid use
Second-generation sulfonylureas	
Glipizide	No dose adjustment
Glimepiride	Start 1 mg daily
Glyburide	Avoid use
Gliclazide	No dose adjustment
Meglitinides	
Repaglinide	Start 0.5 mg with meals if GFR <30 ml/min/1.73 m²
Nateglinide	Start 60 mg with meals if GFR <30 ml/min/1.73 m²
Biguanides	
Metformin	US FDA recommends not to use for SCr ≥1.5 mg/dl for men and 1.4 mg/dl for women British National Formulary and Japanese Society of Nephrology recommends discontinuation for GFR <30 ml/min/1.73 m²
Thiazolidinediones	
Pioglitazone, rosiglitazone	No dose adjustment necessary
Alpha-glucosidase Inhibitors	
Acarbose	Avoid if GFR<30 ml/min/1.73 m²
Miglitol	Avoid if GFR <25 ml/min/1.73 m²
DPP-4 inhibitor	
Sitagliptin	100 mg daily for GFR >50 ml/min/1.73 m²; 50 mg daily for GFR 30–50 ml/min/1.73 m²; 25 mg daily for GFR <30 ml/min/1.73 m²
Saxagliptin	5 mg daily for GFR >50 ml/min/1.73 m²; 2.5 mg daily for GFR ≤50 ml/min/1.73 m²
Linagliptin	No dose adjustment
Vildagliptin	50 mg twice daily for GFR ≥50 ml/min/1.73 m² 50 mg daily for GFR <50 ml/min/1.73 m²
Incretin mimetic	
Exenatide	Not recommended for GFR <30 ml/min/1.73 m²
Liraglutide	Not recommended for GFR <60 ml/min/1.73 m²
Amylin analog	
Pramlintide	No dose adjustment, however not recommended for patients with CKD 4 or greater
Dopamine receptor agonist	
Bromocriptine mesylate	Not studied in patients with reduced GFR

Source: Data from KDOQI [21]

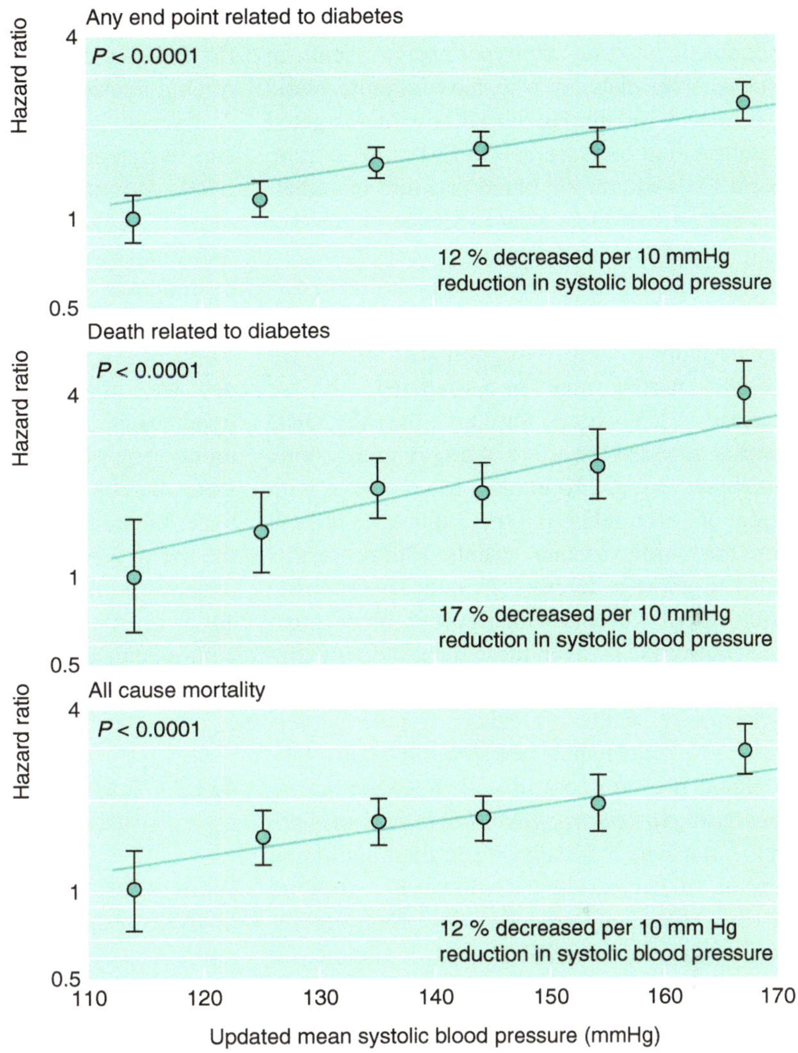

Fig. 4.5 Hazard rates (95 % confidence intervals as floating absolute risks) as estimate of association between category of updated mean systolic blood pressure and any end point related to diabetes, death related to diabetes, and all-cause mortality with log-linear scales (Reproduced from Adler et al. [23], with permission from BMJ Publishing Group Ltd.)

USA. Currently canagliflozin use is not recommended for renal clearance below 45 ml/min with dose adjustment to 100 mg daily for those with GFR between 45 and 60 ml/min. Other potential agents are currently being evaluated for use with their use in those with decreased renal clearances and/or specific effects on diabetic kidney disease being currently investigated.

4.4.2 Blood Pressure Control

Strict blood pressure control in patients with DM reduces onset of both microalbuminuria and macroalbuminuria and improves retinopathy when systolic blood pressure is targeted <130 mmHg. In addition, there is graded and continuous increase in mortality with increasing blood pressure in patients with diabetes across the entire range of levels of systolic blood pressure, including prehypertensive levels (Fig. 4.5). The United Kingdom Prospective Diabetes Study (UKPDS) including 4,801 patients with type 2 DM showed that every 10 mmHg decrease in systolic pressure was associated with a 12 % decrease in risk of diabetic complications [7]. The lowest risk was at a systolic pressure below 120 mmHg. While these data prompted the Seventh Report of the Joint National Committee on Prevention, Detection, Evaluation, and

Treatment of High Blood Pressure (JNC 7) to recommend starting antihypertensive agents in patients with diabetes who have systolic blood pressures of 130 mmHg or higher with a targeted systolic blood pressure below 130 mmHg, more recent trials examining blood pressure in diabetics have provided less clear evidence for a lower limit of systolic blood pressure.

The impact of achieved blood pressure on cardiovascular outcomes in the Irbesartan Diabetic Nephropathy Trial suggested that BP ≤120/85 mmHg may be associated with an increase in CV events. Similarly the ACCORD BP trial assessed the effect of targeting a systolic blood pressure of 120 mmHg, as compared with a goal of 140 mmHg, in type 2 diabetics at high risk for cardiovascular events. Study results failed to show a decrease in rate of composite cardiovascular events with rigorous blood pressure control [15]. Given these data, individualizing blood pressure control to avoid symptomatic hypotension while achieving systolic targets close to 130 mmHg may be appropriate (Box 4.4).

Blood pressure control with RAAS-*blocking agents are particularly favorable in patients with type 1 and type 2 diabetes* given their additional benefits of decreasing intraglomerular pressure and hyperfiltration to reduce urine protein excretion beyond effects on BP. The use of angiotensin converting enzyme inhibitor (ACEI), captopril, in type 1 DM patients decreased urine protein excretion and doubling of serum creatinine independent of the effects of blood pressure. Two major clinical trials, Irbesartan Diabetic Nephropathy Trial (IDNT) and Effects of losartan on renal and cardiovascular outcomes in patients with type 2 diabetes and nephropathy (REENAL), demonstrated renoprotective effects of angiotensin receptor blockers (ARBs) in type 2 diabetic patients with diabetic nephropathy. However, combination therapy with ACEI and ARBs does not seem to add further benefit to use of ACEI or ARB alone and in fact was associated with increased hypotension, syncope, and renal dysfunction. Similarly combination use of a direct renin inhibitor (aliskiren) with either an ACEI or ARB did not preserve kidney function and was associated with increased events of hypotension and hyperkalemia [16]. Thus careful monitoring of blood pressure to avoid hypotension, thereby decreasing kidney perfusion, and hyperkalemia is of paramount importance with the use of RAAS agents particularly for diabetic patients with baseline kidney dysfunction. In addition, the use of ACEI and ARBs is contraindicated during pregnancy because of teratogenicity.

Box 4.4. What the Guidelines Say You Should Do: Blood Pressure Recommendations in DKD

1. Recommended target blood pressure for those with CKD 1–4 is <130/80 mmHg.
2. RAAS blockers with a diuretic are recommended as the first choice if tolerated by the patient.

Source: Data from KDOQI [21]

4.4.3 RAAS Blockers Not for Primary Prevention

While RAAS-blocking agents have shown benefit in decreasing urinary protein excretion, current evidence does not support the use of ACEI and ARB for the primary prevention of microalbuminuria in diabetic patients. With a lack of clinical trial data showing benefit of RAAS in preventing development of microalbuminuria in normoalbuminuric, normotensive patients with either type 1 or type 2 DM, these drugs cannot be recommended for primary prevention for this purpose [17, 18].

4.4.4 Lipid Control

Elevated triglycerides and LDL cholesterol are a common pattern of hyperlipidemia in diabetic patients. Moreover, the tendency for dyslipidemia is further increased by the development of CKD. Since diabetes is considered a coronary artery disease equivalent, *aggressive lipid lowering* becomes *important* in the intensive medical management of all patients with diabetes. Hyperlipidemia is also thought to play a role in the development of glomerulosclerosis in CKD patients (Box 4.5).

Hydroxymethylglutaryl-coenzyme A (*HMG-CoA*) *reductase inhibitors* (statins) remain *first-line agents* in achieving target low-density lipoprotein (LDL) levels in diabetic patients. In addition, statins have anti-inflammatory effects by decreasing inflammatory chemokines, such as MCP-1, VCAM1, and ICAM1, and cytokines TNF and IL1β. Antioxidant effects of statins on mesangial and tubular cells in diabetic rodent models have suggested a decrease in diabetic nephropathy with their use. Studies in diabetic patients suggest a decrease in microalbuminuria with statin use. Secondary analysis of the randomized placebo-controlled Collaborative Atorvastatin Diabetes Study (CARDS Trial) however did not find differences in either the incidence of albuminuria or regression of albuminuria in diabetics though there was a modest benefit in estimated GFR in those treated with statins. Statin-treated group showed a modest benefit in estimated GFR [19].

Box 4.5. What the Guidelines Say You Should Do: Recommended Lipid Lowering in Diabetic Patients with Renal Disease (CKD 1–4)

1. LDL cholesterol (LDLc) <100 mg/dl; <70 mg/dl is a therapeutic option.
   (a) Statin is recommended for those with LDLc >100 mg/dl.
2. ADA recommends HDL levels in men and women older than 50 years of age. No specific recommendations have been made for those with chronic kidney disease.
3. ADA recommends triglyceride levels <150 mg/dl in general. No specific recommendations for triglyceride levels have been made for those with chronic kidney disease.

Sources: Data from KDOQI [21] and American Diabetes Association [22]

The use of fenofibrate in type 2 DM patients is associated with an improvement in lipid profiles in addition to a decrease in the rate of progression from normoalbuminuria to microalbuminuria. Fenofibrates in part mediate clinical effects via PPAR-α activation resulting in a 35–50 % decrease in triglyceride levels and a 5–20 %increase in high-density lipoprotein (HDL) cholesterol. These agents also moderately decrease total and LDL cholesterol. The use of fenofibrates, however, requires dose adjustment for creatinine clearance of <50 ml/min.

The use of statins in combination with fibric acid derivatives does increase risk for myopathy and/or rhabdomyolysis with incidence reported in the literature of 0.12%, particularly in those with comorbidities including diabetes and kidney disease, as well as increased age, female gender, increased exercise habits, alcoholism, thyroid disease, liver disease, or those undergoing surgery. Therefore, caution in weighing benefits with risks, as well as careful follow-up of patients, is required in those with underlying predisposition and specific need for combined therapy.

4.4.5 Weight Control

Weight control remains a crucial part in the management of diabetic patients as an increase in waist circumference is associated with progression of albuminuria in type 2 diabetics [20]. *A reduction in weight has been shown to improve kidney function and decrease urine protein excretion in obese patients with diabetic nephropathy* (Fig. 4.6).

Since the use of anti-glycemic agents such as sulfonylureas, thiazolidinediones, and insulin is often associated with modest weight gain, control of weight in diabetic patients becomes challenging. Therefore, the effect of weight gain and weight control, in addition to blood glucose control with use of anti-glycemic agents, must be carefully balanced in order to optimize the effect of weight in its contribution to diabetic kidney disease.

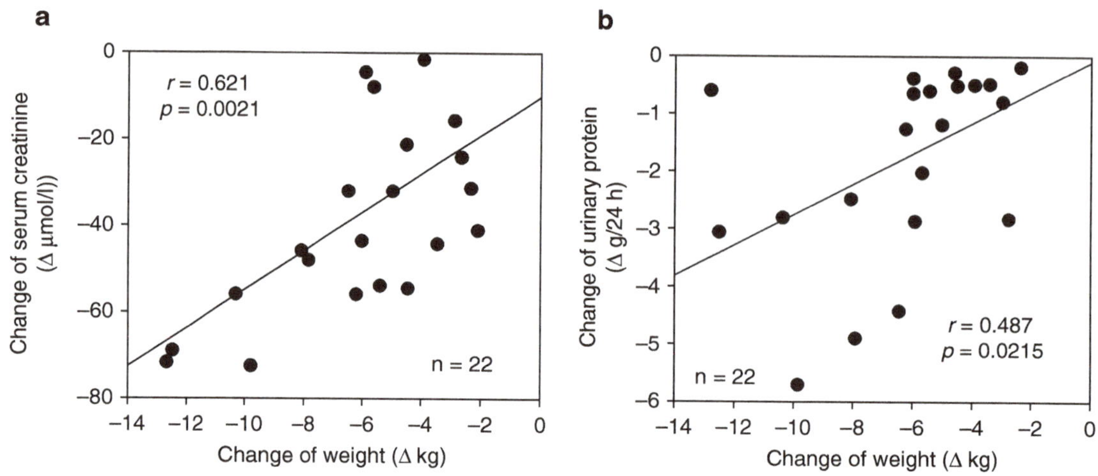

Fig. 4.6 (**a**) Correlation between change of the body weight and change of serum creatinine. Decrease in serum creatinine and weight loss show a significant correlation ($r=0.62$, $P<0.005$). (**b**) Correlation between change of the body weight and change of urinary protein. Decrease in proteinuria correlates with weight loss ($r=0.49$, $P<0.05$) (Reprinted by permission of Macmillan Publishers Ltd: Saiki et al. [24], copyright 2005)

4.4.6 Protein Restriction

Whether dietary protein restriction slows the long-term decline in GFR in diabetic nephropathy is unclear. In addition to the problem of a lack of patient adherence to treatment, protein malnutrition becomes a problem particularly for type 1 diabetics who are at increased risk for protein breakdown from insulin deficiency. A dietary protein intake of 0.8–1.0 g/kg of body weight per day is reasonable though it remains unclear at this time whether careful protein intake adds further in the management of nephropathy given aggressive blood pressure and blood glucose control as well as RAAS inhibition.

Before You Finish: Practice Pearls for the Clinicians

- Early diagnosis of DN is crucial in preventing long-term devastating consequences of kidney failure, and screening for urine albumin excretion should be routine for those with diabetes, particularly for those at high risk.
- Microvascular disease including retinopathy and neuropathy frequently coexists with diabetic kidney disease although the absence of other microvascular diseases does not rule out the presence of diabetic kidney disease.
- As chronic kidney disease from diabetes progresses over decades, a rapid loss of kidney function in those with diabetes or diabetics with active urine sediment suggestive of other glomerular pathologies require further investigation including kidney biopsy if indicated.
- Optimizing blood glucose control, blood pressure, serum lipids, and weight in patients with diabetes is crucial early on to prevent progression to nephropathy and improve cardiovascular mortality.
- Avoidance or minimizing nephrotoxins in those with diabetic kidney disease is necessary.
- The use of RAAS-blocking agents if tolerated has proven particularly beneficial in patients with diabetes in decreasing progression of their diabetic kidney disease.

References

1. Okada R, Yasuda Y, Tsushita K, Wakai K, Hamajima N, Matsuo S. Glomerular hyperfiltration in prediabetes and prehypertension. Nephrol Dial Transplant. 2012;27(5):1821–5.
2. Fioretto P, Mauer M. Histopathology of diabetic nephropathy. Semin Nephrol. 2007;27(2):195–207.
3. UK Prospective Diabetes Study Group. Tight blood pressure control and risk of macrovascular and microvascular complications in type 2 diabetes: UKPDS 38. BMJ. 1998;317(7160):703–13.
4. Duckworth W, Abraira C, Moritz T, et al. Glucose control and vascular complications in veterans with type 2 diabetes. N Engl J Med. 2009;360(2):129–39.
5. Solano MP, Goldberg RB. Management of dyslipidemia in diabetes. Cardiol Rev. 2006;14(3):125–35.
6. The Diabetes Control and Complications Trial Research Group. The effect of intensive treatment of diabetes on the development and progression of long-term complications in insulin-dependent diabetes mellitus. N Engl J Med. 1993;329(14):977–86.
7. UK Prospective Diabetes Study (UKPDS) Group. Intensive blood-glucose control with sulphonylureas or insulin compared with conventional treatment and risk of complications in patients with type 2 diabetes (UKPDS 33). Lancet. 1998;352(9131):837–53.
8. Ohkubo Y, Kishikawa H, Araki E, et al. Intensive insulin therapy prevents the progression of diabetic microvascular complications in Japanese patients with non-insulin-dependent diabetes mellitus: a randomized prospective 6-year study. Diabetes Res Clin Pract. 1995;28(2):103–17.
9. Fioretto P, Steffes MW, Sutherland DE, Goetz FC, Mauer M. Reversal of lesions of diabetic nephropathy after pancreas transplantation. N Engl J Med. 1998;339(2):69–75.
10. Ahmed Z, Simon B, Choudhury D. Management of diabetes in patients with chronic kidney disease. Postgrad Med. 2009;121(3):52–60.
11. Ryan EA, Bigam D, Shapiro AM. Current indications for pancreas or islet transplant. Diabetes Obes Metab. 2006;8(1):1–7.
12. Wagner RT, Lewis J, Cooney A, Chan L. Stem cell approaches for the treatment of type 1 diabetes mellitus. Transl Res. 2010;156(3):169–79.
13. Wang XX, Jiang T, Levi M. Nuclear hormone receptors in diabetic nephropathy. Nat Rev Nephrol. 2010;6(6):342–51.
14. Bakris GL, Fonseca VA, Sharma K, Wright EM. Renal sodium-glucose transport: role in diabetes mellitus and potential clinical implications. Kidney Int. 2009;75(12):1272–7.
15. Cushman WC, Evans GW, Byington RP, et al. Effects of intensive blood-pressure control in type 2 diabetes mellitus. N Engl J Med. 2010;362(17):1575–85.
16. Parving HH, Brenner BM, McMurray JJ, et al. Cardiorenal end points in a trial of aliskiren for type 2 diabetes. N Engl J Med. 2012;367(23):2204–13.
17. The EUCLID Study Group. Randomised placebo-controlled trial of lisinopril in normotensive patients with insulin-dependent diabetes and normoalbuminuria or microalbuminuria. Lancet. 1997;349(9068):1787–92.
18. Bilous R, Chaturvedi N, Sjolie AK, et al. Effect of candesartan on microalbuminuria and albumin excretion rate in diabetes: three randomized trials. Ann Intern Med. 2009;151(1):11–20, W13–14.
19. Colhoun HM, Betteridge DJ, Durrington PN, et al. Effects of atorvastatin on kidney outcomes and cardiovascular disease in patients with diabetes: an analysis from the Collaborative Atorvastatin Diabetes Study (CARDS). Am J Kidney Dis. 2009;54(5):810–9.
20. Rossi MC, Nicolucci A, Pellegrini F, et al. Obesity and changes in urine albumin/creatinine ratio in patients with type 2 diabetes: the DEMAND study. Nutr Metab Cardiovasc Dis. 2010;20(2):110–6.
21. KDOQI. KDOQI clinical practice guidelines and clinical practice recommendations for diabetes and chronic kidney disease. Am J Kidney Dis. 2007;49(2 Suppl 2):S12–154.
22. American Diabetes Association. Standards of medical care in diabetes- 2012. Diab Care. 2012;35 Suppl 1:S11–63.
23. Adler AI, Stratton IM, Neil HA, Yudkin JS, Matthews DR, Cull CA, et al. Association of systolic blood pressure with macrovascular and microvascular complications of type 2 diabetes (UKPDS 36): prospective observational study. BMJ. 2000;321(7258):412–9.
24. Saiki A, Nagayama D, Ohhira M, Endoh K, Ohtsuka M, Koide N, et al. Effect of weight loss using formula diet on renal function in obese patients with diabetic nephropathy. Int J Obes (Lond). 2005;29(9):1115–20.

Hypertension and Chronic Kidney Disease

5

Stephanie Riggen and Rajiv Agarwal

Before You Start: Facts You Need to Know

- Hypertension is the second leading cause of ESRD in the United States.
- Uncontrolled hypertension is associated with accelerated progression to ESRD.
- Recent genetic advances may provide more information on the cause and effect relationship of hypertension and kidney disease.
- Renovascular hypertension and ischemic nephropathy are associated with progressive chronic kidney disease but their diagnosis and treatment remain complex and challenging.
- Treatment of hypertension in CKD patients is important to delay progression of renal function loss and to protect against cardiovascular disease.
- Resistant hypertension is defined as blood pressure that remains above goal (such as 140/90) in spite of the concurrent use of 3 antihypertensive agents of different classes.

Worldwide, hypertension is a major public health problem and is associated with morbidity and mortality due to cardiovascular and kidney diseases. In the United States, hypertension is present in approximately 80–85 % of patients with CKD and is the second leading cause of ESRD in the United States after diabetes. Uncontrolled hypertension is associated with accelerated progression to ESRD. This association was prospectively studied among 332,544 men screened for the Multiple Risk Factor Intervention Trial (MRFIT); among the 814 subjects who either died of or were treated for ESRD, it was found that elevated blood pressure was a strong independent risk factor for ESRD [1].

Although the association of hypertension and ESRD was strong, this study did not prove a cause and effect relationship. In fact, whether hypertension causes CKD or is a result of CKD or both remains debated.

The diagnosis of hypertensive nephrosclerosis is a diagnosis of exclusion; it is a clinical diagnosis based on history, physical examination, urinalysis, and laboratory testing. The diagnosis is typically made in patients with chronic kidney disease who have had long-standing hypertension and subnephrotic range proteinuria without evidence of other kidney disease (based on serologic testing and imaging tests). Few patients diagnosed with hypertensive nephrosclerosis undergo renal biopsy.

Histologic lesions of hypertensive nephrosclerosis are characterized by changes in vascular, glomerular, and tubulointerstitial structures.

S. Riggen, MD • R. Agarwal, MD, FASN, FAHA, FASH (✉)
Department of Medicine, Indiana University School of Medicine, Indianapolis, IN, USA
e-mail: stasteve@iu.edu; ragarwal@iupui.edu

M. Arici (ed.), *Management of Chronic Kidney Disease*,
DOI 10.1007/978-3-642-54637-2_5, © Springer-Verlag Berlin Heidelberg 2014

For example, vascular changes are characterized by afferent arteriolar narrowing and fibrosis, arteriosclerosis and arteriolosclerosis, and intimal fibrosis; glomerular changes by hyalinosis, global glomerulosclerosis, and segmental glomerulosclerosis; and tubulointerstitial changes by atrophy, inflammation, and fibrosis.

To examine the accuracy of the diagnosis of hypertensive nephrosclerosis, an examination of renal biopsies was performed on a subset of patients enrolled in the African American Study of Kidney Disease (AASK) Trial, a trial that was designed to examine the impact of antihypertensive therapies and two levels of blood pressure control on the rate of progression of renal dysfunction in African Americans with presumed hypertensive renal disease. The AASK pilot biopsy study of 39 patients showed 38 patients with arteriosclerosis and/or arteriolosclerosis [2]. This confirmed that renal biopsies in nondiabetic hypertensive African Americans with mild to moderate renal insufficiency in the absence of nephrotic proteinuria are likely to show changes consistent with what we call hypertensive nephrosclerosis as outlined above.

The mechanism by which hypertension causes renal dysfunction is based on animal models, which have demonstrated that autoregulation protects the glomerular microcirculation from high arterial pressures. In certain conditions, such as chronic kidney disease and diabetes, this autoregulation is impaired, which is associated with glomerular injury and glomerulosclerosis. Although some evidence from human studies support the concept of autoregulatory dysfunction at the level of the glomerular microcirculation, the evidence from animals are much stronger.

Just as hypertension may cause CKD, CKD may also cause hypertension. Why this may be so is multifactorial. These factors include sodium retention, increased activity of the renin-angiotensin system and sympathetic nervous system, and impaired nitric oxide synthesis and endothelium-mediated vasodilatation in uremic patients. Patients with CKD frequently have sleep apnea and secondary hyperparathyroidism, both of which can contribute to hypertension with the latter causing increased intracellular calcium concentration leading to vasoconstriction. Besides, the circadian variation in BP is profoundly disturbed. Ambulatory blood pressure monitoring in patients with CKD often identifies a loss of normal decline in blood pressure of 10 % during sleep, such patients are termed "nondippers," which has been associated with an increased risk of left ventricular hypertrophy and cardiovascular events [3].

The diagnosis of hypertensive nephrosclerosis has been called into question with the discovery of the association of specific genes with kidney disease. Molecular genetic advances, particularly mapping by admixture linkage disequilibrium (MALD) analyses, pointed to a cluster of polymorphisms in the *MYH9* gene on chromosome 22 that were strongly associated with African ancestry nondiabetic kidney disease. However, Genovese et al. searched an expanded risk interval and found a statistically stronger genetic association with kidney disease in *APOL1*, the gene encoding apolipoprotein L-1, which is located <20 kb from the 3′ end of *MYH9* [4].

The two *APOL1* risk allele variants, G1 and G2, have been found to be strongly associated with nondiabetic kidney disease, particularly FSGS. It is hypothesized that patients with *APOL1* risk variant alleles have a genetic predisposition to kidney disease and then suffer a "second hit" such as a gene-gene or gene-environment interaction leading to various histologic forms of nondiabetic kidney disease and perhaps many patients who are labeled as having "hypertensive nephrosclerosis" actually have an underlying genetic predisposition to kidney disease [5].

The normal in vivo functions of *APOL1* and the mechanism of kidney injury are unknown. Interestingly, however, *APOL1* risk variants likely rose to high frequency in sub-Saharan Africa due to conferring protection from African sleeping sickness caused by trypanosomes. Genovese et al. found that serum from carriers of *APOL1* risk variants demonstrated a trypanolytic effect on *Trypanosoma brucei rhodesiense* and absence of trypanosomal killing with serum from individuals lacking *APOL1* risk variants [4]. Thus, the *APOL1* risk variants provided a likely selective advantage to carriers against African sleeping sickness, but unfortunately, possession of two *APOL1* risk variants is associated with increased risk of kidney disease. This story is similar to the protection of malaria by HgbS.

As more data emerges regarding genetic and environmental influences on the development of kidney disease, some have proposed that hypertensive kidney disease is a no longer useful term and a more generic term of arterionephrosclerosis should be used.

5.1 Renovascular Hypertension and Ischemic Nephropathy

Renovascular disease is a term used to describe several clinical syndromes resulting from reduced perfusion to the kidney including ischemic renal disease and renovascular hypertension. Ischemic renal disease occurs when renal blood flow falls below the level of renal autoregulation and leads to reduced GFR and renal atrophy. On the other hand, renovascular hypertension (RVH) is defined as a syndrome of elevated blood pressure that is produced as a result of a variety of conditions that cause renal ischemia. The most common cause of RVH is main renal artery stenosis (RAS), either by fibromuscular dysplasia or atherosclerotic renal vascular disease.

Mechanisms responsible for sustained RVH differ according to whether one or both kidneys are affected by significant stenosis. Both situations have impaired renal perfusion, which activates the renin-angiotensin system causing sodium retention. However, when there is still one functioning kidney (in experimental animals this is simulated by one clipped renal artery, with two kidneys present and is termed "two-kidney hypertension"), pressure natriuresis can occur in the functioning kidney eliminating excess sodium. This leads to a sustained decreased perfusion to the stenotic side, leading to sustained activation of the renin-angiotensin system. Hypertension in this situation is angiotensin II-dependent hypertension with secondary aldosterone excess. On the other hand when the vascular lesion involves both kidneys or affects a solitary functioning kidney (termed "one-kidney hypertension"), there is no normal kidney to counteract the increased systemic pressure. Sodium is thus retained and blood volume expanded, which feeds back to inhibit the renin-angiotensin system. However, the renin-angiotensin system activation is inappropriately activated for the degree of sodium retention.

Renovascular disease can have varied presentations. Clinical features that may alert to the presence of renovascular disease include an acute rise of serum creatinine of at least 30 % after administration of ACE inhibitor or ARB (often accompanied by hypotension), a unilateral small kidney, or asymmetry in renal size of more than 1.5 cm that cannot be explained by another reason, moderate to severe hypertension in patients with recurrent episodes of flash pulmonary edema, late onset of severe hypertension (after age of 55 years), or presence of an abdominal bruit.

The diagnosis of RVH requires demonstration of a critical stenotic vascular lesion affecting the renal artery. Luminal occlusion of less than 60 % rarely reduces either pressure or blood flow. RVH usually only occurs when luminal occlusion is relatively severe, usually in the 70–80 % occlusion range.

American College of Cardiology/American Heart Association (ACC/AHA) developed guidelines to assist clinicians with the diagnosis, medical treatment, and revascularization for renal artery stenosis (Box 5.1).

The gold standard for diagnosing renal artery stenosis is renal arteriography but is usually performed only after a less invasive test has increased the likelihood of an accurate diagnosis. Less invasive tests include duplex Doppler ultrasonography, CTA, or MRA. The test of choice should be based on institutional expertise and patient

Box 5.1. What the Guidelines Say You Should Do: Renal Artery Stenosis (RAS) [6]

Clinical Clues to Diagnosis

Class I Recommendations

- The performance of diagnostic studies to identify clinically significant RAS is indicated in patients with the onset of hypertension before the age of 30 years
- The performance of diagnostic studies to identify clinically significant RAS is indicated in patients with the onset of severe hypertension [as defined in the Seventh Report of the Joint National Committee on Prevention, Detection, Evaluation, and Treatment of High Blood Pressure: the JNC-7 report] after the age of 55 years
- The performance of diagnostic studies to identify clinically significant RAS is indicated in patients with the following characteristics: (a) accelerated hypertension (sudden and persistent worsening of previously controlled hypertension), (b) resistant hypertension (defined as the failure to achieve goal blood pressure in patients who are adhering to full doses of an appropriate 3-drug regimen that includes a diuretic), or (c) malignant hypertension (hypertension with coexistent evidence of acute end-organ damage)
- The performance of diagnostic studies to identify clinically significant RAS is indicated in patients with new azotemia or worsening renal function after the administration of an ACE inhibitor or/and angiotensin receptor blocking agent
- The performance of diagnostic studies to identify clinically significant RAS is indicated in patients with sudden, unexplained pulmonary edema (especially in azotemic patients)

Class IIa Recommendations

- The performance of diagnostic studies to identify clinically significant RAS is reasonable in patients with unexplained renal failure, including individuals starting renal replacement therapy (dialysis or renal transplantation)
- *Class IIb*The performance of arteriography to identify significant RAS may be reasonable in patients with multivessel coronary artery disease and none of the clinical clues or PAD at the time of arteriography
- The performance of diagnostic studies to identify clinically significant RAS may be reasonable in patients with unexplained congestive heart failure or refractory angina

Diagnostic Methods for Renal Artery Stenosis

Class I

- Duplex ultrasonography is recommended as a screening test to establish the diagnosis of RAS
- Computed tomographic angiography (in individuals with normal renal function) is recommended as a screening test to establish the diagnosis of RAS
- Magnetic resonance angiography is recommended as a screening test to establish the diagnosis of RAS
- When the clinical index of suspicion is high and the results of the noninvasive tests are inconclusive, catheter angiography is recommended as a diagnostic test to establish the diagnosis of RAS

Class III

- Captopril renal scintigraphy is not recommended as a screening test to establish the diagnosis of RAS
- Selective renal vein renin measurements are not recommended as a useful screening test to establish the diagnosis of RAS
- Plasma renin activity is not recommended as a useful screening test to establish the diagnosis of RAS
- The captopril test (measurement of plasma renin activity after captopril administration) is not recommended as a useful screening test to establish the diagnosis of RAS

Medical Treatment for Renal Artery Stenosis

Class I

- Angiotensin-converting enzyme inhibitors are effective medications for treatment of hypertension associated with unilateral RAS

- Angiotensin receptor blockers are effective medications for treatment of hypertension associated with unilateral RAS
- Calcium-channel blockers are effective medications for the treatment of hypertension associated with unilateral RAS
- Beta-blockers are effective medications for treatment of hypertension associated with RAS

Indications for Revascularization for Renal Artery Stenosis

Asymptomatic Stenosis

Class IIb

- Percutaneous revascularization may be considered for treatment of an asymptomatic bilateral or solitary viable kidney with a hemodynamically significant RAS
- The usefulness of percutaneous revascularization of an asymptomatic unilateral hemodynamically significant RAS in a viable kidney is not well established and is presently clinically unproven

Hypertension

Class IIa

- Percutaneous revascularization is reasonable for patients with hemodynamically significant RAS and accelerated hypertension, resistant hypertension, malignant hypertension, hypertension with unexplained unilateral small kidney, and hypertension with intolerance to medication

Preservation of Renal Function

Class IIa

- Percutaneous revascularization is reasonable for patients with RAS and progressive chronic kidney disease with bilateral RAS or a RAS to a solitary functioning kidney

Class IIb

- Percutaneous revascularization may be considered for patients with RAS and chronic renal insufficiency with unilateral RAS

Congestive Heart Failure and Unstable Angina

Class I

- Percutaneous revascularization is indicated for patients with hemodynamically significant RAS and recurrent, unexplained congestive heart failure or sudden, unexplained pulmonary edema

Class IIa

Percutaneous revascularization is reasonable for patients with hemodynamically significant RAS and unstable angina

factors as radiocontrast and gadolinium are potentially harmful in patients with CKD stage 4 or 5. Captopril renal scintigraphy, selective renal vein renin measurements, and plasma renin activity are not useful as initial diagnostic tests for renal artery stenosis.

It has been suggested that calculation of resistance index by duplex Doppler ultrasonography can identify patients who are likely or not to respond to revascularization. A high resistive index was associated with a poor outcome and may indicate irreversible intrarenal vascular disease.

Once diagnosed, the optimal treatment for the patient is not clear. Patients with atherosclerotic renovascular disease have a high rate of systemic atherosclerosis and are at increased risk for adverse cardiovascular outcomes. The increased cardiovascular risk in patients with atherosclerotic renal artery stenosis may be due to mechanisms activated by the renal artery stenosis or due to the high likelihood that these patients have atherosclerosis in multiple vascular beds. Treatment should address modifiable cardiovascular risk factors, including weight loss, smoking cessation, treatment of hyperlipidemia, and blood pressure and glucose control.

There are no definitive randomized controlled trial data to guide clinicians on specific antihypertensive medical therapies in patients with RAS. It would appear that the first-line therapy should be directed at the principal mechanism thought to be responsible for the elevated blood pressure, activation of the renin-angiotensin-aldosterone system. Although blockade of the renin-angiotensin system is considered fundamental, it is contraindicated in most patients. Antihypertensive agents that block the renin-angiotensin system remove the vasoconstrictive action of angiotensin II (AII) at the efferent arteriole. When pre-glomerular pressures are reduced for any reason, blockade of AII causes the kidney to lose its compensatory ability to preserve glomerular transcapillary filtration pressures by constricting the efferent arteriole. This can lead to "functional acute renal insufficiency." Paying particular importance to volume status and cardiac function and monitoring serum creatinine if ever agents that block the renin-angiotensin system are initiated are important in limiting renal toxicity in these patients.

Whether to treat patients with medical therapy alone or with revascularization has been evaluated in several randomized clinical trials. These trials, including the ASTRAL trial, showed a lack of benefit of revascularization using BP as an endpoint. The ASTRAL trial was a multicenter, randomized, unblinded trial of 806 patients with atherosclerotic renovascular disease assigned to undergo either revascularization in addition to medical therapy or to medical therapy alone with a primary outcome of renal function. During a 5-year period, patients in the group who underwent revascularization had a slightly slower rate of progression of renal impairment; however, the change was too small to offer clinical benefit. In addition there was no significant difference in a secondary endpoint of systolic blood pressure between the two groups. The two groups had similar rates of renal events, major cardiovascular events, and death. Given serious complications associated with revascularization occurred in 23 patients including 2 deaths, the investigators concluded that there was an increased risk but no evidence of significant clinical benefit from revascularization in patients with atherosclerotic renovascular disease. The major limitation of the ASTRAL trial was that the population enrolled only included patients who their own physician was uncertain as to whether revascularization would provide a clinical benefit leaving an unresolved question of whether some patients with severe renal artery stenosis may benefit from revascularization [8].

The CORAL trial, cardiovascular outcomes in renal atherosclerotic lesions, is an ongoing trial that was designed to answer the question if stent revascularization of hemodynamically significant atherosclerotic RAS in hypertensive patients when added upon medical therapy can prevent adverse cardiovascular and renal events. It has been proposed that atherosclerotic renal artery stenosis has many other deleterious effects throughout the body other than causing elevated blood pressure and that treating RAS with revascularization may be beneficial in ways other than lowering blood pressure. The results of this trial may provide guidance for a disease whose diagnosis and treatment remain complex and challenging at present [9].

5.1.1 BP Control in CKD

Treatment of hypertension in CKD patients is important to delay progression of renal function loss and to protect against cardiovascular disease. KDIGO clinical practice guidelines for management of blood pressure in chronic kidney disease are based on quality of evidence (Boxes 5.2 and 5.3).

BP goals should be individualized according to age, coexistent cardiovascular disease and other comorbidities, risk of progression of CKD, presence or absence of retinopathy (in CKD patients with diabetes), and tolerance of treatment. Evidence supports a goal blood pressure ≤140/90 mmHg for CKD patients without proteinuria defined as albuminuria <30 mg/24 h, regardless of diabetes status. Since proteinuria has been associated with worse kidney outcomes, stricter BP control is recommended with goal BP ≤130/80 mmHg in both diabetic and nondiabetic patients with albuminuria >30 mg/24 h.

A meta-analysis by Jafar et al. was performed to determine the levels of blood pressure and urine protein excretion associated with the lowest risk of progression of CKD using antihypertensive therapy with and without ACE inhibitors. Although the data must be interpreted with caution as the clinical trials were not designed to primarily assess this, the meta-analysis on 1860 nondiabetic patients from 11 randomized, controlled trials showed that systolic blood pressure

Box 5.2. What the Guidelines Say You Should Do: Management of Blood Pressure in Non-dialysis-Dependent CKD Patients Without Diabetes Mellitus [10]

- We recommend that nondiabetic adults with non-dialysis-dependent CKD and urine albumin excretion <30 mg per 24 h whose office BP is consistently >140 mmHg systolic or >90 mmHg diastolic be treated with BP-lowering agents to maintain a BP that is consistently ≤140 mmHg systolic and ≤90 mmHg diastolic (1B).
- We suggest that nondiabetic adults with non-dialysis-dependent CKD and urine albumin excretion of 30–300 mg per 24 h whose office BP is consistently >130 mmHg systolic or >80 mmHg diastolic be treated with BP-lowering agents to maintain a BP that is consistently ≤130 systolic and ≤80 mmHg diastolic (2D).
- We suggest that nondiabetic adults with non-dialysis-dependent CKD and urine albumin excretion >300 mg per 24 h whose office BP is consistently >130 mmHg systolic or >80 mmHg diastolic be treated with BP-lowering agents to maintain a BP that is consistently ≤130 systolic and ≤80 mmHg diastolic (2C).
- We suggest that an ARB or ACE-I be used in nondiabetic adults with non-dialysis-dependent CKD and urine albumin excretion of 30–300 mg per 24 h in whom treatment with BP-lowering drugs is indicated (2D).
- We recommend that an ARB or ACE-I be used in nondiabetic adults with non-dialysis-dependent CKD and urine albumin excretion >300 mg per 24 h in whom treatment with BP-lowering drugs is indicated (1B).

Box 5.3. What the Guidelines Say You Should Do: Management of Blood Pressure in Non-dialysis-Dependent CKD Patients with Diabetes Mellitus [10]

- We recommend that adults with diabetes and non-dialysis-dependent CKD and urine albumin excretion <30 mg per 24 h whose office BP is consistently >140 mmHg systolic or >90 mmHg diastolic be treated with BP-lowering agents to maintain a BP that is consistently ≤140 mmHg systolic and ≤90 mmHg diastolic [1B].
- We suggest that adults with diabetes and non-dialysis-dependent CKD urine albumin excretion of >30 mg per 24 h whose office BP is consistently >130 mmHg systolic or >80 mmHg diastolic be treated with BP-lowering agents to maintain a BP that is consistently ≤130 mmHg systolic and ≤80 mmHg diastolic [2D].
- We suggest that an ARB or ACE-I be used in adults with diabetes and non-dialysis-dependent CKD with urine albumin excretion of 30–300 mg per 24 h [2D].
- We recommend that an ARB or ACE-I be used in adults with diabetes and non-dialysis-dependent CKD with urine albumin excretion >300 mg per 24 h [1B].

of 110–129 mmHg and urine protein excretion of less than 2 g/day were associated with the lowest risk for kidney disease progression. The risk of progression increased with urine protein excretion greater than 1 g/day and systolic blood pressures greater than 120–130 mmHg. The results of the meta-analysis, which were consistent with the results of the MDRD and AASK trials, showed that lowering blood pressure is more beneficial in delaying progression of kidney disease in patients with higher levels of proteinuria [11].

Although BP control has been shown to delay progression of kidney disease, more aggressive blood pressure control has not been shown to be better. Three main randomized controlled trials, MDRD, AASK, and REIN2, evaluated lower blood pressure and cardiovascular and renal outcomes.

The Modification of Diet in Renal Disease (MDRD) study was a multicenter clinical trial designed to test the hypotheses that restricting protein intake and controlling BP would delay the progression of chronic kidney disease. The MDRD study consisted of 2 studies. The first study randomized patients with GFR 22–55 mL/min per 1.73 m^2 to usual protein diet or low-protein diet and to a usual BP defined as MAP ≤107 mmHg or low BP defined as MAP ≤92 mmHg. The projected mean decline in GFR at 3 years did not differ significantly between the protein and blood pressure groups. In study 2, patients with GFR 13–24 mL/min per 1.73 m^2 were assigned to low-protein diet or very-low-protein diet and usual BP defined as MAP ≤107 or low BP defined as MAP ≤92. In study 2, the very-low-protein group has a marginally slower decline in GFR but no delay in the time to occurrence of ESRD or death [12].

The African American Study of Kidney Disease and Hypertension (AASK) trial randomized African Americans with hypertension, age 18–70 years old with GFR 20–65 mL/min per 1.73 m^2, and no other identified causes of renal insufficiency to one of the two mean arterial pressure goals, 102–107 mmHg or <92 mmHg, and to initial treatment with one of the three antihypertensive study drugs, metoprolol, ramipril, or amlodipine. The primary outcome measure was rate of change of GFR. Main secondary outcome was composite index of three clinical endpoints including reduction of GFR of >50 % or 25 mL/min/1.73 m^2, ESRD, or death. The study did not find a significant difference in primary or secondary outcomes or CV events or mortality between the two blood pressure groups [13].

Ramipril efficacy in nephropathy 2 (REIN-2) is a multicenter, randomized controlled trial of patients with nondiabetic kidney disease and proteinuria >1 g/day receiving ramipril 2.5–5 mg/day which randomly assigned them to either conventional BP defined as diastolic BP <90 mmHg or intensive BP control defined as BP <130/80 mmHg using add-on therapy with felodipine 5–10 mg/day. The systolic BP difference between the conventional and intensive BP groups was 4.1 mmHg and diastolic BP difference was 2.8 mmHg. The study showed no difference in ESRD rate between the two BP groups [14].

In summary, there is good evidence from the MDRD, AASK, and REIN-2 trials that aggressive BP control is not protective in regard to cardiovascular, renal, or mortality outcomes.

Once BP goals have been identified, aim should focus on the appropriate treatment plan to achieve that goal. Lifestyle modifications should be encouraged in all patients with CKD to lower BP and improve long-term cardiovascular and renal outcomes. KDIGO guidelines on lifestyle modifications are listed in Box 5.4.

Attainment of blood pressure goal generally requires multiple antihypertensive agents. A number of trials have shown that ACE inhibitors

Box 5.4. What the Guidelines Say You Should Do: Lifestyle and Pharmacologic Treatments for Lowering Blood Pressure in Non-dialysis-Dependent CKD Patients [10]

- Individualize BP targets and agents according to age, coexistent cardiovascular disease and other comorbidities, risk of progression of CKD, presence or absence of retinopathy (in CKD patients with diabetes), and tolerance of treatment [not graded]
- Inquire about postural dizziness and check for postural hypotension regularly when treating CKD patients with BP-lowering agents [not graded]
- Encourage lifestyle modification in people with CKD to lower BP and improve long-term cardiovascular and other outcomes
- We recommend achieving or maintaining a healthy weight (BMI 20–25) (1D)
- We recommend lowering salt intake to <90 mmol (<2 g) per day of sodium (corresponding to 5 g of sodium chloride), unless contraindicated (1C)
- We recommend undertaking an exercise program compatible with cardiovascular health and tolerance, aiming for at least 30 min 5 times per week (1D)
- We suggest limiting alcohol intake to no more than two standard drinks per day for men and no more than one standard drink per day for women (2D)

or ARBs can slow the progression of diabetic kidney disease with overt nephropathy. A meta-analysis performed by Jafar et al. that included 11 randomized controlled trials comparing the efficacy of ACE inhibitors to other antihypertensive regimens that did not contain ACE inhibitors in nondiabetic patients with kidney disease showed that ACE inhibitors decreased blood pressure and urinary protein excretion, as well as slowed the increase in creatinine and reduced the incidence of ESRD. The benefit was greater in patients with higher levels of proteinuria [15]. The benefit of ACE inhibitors or ARBs on patients without proteinuria is unknown. KDIGO recommends ARBs or ACE inhibitors as first-line therapy in all CKD patients with albuminuria >300 mg/24 h.

ACE inhibitors generally reduce proteinuria by 30–35 %. The anti-proteinuric effects are generally enhanced when the patient is on a low-sodium diet or taking a diuretic since glomerular microcirculation is more dependent on angiotensin II in relative volume depletion states.

Although ACE inhibitors and ARBs may be particularly beneficial in patients with CKD as noted above, the side effects of these medications, including hyperkalemia, hypotension, and reduction in GFR, make them difficult to use in patients with CKD. Patients who become volume depleted are particularly susceptible to reduction in GFR while taking an ACE inhibitor or ARB. In response to low perfusion pressures, angiotensin II causes increased resistance at the efferent arteriole in an attempt to preserve intraglomerular pressure. This compensatory mechanism is blocked by ACE inhibitors and ARBs. Patients with reduced GFR are more susceptible to elevated potassium levels due to impaired excretion; reducing aldosterone secretion with ACE inhibitors or ARBS blocks the major hormonal stimulus for urinary potassium excretion leading to increased susceptibility to hyperkalemia in patients with CKD. Patients should have their blood pressure, potassium, and creatinine monitored within 1–2 weeks after initiating ACE inhibitor or ARB therapy. Patients at increased susceptibility for adverse effects include elderly patients and those with heart failure, potassium levels >5 mmol/L, advanced CKD with GFR <30 mL/min/1.73m^2, or on high-dose diuretics. Termination of ACE inhibitors should occur if there is a dramatic increase in serum creatinine concentration from the baseline value within the first few weeks of initiation of therapy or if patient experiences uncontrolled hyperkalemia or any other significant adverse effect.

Despite the benefit of ACE inhibitors and ARBs in previous studies, progression of CKD still occurred in a significant number of patients. Based on this finding, combination blockade of the RAAS has been evaluated in several studies to determine if dual therapy can provide additional benefit. The Aliskiren Trial in Type 2 Diabetics Using Cardiorenal Endpoints (ALTITUDE) was an international, randomized, double-blind, placebo-controlled, parallel group study which randomized a large number of type 2 diabetic patients with renal impairment to receive aliskiren 300 mg daily, a direct renin inhibitor, or placebo in addition to conventional therapy with ACE inhibitor or ARB. The study was terminated early due to lack of benefit of aliskiren over placebo in reducing cardiovascular or renal endpoints after approximately 2 years but an increased risk of adverse events including hypotension, hyperkalemia, and renal impairment [16].

The VA NEPHRON-D trial was a recently terminated multicenter, prospective, randomized, double-blind clinical trial to assess the effect of combination losartan and lisinopril compared with losartan alone, on the progression of kidney disease in diabetic patients with overt proteinuria. Those randomized to combination therapy had more adverse events leading to early termination of the trial. Publication is pending [17].

Although ACE inhibitors or ARBs are considered first-line therapy in most patients with proteinuric kidney disease, there are no specific guidelines regarding second and third agents used to control blood pressure in CKD patients. Volume expansion often plays a role in hypertensive CKD patients. Higher doses of diuretics are typically required in CKD patients due to the reduction in kidney function. There is some data that taking at least one antihypertensive at night may improve BP control in CKD patients as many are "nondippers," which is one of the strongest predictors of adverse cardiovascular outcomes.

When treating hypertension in CKD patients, it is most important to individualize therapy.

5.1.2 Resistant HTN

According to the definition endorsed by the American Heart Association, resistant hypertension is defined as blood pressure that remains above goal (such as 140/90) in spite of the concurrent use of 3 antihypertensive agents of different classes. Ideally, one of the three agents should be a diuretic and all agents should be prescribed at optimal doses. The definition also includes patients with normal or elevated BP in the setting of four or more antihypertensive agents [18].

Resistant hypertension is common and the prevalence is increasing. It is seen among 15–30 % of treated hypertensive patients. Older age, obesity, chronic kidney disease, and diabetes are the strongest predictors of resistant hypertension.

Before diagnosing a person with resistant hypertension, pseudoresistance must be excluded. Pseudoresistance is defined as BP above goal in clinic but below goal outside of the clinic, frequently from white coat hypertension. De Nicola prospectively studied 436 hypertensive CKD patients to determine the prevalence and prognostic role of resistant hypertension in chronic kidney disease patients. The study showed that patients with true resistant hypertension were at high risk for cardiovascular and renal events; however, pseudoresistance in CKD patients is also frequent and does not increase the cardiorenal risk [3].

The best way to exclude pseudoresistance is with home blood pressure or ambulatory blood pressure readings. Home blood pressure monitoring has been shown to be useful in predicting target organ damage, CVD mortality, and CVD events. If the home BP is >135/85 mmHg, there is high probability that the ambulatory blood pressure will also be high and treatment should be started. If home BP is <125/76 mmHg, then a patient may be considered a true normotensive and no ambulatory BP is needed. The gray zone between 125–135 mmHg systolic and 76–85 mmHg diastolic requires further evaluation with ambulatory BP [7]. Agarwal and Andersen found that in patients with CKD, ambulatory blood pressures are a stronger predictor of ESRD or death compared to blood pressures obtained in the clinic [19] (Box 5.5).

Once true resistant hypertension is diagnosed, a complete history, physical examination, and laboratory studies should be done to look for contributing factors, as the etiology of resistant hypertension is commonly multifactorial. A careful history focusing on lifestyle factors such as physical activity, dietary salt intake, and heavy alcohol intake should be performed. Sodium restriction can lower blood pressure and enhance the anti-proteinuric effects of drugs that block the renin-angiotensin system in patients with proteinuria. Patients should be educated on interpreting food labels and should be provided feedback by assessing their sodium intake with a 24 h urine collection. Elderly, African Americans, and patients with CKD are particularly salt-sensitive.

A complete medication history is essential as many classes of drugs increase blood pressure including NSAIDS, erythropoietin, oral contraceptives, sympathomimetic agents such as decongestants or diet pills, stimulants, cyclosporine, and natural licorice. Physical examination and laboratory evaluation may reveal signs of organ damage such as retinopathy, cardiovascular disease, or kidney disease.

As part of their complete evaluation, patients with resistant hypertension should be screened for secondary causes of hypertension. CKD and obstructive sleep apnea are the two most common causes of secondary hypertension. Other causes include primary aldosteronism, pheochromocytoma, Cushing's syndrome, and renal artery stenosis.

Box 5.5. What the Guidelines Say You Should Do: Home and Ambulatory BP Monitoring [7]

Technical Aspects of BP Measurement

No tobacco or caffeine for 30 min preceding measurement

After 5 min of rest

With arm at heart level; back supported and feet flat on the ground

On nondominant arm (or arm with highest BP)

BP Monitor

Use a fully automated device with an upper arm cuff that has been validated by British Hypertension Society, Association for the Advancement of Medical Instrumentation, or International Protocol for the Validation of Automated BP

Measuring Devices

Monitors with memory that are able to store measurements are preferred

Training of Patients

Patients should be trained by their healthcare provider, and the monitor readings should be checked against mercury

Education content: hypertension and cardiovascular risk, BP measurement procedure, use of a validated monitor, cuff size, protocols for measuring BP, interpretation of BP readings, and monitor for their use only

Reevaluate patient technique and accuracy of the device annually

Target BP Goal

135/85 mmHg or 130/80 mmHg if patient has diabetes, coronary heart disease, or chronic kidney disease

Frequency and Schedule of Measurement

Initial values (when patients begin HBPM at home):

Base decisions on a 7-day measurement period with 2–3 measurements each morning and 2–3 measurements in the evening at prestipulated times (an average of 12 morning and evening values)

Exclude the first day measurements from the analyses; take advantage of these values as the reference parameter in the subsequent dose-titration phase

Dose-titration phase (titration of initial dose and adjustment therapy):

All measurements should be made under identical conditions and at the same times of the day and the initial values

HBPM data should be ascertained as trough values (i.e., before medication taken) in the morning and again at night

Use the average of BPs measured after 2–4 weeks to assess the effect of treatment

Long-term observation:

For stable normotensive (controlled) patients, patients should conduct HBPM a minimum of 1 week per quarter (an average of 12 morning and evening measurements under conditions described above)

Measurement should be made more frequently in patients with poor compliance.

Even after addressing lifestyle factors, contributing medications, and secondary causes of hypertension, patients often require multiple antihypertensive agents to control blood pressure. There is relatively little data addressing the efficacy of specific combinations of 3 or more drugs. In general, patients with resistant hypertension often have occult volume overload and diuretics may be particularly beneficial and are often underused. Aldosterone antagonists may provide significant antihypertensive benefit when added to other antihypertensive agents in patients with resistant hypertension. This effect may be due to lowering the elevated plasma aldosterone levels in these patients; however, the antihypertensive effect has also been seen in patients with normal aldosterone levels. In addition, spironolactone has anti-proteinuric effects. However, extreme caution must be used when treating patients with resistant hypertension with aldosterone antagonists. These patients are at increased risk for hyperkalemia especially if they also have CKD and/or are also taking an ACE inhibitor or ARB. Given the lack of strong data, combination regimens should be chosen based on prior benefit, adverse events, comorbidities, and financial limitations.

Box 5.6. Relevant Guidelines

1. KDIGO Clinical Practice Guidelines for the Management of Blood Pressure in Chronic Kidney Disease available at: http://kdigo.org/home/guidelines/blood-pressure-in-ckd/
2. ACC/AHA 2005 Practice Guidelines for Management of Patients with Peripheral Arterial Disease (Lower Extremity, Renal, Mesenteric, and Abdominal Aorta) available at: http://circ.ahajournals.org/content/113/11/e463.full.pdf

Before You Finish: Practice Pearls for the Busy Clinician

- There is a strong association between hypertension and ESRD; however, the cause and effect relationship remains debated especially with the recent discovery of specific genes associated with kidney disease.
- The gold standard for diagnosing renal artery stenosis is renal arteriography. However, less invasive screening tests such as duplex Doppler ultrasonography, CTA, or MRA are typically performed first.
- There are no definitive randomized controlled trial data to guide clinicians on specific antihypertensive medical therapies in patients with renal artery stenosis. Despite previous RCT, whether revascularization is beneficial remains unclear. The CORAL trial may provide more data regarding this topic.
- BP goals should be individualized.
- Evidence supports a goal blood pressure ≤140/90 mmHg for CKD patients without proteinuria defined as albuminuria <30 mg/24 h, regardless of diabetes status.
- Since proteinuria has been associated with worse kidney outcomes, stricter BP control is recommended with goal BP ≤130/80 mmHg in both diabetic and nondiabetic patients with albuminuria >30 mg/24 h.
- Home blood pressure and ambulatory blood pressure monitoring should be used to make an accurate diagnosis of resistant hypertension.
- Treatment of resistant hypertension is typically multifactorial and should focus on a detailed history including lifestyle factors and contributing medications, physical examination, and evaluation for secondary causes of hypertension.

References

1. Klag MJ, Whelton PK, Randall BL, Neaton JD, Brancati FL, Ford CE, et al. Blood pressure and end-stage renal disease in men. N Engl J Med. 1996;334(1):13–8.
2. Fogo A, Breyer JA, Smith MC, Cleveland WH, Agodoa L, Kirk KA, et al. Accuracy of the diagnosis of hypertensive nephrosclerosis in African Americans: a report from the African American Study of Kidney Disease (AASK) Trial. AASK Pilot Study Investigators. Kidney Int. 1997;51(1):244–52.
3. De NL, Gabbai FB, Agarwal R, Chiodini P, Borrelli S, Bellizzi V, et al. Prevalence and prognostic role of resistant hypertension in chronic kidney disease patients. J Am Coll Cardiol. 2013;61(24):2461–7.
4. Genovese G, Friedman DJ, Ross MD, Lecordier L, Uzureau P, Freedman BI, et al. Association of trypanolytic ApoL1 variants with kidney disease in African Americans. Science. 2010;329(5993):841–5.

5. Freedman BI, Langefeld CD. The new era of APOL1-associated glomerulosclerosis. Nephrol Dial Transplant. 2012;27(4):1288–91.
6. Hirsch AT, Haskal ZJ, Hertzer NR, Bakal CW, Creager MA, Halperin JL, et al. ACC/AHA 2005 practice guidelines for the management of patients with peripheral arterial disease (lower extremity, renal, mesenteric, and abdominal aortic): a collaborative report from the American Association for Vascular Surgery/Society for Vascular Surgery, Society for Cardiovascular Angiography and Interventions, Society for Vascular Medicine and Biology, Society of Interventional Radiology, and the ACC/AHA Task Force on Practice Guidelines (Writing Committee to Develop Guidelines for the Management of Patients With Peripheral Arterial Disease): endorsed by the American Association of Cardiovascular and Pulmonary Rehabilitation; National Heart, Lung, and Blood Institute; Society for Vascular Nursing; TransAtlantic Inter-Society Consensus; and Vascular Disease Foundation. Circulation. 2006;113(11):e463–654.
7. Pickering TG, Miller NH, Ogedegbe G, Krakoff LR, Artinian NT, Goff D. Call to action on use and reimbursement for home blood pressure monitoring: a joint scientific statement from the American Heart Association, American Society of Hypertension, and Preventive Cardiovascular Nurses Association. Hypertension. 2008;52(1):10–29.
8. Wheatley K, Ives N, Gray R, Kalra PA, Moss JG, Baigent C, et al. Revascularization versus medical therapy for renal-artery stenosis. N Engl J Med. 2009;361(20):1953–62.
9. Cooper CJ, Murphy TP, Matsumoto A, Steffes M, Cohen DJ, Jaff M, et al. Stent revascularization for the prevention of cardiovascular and renal events among patients with renal artery stenosis and systolic hypertension: rationale and design of the CORAL trial. Am Heart J. 2006;152(1):59–66.
10. Kidney Disease: Improving Global Outcomes (KDIGO) Blood Pressure Work Group. KDIGO clinical practice guideline for the management of blood pressure in chronic kidney disease. Kidney Int Suppl. 2013;2(5):337–414.
11. Jafar TH, Stark PC, Schmid CH, Landa M, Maschio G, de Jong PE, et al. Progression of chronic kidney disease: the role of blood pressure control, proteinuria, and angiotensin-converting enzyme inhibition: a patient-level meta-analysis. Ann Intern Med. 2003;139(4):244–52.
12. Klahr S, Levey AS, Beck GJ, Caggiula AW, Hunsicker L, Kusek JW, et al. The effects of dietary protein restriction and blood-pressure control on the progression of chronic renal disease. Modification of Diet in Renal Disease Study Group. N Engl J Med. 1994;330(13):877–84.
13. Wright Jr JT, Bakris G, Greene T, Agodoa LY, Appel LJ, Charleston J, et al. Effect of blood pressure lowering and antihypertensive drug class on progression of hypertensive kidney disease: results from the AASK trial. JAMA. 2002;288(19):2421–31.
14. Ruggenenti P, Perna A, Loriga G, Ganeva M, Ene-Iordache B, Turturro M, et al. Blood-pressure control for renoprotection in patients with non-diabetic chronic renal disease (REIN-2): multicentre, randomised controlled trial. Lancet. 2005;365(9463):939–46.
15. Jafar TH, Schmid CH, Landa M, Giatras I, Toto R, Remuzzi G, et al. Angiotensin-converting enzyme inhibitors and progression of nondiabetic renal disease. A meta-analysis of patient-level data. Ann Intern Med. 2001;135(2):73–87.
16. Parving HH, Brenner BM, McMurray JJ, de Zeeuw D, Haffner SM, Solomon SD, et al. Cardiorenal end points in a trial of aliskiren for type 2 diabetes. N Engl J Med. 2012;367(23):2204–13.
17. Fried LF, Duckworth W, Zhang JH, O'Connor T, Brophy M, Emanuele N, et al. Design of combination angiotensin receptor blocker and angiotensin-converting enzyme inhibitor for treatment of diabetic nephropathy (VA NEPHRON-D). Clin J Am Soc Nephrol. 2009;4(2):361–8.
18. Calhoun DA, Jones D, Textor S, Goff DC, Murphy TP, Toto RD, et al. Resistant hypertension: diagnosis, evaluation, and treatment. A scientific statement from the American Heart Association Professional Education Committee of the Council for High Blood Pressure Research. Hypertension. 2008;51(6):1403–19.
19. Agarwal R, Andersen MJ. Prognostic importance of ambulatory blood pressure recordings in patients with chronic kidney disease. Kidney Int. 2006;69(7):1175–80.

6 Dyslipidemia and Chronic Kidney Disease

Kosaku Nitta

Before You Start: Facts You Need to Know

- CKD is a common cause of CVD and is associated with substantial health and economic costs.
- Kidney dysfunction in CKD patients has been established as a risk factor for cardiovascular events that is independent of conventional cardiovascular risk factors.
- CKD results in profound dysregulation of several key enzymes and metabolic pathways that eventually contributes to disordered high-density lipoprotein (HDL) cholesterol and triglyceride-rich lipoprotein.
- The relationship between dyslipidemia and disease progression in patients with moderate to advanced CKD remains controversial.
- Dyslipidemia treatment is highly effective in preventing cardiovascular events in general population with increased cardiovascular risk. As CKD patients have a very high risk for cardiovascular events, dyslipidemia treatment in CKD patients is also justified.

6.1 Diagnostic Criteria of Dyslipidemia

The first step in the diagnostic procedure is to measure total cholesterol (TC), high-density lipoprotein cholesterol (HDL-C), and triglyceride (TG) levels after overnight fasting. Low-density lipoprotein cholesterol (LDL-C) level is then calculated by the use of the Friedewald equation (LDL-C = TC – HDL-C – TG/5). The LDL-C level may be measured by a homogeneous method especially in the case of postprandial examination or when the TG level is 400 mg/dL or higher.

On the basis of the relationship between serum TC level and mortality due to coronary artery disease (CAD) shown by the MRFIT [1], the National Cholesterol Education Program (NCEP), which is a guideline for lipid measurement in the United States, defines a TC level of 240 mg/dL, at which the relative risk of CAD doubles compared with that at 200 mg/dL, as a criterion of hypercholesterolemia [2].

Results of many epidemiological studies conducted in Western countries, including the Framingham study, have shown that the morbidity and mortality of CAD increase with elevations in serum LDL-C level. A serum LDL-C level of 140 mg/dL, which corresponds to this TC level, is a criterion for high-LDL cholesterolemia.

A significant negative correlation between the HDL-C level and the risk of CAD has been established in Western countries. However, there is no threshold HDL-C level for the relationship

K. Nitta, MD, PhD
Department of Medicine, Kidney Center,
Tokyo Women's Medical University,
8-1 Kawada—cho, Shinjuku-ku, Tokyo 162-8666, Japan
e-mail: knitta@kc.twmu.ac.jp

M. Arici (ed.), *Management of Chronic Kidney Disease*,
DOI 10.1007/978-3-642-54637-2_6, © Springer-Verlag Berlin Heidelberg 2014

Table 6.1 Diagnostic criteria for dyslipidemia (serum sampled after overnight fasting)

LDL cholesterol	≥140 mg/dL
HDL cholesterol	<40 mg/dL
Triglycerides	≥150 mg/dL

Diagnosis of dyslipidemia is made when either type of lipid abnormalities is present
These diagnostic criteria are not intended for the beginning of drug therapy
It is important to consider the indications of drug therapy only after evaluation of other risk factors
LDL-C is evaluated basically by calculation with the Friedewald equation
[LDL-C = TC − HDL-C − TG/5 (when TG is < 400 mg/dL)]
When the TG is ≥400 mg/dL or non-fasting state, the LDL-C should be determined by direct measurement

between serum HDL-C levels and the morbidity of CAD. The NCEP-ATPIII defines as an HDL-C level below 40 mg/dL as low HDL-C [3].

Although there have been a number of reports on the positive correlation between the TG level and morbidity of CAD in Western countries, the issue remains controversial. Particularly, disappearance of the association after correction for the HDL-C level has been reported in a number of studies. In the United States, a TG level of 150 mg/dL or higher is regarded as hypertriglyceridemia on the basis of the Framingham study [4].

The criteria for the diagnosis of dyslipidemia were defined with a greater emphasis on the prevention of CAD (Table 6.1).

6.2 Lipid Profiles in CKD

CKD is one of the major causes of dyslipidemia. Since CKD is diagnosed on the basis of the presence of proteinuria and/or reduced GFR, dyslipidemia secondary to CKD can be discussed separately in proteinuria-dominant CKD and reduced GFR-dominant CKD. The classification of lipoproteins is shown in Fig. 6.1 as a fraction of TC.

Nephrotic syndrome is a representative condition for dyslipidemia in patients without kidney dysfunction [5]. Hepatic production of very-low-density lipoprotein (VLDL) is increased in the nephrotic syndrome because of a nonspecific increase in protein secretion by the liver to compensate for the hypoalbuminemia caused by massive loss of serum proteins in the urine. VLDL is metabolized to LDL-C in a reaction catalyzed by lipoprotein lipase (LPL) in peripheral tissues (Fig. 6.2). Urinary loss of apoC-II, an activator of LPL, decreases LPL activity, and the decrease results in impaired catabolism of TG-rich lipoproteins to LDL-C. HDL-C has been reported to be unchanged or reduced in human nephrotic syndrome.

An increased serum TG level is one of the most common quantitative lipid abnormalities in CKD patients [6]. The serum concentrations of TG-rich lipoproteins such as VLDL start to increase in the early stages of CKD. In addition, CKD patients usually exhibit abnormal increases in serum TG levels after a fat meal. The predominant mechanism responsible for the increased concentration of TG-rich lipoproteins is a low catabolic rate. The reduced catabolic rate is likely attributable to diminished LPL activity as a consequence of the downregulation of the gene that encodes the enzyme and the presence of LPL inhibitors. Apolipoprotein C-III is a potent inhibitor of LPL, whereas apolipoprotein C-II is an activator of LPL. A decrease in apolipoprotein C-II/C-III ratio due to a disproportionate increase in plasma apolipoprotein C-III is a possible cause of LPL inactivation in CKD. Also, it is well known that CKD causes insulin resistance, which results in promotion of hepatic VLDL production, suggesting that the insulin-resistance-driven overproduction of VLDL significantly may contribute to the development of hypertriglyceridemia in CKD patients.

The plasma TC level of CKD patients is usually normal or reduced. The degree of proteinuria besides deterioration in kidney function is another significant factor that determines the levels of plasma cholesterol-rich lipoproteins. LDL-receptor-mediated cholesterol uptake plays an important role in cholesterol homeostasis. CKD in the absence of heavy proteinuria does not significantly affect gene expression either of hydroxyl-3-methylglutaryl-CoA reductase (HMG-CoA reductase), which is the rate-limiting enzyme in cholesterol biosynthesis, or of cholesterol 7α-hydroxylase, which is the rate-limiting enzyme in cholesterol catabolism and conversion

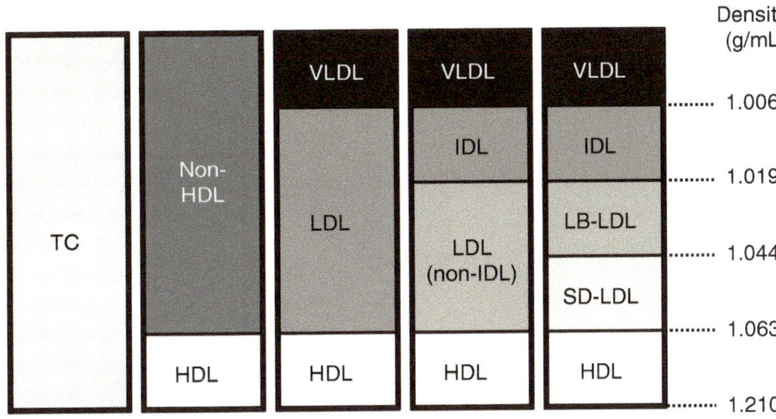

Fig. 6.1 Fraction of serum total cholesterol

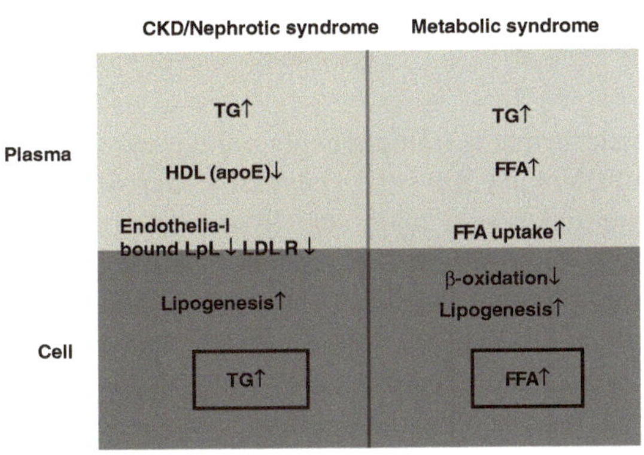

Fig. 6.2 Mechanisms of hypertriglyceridemia and intracellular lipid accumulation in chronic kidney disease (*CKD*)/nephrotic syndrome and metabolic syndrome. *TG* triglyceride, *HDL* high-density lipoprotein, *LpL* lipoprotein lipase, *LDL R* low-density lipoprotein receptor, *FFA* free fatty acid

to bile acids, nor does CKD in the absence of heavy proteinuria or significant glomerulosclerosis alter hepatic LDL receptor gene expression in nephrectomized rats. CKD patients exhibit major qualitative alterations in LDL metabolism. The proportion of small dense LDL particles, which are considered highly atherogenic, is increased in CKD [7]. Small dense LDL is a subtype of LDL that has a high propensity to penetrate the vessel wall, where it becomes oxidized and triggers the atherosclerotic process (Fig. 6.3).

The main function of HDL-C is to transport surplus cholesterol from the arterial wall to the liver for excretion. This process, which is commonly called 'reverse cholesterol transport', is critical for cellular cholesterol homeostasis and protection against atherosclerosis. HDL-C also acts as a potent endogenous inhibitor of inflammation, platelet adhesion, and LDL oxidation, because of a number of HDL-C associated apolipoproteins and lecithin-cholesterol acyltransferase (LCAT) [8]. Several epidemiological studies have demonstrated that HDL-C is a negative risk factor for atherosclerosis. CKD patients have generally lower plasma HDL-C levels than individuals with normal kidney function [9], and as a result patients with impaired kidney function usually have low levels of apolipoproteins AI and AII, the main protein constituents of HDL-C, diminished LCAT activity, and increased cholesteryl ester transfer protein (CETP) activity, which facilitates the transfer of cholesterol esters from HDL to TG-rich lipoproteins and thereby reduces the serum HDL-C concentrations. In addition to their reduced efficiency as cholesterol acceptors, HDL particles from individuals with impaired kidney function have less effective anti-oxidative and anti-inflammatory functions. Moreover, oxidized HDL may be associated with protein-energy wasting in dialysis patients.

6.3 Dyslipidemia as a Risk Factor for CVD in CKD

It is well known that dyslipidemia represents an important risk factor for the development of CVD in the general population. Indeed, large-scale epidemiological studies have revealed a linear relationship between serum total and

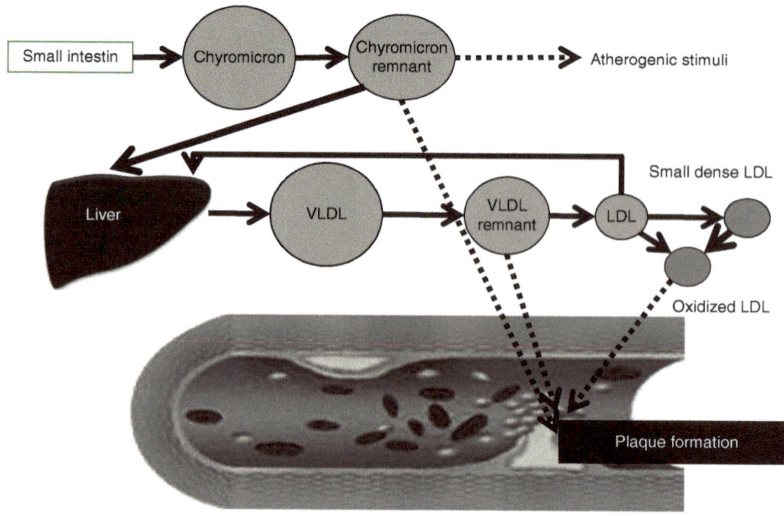

Fig. 6.3 Lipoprotein metabolism and atherogenic process

LDL-C values and the incidence of ischemic events in both primary and secondary prevention individuals, whereas lowering the concentration of their LDL-C values by diet, drug therapy, or surgery is followed by an impressive reduction in future cardiovascular risk [10]. On the other hand, the role of dyslipidemia in the pathophysiology of atherosclerotic disease in patients with impaired kidney function remains a matter of controversy.

A low serum total cholesterol level is known to predict a higher risk of all-cause mortality in dialysis patients. Since hypercholesterolemia is an established risk factor for CVD in the general population, this strange relationship between the risk of death and the risk factor for CVD is called "reverse epidemiology" [11]. Importantly, the endpoints are not incident CVD, but death from CVD or death from any cause. In addition, no adjustment is performed for possible confounders, such as advanced age, nutritional status, and inflammation. Since death from CVD occurred only when a subject experienced incident CVD and died, the risk factors for death from CVD may be different from the risk factors for incident CVD.

The risk of death from CVD is increased in CKD patients, particularly in CKD patients with end-stage renal disease (ESRD). Sarnak et al. listed candidate traditional and nontraditional risk factors that might explain the increased risk of CVD in CKD [12]. The traditional risk factors are older age, male sex, hypertension, higher LDL-C, lower HDL-C, diabetes mellitus, smoking, physical inactivity, menopause, family history of CVD, and left ventricular hypertrophy. They also proposed the following nontraditional risk factors: albuminuria, homocysteine, lipoprotein (a), apolipoprotein (a) isoforms, lipoprotein remnants, anemia, abnormal calcium/phosphate metabolism, extracellular fluid overload, electrolyte imbalance, oxidative stress, inflammation, malnutrition, thrombogenic factors, sleep disturbances, and altered nitric oxide/endothelin balance.

6.4 Dyslipidemia and Progression of CKD

Dyslipidemia may accelerate the progression of established CKD by several mechanisms. Reabsorption of the fatty acids and phospholipids contained in the filtered proteins by tubular epithelial cells stimulates tubulointerstitial inflammation, foam cell formation, and tissue injury. The existence of a link between dyslipidemia and oxidative stress in the pathogenesis of CKD was demonstrated, because dyslipidemia increased glomerular and tubulointerstitial infiltration and aggravated glomerulosclerosis. Accumulation of lipoproteins in glomerular mesangial cells promotes matrix production and glomerulosclerosis with the native and oxidized lipoproteins, particularly LDL-C, which stimulate production of extracellular matrix proteins by cultured mesangial cells and promote generation of proinflammatory cytokines, which can lead to recruitment and activation of circulating and resident macrophages [12].

A secondary analysis of the Modification of Diet in Renal Disease (MDRD) study demonstrated that low serum HDL-C and TG-rich lipoprotein levels were correlated with the progression of CKD [13]. Although the results of experimental studies have tended to support the hypothesis that dyslipidemia accelerates the progression of CKD, the results of clinical studies have been inconsistent.

Statins have been found to be effective in inhibiting the progression of kidney damage in experimental models, mainly through their pleiotropic effects. Possible pathways for the renoprotective action of statins, other than any hypocholesterolemic effect, are cellular apoptosis/proliferation balance, inflammatory cytokine production, and signal transduction regulation [14].

Lipid-lowering therapies may decrease proteinuria and increase or maintain kidney function. Lipid-lowering therapy with statins has been reported to decrease proteinuria and podocyturia in controlled clinical trials. Statin therapy has been found to be associated with increased GFR in comparison with a placebo in post hoc analyses of primary prevention [15] and secondary prevention trials with statins [16], and a meta-analysis showed that statin therapy was associated with decreased albuminuria in comparison with a placebo [17].

6.5 Categorization and Goals of Dyslipidemia

Most recent ACC/AHA Guideline on the Treatment of Blood Cholesterol recommends treating blood cholesterol to reduce atherosclerotic cardiovascular disease risk [18]. This guideline does not make any recommendation for threshold or target cholesterol levels but proposes four major statin benefit groups from whom the atherosclerotic cardiovascular disease (ASCVD) risk reduction clearly outweighs the risk of adverse events. According to this guideline, individuals with (1) clinical atherosclerotic vascular disease (acute coronary syndromes or a history of MI, stable or unstable angina, coronary or other arterial revascularization, stroke, TIA, or peripheral arterial disease presumed to be of atherosclerotic origin), (2) primary elevations of LDL-C ≥190 mg/dL, (3) diabetes aged 40–75 years with LDL– C 70–189 mg/dL and without clinical ASCVD, or (4) without clinical ASCVD or diabetes with LDL–C 70–189 mg/dL and estimated 10-year ASCVD risk >7.5 % should receive statin treatment (Fig. 6.4). The guideline recommends that for the primary prevention of ASCVD in individuals without clinical ASCVD and LDL–C 70–189 mg/dL, the estimated absolute 10-year risk of ASCVD (defined as nonfatal MI, CHD death, nonfatal and fatal stroke) should be used to guide the initiation of statin therapy. The 10-year ASCVD risk should be estimated using the Pooled Cohort Equations (a downloadable spreadsheet enabling estimation of 10-year and lifetime risk for ASCVD and a web-based calculator are available at http://my.americanheart.org/cvriskcalculator and http://www.cardiosource.org/science-and-quality/practice-guidelines-and-quality-standards/2013-prevention-guideline-tools.aspx). This guideline adopts a high-intensity and moderate-intensity statin therapy for use in secondary and primary prevention rather than "a treat-to-cholesterol target" or "lower cholesterol is better" strategy [18].

6.6 Lipid-Lowering Therapy and CVD in CKD

The Work Group for Kidney Disease Outcomes Quality Initiative (K/DOQI) proposed the adoption of Adult Treatment Panel (ATP) III LDL-C targets for individuals with ESRD and recommended aggressive treatment of lipid disorders [3, 19]. However, recent studies have indicated that the lipid-lowering therapy in individuals

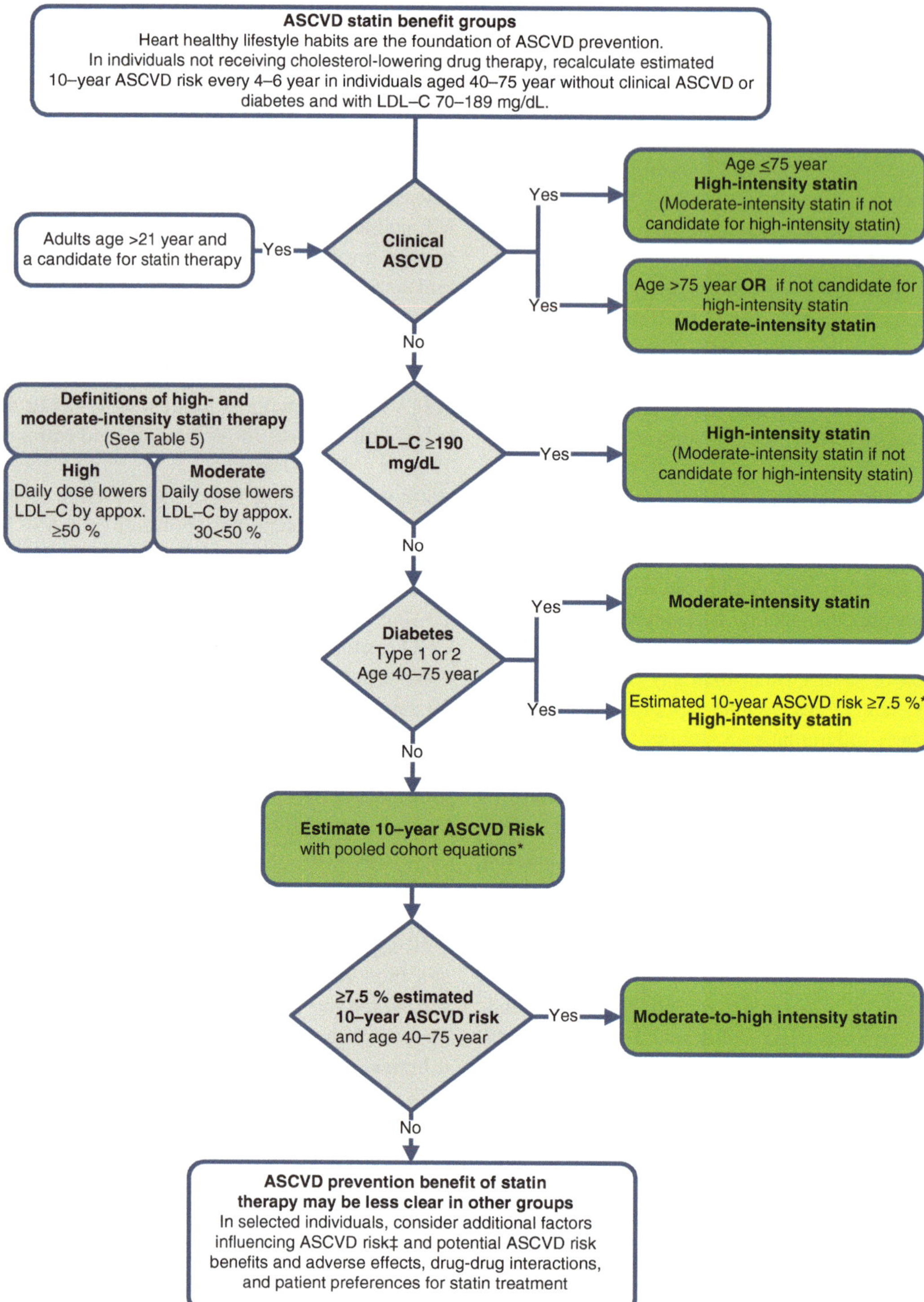

Fig. 6.4 Major recommendations for statin therapy for ASCVD prevention (Reprinted with permission from Stone et al. [18])

with impaired kidney function is limited but that the therapeutic targets are achieved in a small minority of patients with impaired kidney function who are treated with hypolipidemic drugs. The most important factor limiting the use of hypolipidemic drugs for CKD patients may be the contradictory results of the studies that tried to delineate the effects of statins on total and cardiovascular mortality in CKD patients. It is well known that statins are by far the most commonly prescribed hypolipidemic drugs in the general population, and numerous large, randomized, prospective studies have shown that their use is accompanied by an impressive reduction in the incidence of cardiovascular events [20]. The second United Kingdom Heart and Renal Protection (UK-HARP-II) Study is a randomized controlled trial in terms of the biochemical safety and efficacy of adding ezetimibe to simvastatin as initial therapy in CKD patients [21]. This 6-month study shows that the addition of ezetimibe 10 mg/day to simvastatin 20 mg/day produced an additional 21 % decrease in LDL-C levels.

On the other hand, the beneficial effect of statin therapy on cardiovascular morbidity and mortality in CKD patients seems to be related to the severity of the kidney dysfunction (Table 6.2). Indeed, post hoc analyses of subgroups of patients with mild to moderate CKD (stages 1–3) in several large, prospective, placebo-controlled trials of statin have revealed a significant reduction in cardiovascular morbidity and mortality independently of the baseline lipid values or the presence or the absence of diabetes mellitus and coronary artery disease. Similar results were obtained in a study of prespecified subgroups of patients with impaired kidney function in the ASCOT-LLA study [22] treated with simvastatin and atorvastatin, respectively. A recently published meta-analysis of 26 studies (about 25,000 participants) revealed that statin treatment of predialysis CKD patients was associated with a significant reduction in all-cause and cardiovascular mortality by approximately 20 % [23]. Interestingly, the rate of adverse events was similar in the group treated with statins and the placebo group. These findings suggest that the use of statin to prevent ischemic events in patients with early CKD who have dyslipidemia is a safe, valid, and evidence-based approach. The recently released KDIGO clinical practice guideline for lipid management in CKD therefore recommended treatment with a statin or statin/ezetimibe combination in CKD patients aged ≥50 years with eGFR categories G3a to G5 but not on dialysis. KDIGO guideline also adopted a "fire-and-forgot" strategy in cholesterol treatment and did not recommend either a target level or regular follow-up measurements (Box 6.1) (Table 6.3) [24].

Although epidemiological studies have shown that statin therapy for maintenance hemodialysis patients is accompanied by a reduction in cardiovascular mortality, the prospective, randomized trials that tested statins for a beneficial effect in

Box 6.1. What the Guidelines Say You Should Do: Pharmacological Cholesterol-Lowering Treatment in Adults

- In adults ≥50 years with eGFR <60 mL/min/1.73 m^2 but not treated with chronic dialysis or kidney transplantation (GFR categories G3a–G5), we recommend treatment with a statin or statin/ezetimibe combination (1A).
- In adults aged <50 years with CKD and eGFR <60 mL/min/1.73 m^2 (GFR categories G1–G2), we recommend treatment with a statin (1B).
- In adults aged 18–49 years with CKD but not treated with chronic dialysis or kidney transplantation, we suggest statin treatment in people with one or more of the following (2A):
  - Known coronary disease (myocardial infarction or coronary revascularization)
  - Diabetes mellitus
  - Prior ischemic stroke
  - Estimated 10-year incidence of coronary death or nonfatal myocardial infarction >10 %

Source: Kidney Disease: Improving Global Outcomes (KDIGO) Lipid Work Group [25]

Table 6.2 Major lipid trials targeting individuals with CKD

Study	Intervention (vs placebo)	Population	Median follow-up (years)	Primary study outcome			All-cause mortality	
				Definition	Events (%)	Risk	Events (%)	Risk
4D	Atorvastatin, 20 mg, daily	1,255 participants aged 18–80 years with type 2 diabetes treated with HD for <2 years; LDL-C, 80–190 mg/dL	4.0	Composite of death from cardiac causes, fatal stroke, nonfatal MI, or nonfatal stroke	36.5 vs 38.2	HR, 0.92 (0.77–1.10)	48.0 vs 50.3	RR, 0.93 (0.79–1.08)
AURORA	Rosuvastatin, 10 mg, daily	2,776 participants aged 50–80 years treated with HD or hemofiltration for >3 months	3.8	Composite of death from cardiovascular causes, nonfatal MI, or nonfatal stroke	28.5 vs 29.5	HR, 0.96 (0.84–1.11)	45.8 vs 47.7	HR, 0.96 (0.86–1.07)
ALERT	Fluvastatin, 40 mg, daily with dose increase permitted	2,102 participants aged 30–75 years, at least 6 months from kidney transplant, with stable transplant function and no recent MI; total cholesterol, 155–348 mg/dL	5.4	Major adverse cardiac event, defined as cardiac death, nonfatal MI, or coronary revascularization procedure	10.7 vs 12.7	RR, 0.83 (0.64–1.06)	13.6 vs 13.1	RR, 1.02 (0.81–1.30)
SHARP	Simvastatin, 20 mg, daily + ezetimibe, 10 mg, daily	9,270 participants aged ≥40 years with no prior MI or coronary revascularization and creatinine ≥1.7 mg/dL (men) or ≥1.5 mg/dL (women)	4.9	Composite of coronary death, nonfatal MI, ischemic stroke, or any revascularization procedure	11.3 vs 13.4	RR, 0.83 (0.74–0.94)	24.6 vs 24.1	RR, 1.02 (0.94–1.11)
SHARP subgroups								
Nondialysis	As above	6,247 participants	NR	As above	9.5 vs 11.9	RR, 0.78 (0.67–0.91)	NR	NR
HD		2,527 participants			15.2 vs 15.9	RR, 0.95 (0.78–1.15)		
Peritoneal dialysis		496 participants			14.0 vs 19.7	RR, 0.70 (0.46–1.08)		

Abbreviations: *4D* Deutsche Diabetes Dialyse Studie, *ALERT* Assessment of Lescol in Renal Transplantation, *AURORA* A Study to Evaluate the Use of Rosuvastatin in Subjects on Regular Hemodialysis: An Assessment of Survival and Cardiovascular Events, *CHD* coronary heart disease, *CKD* chronic kidney disease, *HD* hemodialysis, *HR* hazard ratio, *LDL-C* low-density lipoprotein cholesterol, *MI* myocardial infarction, *NR* not reported, *RR* risk ratio, *SHARP* Study of Heart and Renal Protection

Table 6.3 Recommended doses (mg/day) of statins in adults with CKD

Statin	eGFR G1–G2	eGFR G3a–G5, including patients on dialysis or with a kidney transplant
Lovastatin	GP	nd
Fluvastatin	GP	80
Atorvastatin	GP	20
Rosuvastatin	GP	10
Simvastatin/Ezetimibe	GP	20/10
Pravastatin	GP	40
Simvastatin	GP	40
Pitavastatin	GP	2

Source: Reprinted by permission from Macmillan Publishers Ltd: from Kidney Disease: Improving Global Outcomes (KDIGO) Lipid Work Group [24], copyright 2013

GP general population, *nd* not done or not studied

this patient population yielded disappointing results. The 4D (Die Deutsche Diabetes Dialyse) trial enrolled 1,255 diabetics who had been on maintenance HD for 4 years, and it randomized them to receive either placebo or 20 mg/day of atorvastatin [25]. After a mean follow-up period of 2.4 years, atorvastatin had not significantly reduced the risk of the composite primary endpoint (cardiovascular death, nonfatal myocardial infarction, and stroke), despite a significant 42 % reduction in serum LDL-C concentration [26].

The results of the AURORA (A Study to Evaluate the Use of Rosuvastatin in Subjects on Regular Hemodialysis: An Assessment of Survival and Cardiovascular Events) study [27] led to the concept of "a point of no return," i.e., a point in the deterioration of kidney function beyond which the beneficial effect of statins on cardiovascular morbidity and mortality is offset by the uremic environment. The AURORA study was a prospective, double-blind trial conducted on 2,775 maintenance hemodialysis patients that randomized them to receive 10 mg of rosuvastatin per day or placebo. After a median follow-up period of 3.8 years, despite impressive reductions in serum LDL-C and CRP concentrations (by 43 and 11.5 %, respectively), rosuvastatin administration had no effect on the primary composite endpoint (nonfatal myocardial infarction, nonfatal stroke, and cardiovascular death) or the individual components of the primary endpoint. Nor was there any significant effect on all-cause mortality, and none of the prespecified secondary outcomes was influenced by active treatment.

SHARP (Study of Heart and Renal Protection) is a randomized double-blind trial enrolling 9,270 participants 40 years of age or older with two or more serum creatinine measurements of at least 1.7 mg/dl for men or 1.5 mg/dl for women and without a prior history of myocardial infarction or coronary revascularization [28]. Participants were assigned to receive simvastatin 20 mg/day plus ezetimibe 10 mg/day daily versus placebo and were followed up for a median of 4.9 years. The primary outcome was a composite of major atherosclerotic events, defined as nonfatal myocardial infarction, coronary death, nonhemorrhagic stroke, or arterial revascularization. Major atherosclerotic events occurred in 11.3 % of participants in the intervention group compared with 13.4 % of participants in the placebo group, corresponding to a 17 % lower rate of events in the intervention group. However, unlike many general population studies, SHARP did not show a benefit of LDL-C lowering for total mortality or coronary deaths, suggesting that many deaths in patients with advanced CKD are from nonatherosclerotic causes, which LDL-C-lowering therapy is unlikely to affect. Nakamura et al. reported that coadministration of ezetimibe enhanced proteinuria-lowering effects of pitavastatin in chronic kidney disease patients partly via a cholesterol-independent manner [29]. Recent KDIGO guidelines do not suggest initiation of statins or statin/ezetimibe combination in patients with dialysis-dependent CKD [24].

Fibrates can reduce triglycerides by 20–50 % and increase HDL cholesterol by 10–35 %. Their effect on LDL cholesterol is variable, yet fibrates can increase the size of LDL particles. The current evidence is insufficient to determine the effect of fibrates on cardiovascular and clinical kidney outcome prevention in CKD patients. The Veterans Affairs Cooperative HDL Cholesterol Intervention Trial (VA-HIT) reported results for only a composite vascular outcome in a small subgroup of participants with diabetes and CKD [30]. In patients with diabetes and albuminuria, fenofibrate treatment increased regression from micro- to normoalbuminuria and from macro- to microalbuminuria compared to placebo. Action to Control Cardiovascular Risk in Diabetes (ACCORD) was designed to address the effect of add-on therapy of fenofibrate to simvastatin in type 2 diabetes patients. However, the combination of fenofibrate and simvastatin did not reduce the rate of fatal cardiovascular events, nonfatal myocardial infarction, or nonfatal stroke, as compared with simvastatin alone [31]. KDIGO clinical practice guideline for lipid management in CKD recommends only lifestyle changes in patients with CKD and hypertriglyceridemia (Boxes 6.2 and 6.3) [24].

Box 6.2. What the Guidelines Say You Should Do: Triglyceride-Lowering Treatment in Adults

- In adults with CKD (including those treated with chronic dialysis or kidney transplantation) and hypertriglyceridemia, we suggest that therapeutic lifestyle changes be advised (2D).

Source: Kidney Disease: Improving Global Outcomes (KDIGO) Lipid Work Group [25]

Box 6.3. Relevant Guidelines

1. *KDIGO Guideline*

   Kidney Disease: Improving Global Outcomes (KDIGO) Lipid Work Group. KDIGO clinical practice guideline for lipid management in chronic kidney disease. Kidney Int Suppl. 2013;3: 259–305.

   http://kdigo.org/home/guidelines/lipids/
2. *ACC/AHA Joint Guidelines*

   2013 ACC/AHA Guideline on the Treatment of Blood Cholesterol to Reduce Atherosclerotic Cardiovascular Risk in Adults http://my.americanheart.org/professional/StatementsGuidelines/ByTopic/TopicsA-C/ACCAHA-Joint-Guidelines_UCM_321694_Article.jsp
3. *NKF KDOQI Guideline*

   KDOQI Clinical Practice Guidelines for Managing Dyslipidemias in Chronic Kidney Disease

   http://www.kidney.org/professionals/kdoqi/guidelines_commentaries.cfm

Before You Finish: Practice Pearls for the Clinician

- CKD patients often have risk factors for death from CVD, including both traditional and nontraditional risk factors.
- One of the traditional risk factors, dyslipidemia, is modifiable. Abnormalities of lipoprotein metabolism are evident even in the early stages of CKD, and they usually follow a downhill course that parallels the deterioration in renal function.
- TG-rich lipoproteins are increased in CKD patients, particularly in advanced stages, the serum non-HDL-C may be a better biomarker for dyslipidemia than the serum LDL-C in this population.
- Lipid-lowering therapy with statins is effective in reducing the risk of CVD in the early stages of CKD, but the benefit of statin therapy may be limited in ESRD patients.

References

1. MRFIT Research Group, personal communication, 1989, as reported in National Cholesterol Education Program. Report of the expert panel on population strategies for blood cholesterol reduction. Circulation. 1991;83:2154–232.
2. National Cholesterol Education Program: second report of the expert panel detection, evaluation, and treatment of high blood cholesterol in adults (Adult Treatment Panel II). Circulation. 1994;89:1333–445.
3. Expert Panel on Detection, Evaluation, and Treatment of High Blood Cholesterol in Adults. Executive Summary of the Third Report of the National Cholesterol Education Program (NCEP) Expert Panel on Detection, Evaluation, and Treatment of High Blood Cholesterol in Adults (Adult Treatment Panel III). JAMA. 2001;285:2486–97.

4. Castelli WP. Lipids, risk factors and ischaemic heart disease. Atherosclerosis. 1996;124(Suppl):S1–9.
5. Kronenberg F. Dyslipidemia and nephrotic syndrome: recent advances. J Ren Nutr. 2005;15:195–203.
6. Wanner C, Quaschning T. Dyslipidemia and renal disease: pathogenesis and clinical consequences. Curr Opin Nephrol Hypertens. 2001;10:195–201.
7. Deighan CJ, Caslake MJ, McConnell M, Boulton-Jones JM, Packard CJ. Atherogenic lipoprotein phenotype in end-stage renal failure: origin and extent of small dense low-density lipoprotein formation. Am J Kidney Dis. 2000;35:852–62.
8. Kontush A, Chapman MJ. Antiatherogenic small, dense HDL-guardian angel of the arterial wall? Nat Clin Pract Cardiovasc Med. 2006;3:144–53.
9. Attman PO, Samuelsson O. Dyslipidemia of kidney disease. Curr Opin Lipidol. 2009;20:293–9.
10. Lewington S, Whitlock G, Clarke R, Sherliker P, Emberson J, Halsey J, et al. Blood cholesterol and vascular mortality by age, sex, and blood pressure: a meta-analysis of individual data from 61 prospective studies with 55,000 vascular deaths. Lancet. 2007;370:1829–39.
11. Kalantar-Zadeh K, Block G, Humphreys MH, Kopple JD. Reverse epidemiology of cardiovascular risk factors in maintenance dialysis patients. Kidney Int. 2003;63:793–808.
12. Sarnak MJ, Levey AS, Schoolwerth AC, Coresh J, Culleton B, Hamm LL, et al. Kidney disease as a risk factor for development of cardiovascular disease: a statement from the American Heart Association Councils on Kidney in Cardiovascular Disease, High Blood Pressure Research, Clinical Cardiology, and Epidemiology and Prevention. Circulation. 2003;108: 2154–69.
13. Vaziri ND. Dyslipidemia of chronic renal failure: the nature, mechanisms, and potential consequences. Am J Physiol Renal Physiol. 2006;290:F262–72.
14. Muntner P, Coresh J, Smith JC, Eckfeldt J, Klag MJ. Plasma lipids and risk of developing renal dysfunction: the atherosclerosis risk in communities study. Kidney Int. 2000;58:293–301.
15. Buemi M, Senatore M, Corica F, Aloisi C, Romeo A, Cavallaro E, et al. Statins and progressive renal disease. Med Res Rev. 2002;22:76–84.
16. Colhoun HM, Betteridge DJ, Durrington PN, Hitman GA, Neil HA, Livingstone SJ, et al. Effects of atorvastatin on kidney outcomes and cardiovascular disease in patients with diabetes: an analysis from the Collaborative Atorvastatin Diabetes study (CARDS). Am J Kidney Dis. 2009;54:810–9.
17. Athyros VG, Mikhailidis DP, Papageorgiou AA, Symeonidis AN, Pehlivanidis AN, Bouloukos VI, et al. The effect of statins versus untreated dyslipidemia on renal function in patients with coronary heart disease. A subgroup analysis of the Greek atorvastatin and coronary heart disease evaluation (GREACE) study. J Clin Pathol. 2004;57:728–34.
18. Stone NJ, Robinson J, Lichtenstein AH, Bairey Merz CN, Lloyd-Jones DM, Blum CB, et al. 2013 ACC/AHA guideline on the treatment of blood cholesterol to reduce atherosclerotic cardiovascular risk in adults: a report of the American College of Cardiology/American Heart Association Task Force on Practice Guidelines. J Am Coll Cardiol. 2013. doi:10.1016/j.jacc.2013.11.002. pii: S0735-1097(13)06028-2.
19. Kidney Disease Outcomes Quality Initiative (K/DOQI) Group. K/DOQI clinical practice guidelines for management of dyslipidemias in patients with kidney disease. Am J Kidney Dis. 2003;41:1–91.
20. Baigent C, Keech A, Kearney PM, Blackwell L, Buck G, Pollicino C, et al. Efficacy and safety of cholesterol-lowering treatment: prospective meta-analysis of data from 90, 056 participants in 14 randomised trials of statins. Lancet. 2005;366:1267–78.
21. Landray M, Baigent C, Leaper C, Adu D, Altmann P, Armitage J, et al. The second United Kingdom Heart and Renal Protection (UK-HARP-II) Study: a randomized controlled study of the biochemical safety and efficacy of adding ezetimibe to simvastatin as initial therapy among patients with CKD. Am J Kidney Dis. 2006;47:385–95.
22. Sever PS, Dahlof B, Poulter NR, Wedel H, Beevers G, Caulfield M, et al. Prevention of coronary and stroke events with atorvastatin in hypertensive patients who have average or lower-than-average cholesterol concentrations, in the Anglo-Scandinavian Cardiac Outcomes Trial – Lipid Lowering Arm (ASCOT-LLA): a multicentre randomised controlled trial. Lancet. 2003;361:1149–58.
23. Navaneethan SD, Pansini F, Perkovic V, Manno C, Pellegrini F, Johnson DW, et al. HMG CoA reductase inhibitors (statins) for people with chronic kidney disease not requiring dialysis. Cochrane Database Syst Rev. 2009;(2) CD007784.
24. Kidney Disease: Improving Global Outcomes (KDIGO) Lipid Work Group. KDIGO Clinical Practice Guideline for Lipid Management in Chronic Kidney Disease. Kidney Int. 2013;3(Suppl):259–305.
25. Wanner C, Krane V, Marz W, Olschewski M, Asmus HG, Kramer W, et al. Randomized controlled trial on the efficacy and safety of atorvastatin in patients with type 2 diabetes on hemodialysis (4D study): demographic and baseline characteristics. Kidney Blood Press Res. 2004;27:259–66.
26. Wanner C, Krane V, Marz W, Olschewski M, Mann JF, Ruf G, et al. Atorvastatin in patients with type 2 diabetes mellitus undergoing hemodialysis. N Engl J Med. 2005;353:238–48.
27. Fellstrom BC, Jardine AG, Schmieder RE, Holdaas H, Bannister K, Beutler J, et al. Rosuvastatin and cardiovascular events in patients undergoing hemodialysis. N Engl J Med. 2009;360:1395–407.
28. Baigent C, Landray MJ, Reith C, Emberson J, Wheeler DC, Tomson C, et al. The effects of lowering LDL cholesterol with simvastatin plus ezetimibe in patients with chronic kidney disease (Study of Heart and Renal Protection): a randomized placebo-controlled trial. Lancet. 2011;377:2181–92.
29. Nakamura T, Sato E, Fujiwara N, Kawagoe Y, Ueda Y, Suzuki T, et al. Co-administration of ezetimibe enhances proteinuria-lowering effects of pitavastatin in chronic kidney disease patients partly via a cholesterol-independent manner. Pharmacol Res. 2010;61:58–61.

30. Tonelli M, Collins D, Robins S, Bloomfield H, Curhan GC. Gemfibrozil for secondary prevention of cardiovascular events in mild to moderate chronic renal insufficiency. Kidney Int. 2004;66:1123–30.
31. Ginsberg HN, Elam MB, Lovato LC, Crouse 3rd JR, Leiter LA, Linz P, et al. Effects of combination lipid therapy in type 2 diabetes mellitus. N Engl J Med. 2010;362:1563–74.

7 Metabolic Acidosis and Chronic Kidney Disease

Richard M. Treger and Jeffrey A. Kraut

Before You Start: Facts You Need to Know

- A reduction in bicarbonate and blood pH (metabolic acidosis) is a common but not inevitable occurrence with CKD.
- Metabolic acidosis usually occurs when the estimated glomerular filtration rate (eGFR) falls below 25–30 mL/min but can occur earlier with certain disorders which affect renal function such as hyporeninemic hypoaldosteronism.
- Major adverse effects of untreated metabolic acidosis include muscle wasting, bone disease, progression of CKD, and increased mortality.
- Acid-base parameters including pH, PCO_2, and serum $[HCO_3^-]$ should be checked upon first evaluation, and then serum bicarbonate should be checked at least annually in stage 3 CKD and approximately every 3 months in stages 4 and 5 CKD.
- Treatment of metabolic acidosis with base leads to slowing of progression of CKD, decreased muscle wasting, and improvement in bone disease.
- Recommendations are to initiate base treatment with serum bicarbonate ≤22 mEq/L, although the precise bicarbonate range to be targeted remains under study.

R.M. Treger, MD
Division of Nephrology, Department of Internal Medicine, VA Greater Los Angeles Healthcare System, 11301 Wilshire Blvd, Los Angeles, CA 90073, USA

David Geffen School of Medicine, UCLA, Los Angeles, CA USA
e-mail: richard.treger@va.gov

J.A. Kraut, MD (✉)
Division of Nephrology, VHAGLA Healthcare System, 11301 Wilshire Boulevard, Los Angeles, CA 90073, USA

UCLA Membrane Biology Laboratory, David Geffen UCLA School of Medicine, Los Angeles, CA, USA
e-mail: jkraut@ucla.edu

7.1 Introduction

A decrease in serum bicarbonate in association with a reduction in blood pH (metabolic acidosis) is a frequent although not inevitable occurrence in progressive chronic kidney disease (CKD) [1]. The hypobicarbonatemia usually develops when glomerular filtration rate (GFR) falls below 25–30 mL/min. It is usually mild in degree with serum bicarbonate ranging from 15 to 23 mmol/L [1]. However, despite being mild, it can be associated with several adverse effects including muscle wasting, bone disease, progression of CKD, and increased mortality [2]. Although traditionally it has been considered to be a high anion gap metabolic acidosis, it can present as a

M. Arici (ed.), *Management of Chronic Kidney Disease*,
DOI 10.1007/978-3-642-54637-2_7, © Springer-Verlag Berlin Heidelberg 2014

nongap, mixed nongap and high anion gap, or high anion gap alone [3, 4]. CKD is the most common cause of chronic metabolic acidosis; therefore, the clinician must know how to recognize this disorder and distinguish it from other causes of metabolic acidosis. This chapter reviews the genesis of the acidosis of CKD, the impact of this acid-base disorder on cellular function, and the present recommendations for its evaluation and treatment.

7.2 Pathophysiology

The serum bicarbonate is normally maintained between 23 and 29 mEq/L (mean, 24 mmol/L) and blood pH between 7.38 and 7.42 (mean, 7.40). As shown in Fig. 7.1, in adults approximately 1 mEq/kg body weight of fixed acid is generated from the combined effects of the metabolism of ingested food stuffs and the absorption of organic anions from the gastrointestinal tract. The kidney must generate equivalent quantities of base to neutralize this endogenous acid load and also reabsorb the large quantity of bicarbonate filtered by the glomerulus (~4,500 mEq/day) to maintain acid-base balance. Excretion of the acid load by the kidneys occurs via urinary excretion of hydrogen ions, both in the form of titratable acid ($H_2PO_4^-$) (approximately 1/3 of the acid load) and as ammonium (approximately 2/3 of the acid load). However, an increase in urinary ammonium excretion (NH_4) accounts for the vast majority of the increased renal acid excretion observed in response to an acid load.

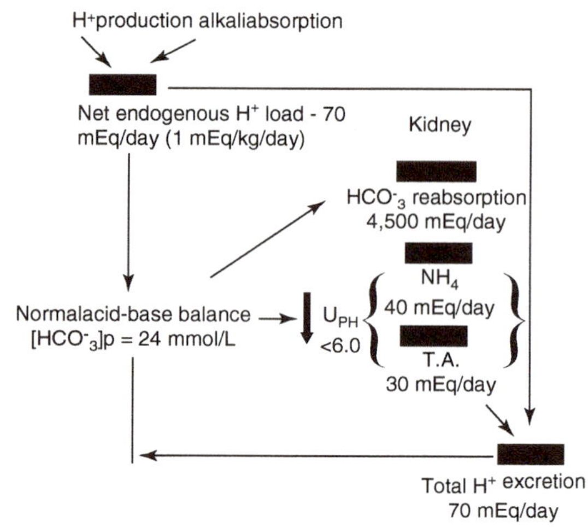

Fig. 7.1 Normal acid-base balance in health. Ingestion of foodstuffs and absorption of base lead to the net production of approximately 1 mEq/kg/day of hydrogen ions in adults. The kidney generates an equivalent quantity of base and also reabsorbs approximately 4,500 mEq of filtered bicarbonate each day to maintain serum bicarbonate concentration at 24 mEq/L. With the development of chronic kidney disease, there is usually a decrease in ammonium excretion leading to positive hydrogen balance and metabolic acidosis. In a small number of patients, there might also be a defect in bicarbonate reabsorption leading to bicarbonaturia

A defect in bicarbonate reabsorption observed in some patients with CKD can contribute to the development of metabolic acidosis [1]. However, the major mechanism producing metabolic acidosis with CKD is decreased ammonium excretion. This decrease in ammonium excretion is primarily a consequence of a reduction in the number of functioning nephrons, as ammonium excretion per residual nephron is actually substantially increased above normal. As a result, net acid excretion falls below acid production leading to positive hydrogen ion balance. Studies in patients with a stable, albeit reduced GFR, have demonstrated that they are actually in continual positive hydrogen balance despite having a stable serum bicarbonate concentration. The stability of serum bicarbonate at any given level of GFR has been attributed to buffering of retained hydrogen by body buffers, primarily those residing in bone [5]. This process might contribute to some of the adverse effects of metabolic acidosis.

In some patients, a superimposed defect in tubular hydrogen secretion and/or ammonia production can lead to a more severe metabolic acidosis or its appearance earlier in the course of CKD. The most common explanation for this exacerbation of metabolic acidosis is a reduction in aldosterone synthesis found with hyporeninemic hypoaldosteronism. However, it can also be due to impaired proton excretion resulting from renal damage to the medullary interstitium in patients with diseases such as sickle cell disease. Hyperkalemia out of proportion to the decrease in GFR accompanying these disorders contributes to the suppression of ammonia production and thereby the development of metabolic acidosis [1].

7.3 Clinical Characteristics

Approximately 80 % of patients with CKD will develop hypobicarbonatemia once GFR falls below 25–30 mL/min [1]. However, a small percentage of patients will maintain a normal serum bicarbonate concentration even in the presence of severe kidney failure (GFR <20 mL/min), findings theoretically consistent with normal acid-base balance. The explanation for this discrepancy is presently unclear. However, it has been recently shown in experimental studies of animals with CKD that acid retention with an increase in interstitial acidity of various tissues can precede an overt fall in serum bicarbonate concentration [6]. These findings might suggest that patients with CKD and normal serum bicarbonate might actually have so-called subclinical metabolic acidosis. Thus, overt metabolic acidosis or so-called subclinical metabolic acidosis might be present in the vast majority of patients with CKD at all stages of renal failure.

When present, the metabolic acidosis is usually mild: serum bicarbonate ranging from 15 to 23 mmol/L and rarely falling below 15 mEq/L in the absence of an increased acid load. There is usually a direct correlation with the severity of kidney failure: the lower the GFR, the more severe the hypobicarbonatemia [1]. However, there can be great variability in the severity of the metabolic acidosis among individuals with similar levels of GFR. This has been attributed, in part, to differences in dietary intake of protein and fruits and vegetables, differences in buffering capacity arising from differences in bone disease, and differences in tubular function [1]. However, the precise explanation for this variability remains to be determined.

Early in the course of CKD, the metabolic acidosis might be of the normal anion gap variety [7]. Subsequently it can evolve into a mixed pattern with both a normal anion gap and a high anion gap metabolic acidosis and then finally a high anion gap metabolic acidosis alone. However, all three patterns can be observed both early and late in the course of CKD [1]. Patients with hyporeninemic hypoaldosteronism or medullary damage and CKD will usually manifest primarily a nongap metabolic acidosis. In addition, serum potassium concentration in these patients will be elevated out of proportion to the decrease in GFR.

Assuming there is no abnormality in renal bicarbonate reabsorption causing urinary bicarbonate wasting, most patients with uncomplicated CKD and hypobicarbonatemia will be able to acidify their urine to a pH <5.5. However, despite the ability to develop a large proton gradient between tubular fluid and blood, urinary ammonium excretion will be low (as reflected by a positive urine anion gap or abnormal urine osmolal gap). This is illustrated in Table 7.1.

Patients with CKD and hyporeninemic hypoaldosteronism will also be able to appropriately acidify their urine making the distinction between these patients and those with CKD alone difficult. On the other hand, those with medullary damage have a defect in urinary acidification with urine pH > 5.5 despite the presence of hypobicarbonatemia [1]. The clinical characteristics of different types of metabolic acidosis observed with CKD are summarized in Table 7.1.

7.4 Assessment of Acid-Base Balance in CKD

Since hypobicarbonatemia is often mild in patients with CKD, it sometimes can be difficult to distinguish the metabolic acidosis of CKD from chronic hypocapnia. Therefore, we recommend blood gases be obtained upon first evaluation of these patients, even if the serum bicarbonate concentration is minimally perturbed.

Table 7.1 Clinical characteristics of disorders associated with metabolic acidosis in patients with chronic kidney disease

Disorder	Electrolyte pattern	Urine NH_4	[a]Urine anion gap and [b]urine osmolal gap	Urine pH	Comments
Chronic kidney disease	Nongap early; mixed pattern, and high anion gap with severe disease	Low	Positive anion gap Low urine osmolal gap	<5.5	Most common cause of metabolic acidosis with kidney disease
Hyporeninemic hypoaldosteronism	Nongap pattern throughout course	Low	Positive anion gap Low urine osmolal gap	<5.5	More frequent in patients with diabetes mellitus, acidosis earlier than predicted on basis of glomerular filtration rate, hyperkalemia common
Renal disorders affecting medullary interstitium	Nongap pattern throughout course	Low	Positive anion gap Low urine osmolal gap	>5.0	Acidosis earlier than predicted based on glomerular filtration rate, hyperkalemia common

[a]Urine anion gap is defined as $Na^+ + K^+ - Cl^-$. In patients with ability to excrete acid appropriately, it is approximately −30 mEq/L, whereas it is positive in patients with impaired ability to excrete acid such as those with CKD
[b]The urine osmolal gap is defined as measured urine osmolality − $2 \times Na^+ + K^+$ + urea nitrogen/2.8 + glucose/18. The difference if divided by 2 gives an approximation of NH^4 excretion. In normal patients it increases from 30 mmol/day to more than 150 mmol/day. It is considerably less in patients with impaired acid excretion

Although arterial blood gases are traditionally utilized for this purpose, recent studies have demonstrated that venous blood gases can suffice [8, 9].

Measurement of urine pH in patients with a reduced serum bicarbonate concentration (obtained immediately upon voiding or collected under oil to prevent dissipation of CO_2) can be helpful in distinguishing patients with CKD alone or in combination with hypoaldosteronism from those with medullary damage. Therefore, it can be worthwhile obtaining a measurement of urine pH in patients with hypobicarbonatemia.

Urinary ammonium excretion will be low in all patients with metabolic acidosis arising from kidney dysfunction, and therefore, estimates of urinary ammonium excretion are helpful in distinguishing the acidosis related to the presence of kidney disease to that caused by nonrenal mechanisms. Either indirect estimates of urinary ammonium excretion, such as urine anion gap or osmolal gap, or direct determination of urinary ammonium excretion can be utilized. However, given the complexity of indirect estimates of urinary ammonium excretion, we have found direct measurement of urinary ammonium excretion to be the most cost-effective [4]. In patients in whom kidney dysfunction is the only mechanism underlying the metabolic acidosis, urine ammonium excretion will be considerably less than the normal value of 40 mmol/day. On the other hand, if there is an increased acid load, urinary ammonium excretion can be greater than this value but substantially less than the 200 mmol/day observed in patients with metabolic acidosis and intact kidney function [4].

Once acid-base parameters have been assessed and the presence of metabolic acidosis has been confirmed, blood gases need not be obtained again, but rather serum bicarbonate alone can be monitored. The recommended appropriate time of assessment for this parameter is shown in Table 7.2. If patients are being treated with base or there is a subsequent reduction in GFR, more frequent determinations of serum bicarbonate might be necessary.

7.5 Adverse Effects of Chronic Metabolic Acidosis and Rationale for Treatment

Although chronic metabolic acidosis in CKD has a number of potential adverse effects as summarized in Box 7.1, arguably the most important are acceleration of the progression of CKD, generation or exacerbation of bone disease, increased protein degradation with muscle wasting, impaired protein synthesis with hypoalbuminemia, and increased mortality (Box 7.1).

Both animal and human studies have documented that metabolic acidosis is associated with the progression of CKD [6, 10]. The potential mechanism(s) underlying this effect has been an area of intense investigation and are summarized in Fig. 7.2. Based on elegant studies performed in

Table 7.2 Recommended frequency of measurement of acid-base parameters in patients with chronic kidney disease

CKD stage (G)	GFR range ($mL/min/1.73\ m^2$)	Frequency of measurements
2	60–90	At least every 12 months
3	30–59	At least every 12 months
4	15–29	At least every 3 months
5	<15	At least every 3 months

Measurement of pH, PCO_2, and $[HCO_3^-]$ should be obtained upon first detection of reduction in serum bicarbonate; subsequently only serum bicarbonate needs be measured

Box 7.1. Major Adverse Effects of Chronic Metabolic Acidosis

- Progression of chronic kidney disease
- Stunted growth in children
- Generation or exacerbation of bone disease
- Muscle wasting with increased protein degradation
- Decreased albumin synthesis with tendency to hypoalbuminemia
- Increased mortality

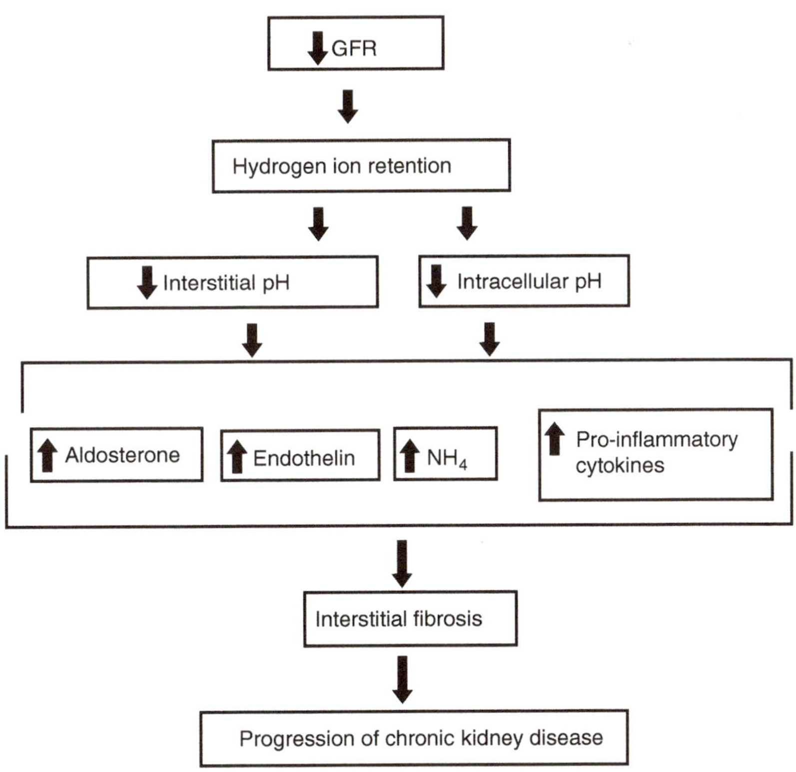

Fig. 7.2 Factors contributing to the progression of chronic kidney disease in patients with metabolic acidosis. Kidney impairment leads to a retention of protons and an increase in interstitial acidity of the kidney, with or without a concomitant fall in serum bicarbonate concentration. The increase in interstitial acidity is associated with a rise in endothelin, aldosterone, and proinflammatory cytokines. There is also stimulation of ammonia production and activation of the complement cascade. All four factors cause tubulointerstitial inflammation and eventual renal fibrosis and decline in GFR

animals and man, it appears that the hydrogen ion retention occurring with CKD leads to an increase in the acidity of the renal interstitium (and presumably intracellular pH of renal tubules) with resultant stimulation of endothelin production [11]. There is also increased production of aldosterone [6, 10] and possibly direct renal synthesis of proinflammatory cytokines [12]. Finally, the increased ammonia production per nephron found with CKD can be associated with activation of the complement cascade. These alterations in hormones, cytokines, and the complement cascade can individually induce tubulointerstitial inflammation and eventually renal fibrosis [10, 13]. Therefore, the composite effects on renal function of the individual changes of these factors are likely to be magnified. Of note, as mentioned previously the alterations in concentrations of endothelin and aldosterone have been reported even when there is little or no change in serum bicarbonate concentration [14]. Whether the changes in proinflammatory cytokines and the activation of the complement cascade noted with enhanced ammonia production are also found without overt hypobicarbonatemia remains unknown. Be that as it may, the data on endothelin and aldosterone suggest that neutralization of the endogenous acid load in patients with CKD might be of value even if serum bicarbonate concentration is normal. As discussed below, the criteria for initiating base therapy remains an area of intense interest.

Recent clinical trials involving small numbers of patients have demonstrated that treatment of the metabolic acidosis complicating advanced CKD with bicarbonate supplementation, sodium citrate, or increased intake of fruits and vegetables appears to slow the progression of CKD [6, 15, 16]. Although these studies support the benefits of base therapy in slowing the progression of CKD, a recent meta-analysis and editorial have called for larger randomized controlled studies to confirm the value of this therapeutic maneuver [17, 18]. At least two such studies are in progress and should provide valuable information about the impact of base therapy on renal progression [18].

Metabolic acidosis of CKD has also been implicated in the stunting of growth in children, as well as the generation of bone disease and/or the exacerbation of preexisting bone disease. The mechanisms underlying this effect are multiple and can include direct buffering of acid by bone, stimulation of parathyroid hormone secretion, or enhancement of the effects of parathyroid hormone on bone [19]. Various types of bone disease can be observed including osteomalacia and osteitis fibrosa cystica. Clinical assessment using x-rays might show changes typical of a specific bone disease, but bone biopsy is the most effective method of confirming the type of bone disease present [5]. Base therapy in individuals with CKD with minimally impaired kidney function and severe CKD receiving chronic dialysis improves growth in children and promotes healing of bone in children and adults [2].

The metabolic acidosis complicating CKD has been shown to result in increased protein degradation and muscle wasting, a process thought to be mediated in part by increased release of cortisol and decreased release of insulin-like growth factor. The muscle wasting associated with metabolic acidosis is improved by alkali therapy, resulting in clinical improvement in muscle strength. However, it is unclear whether reversing muscle wasting and improving muscle strength ultimately translate into improvements in functional status, and this will undoubtedly be a topic of further study. In addition to its effects on lean body mass, administration of base has been demonstrated in some but not all studies to cause an improvement in albumin synthesis and rise in serum albumin concentration.

Many factors affect mortality in patients with CKD. Several studies in patients with CKD, both before and after initiation of chronic maintenance dialysis, have shown a correlation between metabolic acidosis and increased mortality. The mechanism(s) underlying this effect is unclear, but it provides additional reasons for the correction of the metabolic acidosis.

In summary, the development of metabolic acidosis is associated with myriad adverse effects which can have a dramatic effect on the quality of life and mortality of patients with CKD. The clinical studies performed so far indicate base therapy is beneficial in ameliorating many of these adverse effects but further randomized controlled studies are necessary to provide sufficient information for generation of guidelines.

7.6 Treatment of Metabolic Acidosis of CKD

Based on evidence that metabolic acidosis is associated with progression of chronic kidney disease, production or worsening of bone disease, and increased mortality, several experts have suggested administering base to patients with serum bicarbonate concentrations ≤22 mEq/L [2, 20, 21]. No randomized controlled studies have determined whether this criterion is appropriate and this remains an important issue to assess. In addition, the goal of therapy remains elusive with some [2] recommending normalization of acid-base parameters and others being more noncommittal [21].

Both the precise serum bicarbonate at which to initiate therapy and the goal of therapy are extremely important to determine. Given that some studies have suggested that acid retention can be observed early in the course of CKD which can contribute to progression of CKD (and possibly other adverse effects) despite the absence of overt hypobicarbonatemia [14], there could be an inclination to initiate base therapy even with minimal or no reductions in serum bicarbonate. On the other hand, there remains potential risk of base therapy should it rise even slightly above normal. A recent randomized study indicated that although base therapy slowed progression of CKD, a serum bicarbonate above 24 mEq/L even when produced by measures other than base therapy was associated with a higher prevalence of congestive heart failure [22]. Moreover, others have suggested that an increased serum bicarbonate might provide an alkaline milieu that would predispose to deposition of calcium and phosphorus in tissues with resultant organ dysfunction.

Be that as it may, we conclude that until randomized controlled studies which evaluate the risks and benefits of base therapy with CKD allow for the development of evidence-based guidelines for therapy, we recommend that base be given to all patients with any reduction in serum bicarbonate with the goal of approximating mean normal values of 24 mmol/L. The clinician should be very vigilant to assess patients for possible complications such as volume overload with exacerbation of hypertension and congestive heart failure. Also, strong emphasis should be given on control of serum calcium and phosphorus to lessen the risk of calcifications. An increase in serum bicarbonate above normal should be prevented at all costs because of concern for exacerbation of heart failure or promotion of tissue calcifications.

Studies of different forms of base have indicated that sodium bicarbonate, sodium citrate (Shohl's solution), or dietary fruits and vegetables are all effective in raising serum bicarbonate concentration [15, 23]. Sodium bicarbonate is inexpensive, but has the complication of producing excess carbon dioxide which can be uncomfortable for the patient. The use of enteric-coated tablets might lessen this complication. The administration of sodium citrate (Shohl's solution) is effective and relatively inexpensive, but caution should be advised in patients that are taking aluminum binders. Citrate enhances the gastrointestinal absorption of aluminum. Changes in dietary habits rather than administration of supplements might be the most cost-effective means of raising serum bicarbonate concentration. A reduction in protein intake with increased intake of fruits and vegetables has been shown to be very successful in raising serum bicarbonate with little complications [23]. Given the high potassium content of fruits and vegetables, however, one has to be cautious about a possible increase in serum potassium with this regimen.

No matter what regimen is utilized, an estimate of base deficit should be obtained before embarking on therapy. This can easily be accomplished by subtracting the prevailing serum bicarbonate from the desired serum bicarbonate and multiplying this value by the approximate space of distribution of administered bicarbonate, usually 50 % body weight. This calculation will allow the clinician to estimate not only how much base should be given but also how long it will take before the target bicarbonate is reached.

The serum bicarbonate can be raised slowly over a matter of days while observing the patient for evidence of various complications particularly exacerbation of hypertension or congestive heart failure. Once the target serum bicarbonate has been reached, base administration can be reduced to values that approximate the rate of endogenous acid production. This precaution will aid in ensuring the clinician does not overshoot the target serum bicarbonate concentration. Recommendations for therapy of patients with CKD are summarized in Box 7.2.

Box 7.2. Recommendations for Treatment of Acidosis in Chronic Kidney Disease
[2, 8, 11, 21, 23]

Reduce protein intake to decrease acid generation while maintaining sufficient protein to preserve muscle mass.

Increase slightly intake of fruits and vegetables while avoiding hyperkalemia.

In patients with CKD, but not on maintenance dialysis, base can be given in the form of sodium bicarbonate or sodium citrate (Shohl's solution) once serum bicarbonate falls below the normal mean value of 24 mmol/L.

Calculate the bicarbonate deficit prior to administering base to get an estimate of base requirements. Use 50 % body weight as space of distribution for administered bicarbonate.

Correct the base deficit over 3–4 days. Once serum bicarbonate has reached the target value, reduce base administration to the quantity required to neutralize net endogenous acid load.

Be careful not to raise serum bicarbonate above 24 mmol/L.

Monitor patient for adverse effects of bicarbonate administration such as exacerbation of hypertension and congestive heart failure. If these are present, reduce dosage accordingly.

Conclusions

Acid retention is a common complication of chronic progressive kidney disease. This often leads to the development of metabolic acidosis. Although the acidosis can be mild, it can adversely affect several organ systems and thereby be an important contributory factor to the signs and symptoms of CKD. Several important questions remain unanswered that are relevant to the diagnosis and treatment of this disorder. Is base treatment beneficial in patients with early CKD in the absence of a fall in serum bicarbonate concentration? What serum bicarbonate should be targeted? What are the complications of base therapy? The answers to these questions should facilitate the development of evidence-based guidelines for the treatment of metabolic acidosis of CKD and aid in the prevention of progression of CKD and amelioration of some of its complications.

Before You Finish: Practice Pearls for the Clinician

- Alkali therapy should be used to maintain a serum bicarbonate of approximately 24 mEq/L.
- Commonly used alkalis include sodium bicarbonate and sodium citrate.
- Sodium bicarbonate can be given at a daily dose of 0.5–1 mEq/kg/day, although it can cause gastrointestinal discomfort from generated CO_2.
- Sodium citrate (Shohl's solution) can also be used, although it should be avoided in patients taking aluminum-containing antacids.

Acknowledgment This work was supported in part by funds from the Veterans Administration.

References

1. Kraut JA, Kurtz I. Metabolic acidosis of CKD: diagnosis, clinical characteristics, and treatment. Am J Kidney Dis. 2005;45(6):978–93.

2. Kraut JA, Madias NE. Consequences and therapy of the metabolic acidosis of chronic kidney disease. Pediatr Nephrol. 2011;26(1):19–28.
3. Kraut JA, Madias NE. Serum anion gap: its uses and limitations in clinical medicine. Clin J Am Soc Nephrol. 2007;2(1):162–74.
4. Kraut JA, Madias NE. Differential diagnosis of non-gap metabolic acidosis: value of a systematic approach. Clin J Am Soc Nephrol. 2012;7(4): 671–9.
5. Kraut JA. Disturbances of acid–base balance and bone disease in end-stage renal disease. Semin Dial. 2000;13:261–5.
6. Wesson DE, Simoni J. Acid retention during kidney failure induces endothelin and aldosterone production which lead to progressive GFR decline, a situation ameliorated by alkali diet. Kidney Int. 2010;78(11): 1128–35.
7. Widmer B, Gerhardt RE, Harrington JT, Cohen JJ. Serum electrolytes and acid base composition the influence of graded degrees of chronic renal failure. Arch Intern Med. 1979;139:1099–102.
8. Kraut JA, Madias NE. Metabolic acidosis: pathophysiology, diagnosis and management. Nat Rev Nephrol. 2010;6(5):274–85.
9. Kraut JA, Madias NE. Treatment of acute metabolic acidosis: a pathophysiologic approach. Nat Rev Nephrol. 2012;8(10):589–601.
10. Kraut JA. Effect of metabolic acidosis on progression of chronic kidney disease. Am J Physiol. 2011;300(4): F828–9.
11. Goraya N, Wesson DE. Does correction of metabolic acidosis slow chronic kidney disease progression? Curr Opin Nephrol Hypertens. 2013;22(2):193–7.
12. Raj S, Scott DR, Nguyen T, Sachs G, Kraut JA. Acid stress increases gene expression of proinflammatory cytokines in Madin-Darby canine kidney cells. Am J Physiol Renal Physiol. 2013;304(1):F41–8.
13. Scialla JJ, Anderson CA. Dietary Acid load: a novel nutritional target in chronic kidney disease? Adv Chronic Kidney Dis. 2013;20(2):141–9.
14. Wesson DE, Simoni J, Broglio K, Sheather SJ. Acid retention accompanies reduced GFR in humans and increases plasma levels of aldosterone and endothelin. Am J Physiol. 2011;300:F830–7.
15. de Brito-Ashurst I, Varagunam M, Raftery MJ, Yaqoob MM. Bicarbonate supplementation slows progression of CKD and improves nutritional status. J Am Soc Nephrol. 2009;20:2075–84.
16. Goraya N, Simoni J, Jo C, Wesson DE. Dietary acid reduction with fruits and vegetables or bicarbonate attenuates kidney injury in patients with a moderately reduced glomerular filtration rate due to hypertensive nephropathy. Kidney Int. 2012;81(1):86–93.
17. Susantitaphong P, Sewaralthahab K, Balk EM, Jaber BL, Madias NE. Short- and long-term effects of alkali therapy in chronic kidney disease: a systematic review. Am J Nephrol. 2012;35(6):540–7.
18. Kraut JA, Madias NE. Association of serum bicarbonate with clinical outcome in CKD: could an increase in serum bicarbonate be a double edge sword. Am J Kidney Dis. 2013;62(4):647–9.
19. Alpern R, Shakhaee K. The Clinical Spectrum of Chronic metabolic acidosis: homeostatic mechanisms produce significant morbidity. Am J Kidney Dis. 1997;29:291–302.
20. Kovesdy CP. Metabolic acidosis and kidney disease: does bicarbonate therapy slow the progression of CKD? Nephrol Dial Transplant. 2012;27(8):3056–62.
21. Foundation NK. KDOQI clinical practice guidelines for bone metabolism and disease in chronic kidney disease 2003. Am J Kidney Dis. 2003;42:s3–201.
22. Dobre M, Yang W, Chen J, et al. Association of serum bicarbonate with risk of renal and cardiovascular outcomes in chronic kidney disease. A report from the Chronic Renal Insufficiency Cohort (CRIC) study. Am J Kidney Dis. 2013;62(4):670–8.
23. Goraya N, Simoni J, Jo C, Wesson DE. A comparison of treating metabolic acidosis in CKD stage 4 hypertensive kidney disease with fruits and vegetables or sodium bicarbonate. Clin J Am Soc Nephrol. 2013;8(3):371–81.

8 Acute Kidney Injury in Chronic Kidney Disease

Sharidan K. Parr and Edward D. Siew

Before You Start: Facts You Need to Know

- AKI is among the fastest growing kidney diseases.
- CKD and proteinuria are common and overlooked risk factors for developing AKI.
- Patients with a rapid course to ESRD often have nonlinear decline in kidney function involving one or more episodes of AKI.
- Ideally, long-term goals of care (including whether to initiate dialysis) should be discussed *before hospitalization*, particularly among frail and elderly patients with CKD.
- Diagnostic tests such as fractional excretion of sodium (FeNa) may be unreliable in patients with CKD.
- After an episode of moderate to severe AKI or those where recovery to baseline has not occurred, patients should be evaluated within 3 months for resolution or for new onset or worsening of CKD.

8.1 Introduction: The Growing Impact of AKI

8.1.1 Occurrence and Definition

The Centers for Disease Control and Prevention estimate that kidney disease is the eighth leading cause of death in the United States (US), which consumes 23 % of total Medicare expenditures. By 2030, two million people in the United States will develop advanced kidney failure, the prevention of which is a global public health concern. AKI, particularly when severe, has been recognized as an increasingly important risk factor CKD progression [1]. AKI is characterized by an abrupt decline in glomerular filtration rate (GFR). The recent Kidney Disease Improving Global Outcomes (KDIGO) Clinical Practice Guidelines for Acute Kidney Injury suggest that a minimal threshold for defining AKI should include an increase in serum creatinine of at least 0.3 mg/dl (26.5 μmol/l) within 48 h, a 1.5 times increase in the baseline value within 7 days, or urine volume less than 0.5 ml/kg/h for at least 6 h (Table 8.1) [2]. This change in paradigm has been largely driven by observations showing that even without overt kidney failure, smaller changes in serum creatinine independently associate with poor clinical outcomes (Fig. 8.1) [3]. These observations have also led to the recent changing of the term "acute renal failure" to "acute kidney injury." The severity of AKI is further staged by incrementally larger increases in serum creatinine values or the persistence or worsening of

S.K. Parr, MD • E.D. Siew, MD, MSCI (✉)
Division of Nephrology and Hypertension,
Department of Medicine,
Vanderbilt University Medical Center,
Nashville, TN, USA
e-mail: sharidan.k.parr@vanderbilt.edu;
edward.siew@vanderbilt.edu

M. Arici (ed.), *Management of Chronic Kidney Disease*,
DOI 10.1007/978-3-642-54637-2_8, © Springer-Verlag Berlin Heidelberg 2014

oliguria. As these definitions require close monitoring of serum creatinine or urine output, most literature comes from hospitalized populations. Incidence rates for AKI vary with the setting studied, ranging up to 9.6 % of general admissions and up to 45 % in the critically ill [4]. Population-based studies within industrialized countries estimate incidence rates of between 2,147 and 5,000 cases/million population/year [5].

Table 8.1 Staging of AKI

Stage	Serum creatinine	Urine output
1	1.5–1.9 times baseline or ≥0.3 mg/dl (≥26.5 μmol/l) increase	<0.5 ml/kg/h for 6–12 h
2	2.0–2.9 times baseline	<0.5 ml/kg/h for ≥12 h
3	3.0 times baseline or increase in serum creatinine to ≥4.0 mg/dl (≥353.6 μmol/l) or initiation of renal replacement therapy or in patients <18 years, decrease in eGFR to <35 ml/min per 1.73 m²	<0.3 ml/kg/h for ≥24 h or Anuria for ≥12 h

Source: Reprinted with permission from Macmillan Publishers Ltd and Nature Publishing Group: Kidney Disease Improving Global Outcomes [2]

While AKI can be associated with exacerbations of intrinsic kidney disease or systemic diseases that target the kidney (e.g., lupus), the majority of AKI in developed countries occurs as a consequence of an acute illness or procedures that either compromise perfusion (e.g., volume-deplet on, acute blood loss, major vascular surgery) or stimulate profound inflammation (e.g., sepsis) (Box 8.3). Medications directly toxic to the kidney (e.g., nonsteroidal anti-inflammatory drugs (NSAIDS), aminoglycosides, iodinated contrast) also contribute to up to 1/5 of cases [6]. In developing countries, where disease surveillance is not widely implemented, available data indicate a higher prevalence of diarrheal and infectious-related causes of AKI, particularly among children.

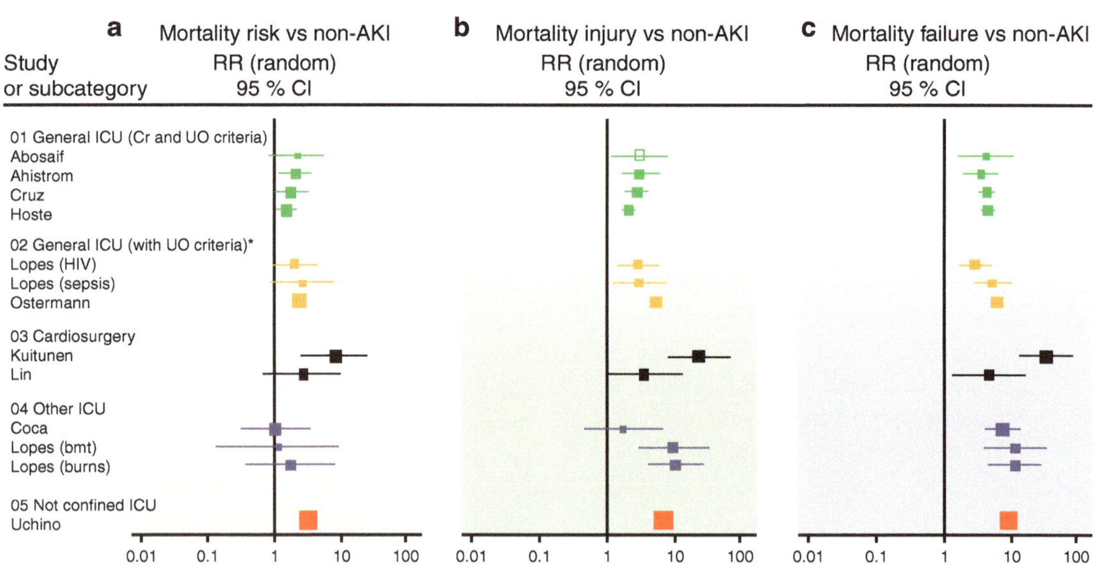

Fig. 8.1 Increased mortality risk associated with AKI extends to milder injury. Systematic review showing consistent increases in mortality risk associated with incrementally larger acute changes in serum creatinine in different acute care settings illustrated by Forrest plot. (**a**) Risk category denoted by a 50 % increase in baseline serum creatinine/25 % decrease in baseline GFR/urine output <0.5 mg/kg/h × 6 h (relative risk = 2.4), (**b**) injury denoted by a doubling in baseline serum creatinine/50 % decrease in GFR/urine output <0.5 ml/kg/h × 12 h (relative risk = 4.15), and (**c**) failure denoted by a tripling of baseline serum creatinine/GFR decrease of >75 %/acute increase in serum creatinine to ≥4 mg/dl with and acute rise of 0.5 mg/dl/urine output <0.3 ml/kg/h × 24 h/anuriax 12 h (relative risk = 6.37) (Reprinted with permission from Macmillan Publishers Ltd: Ricci et al. [3])

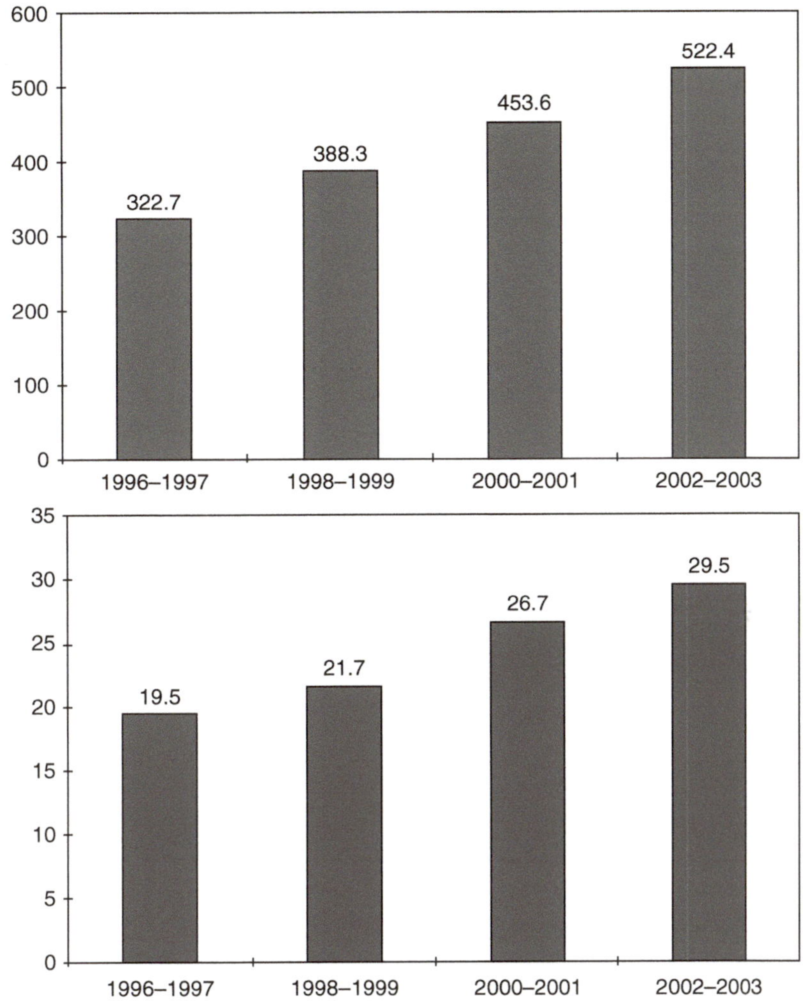

Fig. 8.2 The population incidence of dialysis and non-dialysis-requiring AKI in the United States is increasing. (**a**) Community-based incidence rates (per 100,000 person-years) of non-dialysis-requiring AKI per year. (**b**) Community-based incidence rates (per 100,000 person-years) of dialysis-requiring AKI per year (Reprinted with permission from Macmillan Publishers Ltd: Hsu et al. [5])

8.1.2 Prognosis

AKI is strongly associated with devastating short-term complications with mortality rates ranging from 28.1 % among those with easily recognizable forms of injury up to 60.3 % among critically ill patients who require dialysis [6]. Of greater concern are signals arising from both administrative and laboratory databases that the incidence of AKI is increasing rapidly (Fig. 8.2) [5]. Reasons may include increases in the prevalence of comorbidities including CKD, parallel rises in known precipitants including sepsis, and increasing use of medications or invasive procedures that place patients at increased risk for developing AKI.

Studies focused on the long-term impact of this disease indicate that AKI strongly associates with CKD progression, particularly in severe cases or when superimposed on underlying CKD. Combined with ongoing increases in disease incidence, these observations imply a growing population of survivors of AKI at risk for the development or acceleration of CKD and its complications.

In this chapter, we will examine the bidirectional nature of the interaction between AKI and CKD. Specifically, we will detail how the growing population of patients with CKD may be especially vulnerable to developing AKI and its complications. In addition, we will discuss emerging literature suggesting that AKI is an important contributor to both the development and progression of CKD. Lastly, we will review recent practice guidelines to the diagnostic approach and management of this disease (Boxes 8.1 and 8.2).

Box 8.1. Relevant Guidelines

1. *KDIGO Guideline*
   Kidney Disease: Improving Global Outcomes (KDIGO) Acute Kidney Injury Work Group. KDIGO clinical practice guideline for acute kidney injury. Kidney Int. 2012;2(Suppl):1–138.
   http://kdigo.org/home/guidelines/acute-kidney-injury/ [2]
2. *European Renal Best Practice Guideline*
   A European Renal Best Practice (ERBP) Position Statement on the Kidney Disease Improving Global Outcomes (KDIGO) Clinical Practice Guidelines on Acute Kidney Injury.
   Nephrol Dial Transplant. 2012;27(12): 4263–72 [7].
   Nephrol Dial Transplant. 2013;28(12): 2940–45 [8].
   http://www.european-renal-best-practice.org/content/position-statement-and-update-kdigo-aki-guidelines-now-available-erbp-website
3. *The Renal Association Guideline*
   Acute Kidney Injury – Final Version (08 March 2011) [9].
   http://www.renal.org/clinical/guidelines-section/AcuteKidneyInjury.aspx
4. *National Institute for Health and Clinical Excellence (NICE) Guideline*
   CG169 Acute kidney injury: Prevention, detection and management of acute kidney injury up to the point of renal replacement therapy. Issued: August 2013
   http://publications.nice.org.uk/acute-kidney-injury-cg169 [10]
5. *Canadian Society of Nephrology Guideline:*
   Canadian Society of Nephrology Commentary on the 2012 KDIGO clinical practice guideline for acute kidney injury. Am J Kidney Dis. 2013;61(5): 673–85 [11]
6. *NKF KDOQI Guideline:*
   KDOQI US Commentary on the 2012 KDIGO clinical practice guideline for acute kidney injury. Am J Kidney Dis. 2013;61(5):649–72.
   http://www.kidney.org/Professionals/kdoqi/pdf/AKI-Commentary-2013.pdf [12]

Box 8.2. What the Guidelines Say You Should Do in AKI

- The cause of AKI should be determined whenever possible, paying special attention to reversible causes.
- Patients should be risk stratified for AKI according to their susceptibilities and exposures.
- Test patients at increased risk for AKI with measurements of SCr and urine output to detect AKI, with frequency and duration of monitoring based on patient risk and clinical course.
- In the absence of hemorrhagic shock, use isotonic crystalloids rather than colloids as initial management for expansion of intravascular volume.
- Avoid restriction of protein intake for preventing or delaying initiation of RRT.
- Diuretics should not be used to prevent AKI.
- Diuretics should not be used to treat AKI, except in the management of volume overload.
- Low-dose dopamine should not be used to prevent or treat AKI.

Source: Data from Ref. [2]

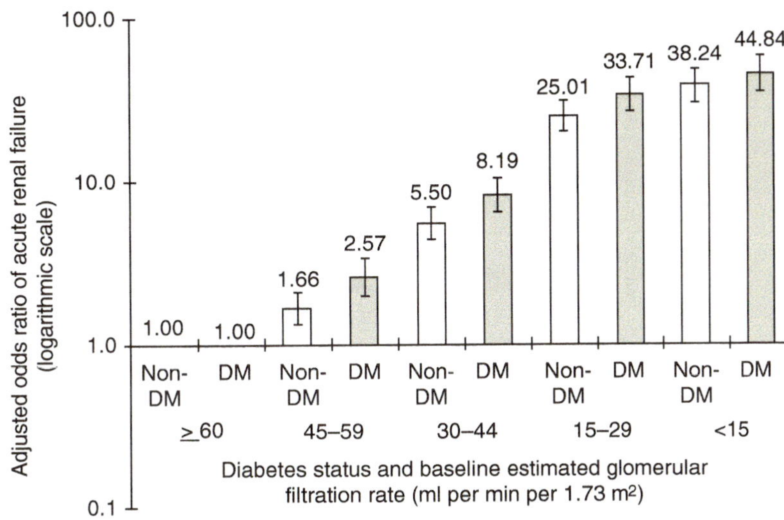

Fig. 8.3 Multivariable association of baseline estimated GFR and dialysis-requiring ARF stratified by the presence or absence of diabetes mellitus (*DM*). Each model adjusted for age, sex, race/ethnicity, diagnosed hypertension, and documented proteinuria (Reprinted with permission from Macmillan Publishers Ltd: Hsu et al. [13])

8.2 CKD as a Risk Factor for AKI

Administrative data have consistently identified CKD as a risk factor for AKI across different clinical settings. However, as many of these early studies used diagnostic coding to identify the occurrence of AKI, concerns over potential biases in detection (e.g., AKI is more likely to be recognized in patients with underlying CKD) prompted additional studies using serum creatinine to define AKI. A population-based study using an integrated health-care database in Northern California observed an adjusted odds of developing dialysis-requiring AKI of up to 20- to 30-fold higher in those with advanced stage III and stage IV CKD compared to non-CKD patients (Fig. 8.3) [13]. Subsequent studies have demonstrated a graded relationship between the severity of CKD and the risk for AKI, indicating that the risk for AKI begins at even earlier stages of CKD [14]. More recently, studies have observed an association between proteinuria and the risk for AKI that appear independent from the effects of eGFR. A recent prospective study of 11,200 in the Atherosclerosis Risk in Communities (ARIC) cohort detected a stepwise increase in risk for AKI with increasing degrees of albuminuria. After adjusting for age, gender, race, cardiovascular risk factors, and categories of eGFR, the ORs for AKI were 1.9 (95 % CI, 1.4–2.6), 2.2 (95 % CI, 1.6–3.0), and 4.8 (95 % CI, 3.2–7.2) for urine albumin-to-creatinine ratio groups of 11–29, 30–299, and ≥300 mg/g, respectively [14]. Another population-based cohort of nearly one million patients in Canada also confirmed a robust association between proteinuria and the risk for hospitalization with AKI, death, and the composite endpoint of doubling of serum creatinine or ESRD. Across all stages of CKD, increasing levels of proteinuria measured by urine dipstick carried an increased adjusted risk for hospitalization for AKI. Even among those with preserved eGFR, mild to heavy proteinuria carried a graded 2.5 (95 % CI: 2.3–2.7)- to 4.4 (95 % CI: 3.7–5.2)-fold risk of hospitalization for AKI (Fig. 8.4) [15].

In summary, these studies reinforce the link between underlying structural or functional impairment of the kidney and the risk for AKI. Whether reducing proteinuria modifies the risk for AKI is an important question that remains to be tested. While the intuitive notion that lower functional reserve in any organ might lower the threshold for injury, the presence of CKD and/or proteinuria remains an important marker to help clinicians identify patients at highest risk for developing AKI. Therefore, we recommend measuring proteinuria and serum creatinine prior to procedures or drug exposures carrying intrinsic risk for AKI (e.g., iodinated contrast procedures)

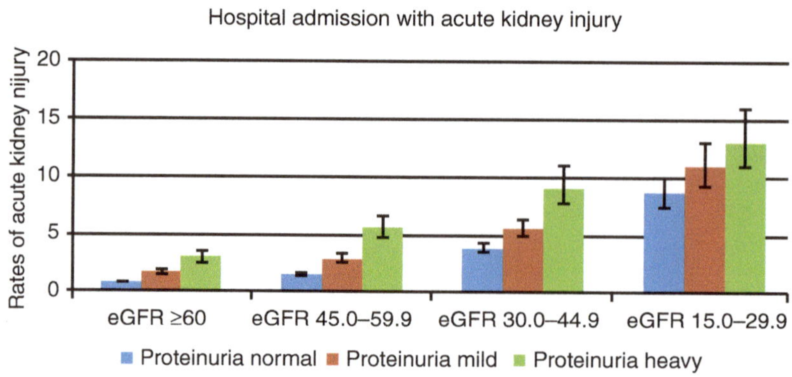

Fig. 8.4 Estimated glomerular filtration rate and proteinuria independently associate with acute kidney injury. Adjusted for means (and frequencies) of covariates for age, sex, aboriginal status, low income, social assistance, and comorbidities (HIV/AIDS, history of cancer, cerebrovascular disease, congestive heart failure, chronic pulmonary disease, dementia, diabetes mellitus, hypertension, metastatic solid tumor, mild liver disease, moderate or severe liver disease, myocardial infarction, paralysis, peptic ulcer disease, peripheral vascular disease, rheumatic disease). In this analysis, dipstick urinalysis was used to classify participants with respect to proteinuria: normal (urine dipstick negative), mild (urine dipstick trace or 1+), or heavy (urine dipstick ≥2+). The tests for linear trend across eGFR categories and across proteinuria categories were all significant at the $p < 0.0001$ level (Data from James et al. [15])

among patients with CKD or other high-risk groups (e.g., elderly, diabetics, hypertension) to better weigh the risks and benefits of a given procedure and to guide use of preventative strategies.

8.3 AKI as a Risk Factor for CKD

Early studies nearly a half-century ago suggested that patients with normal kidney function before severe dialysis-requiring AKI were often able to return to active lives independent of dialysis. However, small but detailed physiologic studies detected subtle decreases in clearance as well as an inability to concentrate and dilute urine among patients whose serum creatinine values appeared to recover. More recently, large observational cohort studies have demonstrated that AKI, particularly when severe, often fails to recover completely, with potential outcomes illustrated in Fig. 8.5. For some patients, there may appear to be a complete or near-complete recovery. In other patients, an incomplete recovery of AKI may occur resulting in the development of incident CKD. Lastly, among those with previous CKD, AKI may serve to accelerate the progressive loss of kidney function over time, yet the mechanisms that lead to decline and potential interventions to attenuate disease progression have not been fully established.

Animal studies have demonstrated that beyond the initial tubular injury and nephron loss, ischemic insults to the kidney also result in endothelial damage to the microvasculature, which has less regenerative capacity than tubules. The loss of vascularity may lead to chronic regional ischemia that promotes downstream hypoxic signaling, inflammation, and fibrosis (Fig. 8.6) [16]. Even after apparent recovery, affected animals can develop proteinuria and are less able to excrete sodium in the urine leading to salt-sensitive hypertension, which may contribute to further loss of kidney function. Further, nephron loss in other experimental models of CKD has also been observed to lead to compensatory adaptations including hyperfiltration that result in glomerular hypertension and cellular proliferation. Whether the latter also occurs following AKI is not clear.

Prospective studies of children who recover from AKI associated with the hemolytic-uremic syndrome (HUS) found survivors were more likely to develop microalbuminuria and lower eGFR values using cystatin C levels relative to a group of control patients during 5 years of

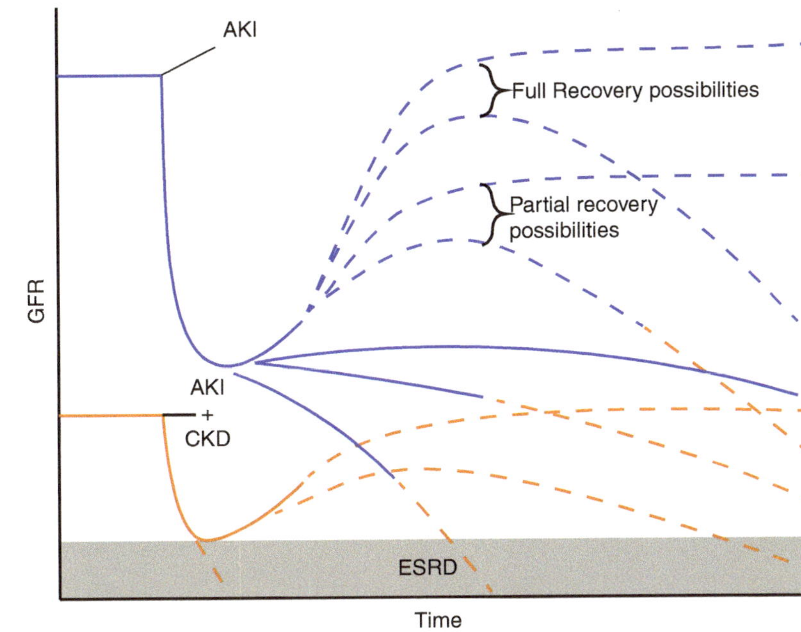

Fig. 8.5 Potential kidney outcomes following AKI

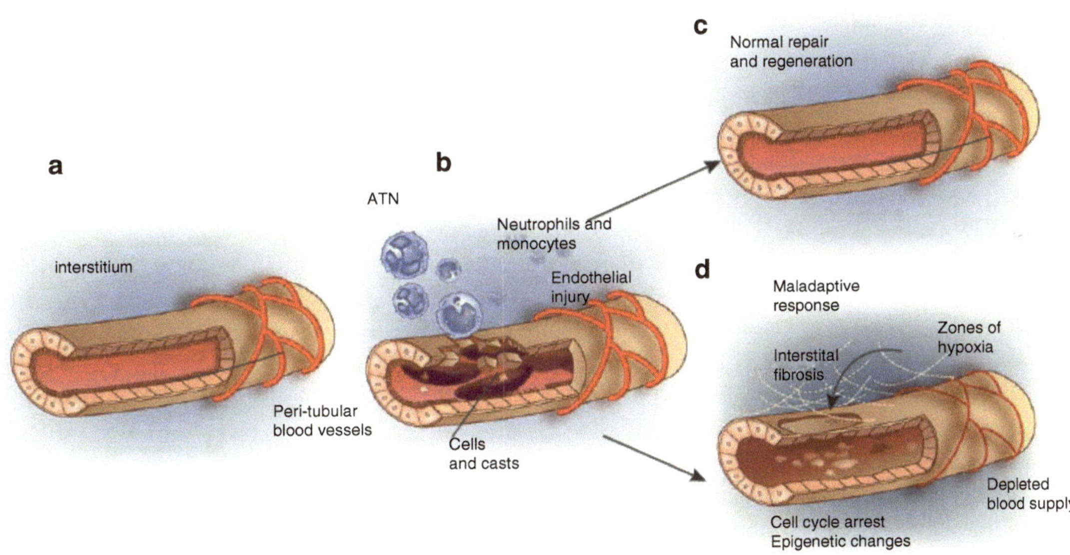

Fig. 8.6 Potential mechanisms of how AKI can lead to irreversible loss of kidney function. Tubule cross section. (**a**) Cross section of normal renal tubule with intact epithelial cells, renal interstitium, and peritubular blood vessels. (**b**) Cross section of renal tubule with acute tubular necrosis (*ATN*) with epithelial cell necrosis, intratubular cast formation, endothelial injury of peritubular blood vessels, and migration of monocytes and macrophages into renal interstitium. (**c**) Cross section of renal tubule after normal repair and regeneration showing restoration of normal renal architecture. (**d**) Cross section of renal tubule after severe episode of AKI, resulting in maladaptive repair. Epithelial cells have evidence of cell cycle arrest and epigenetic changes that favor a fibrosis phenotype. Renal interstitium shows evidence of fibrosis. Post-injury vascular supply is less dense than baseline. The combination of decreased blood supply and fibrosis leads to zones of hypoxia wherein the combination of decreased vascular supply and fibrosis can initiate a vicious cycle leading to ongoing fibrosis (Reprinted with permission from Macmillan Publishers Ltd: Chawla and Kimmel [16])

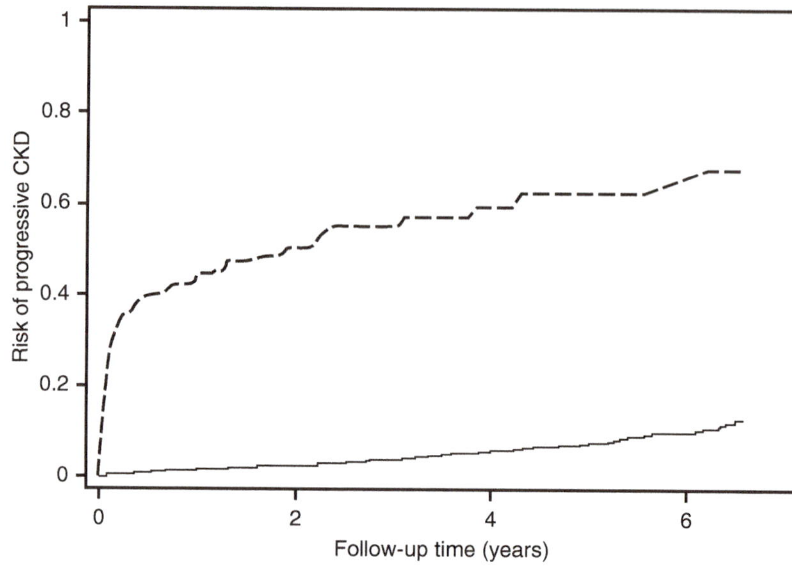

Fig. 8.7 Severe AKI increases the risk of developing advanced kidney disease. Kaplan-Meier curves showing the long-term risk of CKD stage IV or worse among patients with well-preserved kidney function who did (*dashed line*) or did not (*solid line*) suffer and recovered at least partially from dialysis-requiring AKI (Reprinted with permission from Macmillan Publishers Ltd: Lo et al. [19])

follow-up [17]. The extension of these findings to adults has been noted in multiple observational studies [1]. A study using administrative data examined 233,803 hospitalized Medicare beneficiaries found that among those with a discharge diagnosis of AKI, there was a 7 % chance of initiating treatment for ESRD within 2 years of follow-up, with a nearly twofold increase in adjusted risk compared with CKD patients hospitalized without AKI [18]. The likelihood of a patient with CKD experiencing AKI to need treatment for ESRD was 14 %, with an over fourfold adjusted risk compared to CKD patients without an AKI diagnosis.

Subsequent studies anchored by baseline kidney function have found similar results. In a population-based study in Northern California in patients whose eGFR before hospitalization was >45 ml/min/1.73 m^2, patients experiencing dialysis-requiring AKI were 28 times more likely to develop advanced CKD compared to other hospitalized patients without AKI after adjustment and matching for potential confounders (Fig. 8.7) [19]. The risk for incident CKD appears to be increased 1.9-fold even among patients with reversible AKI in whom eGFR returns to within 10 % of their pre-hospitalization baseline [20]. Meta-analyses have estimated pooled adjusted hazard ratios for CKD, ESRD, and mortality following AKI of 8.8 (95 % CI: 3.1–25.5), 3.1(95 % CI: 1.9–5.0), and 2.0 (95 % CI: 1.3–3.1), respectively, compared to hospitalized patients without AKI [1].

Identifying patients at highest risk for developing CKD following AKI has become a high priority. One of the most potent risk factors identified is the severity of AKI [21]. Another potential harbinger of poor outcomes includes the duration of injury. Recent studies in surgical patients found higher long-term mortality rates among those with injury that persists for multiple days, even among those with mild injury [22]. Other risk factors for long-term loss of kidney function following AKI include advancing age; African American race; baseline kidney function; comorbidity burden including the presence of diabetes, hypertension, or congestive heart failure; and serum albumin levels during hospitalization [23].

Lastly, recent attempts have begun to examine the impact of subsequent AKI events on long-term loss of kidney function. Thakar et al. [24] followed a high-risk cohort of 3,679 diabetic patients, 62 % with baseline proteinuria, within an integrated health-care system for the development of stage IV CKD over a mean of 5 years. Despite overall preserved baseline kidney function (mean eGFR 81 ± 26 ml/min/1.73 m^2), fourteen percent of the population experienced an AKI event. Patients experiencing an AKI event were twice as likely to reach stage IV CKD as those who did not

(24.6 % versus 12.9 %, $p < 0.01$). Multivariate Cox regression analysis identified the presence of any AKI to be associated with an adjusted hazard ratio of 3.5 (95 % CI: 2.7–4.6) with each subsequent episode of AKI further doubling that risk (HR 2.02: 95 % CI: 1.78–2.30).

In spite of the accumulating biological and epidemiologic evidence, debate remains over whether the relationship between AKI and the subsequent risk for de novo CKD is a causal one. For example, there is considerable overlap between the risk factors for both CKD and AKI including age, diabetes, hypertension, and cardiovascular disease that can confound this relationship, leading to the hypothesis that AKI is simply a marker for patients who were likely destined to develop CKD. Prospective studies to address these limitations and better identify those likely to have poor longitudinal outcomes have been launched that should shed further light on these issues. In the interim, it is clear that AKI is, at minimum, an important marker for long-term loss of kidney function, particularly among those with preexisting CKD. Therefore, we recommend that an episode of AKI be documented in the electronic medical record and that routine evaluation of all patients with CKD include inquiring about past history of AKI.

8.4 Prevention and Management of AKI in CKD

8.4.1 Before and Early During Hospitalization: Recognizing High-Risk Patients and Situations

As the interaction between AKI and CKD becomes clearer, we will need to improve our understanding of how to optimally care for this growing population. An important first step is for clinicians to recognize how different patients and clinical situations combine to increase the risk for developing AKI in patients with CKD. Among the fastest growing populations experiencing AKI are the elderly, who, like those with CKD, are also less likely to recover and more likely to progress to ESRD following an episode of AKI. Age-related changes in both structure and function of the kidneys and a higher comorbidity burden combine to reduce the threshold for injury. Additionally, these patients are at increased risk for inappropriate drug dosing and polypharmacy that increase the risk of drug interactions and/or nephrotoxicity.

Certain medication classes of proven benefit in the chronic setting can also lower the threshold for AKI during acute illness. For example, the normal response to decreases in kidney perfusion include increases in post-glomerular (i.e., efferent arteriolar) vascular tone, which helps to maintain glomerular perfusion pressure and adequate filtration. However, the increased use of medications in the CKD population, including angiotensin-converting enzyme inhibitors (ACE-I) and angiotensin receptor blockers (ARBs), blunts the compensatory response that maintains glomerular perfusion pressure. When coupled with diuretics or antihypertensive agents that decrease effective circulating volume or reduce perfusion pressure, the threshold for kidney injury can be lowered. While this risk is presumed to be low in the chronic stable setting, an important component of management is to consider temporary suspension of these medications when the risk for AKI is more dynamic. We recommend educating patients to withhold ACE-I, ARBs, and diuretics during prolonged heat exposure or volume-depleting illnesses such as diarrhea or vomiting, especially if intake of solute and fluids is impaired. Patients should also be especially cautioned to avoid NSAIDs alone or in combination with the aforementioned antihypertensives and/or diuretics. The normal response of the afferent arteriole in states of reduced glomerular perfusion is to dilate in order to maintain glomerular perfusion. However, NSAIDs compromise prostaglandin-mediated dilation of the afferent arterioles during decreased perfusion, which further impairs perfusion to the kidneys in patients with CKD. Health-care providers should have a low threshold for suspending these medications when the risk for AKI is more dynamic such as during hospitalization or before anticipated procedures known to increase risk for

AKI including major surgery or contrast exposure. Communication with procedural teams should be pursued to ensure that risk is minimized (i.e., avoiding contrast load such as ventriculogram or "add-on" vascular studies) and that adequate prophylaxis is given (see Chap. 3 for contrast-induced nephropathy).

Finally, facilitating communication with patients or their surrogates regarding the long-term goals of care *before hospitalization* is a much-needed area for improvement, particularly among frail and elderly patients with CKD. Recent studies have demonstrated that among patients with diminished functional status, such as nursing home residents, nearly two-thirds of patients die within a year of initiating chronic dialysis and premorbid functional status is maintained only in 13 % of patients [25]. Therefore, attempts to ascertain patient goals of care in the context of chronic disease and functional status should occur prior to hospitalization. This will enable patients and physicians with an established relationship to develop a plan of action should hospitalization with AKI occur (e.g., advance directive) and help patients better balance the risk of AKI and its consequences with the benefit of procedures that carry an intrinsic risk for AKI (e.g., major vascular surgery). The possibility of a more conservative approach to care should be presented as a viable option early in the course of conversation, and the joint input of both the patient's primary provider and nephrologist should be sought.

8.4.2 Determining the Time Course and Diagnosis of AKI

A simplified algorithm of the evaluation and treatment of AKI is depicted in Fig. 8.8. In evaluating patients with suspected AKI, effort should be made to determine whether the pattern of kidney injury is acute, acute on chronic, or chronic. This discrimination is important, as some forms of AKI are reversible if the inciting event is removed. Clinicians should elicit a history of CKD including obtaining pre-hospitalization serum creatinine values, if available. Baseline serum creatinine obtained during chronic steady state can provide insight into the acuity of change in kidney function, more accurately gauge the severity of AKI, and provide prognostic information. Any abrupt rise from the baseline creatinine in patients with CKD should prompt evaluations for AKI. Radiographic evidence of small, scarred kidneys would suggest underlying CKD. However, in some cases of CKD, the kidney size may be normal or increased such as in HIV-associated nephropathy, polycystic kidney disease, or infiltrative diseases such as amyloidosis. Additional findings that may suggest underlying CKD include anemia, hyperphosphatemia, hypocalcemia, and hyperparathyroidism.

8.4.3 History, Physical Exam, and the Differential Diagnosis of AKI

Once a diagnosis of AKI has been made, steps should be taken to determine the etiology. Classically, underlying causes are grouped into prerenal, intrinsic, or postrenal categories (Box 8.3). However, many cases of AKI are multifactorial, and multiple contributors should be considered.

Prerenal AKI most often results from impaired perfusion to the kidney and is the most common cause of community-acquired AKI. Early in the course of injury, net filtration is diminished. However, compensatory hemodynamic and hormonal adaptations occur within the kidney that increase the efficiency of filtration and promote sodium and water retention that maintain blood volume and minimize the development of tissue injury *if adequate perfusion can be restored quickly*. Therefore, the diagnosis of prerenal AKI is made retrospectively only after a successful intervention is applied (e.g., creatinine decreases with IV fluid resuscitation). However, deciding which intervention to apply can be challenging as prerenal physiology can be seen in both states of absolute volume depletion (e.g., diarrhea, vomiting, overdiuresis, dehydration, bleeding) and diseases with decreased effective circulating volume (e.g., nephrotic syndrome, liver disease, congestive heart failure) which often present with signs of fluid accumulation (i.e., edema). In patients with underlying CKD, diminished renal reserve

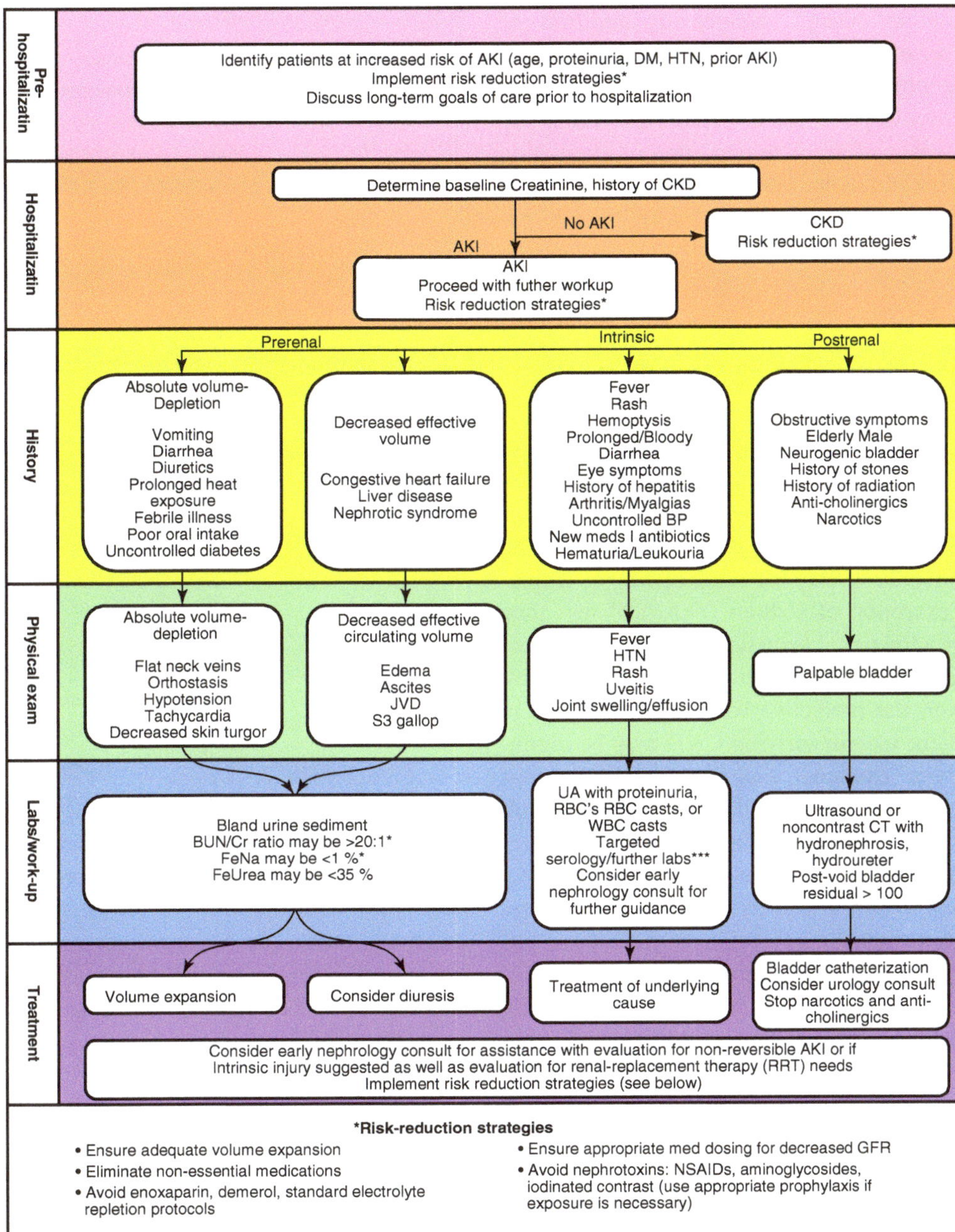

* In CKD, FeN-a may not be <1 % even in pre-renal states. ***CPK. complements, serum and urine protein electrophoresis. ANA. ANCA. anti-GBM Ab

Fig. 8.8 Algorithm for evaluation and treatment of AKI

and blunted ability to adapt to decreased perfusion may lower the threshold for progression to true parenchymal injury, underscoring the importance of a timely diagnosis.

A rapid historical assessment for volume-depleting illness including bleeding, vomiting, diarrhea, febrile illness, infection, or prolonged heat exposure should be elicited. Information on comorbid disease states including poorly controlled diabetes (osmotic diuresis) or those associated with effective arterial volume depletion including congestive heart failure or cirrhosis should also be sought. Additionally, contributing medications should be identified paying particular attention to recent changes or addition of antihypertensives, diuretics, cathartics, NSAIDs/COX-2 inhibitors, and ACE-I/ARB use. Physical exam should prioritize determining volume status. In cases of absolute depletion of circulating volume, patients may have orthostatic hypotension, flat neck veins, decreased skin turgor, hypotension, or tachycardia. In contrast, patients with decreased effective circulating volume (i.e., cirrhosis or CHF) may have evidence of volume overload including jugular venous distension, S3 gallop, edema, or ascites.

Several laboratory tools have traditionally been used to reflect appropriate tubular response to diminished perfusion, supporting the diagnosis of prerenal azotemia rather than intrinsic causes of AKI during oliguric kidney injury. Among these include a BUN/Cr ratio of >20:1, a fractional excretion of sodium (FeNa) of less than 1 %, or a fractional excretion of urea (FeUrea) of less than 35 % in patients exposed to diuretics. However, the predictive value of these tools in the patient with underlying CKD may be diminished. For example, a lower filtered load of sodium and impaired tubular function may result in a higher FeNa at baseline. Therefore, the predictive value of FeNa levels >1 % for indicating the presence of tubular dysfunction may be less reliable, although a low FeNa of <1 % in the oliguric CKD patient still suggests prerenal azotemia. These caveats place a greater emphasis on history and physical exam findings and other supplemental laboratory data to establish the diagnosis and nature of prerenal AKI (Table 8.2).

A diagnosis of intrinsic kidney injury is made when tissue damage to one or more portions of the kidney (glomerulus, vasculature, tubules, or interstitium) has occurred. A discussion of the vast etiologies of intrinsic AKI is beyond the scope of this chapter; however, ATN is considered to be among the most common injuries in hospitalized patients. Kidney perfusion is estimated to account for 25 % of cardiac output with portions of the tubular epithelium being particularly vulnerable to decreases in perfusion due to high metabolic activity and relative low tissue oxygen content. For this reason, many consider

Table 8.2 Urinalysis findings in AKI

Normal or hyaline casts	Prerenal azotemia Postrenal/obstruction
Dysmorphic RBCs/RBC casts	Glomerulonephritis Malignant hypertension Thrombotic microangiopathy Vasculitis
WBCs/WBC casts	Glomerulonephritis Acute interstitial nephritis (AIN) Pyelonephritis
"Muddy-brown casts" or pigmented casts	Acute tubular necrosis (ATN) Myoglobinuria Hemoglobinuria
Eosinophiluria	AIN Atheroembolic disease
Crystals	Uric acid Calcium oxalate (can be seen in ethylene glycol ingestion) Calcium phosphate Triple phosphate Cystine Crystal caused by drugs or toxins (indinavir, acyclovir, amoxicillin)

ATN and prerenal azotemia to represent different points on the same spectrum of response to acute ischemia within the kidneys. However, in addition to diminished perfusion, direct tubular injury can result from inflammation from sepsis or nephrotoxic medications including iodinated contrast, NSAIDs, aminoglycosides, and amphotericin (Table 8.3).

Certain specific diseases can also contribute directly to tubular injury. For example, in some patients with multiple myeloma, monoclonal urinary immunoglobulin light chains (Bence Jones proteins) that are freely filtered can precipitate in the tubular lumen causing intraluminal cast formation and also incite a strong inflammatory reaction that injures tubular epithelia. Clinically, this can mimic ATN, especially since conditions that result in volume depletion can predispose to cast formation. Urinalysis typically shows bland urine sediment and standard urine dipsticks, which detect albumin, do not typically detect light chains. Features

Table 8.3 Drugs associated with AKI

ATN	Antibiotics/antivirals
	Aminoglycosides
	Amphotericin B
	Acyclovir (can also cause crystal formation)
	Indinavir (can also cause crystal formation), tenofovir, cidofovir, adefovir
	Foscarnet
	Pentamidine
	Anti-inflammatory agents
	NSAIDs (including COX-2 inhibitors)
	Immunosuppressive agents
	Cyclosporine
	Tacrolimus
	Chemotherapeutic agents
	Ifosfamide
	Cisplatin
	Organic solvents
	Ethylene glycol (can also cause crystal formation)
	Toluene
	Radiocontrast agents
	Other
	Herbal remedies, acetaminophen
AIN	Antibiotics
	Penicillins
	Cephalosporins
	Sulfamethoxazole
	Ciprofloxacin
	NSAIDs/COX-2 inhibitors
	Loop and thiazide diuretics
	Allopurinol
	Omeprazole
	Phenytoin

that may increase suspicion of myeloma cast nephropathy include ATN without a clear precipitant or out of proportion to the presumed insult in a middle-aged or elderly patient. Accompanying hypercalcemia or anemia, back pain, and/or a history of unexplained CKD should raise suspicion. In these patients, further testing including serum/urine protein electrophoresis, immunofixation, and free light chain assays should be considered. Rhabdomyolysis and gross hemolysis can also cause direct tubular injury due to the release of contents of damaged muscle or red blood cells into the circulation, resulting from trauma, overexertion, autoimmune disease, or associated with medications (e.g., statins). Heme-pigments including myoglobin or hemoglobin are filtered by the glomerulus and degraded with the subsequent release of heme-pigment that can cause direct tubular injury, tubular obstruction, and vasoconstriction. Concurrent volume depletion is an important risk factor in both cases with clinical and laboratory manifestations including decreased urine output, dark urine, elevated creatinine kinase levels (rhabdomyolysis), elevated LDH, low haptoglobin levels (hemolysis), and a urine dipstick that is positive for blood but without obvious red blood cells on microscopy.

Acute interstitial nephritis (AIN) is another subclass of intrinsic kidney injury. AIN is an inflammatory reaction that involves the interstitium of the kidney, the tissue that resides between the tubules. The inflammatory infiltrates generally consist of lymphocytes and monocytes, but plasma cells, eosinophils, and neutrophils may also be present. There is also interstitial edema in sites of inflammatory infiltrate. Medications account for the vast majority of cases of AIN (Table 8.3), with NSAIDs, penicillin antibiotics, and proton-pump inhibitors being common offenders. AIN is also seen rarely as a consequence of infection or systemic disease such as sarcoidosis or Sjögren's syndrome. Physical and laboratory findings consistent with AIN include rash, fever, leukouria, and/or the presence of eosinophils in the blood or urine, though their presence is often variable, as are estimates of their relative and combined diagnostic performance. These observations often make AIN a diagnosis of exclusion. The main treatment of AIN is removal of the offending medication, though steroids may have a limited role. In patients without an obvious cause for AKI, it is important to have a high index of suspicion and a low threshold for discontinuing nonessential medications or using alternatives with less nephrotoxic potential.

Though less common, processes that cause rapid and severe injury to the glomerulus can result in progressive loss of kidney function over days to weeks and constitute a nephrologic emergency. Acute glomerulonephritis (GN) can be caused by numerous different etiologies including autoimmune and infectious contributions (Box 8.3). History should focus on symptoms of vasculitis including arthritis, rash, hemoptysis, serositis, or risk factors for blood-borne viral infections like hepatitis B, C, and human immunodeficiency virus, or endocarditis. Exam findings of uveitis, arthritis, rash, or embolic phenomenon should increase suspicion for potential for glomerulonephritis. On urinalysis, hematuria and/or proteinuria should prompt examination of the urine sediment for dysmorphic red blood cells or red cell casts (Table 8.2), which suggest glomerulonephritis. If proteinuria is detected, a urine spot protein-to-creatinine ratio (PCR) or 24-h protein excretion should be directly quantified. In general, proteinuria >3.5 g/24 h is considered "nephrotic." If a diagnosis of acute GN is being considered, early nephrology consultation should be considered to guide further serologic testing and to facilitate timely tissue diagnosis and treatment.

The constellation of thrombocytopenia, anemia, and kidney dysfunction, with or without fever and central nervous system (CNS) manifestations, should prompt consideration of thrombotic microangiopathy (TMA). TMA is characterized by microangiopathic hemolytic anemia and thrombocytopenia, with kidney dysfunction and CNS symptoms being variable depending on the degree of platelet thrombosis in the microcirculation. Thrombocytopenia occurs from platelet aggregation in

Box 8.3 AKI: Prerenal, Intrinsic, and Postrenal Causes

Prerenal Causes

Intravascular Volume Depletion

Hemorrhage

Renal losses—aggressive diuresis, osmotic diuresis (hyperglycemia)

Increased insensible losses—sweating, burns

GI losses

"Third spacing"—pancreatitis, rhabdomyolysis

Hypercalcemia (also causes renal vasoconstriction)

Decreased Perfusion

Congestive heart failure

Sepsis

Liver failure

Systemic vasodilation/anaphylaxis

Drugs

Antihypertensives

Diuretics

Anesthetics

Vasopressors

Ergotamine

ACE-I or ARBs—in renal artery stenosis or other causes of hypoperfusion

NSAIDs—during kidney hypoperfusion

Vascular

Renal Artery Stenosis

Intrinsic

Acute Tubular Necrosis

Acute Interstitial Nephritis

Medications

Infections

Small-Vessel Disease

Thrombotic microangiopathy, vasculitis, atheroemboli

Glomerular Disease

Lupus

Anti-GBM disease

Membranoproliferative glomerulonephritis (GN)

Postinfectious GN

Infective endocarditis

IgA nephropathy/Henoch-Schonlein purpura

Tubular Obstruction

Cast nephropathy (multiple myeloma)

Stones or crystals

Postrenal

Bladder outlet obstruction

Calculi

Tumors

Retroperitoneal fibrosis

microcirculation. Hemolytic anemia occurs from mechanical stress and fragmentation of RBCs during transit through narrowed vessels. In addition to thrombocytopenia and anemia, other lab findings include elevated bilirubin, elevated LDH, reticulocytosis, and low haptoglobin. Schistocytes are seen on peripheral smear. Hemolytic-uremic syndrome (HUS) predominantly affects children and is characterized by AKI, often associated with diarrheal illness and usually with minimal or no CNS symptoms. Thrombotic thrombocytopenic purpura (TTP) does occur in adults and generally has CNS involvement with variable kidney involvement. Scleroderma and malignant hypertension can also present with TMA.

Lastly, postrenal AKI refers to obstruction to urine flow within the collecting system (kidney, ureters, bladder, or urethra). Obstruction to urine flow can occur via intraluminal (stones, crystals, urethral stricture) or extraluminal (prostate, retroperitoneal fibrosis) causes. Common causes of postrenal AKI in patients with CKD are prostatic obstruction and defects of bladder emptying such as in neurogenic bladder with long-standing diabetes. Additionally, the use of narcotics or antihistamines (which impair bladder emptying) can be problematic in the elderly. In addition to inquiring about symptoms of urinary difficulty (type and duration) and urinary tract infections or nephrolithiasis, providers should also consider recent exposure to medications that can cause urine crystal formation (intravenous acyclovir or indinavir). In patients with a known history of malignancy, a history of prior radiation to the abdomen or pelvis might suggest the possibility of retroperitoneal fibrosis. It is important to note that the absence of oliguria does *not* rule out significant obstruction. Furthermore, bilateral obstruction is not necessary to have significant worsening of kidney function in patients with CKD, as unilateral obstruction can cause significant decline in kidney function when there is underlying parenchymal disease in the contralateral kidney. In addition to physical exam findings of a distended or palpable bladder, noninvasive renal imaging including ultrasound or noncontrasted CT may reveal a dilated collecting system (i.e., hydronephrosis). Imaging should be obtained whenever there is suspicion of obstruction or if AKI is worsening without an obvious cause. However, imaging may not show evidence of obstruction in patients early in the course of obstruction, with concomitant volume depletion, or those with retroperitoneal fibrosis. A simple measure that can be conducted at the bedside is a bladder scan or post-void urine residual. Urine volume greater than 400 ml on a routine bladder scan or a post-void residual volume of greater than 100 ml should prompt workup and management for outflow obstruction. Prompt relief of outflow obstruction can result in rapid improvement in kidney function if addressed early.

8.4.4 General Management Principles

An exhaustive discussion of specific management strategies across the broad spectrum of AKI is beyond the scope of this chapter. However, once the diagnosis of AKI is made, the search for the underlying cause(s) should be accompanied by a simultaneous assessment for evolving complications. Among these include electrolyte abnormalities (e.g., hyperkalemia, hyperphosphatemia, hypocalcemia), acidosis, volume overload, and signs or symptoms of uremia, such as decline in mental status or pericarditis. We recommend early consultation with a nephrologist in patients with evidence of evolving AKI or evidence of complications, as dialytic therapy may soon be required. Concomitantly, interventions to address potentially reversible causes should be applied. In the absence of obvious volume overload, a trial of volume expansion is often reasonable. While both crystalloid and colloid solutions can be used, isotonic crystalloids are recommended except in cases of hemorrhagic shock [2]. We recommend avoiding starch-based solutions given evolving evidence that they may be associated with the development of AKI. There is no established role for the use of diuretics in *prevention* of AKI. However, if volume overload is thought to be

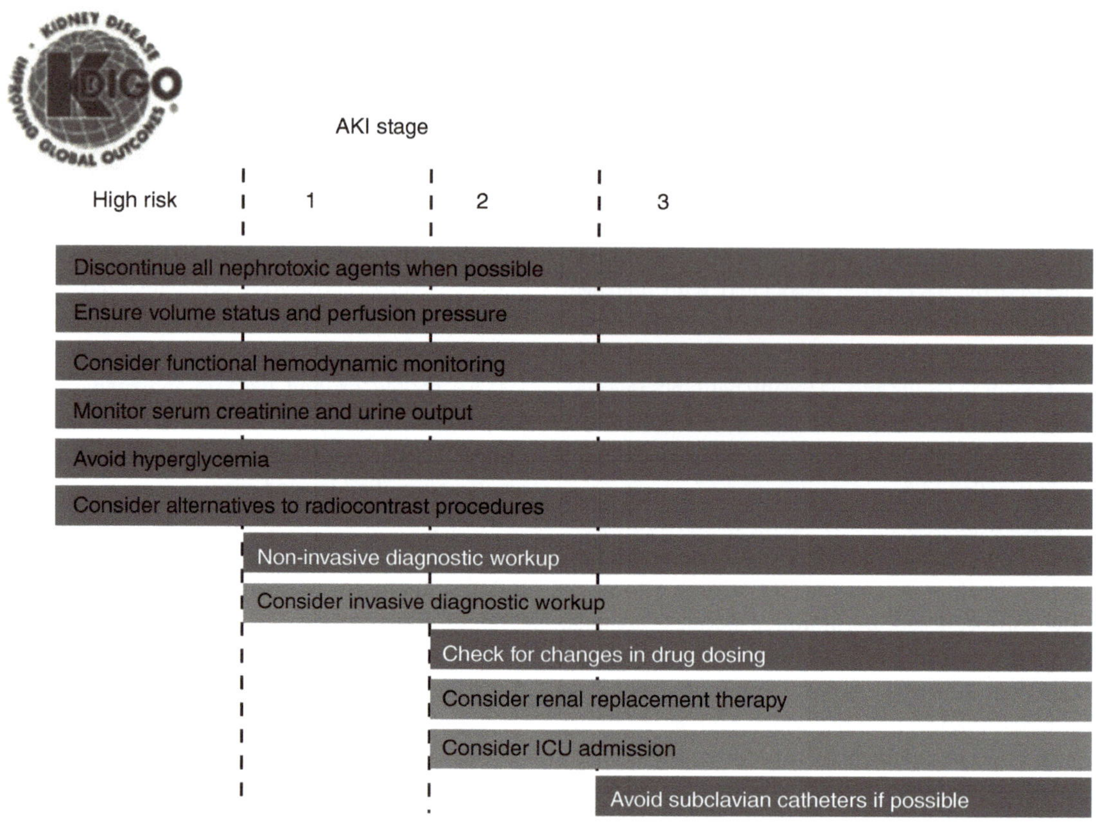

Fig. 8.9 Stage-based management of AKI. *Shading of boxes* indicates priority of action—*solid shading* indicates actions that are equally appropriate at all stages, whereas *graded shading* indicates increasing priority as intensity increases. *AKI* acute kidney injury, *ICU* intensive care unit (Reprinted with permission from Macmillan Publishers Ltd: Kidney Disease: Improving Global Outcomes (KDIGO) [2])

contributing to or complicating the AKI (e.g., congestive heart failure), loop diuretics can be used and are more effective than monotherapy with thiazide diuretics. KDIGO proposes a stage-based approach to the management of AKI, shown in Fig. 8.9. However, we would add that consideration for dose adjustment of drugs as well as the need for renal replacement therapy (RRT) should occur at all stages of AKI and be individualized to each patient. Further, as the optimal care of patients following AKI has not been established, we feel that greater attention for follow-up of patients with AKI shortly after discharge should focus on patients with persistent or moderate to severe injury (KDIGO stages II and III).

It is important to note that estimation of eGFR assumes a "steady state" of glomerular filtration. Thus, eGFR during acute changes in kidney function can misrepresent true GFR. The elevation in creatinine lags behind initial changes in eGFR. Consequently, the trend in creatinine should be considered when interpreting GFR, and if the creatinine trend is increasing, there should be an understanding that the actual GFR is less than the calculated GFR. This is important to keep in mind with medication dosing, particularly with potentially nephrotoxic medications such as vancomycin and aminoglycosides. We would recommend conservative dosing of potentially nephrotoxic medications, cautious use of scheduled dosing in drugs with a narrow therapeutic window, and more frequent measurement of drug levels to guide additional dosing. Some common medications that accumulate with compromised kidney function are listed in Table 8.4.

Table 8.4 Drugs with potentially toxic accumulation in AKI or CKD

Drug	Clinical manifestations of accumulation
Allopurinol	Leukopenia, increased risk for immune-mediated hypersensitivity reaction
Codeine/morphine	Respiratory depression, CNS depression
Propoxyphene	Dysrhythmia
Midazolam	Drowsiness, sedation, apnea
Meperidine	Tremor, agitation, anxiety, myoclonus, seizure
Enoxaparin	Increased risk of bleeding
Succinylcholine	Hyperkalemia

8.4.5 Renal Replacement Therapy (RRT)

Patients whose injury appears progressive or not readily reversible may require dialysis. The optimal timing for initiation of dialysis in patients with AKI is not defined. Currently, the decision to initiate RRT is based on averting or treating complications of AKI including azotemia, hyperkalemia, metabolic acidosis, and volume overload. The process of dialysis itself carries the risk of hypotension and arrhythmia. The anticoagulation process for RRT with heparinization carries bleeding risk, and anticoagulation with regional citrate introduces risk of significant electrolyte abnormalities. Temporary vascular access via catheter for RRT carries risk of bleeding, infection, pneumothorax (with internal jugular catheters), and subsequent central venous stenosis. Balancing the risks and benefits is complex, and we recommend early consultation with a nephrologist to facilitate decision-making.

8.4.6 Special Considerations for the Hospitalized Patient with AKI or CKD

There are some special considerations that should be given to patients with CKD who experience AKI. It is preferable to avoid nephrotoxins including IV contrast dye (e.g., CT with iodinated contrast) in patients with CKD. Additionally, in patients with significantly impaired kidney function (GFR <30 ml/min/1.73 m^2), MRI with gadolinium contrast should be avoided due to the rare but serious potential consequence of nephrogenic systemic fibrosis. Standard electrolyte repletion protocols should be avoided in patients with CKD and with AKI in CKD, as they can result in overcorrection in patients with impaired excretion. In patients with advanced CKD who may need future permanent vascular access for dialysis, an assessment of the patient's nondominant arm should be ascertained. Per KDOQI Guidelines for Vascular Access, permanent vascular access is preferably placed in the patient's nondominant arm to minimize negative impact on quality of life. Full discussion of access planning is beyond the scope of this chapter, but prior central venous access placement resulting in central venous stenosis (e.g., extremity edema or evidence of collateral veins) or presence of cardiac pacemaker device on the nondominant side may preclude vascular access placement in the nondominant arm. In general, we recommend avoiding blood pressure measurement, blood draws, peripheral intravenous access, or peripherally inserted central catheters (PICC) in the arm in which vascular access is planned, as vascular trauma can decrease the likelihood of successful dialysis access placement in the future. Additionally, subclavian central catheters should generally be avoided due to the risk for subsequent central venous stenosis, which can hinder successful creation of arteriovenous fistula or graft placement on the ipsilateral side. Lastly, transfusion of blood products, while often necessary, should be carefully considered in patients who may be eligible for renal transplantation in the future as exposure to and development of preformed antibodies targeting human leukocyte antigen may hinder future organ matching.

8.4.7 Following AKI: At the Time of Discharge and Beyond

As AKI is an important risk factor for both subsequent AKI and accelerated progression of CKD, determining how to best care for these patients will become increasingly important. Per the KDIGO Clinical Practice Guidelines for Acute Kidney Injury, "patients should be evaluated 3 months after AKI for resolution, new onset or worsening of pre-existing CKD [2]". Recent data have indicated that patients with persistent kidney dysfunction following an AKI event are infrequently seen by nephrologists in the year following AKI. Whether this results in lack of receipt of established standards of care such as timely vascular access for dialysis or transplant referral or risk factor management is unknown. Until we can reliably predict which AKI survivors will develop CKD, we recommend that patients who survive an episode of AKI, particularly if severe or sustained, be followed regularly to assess for early evidence of CKD (i.e., development of hypertension, proteinuria, or reduced eGFR) and to determine if the risk for future injury can be reduced.

8.4.8 Novel Biomarkers in the Diagnosis of AKI

The current gold standard for diagnosis of AKI is based on changes in serum creatinine, making the diagnosis of AKI retrospective. Creatinine alone does not distinguish between prerenal azotemia and true parenchymal damage, nor does it segregate the critical aspects of injury—type of injury, onset, and causation. These limitations have prompted the American Society of Nephrology (ASN) to deem the discovery and standardization of AKI biomarkers with early diagnostic and prognostic potential a *top-priority* research area [26]. Several urine and serum candidate biomarkers have shown promise in specific patient populations with defined cause and timing of injury. Preclinical models have identified these candidate markers as serving a functional (i.e., enzymatic or inflammatory) and/or structural role within renal tubular epithelia, or as low molecular weight proteins filtered by the glomerulus and/or metabolized by healthy tubular epithelia. The native functions of these markers situate them in various intracellular locations or on the plasma membrane. In commonly used animal models of AKI including ischemia-reperfusion or nephrotoxic injury, these markers are actively released or shed in either free or membrane bound form (exosomes) into the urine following tubular damage. Serum/plasma markers, particularly low molecular weight proteins normally filtered by the kidney, have also been studied. Their usefulness in diagnosing and predicting the course of AKI in different patient populations is being investigated. At present, there is insufficient evidence to recommend their routine use in the clinical care of patients.

Conclusion

In summary, the incidence of AKI is increasing and associated with increased morbidity and mortality. AKI is now recognized as a risk factor for progressive CKD. Additionally, patients with CKD are at increased risk for development of AKI due to structural and functional abnormalities, comorbidities, need for invasive procedures, and multiple medications. Patients with rapid progression to ESRD often have courses marked by decline in kidney function due to one or more episodes of AKI. It is important to identify and counsel patients at risk for AKI and to employ risk reduction measures *prior* to the development of AKI. A rapid assessment for reversible causes of AKI should occur, especially in patients with CKD, and treatment aimed at timely optimization of volume and hemodynamic status should be pursued. Early consultation with a nephrologist is indicated if the cause is not immediately clear, evidence of progressive AKI or the complications emerge, or if a tissue diagnosis is required. Finally, patients who experience AKI should be followed for the resolution of AKI and evaluated for development or progression of CKD.

Before You Finish: Practice Pearls for the Clinician

- Check eGFR and proteinuria before exposures to nephrotoxins and high-risk procedures to better identify patients at risk for AKI in whom risk reduction strategies may be helpful.
- Discuss long-term goals of care (including whether to initiate dialysis) *before hospitalization*.
- Obtain pre-hospitalization "baseline" serum creatinine, if possible, to better define kidney function.
- As the rise in creatinine tends to lag behind the inciting injury, focus your search for the underlying cause in the hours to days before creatinine starts to rise.
- The trend in eGFR during evolving or recovering AKI will be more useful for guiding drug dosing than a single eGFR value.
- A high FeNa may not exclude prerenal azotemia in the patient with CKD and AKI.
- Starch-based crystalloid solutions, phosphate-containing cathartics, NSAIDS, and meperidine should be avoided in patients with CKD or AKI.
- Avoid subclavian lines and peripherally inserted central catheters (PICC) to preserve future dialysis access in hospitalized patients with CKD or severe AKI.
- As patients with CKD who experience AKI may be at high risk for progression to ESRD, prior episodes of AKI in the patient's medical history should be documented.
- After an episode of moderate to severe AKI or those where recovery to baseline has not occurred, patients should be evaluated within 3 months for resolution or for new onset or worsening of CKD.

Conflict of Interest Dr. Edward Siew has consulting agreements with Abbvie and Alere, Inc.

References

1. Coca SG, Singanamala S, Parikh CR. Chronic kidney disease after acute kidney injury: a systematic review and meta-analysis. Kidney Int. 2011;81(5):442–8.
2. Kidney Disease: Improving Global Outcomes (KDIGO). KDIGO clinical practice guideline for acute kidney injury. Kidney Int Suppl. 2012;2:1–138.
3. Ricci Z, Cruz D, Ronco C. The RIFLE criteria and mortality in acute kidney injury: a systematic review. Kidney Int. 2007;73(5):538–46.
4. Lafrance JP, Miller DR. Acute kidney injury associates with increased long-term mortality. J Am Soc Nephrol. 2010;21(2):345–52.
5. Hsu CY, McCulloch CE, Fan D, Ordoez JD. Community-based incidence of acute renal failure. Kidney Int. 2007;72(2):208–12.
6. Uchino S, Kellum JA, Bellomo R, Doig GS, Morimatsu H, Morgera S, et al. Acute renal failure in critically ill patients: a multinational, multicenter study. JAMA. 2005;294(7):813–8.
7. Fliser D, Laville M, Covic A, Fouque D, Vanholder R, Juillard L, Van Biesen W' ad-hoc working group of ERBP. A European Renal Best Practice (ERBP) position statement on the Kidney Disease Improving Global Outcomes (KDIGO) Clinical Practice Guidelines on Acute Kidney Injury. Nephrol Dial Transplant. 2012;27(12):4263–72.
8. Jörres A, John S, Lewington A, ter Wee PM, Vanholder R, Van Biesen W, Tattersall J. ad-hoc working group of ERBP. Position statement and update of the KDIGO AKI guidelines now available on ERPB website. Nephrol Dial Transplant. 2013;28(12):2940–45. Available at: http://www.european-renal-best-practice.org/content/position-statement-and-update-kdigo-aki-guidelines-now-available-erbp-website.
9. Lewington A, Kanagasundaram S. The Renal Association Guideline. Acute kidney injury – final version (8 Mar 2011). Available at: http://www.renal.org/clinical/guidelinessection/AcuteKidneyInjury.aspx.
10. National Institute for Health and Clinical Excellence (NICE) guideline CG169 acute kidney injury: prevention, detection and management of acute kidney injury up to the point of renal replacement therapy. Issued: Aug 2013. Available at: http://publications.nice.org.uk/acute-kidney-injury-cg169.
11. James M, Bouchard J, Ho J, Klarenbach S, LaFrance JP, Rigatto C, Wald R, Zappitelli M, Pannu N. Canadian Society of Nephrology commentary on the 2012 KDIGO clinical practice guideline for acute kidney injury. Am J Kidney Dis. 2013;61(5):673–85.

12. Palevsky PM, Liu KD, Brophy PD, Chawla LS, Parikh CR, Thakar CV, Tolwani AJ, Waikar SS, Weisbord SD. KDOQI US commentary on the 2012 KDIGO clinical practice guideline for acute kidney injury. Am J Kidney Dis. 2013;61(5):649–72. Available at: http://www.kidney.org/Professionals/kdoqi/pdf/AKI-Commentary-2013.pdf.
13. Hsu CY, Ordonez JD, Chertow GM, Fan D, McCulloch CE, Go AS. The risk of acute renal failure in patients with chronic kidney disease. Kidney Int. 2008;74(1):101–7.
14. Grams ME, Astor BC, Bash LD, Matsushita K, Wang Y, Coresh J. Albuminuria and estimated glomerular filtration rate independently associate with acute kidney injury. J Am Soc Nephrol. 2010;21(10):1757–64.
15. James MT, Hemmelgarn BR, Wiebe N, Pannu N, Manns BJ, Klarenbach SW, et al. Glomerular filtration rate, proteinuria, and the incidence and consequences of acute kidney injury: a cohort study. Lancet. 2010;376(9758):2096–103.
16. Chawla LS, Kimmel PL. Acute kidney injury and chronic kidney disease: an integrated clinical syndrome. Kidney Int. 2012;82(5):516–24.
17. Garg AX, Salvadori M, Okell JM, Thiessen-Philbrook HR, Suri RS, Filler G, et al. Albuminuria and estimated GFR 5 years after Escherichia coli O157 hemolytic uremic syndrome: an update. Am J Kidney Dis. 2008;51(3):435–44.
18. Ishani A, Xue JL, Himmelfarb J, Eggers PW, Kimmel PL, Molitoris BA, et al. Acute kidney injury increases risk of ESRD among elderly. J Am Soc Nephrol. 2009;20(1):223–8.
19. Lo LJ, Go AS, Chertow GM, McCulloch CE, Fan D, Ordo JD, et al. Dialysis-requiring acute renal failure increases the risk of progressive chronic kidney disease. Kidney Int. 2009;76(8):893–9.
20. Bucaloiu ID, Kirchner HL, Norfolk ER, Hartle 2nd JE, Perkins RM. Increased risk of death and de novo chronic kidney disease following reversible acute kidney injury. Kidney Int. 2012;81(5):477–85.
21. Ishani A, Nelson D, Clothier B, Schult T, Nugent S, Greer N, et al. The magnitude of acute serum creatinine increase after cardiac surgery and the risk of chronic kidney disease, progression of kidney disease, and death. Arch Intern Med. 2011;171(3):226–33.
22. Coca SG, King Jr JT, Rosenthal RA, Perkal MF, Parikh CR. The duration of postoperative acute kidney injury is an additional parameter predicting long-term survival in diabetic veterans. Kidney Int. 2010;78(9):926–33.
23. Chawla LS, Amdur RL, Amodeo S, Kimmel PL, Palant CE. The severity of acute kidney injury predicts progression to chronic kidney disease. Kidney Int. 2011;79(12):1361–9.
24. Thakar CV, Christianson A, Himmelfarb J, Leonard AC. Acute kidney injury episodes and chronic kidney disease risk in diabetes mellitus. Clin J Am Soc Nephrol. 2011;6(11):2567–72.
25. Kurella Tamura M, Covinsky KE, Chertow GM, Yaffe K, Landefeld CS, McCulloch CE. Functional status of elderly adults before and after initiation of dialysis. N Engl J Med. 2009;361(16):1539–47.
26. American Society of Nephrology. American Society of Nephrology Renal Research Report. J Am Soc Nephrol. 2005;16(7):1886–903.

9 Preventing Progression of Chronic Kidney Disease: Diet and Lifestyle

Merlin C. Thomas

Before You Start: Facts You Need to Know

- Patients with chronic kidney disease are often recommended to undergo a comprehensive assessment of their diet and lifestyle as part of their overall management strategy.
- Diet and lifestyle modifications are considered to be the cornerstone for the prevention and management of diabetes and hypertension.
- Most patients believe that changes in their diet and lifestyle are among the most important interventions for the management of their kidney disease.
- Most nephrologists are not trained in diet and lifestyle management and are unfamiliar with techniques to institute sustained and effective changes and the potential for adverse outcomes.

M.C. Thomas, MBChB, PhD, FRACP
Department of Biochemistry of Diabetes Complications, Baker IDI Heart and Diabetes Institute, St Kilda Rd Central, 6492, Melbourne, VIC 8008, Australia
e-mail: mthomas@bakeridi.edu.au

9.1 Diet and Lifestyle in the Management of Chronic Kidney Disease

All the major forms of chronic kidney disease contain elements of diet and lifestyle in their pathogenesis. The most obvious is kidney damage caused by type 2 diabetes, the major single cause of end-stage renal disease (ESRD) in western countries and rapidly growing in developing countries as the epidemic of diabetes extends across the world. Fundamentally, diabetic nephropathy cannot occur in the absence of diabetes, which can be placed into remission (or possibly cured) by sustained weight loss associated with very low-calorie diets or bariatric surgery. This should prevent nephropathy or at the very least slow its progression as is suggested by the reduction in urinary albumin excretion observed in some patients following bariatric surgery. Similarly, the development and progression of hypertension are strongly associated with diet and lifestyle factors including caloric excess, inactivity and smoking. Moreover, improvements in these factors (e.g. with the DASH programme) are associated with improvements in both blood pressure control and reductions in markers of kidney damage.

But while the efficacy of diet and lifestyle is established for the primary prevention of diabetes and hypertension, their effects are more modest than first hoped. Indeed the recent Look AHEAD trial was stopped because of futility. It is even less clear what the best strategy is for patients

M. Arici (ed.), *Management of Chronic Kidney Disease*,
DOI 10.1007/978-3-642-54637-2_9,

with established kidney damage. Moreover, the restrictions imposed by adherence may be associated with unwanted side effects and a reduced quality of life in precisely those patients who have the worst life expectancy. This chapter reviews some of the manoeuvres that are often recommended to patients with CKD, including their possible benefits and disadvantages. The specific dietary management of kidney stone disease is beyond the scope of this chapter.

9.2 Should Patients with CKD Restrict Their Intake of Protein?

When considering slowing the progression of kidney disease by dietary intervention, protein restriction is traditionally the first that comes to mind for most nephrologists. Dietary protein has a range of actions on kidney function. In particular, a high protein intake induces preglomerular (afferent) arteriolar vasodilatation and hyperfiltration, possibly by activating tubuloglomerular feedback as a result of increased proximal tubular sodium reabsorption. By restricting protein intake, it is hoped to increase afferent arteriolar tone and protect the kidney from haemodynamic stress. At a time when there was little or no RAAS blockade available, this was perceived as the best way to target renal haemodynamics and their role in progressive kidney damage.

But while renoprotective effects are clearly observed in experiential models of kidney disease, the effects of dietary protein restriction in patients with CKD remain controversial. Some studies have observed a modest but significant effect on proteinuria and slowing of the rate of decline in kidney function, especially but not only in patients with type 1 diabetes [1]. Whether low-protein diets also improve hard kidney outcomes remains to be established. One trial in patients with type 1 diabetes suggested a reduction in mortality [2], although this may be more of a reflection of dietary compliance or other changes in the composition of the diet than protein restriction itself.

At the same time, long-term adherence to a low-protein diet can be difficult outside of a trial setting, especially if fat content is also restricted (see below), meaning that such diets must be high in carbohydrate (which has its own challenges especially in patients with CKD and diabetes). Alternatively, all elements must be reduced which increases the risk of malnutrition, especially in catabolic patients with uraemia. The utility of protein restriction is also problematic as it is unusual for patients with CKD to be consuming high-protein diets, outside of fad weight loss diets which should be discouraged in patients with CKD. In fact it may be that protein intake is naturally reduced with progressive kidney disease as part of a homeostatic response to CKD on appetite control centres. Intake of protein in the normal range does not appear to be associated with the development or progression of CKD. In the absence of definitive data, protein restriction is not currently recommended to most patients with CKD.

There is also a widely held belief that eating vegetable protein is better than animal protein in patients with CKD. This is not because of the protein itself, but rather the other food components including fat, fibre, minerals and vitamins which also potentially impact on health and wellbeing. One crossover study suggested that the addition of vegetable protein was not associated with GFR decline while animal protein intake was associated with progressive decline in kidney function [3]. At the same time many plant protein sources can be high in potassium and/or phosphorus, meaning every diet must be individualised.

9.3 Should Patients with CKD Restrict Their Intake of Phosphorus?

Disturbances of mineral metabolism are commonplace in patients with CKD, including increased phosphorus retention and hyperphosphataemia which generally occurs as the GFR falls below 20 ml/min/1.73 m^2. That it does not occur before this is due to activation of compen-

Box 9.1. Foods Naturally High in Phosphate (Which Should Be Avoided or Eaten in Small Amounts in Patients with CKD When Serum Phosphate or PTH Levels Are Elevated?)

Drinks: beer, milk, cocoa, cola

Dairy products: cheese, custard, yogurt, ice cream

High-protein foods: meat, liver, shellfish, legumes (beans and peas), nuts and seeds, whole-grain products

satory pathways that promote phosphate loss, including secondary hyperparathyroidism and activation of fibroblast growth factor 23 (FGF23). Restriction of dietary phosphate in proportion to the reduction in GFR in patients with CKD can prevent the development of excessive parathyroid hormone (PTH) levels, and phosphate restriction (to less than 1 g a day) is generally recommended to most patients with CKD when serum phosphate or PTH levels are elevated. This is usually achieved by restriction of dairy products and protein intake (Box 9.1). However, it is possible to restrict protein without fully restricting phosphorus, so careful selection of protein sources must also be undertaken. The rationale for phosphate restriction in the absence of disturbances of mineral metabolisms is unclear and is not generally recommended in patients with early-stage CKD.

Box 9.2. Foods Naturally High in Potassium (Which Should Be Avoided or Eaten in Small Amounts in Patients with CKD at Risk of Hyperkalaemia?)

Grains
- Whole-grain breads, wheat bran, granola and granola bars

Dairy products
- Milk and milk products

Drinks
- Sports drinks, energy drinks, vegetable juices, soy milk

Snack foods/sweets
- Peanut butter, nuts or seeds, chocolate, dried fruit

Fruits
- Stone fruit (e.g. apricots, avocado, dates, prunes, mango, papaya, cherries), bananas, kiwifruit, coconut, melon, nectarines, oranges, pears, pomegranate

Vegetables
- Tomatoes and tomato products, raw brassica (e.g. broccoli, Brussels sprouts, cabbage greens), carrots, olives, legumes (e.g. pinto beans, kidney beans, black beans, baked beans, peas) potatoes, pumpkins, parsnips

Seafood
- Shellfish, lobster, whitefish, salmon

Beef
- Ground beef, sirloin steak (and most other beef products)

9.4 Should Patients with CKD Restrict Their Intake of Potassium?

Hyperkalaemia is a common finding in patients with chronic kidney disease, especially in those with diabetes and those using beta blockers or RAAS blockers alone or in combination. Excessive levels of potassium may contribute to bradycardia, severe muscle weakness, paralysis or even sudden death in some patients. However, it is also argued that an elevation in potassium may be an adaptive response to renal impairment, to augment renal potassium excretion and thereby reduce its accumulation. Moreover, some studies suggest that patients with a potassium in mild to moderate hyperkalaemia (5–5.5 mol/l) may have a lower risk of dying than those with low or even low-normal potassium levels (<4 mmol/l) [4]. Most patients with CKD are advised to reduce their intake of foods that are rich in potassium (Box 9.2) and aim to eat less than 2.4 g of potassium per day as a means to avoid dangerous hyperkalaemia. This is usually achieved by choosing lower-potassium fruit and vegetables and their juices (Box 9.3)

Box 9.3. Foods Naturally Low in Potassium (Which Should Be Preferred in Patients with CKD at Risk of Hyperkalaemia?)

Foods prepared with white flour (e.g. pasta, bread)
White rice
Fruits: apples, watermelon, berries (e.g. blackberries, blueberries, cranberries, raspberries, strawberries)
Vegetables: cauliflower, asparagus, zucchini, spinach, corn, onions
Meat: chicken, turkey, tuna, eggs
Dairy products: Cheddar, Swiss or cottage cheese

and limiting the intake of milk, legumes, nuts, tomatoes and stone fruit. Many products now provide potassium content as part of their nutritional information, allowing patients to choose the lower-potassium alternatives.

9.5 Should Obese Patients with CKD Lose Weight (Through a Reduced Calorie Diet)?

The majority of adult patients with CKD are overweight or obese, reflecting the key role of the accumulation of ectopic fat in the development of diabetes, hypertension and atherosclerotic vascular disease, the major causes of CKD. But even outside these obvious settings, more and more of our patients with glomerular diseases and other renal pathology are overweight or obese. This may be considered part of a global trend for all adults to progressively gain weight over their lifetime, amplified by the reduced physical activity associated with chronic illness (see below). Put together, obesity is now an everyday companion for the nephrologist. But should we be doing something about it?

Obesity itself may be associated with focal and segmental glomerulosclerosis, possibly due to changes in intraglomerular haemodynamics induced by obesity. In observational studies, weight gain is independently associated with incident CKD, even after adjusting for blood pressure and incident diabetes [5]. In clinical trials, weight loss clearly results in reduction in blood pressure, especially in patients already taking antihypertensive drug treatment like many of those with CKD. Moreover, amongst overweight patients with chronic kidney disease, weight loss interventions may be associated with a decrease in albuminuria. In a cohort of Dutch patients from the Prevention of Renal and Vascular Endstage Disease (PREVEND) study, weight loss was associated with a reduction in urinary albumin excretion [6]. None of these studies provide sufficient evidence that weight loss diets should be recommended to obese patients with CKD to protect kidney function. However, broad effects of obesity on cardiovascular health, sleep, cancer, mood, wound healing, self image and a myriad of other areas means that most obese patients with CKD should be encouraged to lose weight, chiefly through dieting.

Fundamentally, weight loss diets aim to provide less food energy (measured as calories or kilojoules) than is required for metabolism and daily energy expenditure (known as a negative energy balance). The daily energy requirement can be roughly calculated (Box 9.3). To lose weight, the energy intake must be less than that of the daily energy requirement. Most weight loss diets start at an energy deficit of about 500 kcal/day. For example, if you calculate your patient's energy requirement as 8,000 kJ a day, to slowly lose weight, they can target 7,500 kJ/day. This will generally achieve a weight loss rate of approximately 1 lb (~0.5 kg) per week.

Reducing the amount of energy obtained from the diet can be achieved in any number of different ways. There is no 'one size fits all' approach, which means a comprehensive diet and lifestyle assessment by a trained dietician is an important first step. Sometimes only minor changes are required to reduce the energy content of a diet. For example, the energy in a can of Coke is around 500 kJ. So to lose the weight, subtracting a can a day may be all that it takes.

The most common way to reduce energy intake is to go on a diet. This means regulating some or all of food intake according to a formula, recipe book or strategy. Whether the composition of a diet affects how well it produces weight loss remains highly contentious. Rigorous head-to-head studies of different diets have failed to show any superiority of one over another. On average they all achieve about the same amount of weight loss of 2–4 kg. It may be that what they are eating is probably not as important as the fact that they are adhering to some sort of plan for what they eat. It is likely that the mere process of embracing any dietary restrictions, thinking about and coordinating the foods they eat, makes them tend to eat less (energy) and eat better.

Diets that promote weight loss can be broadly divided into four categories, which restrict one element while at the same time ignoring all others (for the sake of simplicity and compliance):

Low-fat diets – (e.g. STEP, Pritikin and Ornish diets) reduce energy from fat, without reducing meals. Reducing the fat in the diet can also improve lipid levels (see below). However, reducing fat often means increasing the content of carbohydrate and/or protein in the diet which may have drawbacks in insulin-resistant patients with CKD.

Low-carbohydrate diets (e.g. Atkins diet) – are popular for the management of type 2 diabetes, because of their beneficial effects on glucose control as well as caloric intake. There are a range of other diets that share roughly the same principles with respect to carbohydrate but vary in regard to other nutrients (e.g. fat or protein). For example, the Atkins diet does not restrict the (animal) fat you eat, while the CSIRO Total Wellbeing Diet and the 'Zone diet' reduce both fat and carbohydrate in your diet, so the relative proportion of energy from protein goes up. While this can have the added effect of suppressing hunger and promoting your sense of fullness earlier in the meal, it may also have adverse effects in the kidney and is therefore not generally recommended to patients with CKD.

Low-energy diets (e.g. DASH diet and Weight Watchers) – specifically target the problem of too much energy in the diet, by focusing on reducing the intake of processed 'energy-dense' foods exchanging them for low-calorie substitutes without focusing on diet composition. This strategy is generally preferred in obese patients with CKD and can be readily achieved by calorie counting, meal substitutes or following recipe plans.

Low-GI diets – (e.g. New Glucose Revolution, South Beach diet) have also become popular as a means to both slow the delivery of carbohydrate for meals and induce weight loss. How quickly will food cause a rise in blood glucose levels (called the glycaemic index (GI)), when compared to just eating straight glucose (which has a GI of 100)? High-GI (>70) foods such as white bread, potatoes or corn flakes break down their sugars quickly during digestion requiring insulin to surge in response to the extra demand. Over and above the extra energy they contain, a diet rich in high-GI foods is strongly associated with weight gain. By contrast, low-GI (<55) foods deliver their sugar load more slowly, so the demands on the pancreas are not so steep and fat accumulation is reduced. It is thought that low-GI diets may assist weight control by improving satiety and hunger between meals as slow sugars continue to be absorbed well after a meal.

9.6 Should All Patients with CKD Be on a Low-Fat Diet?

There is strong evidence that the presence and severity of dyslipidaemia is associated with the risk of progressive kidney disease in both diabetic and nondiabetic kidney diseases. Whether dyslipidaemia is a marker of kidney dysfunction or a mediator of progressive damage remains to be firmly established. Certainly a renal phenotype is not seen in familial hypercholesterolemia or familial mixed dyslipidaemia that would suggest its primary role in kidney injury. However, treatment with statins may reduce urinary albumin excretion and has been shown to slow the rate of decline of GFR (in some but not all studies and with some but not all agents). In each case, these renal benefits were not correlated with improvements in lipid levels leading to the argument that any renal actions are pleiotropic effects of statins rather than the result of lipid lowering. Yet, because of the high cardiovascular risk and clear benefits of lipid lowering on cardiovascular outcomes in patients with CKD (not on dialysis), most patients will be recommended to reduce their lipid levels. This usually takes the form of statin therapy in combination with dietary modification whether or not patients are overweight.

There is some observational data to suggest dietary fat may be associated with progressive kidney disease. For example, in one study the nutritional pattern of diabetic patients progressing from normoalbuminuria from microalbuminuria was characterised by greater intake of saturated fat and a reduced intake of polyunsaturated and monounsaturated fat [7]. Moreover, these lipid differences are also characteristic of diets associated with hypertension, weight gain and insulin resistance, all of which may contribute to progressive kidney disease. Ultimately, all patients with CKD may be considered at significant risk of CVD, meaning that regardless on any kidney effects, a reduced intake of saturated fat should be recommended for vasculoprotection.

9.7 Should Patients with CKD Restrict Their Intake of Salt?

Urinary sodium retention is a major contributor to hypertension in patients with chronic kidney disease. Consequently, limiting the dietary intake of sodium appears a logical and appealing intervention for the prevention and management of hypertension in patients with CKD. Most guidelines suggest patients should target an intake of <60 mmol/day, equivalent to about one third or normal salt intake in the general public. However, this target remains controversial. The dietary intake of sodium represents only a small fraction of the filtered sodium load (<1 %), so its effects on renal load are minimal. Any reduction in sodium intake is also associated with activation of sodium retention pathways including the RAAS and sympathetic nervous system, which may be counterproductive in the setting of CKD. The anticipated reduction in blood pressure from sodium restriction (1–3 mmHg in a trial setting) is also much lower and more variable than that achieved by antihypertensive therapy, and if blood pressure control is desired, it may be more effectively achieved by medications. Finally, the long-term benefits of sodium restriction in patients with CKD remain unclear. One study in patients with type 1 diabetes and macroalbuminuria suggested that a low sodium intake was associated with an increased risk of progression to ESRD [8]. By contrast, short-term studies have suggested clear additive benefits on both blood pressure and albuminuria when sodium restriction is added to patients with CKD already on RAAS blockers [9]. This may be because the RAAS is the chief counter-regulatory response to sodium restriction, and blocking it prevents escape. Consequently, it is reasonable to consider that RAAS blockade should be given to any patients adhering to a low-salt diet and a low-salt diet be considered for any patient on RAAS blockade, because of this synergism. In practice this means a low-sodium diet is appropriate for most patients with CKD.

9.8 Should Patients with CKD Be Undertaking Regular Physical Activity?

Inactive people have an increased risk of developing kidney disease compared with very active people. Most patients with CKD are sedentary, undertaking little physical activity on a regular basis. Although physical activity can improve blood pressure, lipid, glucose and weight control and alleviate their mood status, it is seldom stressed as an intervention in patients with CKD. This is most because of reduced exercise tolerance and comorbidity, such as hypoglycaemia, anaemia, postural dizziness, foot disease and cardiovascular disease. Indeed so many patients with CKD have established CVD or risk factors for it that vigorous activity is usually contraindicated. However, this does not mean that moderate activity is inappropriate or unhelpful. Indeed even in patients with established CVD, a programme of regular moderate physical activity is associated with improved clinical outcomes.

Unfortunately, only limited research has been undertaken on the effects of exercise in the management of patients with CKD. Some trials have reported improvement in albuminuria following initiation of exercise programmes [10], implying kidney benefits, although this could reflect better haemodynamic control. Particular advantages have also been ascribed to resistance exercise programmes and swimming. However, patients must be carefully selected, given their often extensive comorbidity.

9.9 Should Patients with CKD Give Up Drinking Alcohol?

Many patients believe that excessive alcohol intake is a common cause of chronic kidney disease (largely because of its obvious polyuric effects). Indeed, many patients believe that moderating or giving up their drinking is the most important way to protect kidney function. Certainly, a high intake of alcohol (>5 units per day in men) is associated with an increased risk of cardiovascular disease, hypertension, cancer and other health problems including chronic kidney disease. However, whether this association is confounded by the adverse lifestyle of heavy drinkers remains to be fully established. Moreover, any independent link between alcohol intake and kidney impairment has not been observed in all studies, with some reporting an inverse association between GFR and alcohol intake. Overall, the J-shaped association between alcohol intake and adverse health outcomes (such that abstainers have an increased risk of some health problems compared to those who regularly drink 1–3 units every day) means that abstinence need not be recommended to patients with CKD. So where patients can maintain control of their drinking, this habit should not be discouraged. However, binge drinking may be potentially more dangerous in patients with CKD [11], in whom distinguishing illness from drunken behaviours can be life-saving. So sometimes it is better to quit while you are ahead.

9.10 All Smokers with CKD Should Be Encouraged to Stop Smoking

There is clear evidence that smoking is a risk factor for progressive kidney disease. Inhaled toxins and generated reactive oxygen species pass to the kidney as well as to other parts of the body where they are both directly injurious and amplify injurious processes including inflammation and fibrosis in the kidney. Smoking also results in neurohormonal surges that may be particularly injuries to stiff vascular architecture that characterises patients with CKD. There is some data to suggest that smoking cessation reduces the rate of loss of kidney function amongst patients with progressive kidney disease [10]. At the same time, some studies have reported acute increases in urinary albumin excretion 6 months after quitting [12]. This may be similar to the increase in diabetes and weight gain also observed with smoking cessation, which abates and ultimately leads to reduction in the long term. The long-term effects of smoking cessation on kidney function remain to be established but appear to be positive [13]. However, the heightened cardiovascular risk in patients with CKD means that smoking cessation should be recommended in all cases regardless of its potential renal actions.

9.11 Does Lifestyle Matter at All in Patients with CKD?

More evidence is needed regarding the best approach to diet and lifestyle in patients with CKD. This cannot be simply extrapolated from patients without CKD, as the complex effects of comorbid illness, polypharmacy and the uremic milieu itself each present their own challenges. Overall there is little data that initiating comprehensive changes in diet and lifestyle is able to protect kidney function while at the same time exposing patients to significant restrictions associated with compliance (Box 9.4). Many of these patients can anticipate very poor clinical outcomes, so quality of life is also often an important consideration. Stopping alcohol and changing the composition of the diet remove some of life's pleasures and need not be instituted in every patient. By contrast, smoking cessation should be reiterated for cardio-protection and cancer risk as these remain the major causes of death in patients with CKD (Boxes 9.5 and 9.6).

Box 9.4. Estimating Energy Intake in Adults

Women:

[655.1 + (9.56 × weight in kg) + (1.85 × height in cm) − (4.68 × age in years)] × 4.2 × activity factor

Men:

[664.7 + (13.75 × weight in kg) + (5 × height in cm) − (6.76 × age in years)] × 4.2 × activity factor

The activity factor in each equation (which adjusts for how active you are) is:

- For those who do little or no exercise each day, multiply by 1.2.
- For those who do light exercise on 1–3 days a week, multiply by 1.375.
- For those who do moderate exercise on 3–5 days a week, multiply by 1.55.
- For those who do hard exercise on 6–7 days a week, multiply by 1.725.
- For those who do daily exercise, a physical job or hard training, multiply by 1.9.

Box 9.5. What the KDIGO Guidelines Say You Should Do [14]

We recommend that individuals with CKD receive expert dietary advice and information in the context of an education programme, tailored to severity of CKD and the need to intervene on salt, phosphate, potassium and protein intake where indicated.

Restriction of Dietary Salt Intake in Patients with CKD

We recommend lowering salt intake to <90 mmol (<2 g) per day of sodium (corresponding to 5 g of sodium chloride) in adults, unless contraindicated.

Restriction of Dietary Protein Intake in Patients with CKD

We suggest lowering protein intake to 0.8 g/kg/day in adults with diabetes or without diabetes and GFR <30 ml/min/1.73 m^2 with appropriate education. We suggest avoiding high protein intake (41.3 g/kg/day) in adults with CKD at risk of progression.

Lifestyle in Patients with CKD

We recommend that people with CKD be encouraged to undertake physical activity compatible with cardiovascular health and tolerance (aiming for at least 30 min 5 times per week), achieve a healthy weight (BMI 20 to 25, according to country-specific demographics) and stop smoking.

Box 9.6. Relevant Guidelines

1. *KDIGO Guideline*
   Kidney Disease: Improving Global Outcomes (KDIGO) CKD Work Group. KDIGO 2012 clinical practice guideline for the evaluation and management of chronic kidney disease. Kidney Int Suppl. 2013;3:1–150.
   http://www.kdigo.org/clinical_practice_guidelines/pdf/CKD/KDIGO_2012_CKD_GL.pdf
2. *CARI Guideline*
   Clinical Practice Guidelines for Nutrition in Chronic Renal Failure.
   http://www.kidney.org/professionals/kdoqi/guidelines_updates/doqi_nut.html
3. *The Renal Association Guideline*
   Nutrition in CKD.
   http://www.renal.org/clinical/guidelines-section/NutritionInCKD.aspx
4. *Japanese Society of Nephrology Guideline*
   Evidence-based Practice Guideline for the Treatment of CKD. Clin Exp Nephrol. 2009;13:533–66.
   http://www.jsn.or.jp/en/guideline/pdf/guideline2009.pdf
5. *National Institute for Health and Clinical Excellence (NICE) Guideline*
   Chronic Kidney Disease. National clinical guideline for early identification and management in adults in primary and secondary care. 2008, Royal College of Physicians.
   http://www.nice.org.uk/nicemedia/live/12069/57614/57614.pdf
6. *Canadian Society of Nephrology Guideline*:
   Guidelines for the management of chronic kidney disease. CMAJ. 2008;179(11): 1154–62.
   http://www.cmaj.ca/content/suppl/2008/11/17/179.11.1154.DC1
7. *National Kidney Foundation Kidney Disease Outcomes Quality Initiative (KDOQI)*
   KDOQI US Commentary on the 2012 KDIGO clinical practice guideline for acute kidney injury. Am J Kidney Dis. 2013;61(5):649–72. Available at: http://www.kidney.org/Professionals/kdoqi/pdf/AKI-Commentary-2013.pdf.

Before You Finish: Practice Pearls for the Clinician

- There is little evidence that modification of diet and lifestyle improves kidney or cardiovascular outcomes in patients with chronic kidney disease.
- In obese patients, weight loss may improve cardiovascular health, mood, healing, sleep and a myriad of other outcomes and should be encouraged.
- It is likely that the mere act of adhering to dietary restrictions is as important for weight loss as changing the composition of the diet.
- Nephrologists should engage in their patients' weight loss plans to ensure that their safety is not compromised and its potential for success is reinforced.
- A more liberal approach to diet and lifestyle should be considered in patients with advanced CKD in keeping with their poor prognosis and comorbidity and the overall goal of palliation.

References

1. Robertson L, Waugh N, Robertson A. Protein restriction for diabetic renal disease. Cochrane Database Syst Rev. 2007;(4):CD002181.
2. Hansen HP, Tauber-Lassen E, Jensen BR, Parving HH. Effect of dietary protein restriction on prognosis in patients with diabetic nephropathy. Kidney Int. 2002;62:220–8.
3. Kitazato H, Fujita H, Shimotomai T, Kagaya E, Narita T, Kakei M, Ito S. Effects of chronic intake of vegetable protein added to animal or fish protein on renal hemodynamics. Nephron. 2002;90:31–6.
4. Korgaonkar S, Tilea A, Gillespie BW, Kiser M, Eisele G, Finkelstein F, Kotanko P, Pitt B, Saran R. Serum potassium and outcomes in ckd: insights from the rri-ckd cohort study. Clin J Am Soc Nephrol. 2010;5:762–9.
5. Ryu S, Chang Y, Woo HY, Kim SG, Kim DI, Kim WS, Suh BS, Choi NK, Lee JT. Changes in body weight predict ckd in healthy men. J Am Soc Nephrol. 2008;19:1798–805.
6. Bello AK, de Zeeuw D, El Nahas M, Brantsma AH, Bakker SJ, de Jong PE, Gansevoort RT. Impact of weight change on albuminuria in the general population. Nephrol Dial Transplant. 2007;22:1619–27.
7. Cardenas C, Bordiu E, Bagazgoitia J, Calle-Pascual AL, Diabetes, Nutrition Study Group SDA. Polyunsaturated fatty acid consumption may play a role in the onset and regression of microalbuminuria in well-controlled type 1 and type 2 diabetic people: a 7-year, prospective, population-based, observational multicenter study. Diabetes Care. 2004;27:1454–7.
8. Thomas MC, Moran J, Forsblom C, Harjutsalo V, Thorn L, Ahola A, Waden J, Tolonen N, Saraheimo M, Gordin D, Groop PH, FinnDiane Study G. The association between dietary sodium intake, esrd, and all-cause mortality in patients with type 1 diabetes. Diabetes Care. 2011;34:861–6.
9. Slagman MC, Waanders F, Hemmelder MH, Woittiez AJ, Janssen WM, Lambers Heerspink HJ, Navis G, Laverman GD, Group HONS. Moderate dietary sodium restriction added to angiotensin converting enzyme inhibition compared with dual blockade in lowering proteinuria and blood pressure: randomised controlled trial. BMJ. 2011;343:d4366.
10. Chadban S, Howell M, Twigg S, Thomas M, Jerums G, Cass A, Campbell D, Nicholls K, Tong A, Mangos G, Stack A, MacIsaac RJ, Girgis S, Colagiuri R, Colagiuri S, Craig J, CARI. The cari guidelines. Prevention and management of chronic kidney disease in type 2 diabetes. Nephrol. 2010;15 Suppl 1:S162–94.
11. Cecchin E, De Marchi S. Alcohol misuse and renal damage. Addict Biol. 1996;1:7–17.
12. Klarlund M, Prieme H, Loft S, Enghusen PH. Smoking cessation does not change urinary albumin excretion in normal subjects. Scand J Clin Lab Invest. 1997;57:513–20.
13. Voulgari C, Katsilambros N, Tentolouris N. Smoking cessation predicts amelioration of microalbuminuria in newly diagnosed type 2 diabetes mellitus: a 1-year prospective study. Metabolism. 2011;60:1456–64.
14. Kidney Disease: Improving Global Outcomes (KDIGO) CKD Work Group. KDIGO 2012 clinical practice guideline for the evaluation and management of chronic kidney disease. Kidney Int. 2013;3(Suppl):1–150. http://www.kdigo.org/clinical_practice_guidelines/pdf/CKD/KDIGO_2012_CKD_GL.pdf.

10 Preventing Progression of Chronic Kidney Disease: Renin–Angiotensin–Aldosterone System Blockade Beyond Blood Pressure

Merlin C. Thomas

Before You Start: Facts You Need to Know

- Activation of the renin–angiotensin–aldosterone system (RAAS) contributes to the development of hypertension in patients with chronic kidney disease.
- Blockade of the RAAS is the most widely used strategy to prevent progression of chronic kidney disease, both in the presence and absence of diabetes.
- Blockade of the RAAS has also been suggested to have pleiotropic effects in the kidney beyond blood pressure lowering, consistent with the role of the RAAS in renal pathophysiology.
- Clinical trials have demonstrated reduction in proteinuria in patients with chronic kidney disease, beyond that seen with other antihypertensive classes despite comparable efficacy with respect to blood pressure lowering.

10.1 The Renin–Angiotensin–Aldosterone System (RAAS)

The renin–angiotensin–aldosterone system (RAAS) is a fundamental regulator of vascular homeostasis, mediated directly through its myriad effects on vascular structure and function and indirectly through its effects in the kidney, including sodium and water handling, glomerular filtration pressure, renal blood flow and tubular growth (Box 10.1). The RAAS is a complex multienzymatic hormonal cascade (Fig. 10.1) whose activity is regulated on many levels, with both positive and negative feedback pathways that ensure optimal responsiveness to both physiological and pathogenic stimuli. At its most simplistic, angiotensinogen, the major

Box 10.1. Some of the Non-haemodynamic Actions of Angiotensin II in the Kidney

Increased sodium retention
Tubular hypertrophy and atrophy
Epithelial to mesenchymal transition
Myofibroblast accumulation
Mesangial contraction
Foot process effacement (dedifferentiation)
Fibrogenesis
Renal tubular acidosis
NADPH-dependent generation of reactive oxygen species
Mitochondrial dysfunction
Macrophage accumulation

M.C. Thomas, MBChB, PhD, FRACP
Department of Biochemistry of Diabetes Complications, Baker IDI Heart and Diabetes Institute, St Kilda Rd Central, 6492, Melbourne, VIC 8008, Australia
e-mail: mthomas@bakeridi.edu.au

M. Arici (ed.), *Management of Chronic Kidney Disease*,
DOI 10.1007/978-3-642-54637-2_10, © Springer-Verlag Berlin Heidelberg 2014

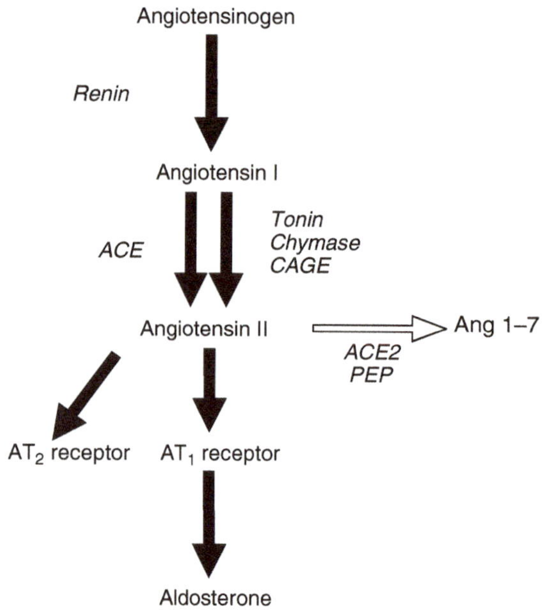

Fig. 10.1 The renin–angiotensin system

substrate, is processed in a two-step proteolytic reaction by renin and angiotensin-converting enzyme (ACE), resulting in the generation of angiotensin (Ang) II, the major effector molecule. Other enzymes can also generate Ang II via different enzymatic processing of angiotensinogen (so-called *non-ACE* pathways) which are more or less important in different tissues and in different states. Ang II is then degraded predominantly by ACE2 and prolylendopetidase (PEP) in the kidney to generate smaller peptides including Ang 1–7 which have vascular and renal actions antagonistic to those of Ang II. The coordinated actions of these opposing pathways provide exquisite control of Ang II levels and its downstream metabolites, allowing for the dynamic responsiveness required to ensure a rapid return to homeostasis.

The most commonly used RAAS blockers inhibit ACE to reduce the synthesis of Ang II or antagonise its actions at the type 1 angiotensin (AT_1) receptors (known as angiotensin receptor blockers or ARBs; Fig. 10.2). Both strategies also increase production of Ang 1–7, by reducing its degradation by ACE or AT_1-receptor-dependent internalisation, respectively. More recently agents that directly inhibit the enzymatic action of renin or antagonise the effects of aldosterone at the mineralocorticoid receptor have also gained popularity, usually in combination with ACE inhibitors or AT_1-receptor blockers. Agents that augment signalling through the AT_2 receptor or mimic the actions of Ang 1–7 via the mas receptor or increase ACE2 are also in clinical development for the management of CKD.

The levels of Ang II and other angiotensin peptides are higher in the kidney than in any other tissue in the body, reflecting its key role in maintaining healthy kidney function. In patients with chronic kidney disease, activity of the intrarenal RAAS is inappropriately elevated for the elevated volume status of most patients, which under normal circumstances should see suppression of the RAAS and natriuresis. It is thought that this compensation is an adaptation to maintain kidney function in the acute setting but is ultimately maladaptive in the long term. Some patients (especially those with diabetes) may manifest no increase or even suppression of the systemic RAAS, possible because of excessive local activation of the RAAS in the kidney.

It is well established that activation of the RAAS promotes the development and maintenance of hypertension in CKD (see Chap. 5). This is partly mediated by the direct vasoconstrictor actions of Ang II on smooth muscle to increase peripheral vascular resistance. However, salt and water retention, tubular hypertrophy, augmented activation of the sympathetic nervous system, and sensitivity to the effects of noradrenaline in the kidney also play a role [1]. In addition, T-cell activation also appears to be an important driver of angiotensin-dependent hypertension, as the induction of hypertension in mice is prevented by removing the AT_1 receptor from T cells.

The key role played by the RAAS in the development of hypertension has meant that blockade of the RAAS has become the most widely used antihypertensive strategy in patients with progressive kidney disease (see Chap. 5). But while the RAAS plays a key role in the pathogenesis of hypertension, it is also recognised that inappropriate or persistent activation can lead to kidney

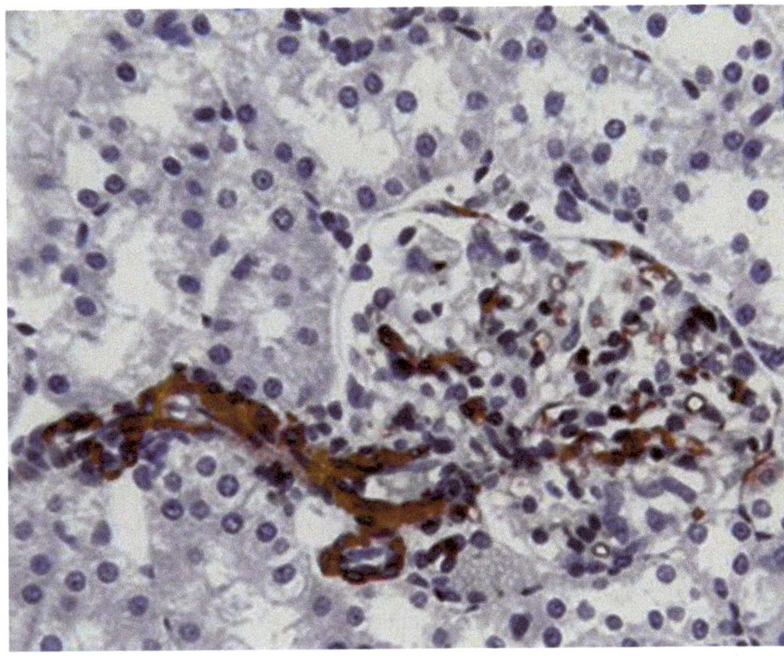

Fig. 10.2 Localisation of AT_1-receptor expression in the kidney with dense staining in the juxtaglomerular apparatus, glomerular capillaries and along the efferent glomerular arteriole

damage over and above its effects on blood pressure. Moreover, it is often suggested that RAAS blockade offers unique renoprotective benefits in patients with chronic kidney disease, beyond blood pressure lowering. These actions are the subject of this chapter.

10.2 Is It Just Because the Blood Pressure Is Better Controlled when Blocking the RAAS?

Blood pressure control is important to prevent the development and progression of kidney damage. There is no doubt that drugs that block the RAAS are effective antihypertensive agents. However, when used as monotherapy, RAAS blockers achieve blood pressure reductions that are similar to that achieved by other antihypertensive agents. If then additional benefits are observed when using RAAS blockers despite similar blood pressure control, it is common to invoke its many pleiotropic actions. However, RAAS blockers may be different to other strategies in other aspects of blood pressure control, even for the same achieved reduction in mean or systolic blood pressure levels. For example, some researchers have argued that the antiproteinuric benefits of RAAS blockade observed in the micro-HOPE study may simply have reflected the better 24-h and/or night-time control of blood pressure achieved with ramipril rather than any pleiotropic effects arising from RAAS blockade [2].

Another key difference between blood pressure-lowering strategies may be their effects on blood pressure variability, beyond simply lowering of mean blood pressure levels. For example, it is known that visit-to-visit variability in blood pressure is independently associated with the risk of progressive kidney disease, over and above mean blood pressure control [3]. Indeed in the DCCT study, visit-to-visit variability in blood pressure explained as much of the variability in incident nephropathy as differences in mean blood pressure [3]. Notably, some antihypertensive combinations, including some that contain RAAS blockers, result in the lower blood pressure variability than other combinations. This may partly explain why additional renoprotective advantages of RAAS blockade have been largely reported in studies of hypertensive patients, where RAAS blockade is one of usually three or four different antihypertensive agents. Indeed, it may be that the better, more sustained and less variable effects of RAAS blockade on blood pressure may partly explain the so-called 'independent' benefits with respect to kidney disease.

10.3 Is RAAS Blockade Better Because the Patients Take the Pills?

The other key advantage of conventional RAAS blockade is its tolerability and compliance [4]. ARBs appear to be, on average, the best tolerated of all antihypertensive agents. ACE inhibitors are not far behind. Although cough from ACE inhibitor may be troublesome for some individuals, its impact on adherence and compliance is more favourable than seen with oedema and frequency observed with calcium channel blockers and diuretics, respectively. RAAS blockers are generally long acting, taken once a day and can be easily combined with other agents in fixed dose formulations. Taken together, these effects mean that patients prescribed RAAS blockers are generally more likely to be taking them [4]. Again this ultimately translates into better blood pressure control on an intention to treat basis and potentially better kidney outcomes.

10.4 How Might RAAS Blockade Actually Slow the Progression of CKD Beyond BP?

An infusion of angiotensin II, even in sub-pressor doses, results in tubular hypertrophy, apoptosis and progressive glomerulosclerosis. The dominant mechanisms by which this occurs include both haemodynamic and non-haemodynamic effects of Ang II (Box 10.1).

The RAAS and renal haemodynamics – Among the earliest changes in the injured kidney is an increase in efferent arteriolar tone leading to an increase in intra-capillary pressure and a loss of auto-regulation. Activation of the RAAS increases the filtration fraction as Ang II constricts the post-glomerular (efferent) arterioles to a greater extent than at the afferent arteriole resulting in an increase intraglomerular pressure (Fig. 10.3). By contrast, blockade of the RAAS with ACE inhibitors or AT_1-receptor blockers alleviates hydrostatic 'stress' on the glomerulus by causing preferential vasodilatation of the same (post-glomerular) efferent arterioles. This effect on glomerular haemodynamics is most often used to explain why RAAS blockade appears to be more efficacious in preventing proteinuria and renal injury when compared to similar blood pressure reduction using other agents. Moreover, the finding that the slight drop in GFR observed

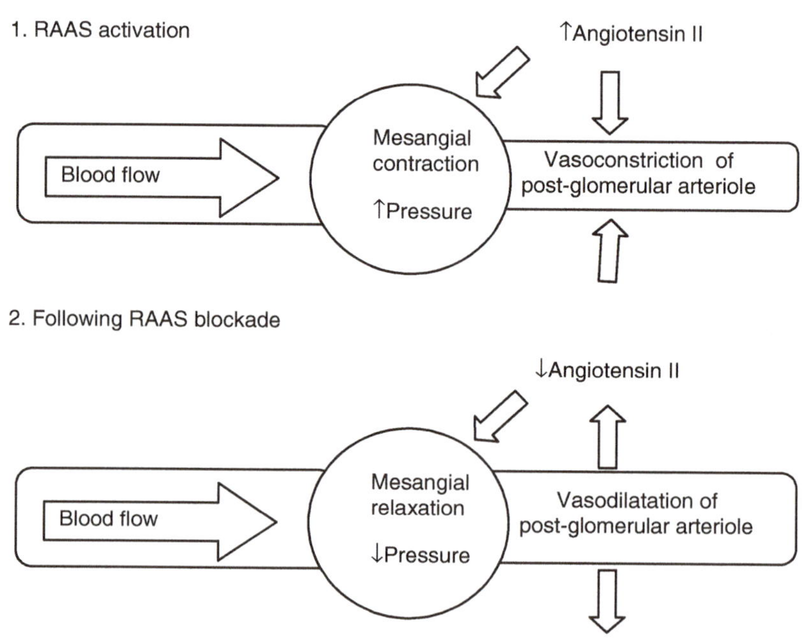

Fig. 10.3 The actions of angiotensin II and RAAS blockade on intraglomerular pressure

in some patients following the commencement of RAAS blockade (see below) is also associated with a slower decline in renal function suggests that a reduction in intraglomerular pressure plays a key role in both phenomena.

Antiproteinuric effects of RAAS blockade – Proteinuria is not only a marker of renal injury, but also a mediator of progressive renal damage as reabsorption of filtered proteins can injure the tubulointerstitium of the kidney by activating intrACEllular events leading to the release of vasoactive, profibrotic and proinflammatory mediators. In controlled trials in patients with CKD, ACE inhibitors and ARBs reduce urinary protein excretion by approximately 35–40 %, which is greater than other antihypertensive agents, even when the effect of blood pressure reduction on urinary protein excretion has been taken into account. This effect is partly mediated through effects on blood pressure and renal haemodynamics (detailed above), as well as antagonising the direct effects of Ang II on glomerular permselectivity, podocyte structure and function tubular protein handling and the contraction of mesangial cells to decrease the glomerular capillary ultrafiltration coefficient. Post hoc analyses from the RENAAL and IDNT trials showed that the ARB-induced reduction in albuminuria explained most of the long-term renal and cardioprotective effects of ARBs in patients with type 2 diabetes and advanced nephropathy. So important is the antiproteinuric effect of RAAS blockade, that current guidelines strongly recommend the use of RAAS blocker in all forms of proteinuric renal disease, even in the absence of hypertension (Boxes 10.2, 10.3, 10.4, and 10.5). By contrast, the potential utility of RAAS blockade in non-proteinuric renal disease, beyond blood pressure lowering, remains controversial.

Box 10.2. What Do the CARI Guidelines (Australia) Say? [5]

ARB or ACEI should be considered as antihypertensive agents of first choice.

In people with type 2 diabetes and microalbuminuria or macroalbuminuria, angiotensin receptor blocker or angiotensin-converting enzyme inhibitor antihypertensives should be used to protect against progression of kidney disease.

In patients with hypertension associated with renovascular disease, pharmacological inhibition of the renin–angiotensin system effectively and safely lowers blood pressure in most patients (level II evidence).

Box 10.3. K/DOQI Clinical Practice Guidelines on Hypertension and Antihypertensive Agents in Chronic Kidney Disease [6]

ACE inhibitors and ARBs can be used safely in most patients with CKD.

ACE inhibitors and ARBs should be used at moderate to high doses, as used in clinical trials (A).

ACE inhibitors and ARBs should be used as alternatives to each other, if the preferred class cannot be used (B).

ACE inhibitors and ARBs can be used in combination to lower blood pressure or reduce proteinuria (C).

Patients treated with ACE inhibitors or ARBs should be monitored for hypotension, decreased GFR and hyperkalaemia (A).

The interval for monitoring blood pressure, GFR and serum potassium depends on baseline levels (B).

In most patients, the ACE inhibitor or ARB can be continued if:

GFR decline over 4 months is <30 % from baseline value (B).

Serum potassium is ≤5.5 mEq/l (B).

ACE inhibitors and ARBs should not be used or used with caution in certain circumstances, including women not practising contrACEption, concomitant use of drugs causing hyperkalaemia and bilateral renal artery stenosis.

Box 10.4. UK Guidelines for Identification, Management and Referral [7]

ACEIs should be included in the regimen for all patients with proteinuria (urine protein: creatinine ratio >100 mg/mmol), diabetic patients with microalbuminuria, and for patients with heart failure; ARBs may be used as alternatives to ACEIs.

Serum creatinine and potassium concentration should be checked prior to starting ACEIs and/or ARBs, within 2 weeks of starting and within 2 weeks after subsequent increases in dose; during severe intercurrent illness, particularly if there is a risk of hypovolaemia; and at annual intervals thereafter, or more frequently if indicated, according to kidney function. A rise of serum creatinine concentration of >20 % or fall in estimated GFR of >15 % after initiation or dose increase should be followed by further measurements within 2 weeks; if deterioration in kidney function is confirmed, a specialist opinion should be sought (not necessarily by formal referral) on whether the drug treatment should be stopped or the patient subjected to investigation for renal artery stenosis.

Hyperkalaemia (serum potassium >6.0 mmol/l) should result in stopping of concomitant nephrotoxic drugs (e.g. NSAIDs), reduction or cessation of potassium-retaining diuretics (amiloride, triamterene, spironolactone) and reduction of loop diuretic dosage if there is no sign of congestion. If hyperkalaemia persists, the ACEI or ARB should be stopped.

'Dual blockade' with combinations of ACEIs and ARBs should usually only be initiated under specialist supervision.

Box 10.5. KDIGO 2012 Clinical Practice Guideline for the Evaluation and Management of Chronic Kidney Disease [8]

BP and RAAS Interruption

Individualise BP targets and agents according to age, coexistent cardiovascular disease and other comorbidities, risk of progression of CKD, presence or absence of retinopathy (in CKD patients with diabetes) and tolerance of treatment

We suggest that an ARB or ACEI be used in diabetic adults with CKD and urine albumin excretion 30–300 mg/24 h (or equivalent).

We recommend that an ARB or ACEI be used in both diabetic and nondiabetic adults with CKD and urine albumin excretion >300 mg/24 h (or equivalent).

There is insufficient evidence to recommend combining an ACEI with ARBs to prevent progression of CKD.

We recommend temporary discontinuation of potentially nephrotoxic and renally excreted drugs in people with a GFR <60 ml/min/1.73 m^2 who have serious intercurrent illness that increases the risk of AKI. These agents include, but are not limited to, RAAS blockers (including ACEIs, ARBs, aldosterone inhibitors, direct renin inhibitors).

Interactions with kidney disease pathways – Ang II is also an important stimulus for inflammation, oxidative stress and fibrogenesis in the kidney (Box 10.1). Each of these represents important pathogenic pathways involved in the development and progression of CKD. For example, the formation of reactive oxygen species (ROS) as a result of oxidative stress is recognised as a key component in the progression of chronic kidney disease. ROS are directly cytotoxic and up-regulate inflammation and fibrosis. The expression and activity of NADPH oxidase represents the major source of ROS in the kidney and NADPH oxidase is directly stimulated by Ang II via activation of the AT_1 receptor. This pro-oxidant action may independently contribute to the renal consequences of activation of the AT_1 receptor and therein the benefits arising from its blockade in the setting of kidney disease. Ang II is also able to modulate immune responses relevant to scarring, inflammation and hypertension in progressive kidney disease. Indeed, immunosuppression during Ang II-induced hypertension is able to reduce albuminuria, inflammatory cell infiltration and structural damage in the kidney, suggesting that changes in immune functioning play a vital role in determining the actions of RAAS activation.

10.5 Is There Evidence that Blocking the RAAS Really Prevents Kidney Disease Beyond BP?

Although there is a strong physiological rationale for early blockade of the RAAS in patients at risk of kidney disease, the utility of RAAS blockade for primary prevention beyond blood pressure lowering continues to be debated. Certainly, lowering blood pressure is effective in preventing diabetic kidney disease (see Chap. 6) and many trials have demonstrated renal benefits using RAAS blockers in hypertensive patients while at the same time lowering blood pressure levels. However, the utility of RAAS blocker in normotensive individuals is variable at best. For example, the ACE inhibitor ramipril (10 mg/day) did not reduce the incidence of new onset microalbuminuria in normotensive patients with type 2 diabetes from the micro-HOPE study [9]. Similarly, in type 2 diabetic patients enrolled in the DIRECT study, the ARB, candesartan (16 mg/day), failed to reduce the development of microalbuminuria, despite lower blood pressure levels in the candesartan-treated group [10].

A number of trials have attempted to specifically explore the unique renoprotective utility of RAAS blockade beyond blood pressure lowering in patients with diabetes. However, with few exceptions these studies have largely failed to demonstrate a clear and independent efficacy for the primary prevention of microalbuminuria. Put together with observational findings in a meta-analysis, Casas et al. controversially concluded that ACE or ARBs provided no renoprotective effect beyond BP control [11]. This study has been widely criticised because of 'methodological flaws' and, in particular, the inclusion of post hoc renal data from the ALLHAT study, which because of its size, dominated the outcome analysis. This study included a large proportion of black patients in whom RAAS blockade is often considered to be less effective, and patients in the RAAS treatment arm were limited in their access to diuretics.

Although some subsequent clinical studies have observed some renoprotective effects from RAAS blockade, many of these studies deliberately included hypertensive patients and/or achieved greater blood pressure lowering with the RAAS blocker. Consequently, whether RAAS blockade truly offers additional benefits for primary prevention over and above blood pressure control remains contentious. At best, any 'independent effects' on primary prevention achieved by RAAS blockers beyond blood pressure lowering are modest, and certainly not the panACEa envisaged by many practitioners.

10.6 Does Blocking the RAAS Slow the Progression of Established Kidney Disease Beyond BP Lowering?

While data in primary prevention are controversial, there is unequivocal evidence that blocking the RAAS has beneficial actions in the kidney in patients with incipient or established kidney disease, beyond its effects to lower pressure. In patients with diabetes, there is strong evidence that RAAS blockade reduce the risk of progression from microalbuminuria to macroalbuminuria by at least one third and increased likelihood of regression from microalbuminuria to normoalbuminuria by two- to threefold when compared to standard (non-RAAS) antihypertensive therapy [12]. Doubling of serum creatinine and/or progression to end-stage renal disease (ESRD) is also reduced by RAAS blockade. Importantly, in each case, these renoprotective benefits in the response to RAAS blockade is independent on baseline blood pressure levels such that relative efficacy is similar in hypertensive and normotensive patients.

10.7 Is the Effect of RAAS Blockade on the Kidneys Sustained?

Although RAAS blockade is effective in patients with CKD, most of the separation in outcomes between patients on RAAS blockers and those receiving standard therapy occurs early, within the first 18 months. After this time, the (time-to-event) lines appear to run in parallel. Moreover, if or when RAAS blocking agents are discontinued, albuminuria often increases. These observations call into question the durability of the treatment effect on the RAAS and/or the underlying disease processes. This may be because the RAAS relies on feedback regulation to achieve and sustain the delicate balance required for vascular function and this feedback regulation is intrinsically antagonistic to the therapeutic goal of blocking the RAAS (Fig. 10.3). The blockade achieved by ACE inhibitors and ARBs is only partial and short lived, even when used in combination [13]. In fact, in a third to a half of all patients treated with ACE inhibitors, there is a paradoxical overshoot in aldosterone concentrations after 12 months of treatment (known as aldosterone escape). This escape phenomenon also occurs with ARBs possibly due to activation of the AT_2 receptor [13]. Indeed equal rates of elevated aldosterone levels are observed among subjects on ACE inhibitors, ARBs, or a combination of both [13], which may explain the lack of additive effect observed in some clinical studies.

10.8 Are ACE Inhibitors Better Than ARBs, or Is It the Other Way Round?

The antihypertensive effects of ACE inhibitors and ARBs are not significantly different, although individuals' responses vary. Similarly, the antiproteinuric response appears to be roughly equivalent in magnitude. It has been argued that ARBs may have several advantages for renoprotection in kidney disease, as compared to ACE inhibitors. Although both agents attenuate signalling through the RAAS, by directly antagonising AT_1 receptors, ARBs also block the signalling of angiotensin II generated via non-ACE-dependent pathways (e.g. chymase). ARBs also lead to the preferential stimulation of the unblocked AT_2 receptor, which may contribute to the prevention of hypertrophic effects of RAAS activation and might provide further end-organ protection [14]. However, in head-to-head trails, similar effects have been observed when using ACE inhibitors and ARBs. Data from the Diabetics Exposed to Telmisartan and Enalapril (DETAIL) study also supports this assertion, finding that enalapril and telmisartan had similar renoprotective actions in patients with type 2 diabetes and early kidney disease [15]. However, a most recent meta-analysis suggested that while ACE inhibitors reduced the risk of new onset of microalbuminuria, macroalbuminuria or both by 29 % when compared to plACEbo (RR 0.71, 95 % CI 0.56–0.89), no effect was observed for angiotensin receptor blockers (RR 0.90, 95 % CI 0.68–1.19). Controversially, this led some guidelines to the recommendation that ACE inhibitors and not ARBs be used for renoprotection, despite a higher incidence of side effects and comparable BP control. However, the confidence intervals overlap significantly, and it is more likely that each produces a similar, albeit modest effect on renal progression.

10.9 What Is the Best Dose to Use?

Although therapy should be initiated at a low dose to reduce the risk of side effects, the best renoprotective outcomes appear to be achieved by titration up to maximum approved dose of ACE inhibitors and ARBs, even without additional blood pressure-lowering efficacy. There also is some evidence that megadoses of ACE inhibitors or ARBs exceed the effectiveness of conventional doses in experimental models of chronic kidney disease and clinical observations have suggested that conventional doses should be exceeded if proteinuria remains substantial. This paradigm remains to be formally tested clinical trials.

10.10 What Are the Potential Drawbacks of RAAS Blockade?

Although RAAS blockers have many potential benefits, treatment with ACE inhibitors and ARBs may also result in adverse effects, which are more common in patients with CKD (Box 10.6). Apart from cough with ACE inhibitors, the most common side effects leading to modification or discontinuation of therapy include an early decrease in GFR, hyperkalaemia and hypotension.

Box 10.6. Side Effects Arising from Blockade of the RAAS

Related to RAAS Blocking Activities

Hypotension

Acute decline in GFR/kidney failure

Hypokalaemia

Foetal toxicity

Unrelated to RAAS Blocking Activity

Cough (10–20 % of those taking ACE inhibitors, minimal with ARBs)

Rash/urticaria/itch (especially with captopril)

Angioedema

Neutropaenia/agranulocytosis

Dysgeusia (abnormal taste sensation; especially with captopril)

Many clinicians are concerned that RAAS blockade might be contraindicated in the presence of CKD or might cause kidney damage because of an acute decline in glomerular filtration rate observed with both ACE inhibitors and/or ARBs. In fact, this fall is a common dose-related adverse effect related to reduce efferent arterial tone following blockade of the RAAS. In all patients starting RAAS blockers, renal function should be checked 4 weeks after initiation. An acute fall in estimated GFR of more than 15 % occurs in approximately 10 % of patients following initiation of RAAS blockade. It is not diagnostic of bilateral renal artery stenosis, which may be present only in a very small number of cases. It is more commonly related volume status, dose at initiation and pressure dependence of renal function in any one individual. This risk of declining renal function should be reduced by optimised volume status prior to initiation (e.g. reducing diuretics, controlling hyperglycaemia or heart failure) and slow dose titration. Nonetheless, an acute fall in GFR that stabilises within the first 2 months actually predicts a slower decrease in long-term renal function. If GFR decreases by more than 30 % over baseline, the dose of ACE inhibitor or ARB should be reduced, and the GFR reassessed frequently until kidney function has stabilised. In many cases, the ACE inhibitor or ARB can be managed without discontinuation.

It is well known that RAAS blockade may precipitate acute renal failure in patients with bilateral critical renal vascular disease, as GFR is maintained in this state by heightened activity of the intrarenal RAAS. However, such events are uncommon and reversible (if detected early). Most patients with established renovascular disease do not experience acute renal failure when treated with a RAAS blocker. Even amongst patients with known renal vascular disease, the use of RAAS blockade is actually associated with an improved kidney and cardiovascular outcomes.

Hyperkalaemia may also be induced following RAAS blockade in patients with CKD due to inhibition of aldosterone production. It may be modestly more common with ACE inhibitors than ARBs. Increases in serum potassium are also more common in kidney patients with diabetes, interstitial nephritis, heart failure and acidosis and those taking NSAIDs, beta-blockers, potassium-sparing diuretics or potassium supplements. Again, this can usually be managed without discontinuation with dose reduction, initiating a 'low-potassium diet' of ≤2–3 g/day (approximately 50–75 mEq/day), loop diuretics and alkali replACEment (if metabolic acidosis, serum bicARBonate concentration <21 mEq/l) or using binding resins like sodium polystyrene sulfonate.

10.11 Is There Any Advantage for Combined RAAS Blockade?

Direct renin inhibition – The feedback induction of prorenin may provide one explanation why renal function and/or albuminuria may still deteriorate in the face of maximally recommended doses of RAAS blockade. As a result, renin inhibition had emerged as a possible target for the management of CKD, both as a means for reducing escape from conventional RAAS blockade and amplifying the clinical response to these agents. Despite exciting data suggesting an additive antiproteinuric effect, the prospective, randomised Aliskiren Trial in Type 2 Diabetes Using Cardio-Renal Disease Endpoints (ALTITUDE) study was stopped by the Data Monitoring Committee in late 2011, because of futility (i.e. no prospect of demonstrating the treatment benefit anticipated in the protocol) as well as safety concerns including an excess of renal dysfunction, hyperkalaemia, hypotension and strokes [16].

Combined ACE inhibition and angiotensin receptor blockade – Another potential strategy to achieve better inhibition of RAAS has been to combine ACE inhibition with angiotensin receptor blockade in so-called dual therapy. A number of studies have reported additive antiproteinuric effects of combination therapy, although this may partly reflect the suboptimal doses used of either or both components when used on their own. More recently, the ONTARGET trial, which used high doses of one or both ramipril and/or telmisartan, did demonstrate that albuminuria fell more from baseline with dual therapy compared with monotherapy at 2 years. But again whether this was due to blood pressure lowering or better blockade is uncertain. Moreover, combination therapy was associated with an increased risk of hyperkalaemia and kidney failure.

Mineralocorticoid receptor blockade – The addition of a mineralocorticoid receptor antagonist to an ACE inhibitor or ARB has also been studied as a potential means to achieve better RAAS blockade. Some (but not all) short-term studies have suggested additive antiproteinuric effects, but it is unclear whether the benefits of combination therapy are specifically enhanced in patients with aldosterone escape, or simply because of better blood pressure control with enhanced diuresis. The long-term effects of combination therapy on hard clinical end points remain unknown. Moreover, hyperkalaemia is a significant risk with this strategy in patients with CKD. There may also be unforeseen problems with combination therapy, with one study reporting higher levels of Ang II and an increased incidence of escape in patients receiving spironolactone in combination with conventional RAAS blockade [17].

10.12 Does an Effect Beyond BP Really Matter?

Although it is widely publicised that RAAS blockade has unique renoprotective benefits for patients with CKD, in modern clinical practice such arguments are largely moot. Given the better tolerability, efficacy and side-effect profile of RAAS blockers over other antihypertensive agents [4], as well as added beneficial effects on retinal and cardiovascular disease [18], heart failure and other end-organ damage [10], most patients with or at risk of CKD currently receive RAAS blockers as first-line antihypertensive agents. Indeed, most patients will initially or ultimately need combination antihypertensive therapy to control their blood pressure, in which case RAAS blockade will almost always be utilised in routine clinical practice. Patients without hypertension or proteinuria generally have a low risk of adverse renal outcomes such that even if there was some renoprotective effect in these patients the number need to treat would be large to afford any benefit while at the same time exposing patients to unnecessary treatment.

Finally, it is important to note that despite its benefits, RAAS blockade even in optimal combination with other interventions is not enough to prevent progressive kidney disease. At its best it achieves a modest and temporary slowing of renal decline in some patients. So while it important to use RAAS blockade in our patients, it is also important to acknowledge that more must be done to preserve kidney function and health in our patients with CKD (Box 10.7).

Box 10.7. Relevant Guidelines

1. *KDIGO Guideline*
   Kidney Disease: Improving Global Outcomes (KDIGO) CKD Work Group. KDIGO 2012 clinical practice guideline for the evaluation and management of chronic kidney disease. Kidney Int. 2013;3(Suppl):1–150.
   http://www.kdigo.org/clinical_practice_guidelines/pdf/CKD/KDIGO_2012_CKD_GL.pdf
2. *CARI Guideline*
   CARI Guidelines. Concord, NSW: Caring for Australasians with Renal Impairment; 2004. Updated 9 Jan 2013, cited 12 Aug 2013. Available from: http://www.cari.org.au
3. *The Renal Association Guideline*
   Clinical Practice Guidelines for the Care of Patients with Chronic Kidney Disease
   http://www.renal.org/Libraries/Old_Guidelines/Module_1_-_Chronic_Kidney_Disease_CKD_-_4th_Edition.sflb.ashx
4. *Japanese Society of Nephrology Guideline*
   Evidence-based practice guideline for the treatment of CKD. Clin Exp Nephrol. 2009;13:533–66.
   http://www.jsn.or.jp/en/guideline/pdf/guideline2009.pdf
5. *National Institute for Health and Clinical Excellence (NICE) Guideline*
   Chronic Kidney Disease. National clinical guideline for early identification and management in adults in primary and secondary care. 2008, Royal College of Physicians.
   http://www.nice.org.uk/nicemedia/live/12069/57614/57614.pdf
6. *Canadian Society of Nephrology Guideline*
   Guidelines for the management of chronic kidney disease. CMAJ. 2008;179:1154–62 [15].
   http://www.cmaj.ca/content/suppl/2008/11/17/179.11.1154.DC1
7. *National Kidney Foundation Kidney Disease Outcomes Quality Initiative (NKF KDOQI) Clinical Practice Guidelines*
   NKF KDOQI guidelines on hypertension and antihypertensive agents in chronic kidney disease [internet]. New York: National Kidney Foundation; 2013. Cited 12 Aug 2013.
   http://www.kidney.org/professionals/kdoqi/guidelines_bp/guide_11.htm

Before You Finish: Practice Pearls for the Clinician

- Blockade of the RAAS is an effective strategy to reduce blood pressure in patients with CKD, but no more so than other antihypertensive strategies.
- RAAS blockers have a more favourable side-effect profile than other antihypertensive agents, meaning that patients are generally more likely to be taking them.
- Any 'independent' effect of RAAS blockade for the primary prevention of diabetic nephropathy, beyond blood pressure control, remains to be clearly established.
- Clear benefits have been observed in proteinuric renal disease, while renoprotective actions in the absence of proteinuria remain controversial.
- Combination strategies using dual blockade, renin inhibitors or aldosterone antagonists to achieve a more complete RAAS blockade have not improved renal outcomes in patients with diabetes.

References

1. Price DA, De'Oliveira JM, Fisher ND, Williams GH, Hollenberg NK. The state and responsiveness of the renin-angiotensin-aldosterone system in patients with type II diabetes mellitus. Am J Hypertens. 1999;12: 348–55.
2. Effects of ramipril on cardiovascular and microvascular outcomes in people with diabetes mellitus: results of the hope study and micro-hope substudy. Heart outcomes prevention evaluation study investigators. Lancet. 2000;355:253–259.
3. Kilpatrick ES, Rigby AS, Atkin SL. The role of blood pressure variability in the development of nephropathy in type 1 diabetes. Diabetes Care. 2010;33: 2442–7.
4. Kronish IM, Woodward M, Sergie Z, Ogedegbe G, Falzon L, Mann DM. Meta-analysis: impact of drug class on adherence to antihypertensives. Circulation. 2011;123:1611–21.
5. CARI Guidelines [internet]. Concord: caring for Australasians with renal impairmen; 2004. Available from: http://www.cari.org.au. Updated 9 Jan 2013, cited 12 Aug 2013.
6. National Kidney Foundation: Kidney Disease Outcomes Quality Initiative (NKF KDOQI) clinical practice guidelines on hypertension and antihypertensive agents in chronic kidney disease [internet]. New York: National Kidney Foundation; 2013. Available from: http://www.kidney.org/professionals/kdoqi/guidelines_bp/guide_11.htm. Cited 12 Aug 2013.
7. Royal College of Physicians of London. Chronic kidney disease in adults: UK guidelines for identification, management and referral [internet]. London: Royal College of Physicians of London; 2006. Available at: http://www.renal.org/CKDguide/full/CKDprintedfullguide.pdf. Cited 12 Aug 2013.
8. Kidney Disease: Improving Global Outcomes (KDIGO) CKD Work Group. KDIGO 2012 clinical practice guideline for the evaluation and management of chronic kidney disease. Kidney Int. 2013;3(Suppl):1–150. http://www.kdigo.org/clinical_practice_guidelines/pdf/CKD/KDIGO_2012_CKD_GL.pdf.
9. Gerstein HC, Mann JF, Pogue J, Dinneen SF, Halle JP, Hoogwerf B, Joyce C, Rashkow A, Young J, Zinman B, Yusuf S. Prevalence and determinants of microalbuminuria in high-risk diabetic and nondiabetic patients in the heart outcomes prevention evaluation study. The hope study investigators. Diabetes Care. 2000;23 Suppl 2:B35–9.
10. Bilous RCN, Sjølie AK, Fuller J, Klein R, Orchard T, et al. Effect of candesartan on microalbuminuria and albumin excretion rate in diabetes. Three randomized trials. Ann Intern Med. 2009;151:11–20.
11. Casas JP, Chua W, Loukogeorgakis S, Vallance P, Smeeth L, Hingorani AD, MacAllister RJ. Effect of inhibitors of the renin-angiotensin system and other antihypertensive drugs on renal outcomes: systematic review and meta-analysis. Lancet. 2005;366:2026–33.
12. Strippoli GF, Craig M, Deeks JJ, Schena FP, Craig JC. Effects of angiotensin converting enzyme inhibitors and angiotensin ii receptor antagonists on mortality and renal outcomes in diabetic nephropathy: systematic review. BMJ. 2004;329:828.
13. Horita Y, Taura K, Taguchi T, Furusu A, Kohno S. Aldosterone breakthrough during therapy with angiotensin-converting enzyme inhibitors and angiotensin ii receptor blockers in proteinuric patients with immunoglobulin a nephropathy. Nephrology (Carlton). 2006;11:462–6.
14. Hollenberg NK. Renal implications of angiotensin receptor blockers. Am J Hypertens. 2001;14:237S–41.
15. Barnett AH, Bain SC, Bouter P, Karlberg B, Madsbad S, Jervell J, Mustonen J. Angiotensin-receptor blockade versus converting-enzyme inhibition in type 2 diabetes and nephropathy. N Engl J Med. 2004;351: 1952–61.
16. Parving HH, Brenner BM, McMurray JJ, de Zeeuw D, Haffner SM, Solomon SD, Chaturvedi N, Persson F, Desai AS, Nicolaides M, Richard A, Xiang Z, Brunel P, Pfeffer MA. Cardiorenal end points in a trial of aliskiren for type 2 diabetes. N Engl J Med. 2012;367:2204–13.
17. van de Wal RMPH, Lok DJ, Boomsma F, van der Horst FA, van Veldhuisen DJ, van Gilst WH, Voors AA. Determinants of increased angiotensin II levels in severe chronic heart failure patients despite ACE inhibition. Int J Cardiol. 2006;106:367–72.
18. Strippoli G. Angiotensin-converting enzyme inhibitors, angiotensin receptor blockers and combined therapy in patients with micro- and macroalbuminuria and other cardiovascular risk factors: a systematic review of randomized controlled trials. Nephrol Dial Transplant. 2011;26:2827–47.

Part III

Chronic Kidney Disease and Cardiovascular Diseases

11 Chronic Kidney Disease and the Cardiovascular Connection

Peter A. McCullough and Mohammad Nasser

Before You Start: The Facts You Need to Know

- The heart and kidneys are linked via hemodynamic, neurohormonal, and cell signaling systems.
- Chronic kidney disease bone and mineral disorder results in acceleration in calcification of atherosclerosis, particularly in the vascular media.
- Heart failure is the most common symptomatic manifestation of cardiovascular disease requiring hospitalization in patients with chronic kidney disease.
- Myocardial disease, electrolyte imbalance, and acid-base disturbances can lead to arrhythmias in patients with renal failure.

P.A. McCullough, MD, MPH
Department of Cardiovascular Medicine, Baylor Heart and Vascular Institute, Baylor University Medical Center, Baylor Jack and Jane Hamilton Heart and Vascular Hospital, Dallas, TX, USA

The Heart Hospital, Plano
e-mail: peteramccullough@gmail.com

M. Nasser, MD (✉)
Department of Internal Medicine, Providence Hospitals and Medical Centers, 16001 West Nine Mile Rd, Southfield, MI 48075, USA
e-mail: mnasser23@yahoo.com

11.1 Introduction

The heart and the kidneys are inextricably linked via vascular, neurological, hormonal, and cellular signaling systems. The kidneys are the most vascular organ in the body receiving a quarter of cardiac output at rest. Thus, it is no surprise as we explore the extent of the cardiovascular system that kidney disease is strongly associated with cardiovascular disease and, in fact, may reflect the state of vascular health or disease at any time. Additionally, when either organ has injury or begins to fail, there appears to be a sequential effect on the other organ in either an adaptive or maladaptive response, which we now recognize as a "cardiorenal syndrome(s)" [1]. This chapter will review the connections between the heart and the kidneys from epidemiological, biological, and clinical perspectives with the aim of gaining greater appreciation for this important interface in both acute and chronic care.

11.2 Why Does Chronic Kidney Disease Convey Increased Cardiovascular Risk?

The Chronic Kidney Disease Prognosis Consortium (CKD-PC) was established in 2009 by Kidney Disease Improving Global Outcomes (KDIGO) organization in an attempt to understand the risks of declining renal filtration function represented by the estimated glomerular filtration rate (eGFR) and the presence of albu-

M. Arici (ed.), *Management of Chronic Kidney Disease*,
DOI 10.1007/978-3-642-54637-2_11, © Springer-Verlag Berlin Heidelberg 2014

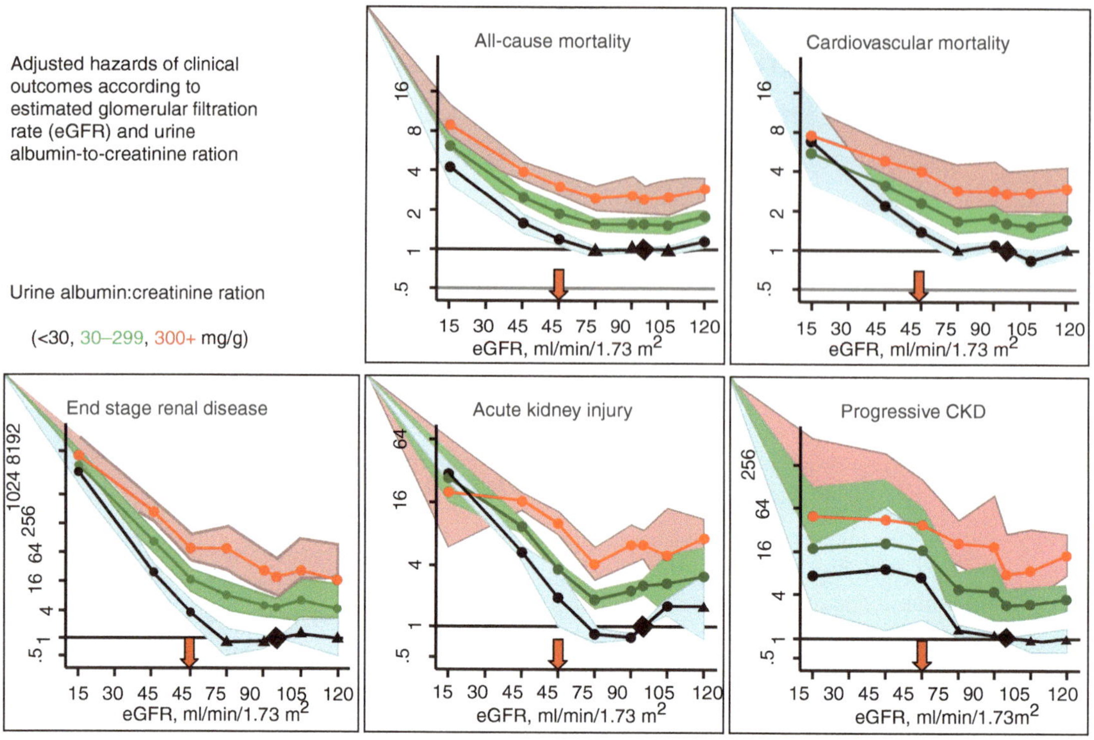

Fig. 11.1 Risks of fatal and nonfatal kidney outcomes from the Chronic Kidney Disease Prognosis Consortium (CKD-PC) (Adapted by permission from Macmillan Publishers Ltd: Levey et al. [2]. Available from: http://www.nature.com/ki/journal/v80/n1/full/ki2010483a.html)

min in the urine indexed to the filtered creatinine concentration (urine albumin/creatinine ratio [ACR]). In a series of manuscripts, this group demonstrated in a very large, pooled database (1,555,332 in 45 cohorts) that the severity of chronic kidney disease (CKD) was related to the risks of all-cause mortality, cardiovascular death, acute kidney injury, progressive CKD, and end-stage renal disease (ESRD) as shown in Fig. 11.1 [2]. These relationships can also be shown in a colored "heat map" of risk as demonstrated in Fig. 11.2. It is important to understand that when both eGFR and elevated ACR overlap, there appears to be magnified risks for all outcomes. Data from the National Kidney Foundation Kidney Early Evaluation Program (KEEP) and the National Health and Nutrition Examination Survey suggest that the majority of individuals with CKD in the younger age groups are identified by albuminuria, while those in the older age strata have reduced eGFR (<60 ml/min/1.73 m^2) as the CKD marker (Fig. 11.3) [3]. Importantly, the overlap between the two markers is less common than one alone in these large populations. However, when both reduced eGFR and albuminuria are present in the same patient, the predicted and observed rates of cardiovascular events are markedly increased over a relatively short (<5 years) duration. Thus, it is critical that, in every patient, both the eGFR be calculated from the age, gender, race, and serum creatinine using standardized equations and the urine ACR be checked using the first morning-voided specimen. Structural kidney disease detected by imaging studies including polycystic kidney disease also are characterized as CKD in the absence of eGFR and ACR abnormalities. The CKD-PC was limited in terms of nonfatal cardiovascular outcomes; therefore, we must turn our attention to other sources of information to understand the connections to coronary atherosclerosis, myocardial disease, valvular disease, and arrhythmias.

Adjusted hazards of clinical outcomes according to estimated glomerular filtration rate (eGFR) and urine albumin-to-creatinine ratio (ACR)

eGFR in ml/min/1.73 m^2
ACR in mg/g

All-cause mortality

	ACR <10	ACR 10–29	ACR 30–299	ACR ≥300
eGFR > 105	1.1	1.5	2.2	5.0
eGFR 90–105	Ref	1.4	1.5	3.1
eGFR 75–90	1.0	1.3	1.7	2.3
eGFR 60–75	1.0	1.4	1.8	2.7
eGFR 45–60	1.3	1.7	2.2	3.6
eGFR 30–45	1.9	2.3	3.3	4.9
eGFR 15–30	5.3	3.6	4.7	6.6

Cardiovascular mortality

	ACR <10	ACR 10–29	ACR 30–299	ACR ≥300
eGFR > 105	0.9	1.3	2.3	2.1
eGFR 90–105	Ref	1.5	1.7	3.7
eGFR 75–90	1.0	1.3	1.6	3.7
eGFR 60–75	1.1	1.4	2.0	4.1
eGFR 45–60	1.5	2.2	2.8	4.3
eGFR 30–45	2.2	2.7	3.4	5.2
eGFR 15–30	14	7.9	4.8	8.1

Kidney failure (ESRD)

	ACR <10	ACR 10–29	ACR 30–299	ACR ≥300
eGFR > 105	Ref	Ref	7.8	18
eGFR 90–105	Ref	Ref	11	20
eGFR 75–90	Ref	Ref	3.8	48
eGFR 60–75	Ref	Ref	7.4	67
eGFR 45–60	5.2	22	40	147
eGFR 30–45	56	74	294	763
eGFR 15–30	433	1,044	1,056	2,286

Acute kidney injury (AKI)

	ACR <10	ACR 10–29	ACR 30–299	ACR ≥300
eGFR > 105	Ref	Ref	2.7	8.4
eGFR 90–105	Ref	Ref	2.4	5.8
eGFR 75–90	Ref	Ref	2.5	4.1
eGFR 60–75	Ref	Ref	3.3	6.4
eGFR 45–60	2.2	4.9	6.4	5.9
eGFR 30–45	7.3	10	12	20
eGFR 15–30	17	17	21	29

Progressive CKD

	ACR <10	ACR 10–29	ACR 30–299	ACR ≥300
eGFR >105	Ref	Ref	0.4	3.0
eGFR 90–105	Ref	Ref	0.9	3.3
eGFR 75–90	Ref	Ref	1.9	5.0
eGFR 60–75	Ref	Ref	3.2	8.1
eGFR 45–60	3.1	4.0	9.4	57
eGFR 30–45	3.0	19	15	22
eGFR 15–30	4.0	12	21	7.7

Fig. 11.2 Adjusted risk of outcomes according to eGFR and urine ACR (Adapted with permission from Macmillan Publishers Ltd: Levey et al. [2]. Available from: http://www.nature.com/ki/journal/v80/n1/full/ki2010483a.html)

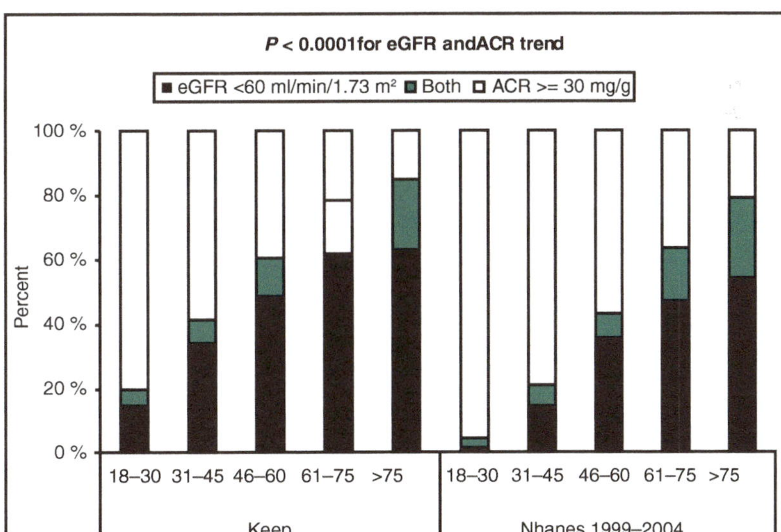

Fig. 11.3 Identification of CKD by eGFR and urine ACR in KEEP, $N = 40{,}013$, and NHANES, $N = 10{,}486$ (Adapted from McCullough et al. [3])

The term "reverse epidemiology" has been applied to patients with ESRD for many risk factors, particularly body weight. What this means is that in the general population, increased adiposity as expressed with the body mass index (BMI) is consistently associated with cardiovascular events and reduced survival. However, in ESRD, increased BMI confers improved survival.

This suggests that increased adiposity is the inverse of cachexia. That is, as chronic disease progresses, cachexia and reduction in weight are a common pathway towards death. Thus, retention of adiposity is associated with survival. Reverse epidemiology has also been observed with total cholesterol and albumin, which are proxies for nutritional intake, which, again, is inversely related to the degree of cachexia.

11.3 Does Kidney Disease Promote Coronary Atherosclerosis Calcification?

Data from many studies suggests that the CKD milieu promotes the early initiation and accelerated course of coronary atherosclerosis. Because CKD is strongly associated with traditional coronary risk factors including hypertension, diabetes, dyslipidemia, and smoking, the combination of these factors may be reflected by CKD, and thus its relationship is amplified by positive confounding. However, when adjusting for these factors, CKD has been consistently associated with nonfatal myocardial infarction and cardiovascular death [3]. A prominent feature of coronary atherosclerosis in patients with CKD and ESRD is accentuated calcification which occurs in all cases of atherosclerosis when reviewed at necropsy. Initially, calcium deposits on cholesterol crystals in the subendothelial space [4]. However, the progression of atherosclerosis involves a multitude of local and systemic factors which stimulate vascular smooth muscle cells to undergo osteoblastic transformation into osteocyte-like cells which deposit calcium hydroxyapatite crystals into both the subendothelial and medial compartments of blood vessels. Many factors have been implicated in CKD to accelerate this process including low-density lipoprotein cholesterol (LDL-C), non-high-density lipoprotein cholesterol, vascular calcification factor, osteoprotegerin, and most notably phosphorus [5]. As eGFR falls, there is retention of phosphate, which can stimulate the Pit-1 receptor on vascular smooth muscle cells thereby facilitating the osteoblastic transformation. Of note, neither the local calcium concentration nor the blood levels of calcium have been independently associated with atherosclerotic calcification in the coronary arteries. As CKD progresses, coronary artery disease is commonly identified on a variety of clinical studies, frequently as longer lesions and in more proximal vessels [6]. Fortunately more extensive calcification, while it is related to the burden of coronary disease, is also associated with more stable lesions; thus, CKD patients often have stable but extensive CAD leading to episodes of both silent and symptomatic coronary ischemia.

It has been suggested that there are both traditional and nontraditional risk factors that may contribute to more accelerated atherosclerosis in persons with CKD. The traditional risk factors include elevated LDL-C, hypertension, diabetes mellitus, smoking, and family history of premature coronary disease (first-degree relative female before age 55 and male before age 45 years). Nontraditional risk factors in CKD have been variously mentioned in the literature and include blood markers of mineral and bone disorder (hyperphosphatemia, elevated calcium-phosphorus product, osteopontin, hyperparathyroidism), C-reactive protein, uremia, asymmetric dimethylarginine and reduced nitric oxide availability, anemia, increased unbound iron (catalytic or poorly liganded iron), homocysteine, fibrinogen, and increased coagulation proteins. None of these factors have been sufficiently tested in prospective studies to be considered a therapeutic target for prevention in CKD patients with atherosclerosis.

11.4 Why Does the Heart Fail as a Pump in Kidney Patients?

Chronic kidney disease promotes the three major pathophysiologic mechanisms by which the left ventricle can fail: pressure overload, volume overload, and cardiomyopathy. Because hypertension is both a determinant and a consequent of CKD, the vast majority of CKD patients have long-standing histories of elevated blood pressure and increased cardiac afterload resulting in

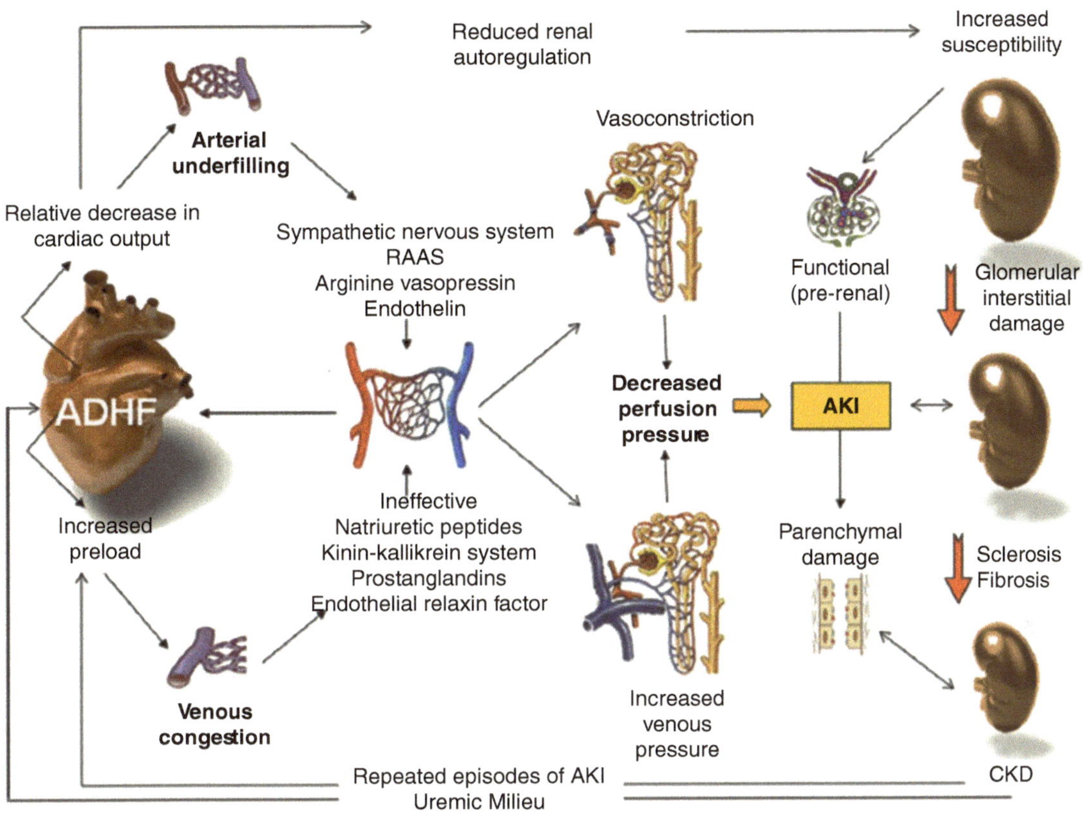

Fig. 11.4 Pathophysiology of cardiorenal syndrome type 1. *ADHF* acutely decompensated heart failure. *AKI* acute kidney injury (Reproduced with permission from Ronco et al. [10]. Copyright 2012, with permission from Elsevier)

left ventricular hypertrophy and increased left ventricular mass [7]. Salt and water retention result in chronic volume overload. Nephrotic syndrome and loss of oncotic forces results in worsened fluid retention and edema. Uremia and retention of many substances (indoxyl sulfate and p-cresol) results in impaired myocyte function in both systole and diastole. It has become recently understood that production of fibroblast growth factor-23 from bone in response to CKD phosphate retention has off-target effects on the left ventricular myocardium resulting in increased left ventricular mass and cardiac fibrosis. The resultant myocardial tissue has a reduced capillary density compared to that of persons with normal renal function. Considerable evidence is accumulating that "CKD cardiomyopathy" is manifest by impaired systole and diastole with biomarker and imaging evidence of cardiac fibrosis. The observation that galectin-3 levels correlate with type III aminoterminal propeptide of procollagen, matrix metalloproteinase-2, and tissue inhibitor of metalloproteinase-1 suggests that myocardial macrophage infiltration enhances turnover of extracellular matrix proteins in patients with CKD [8]. Thus, patients with CKD are at very high risk for the development of heart failure associated with markedly impaired cardiorespiratory function and the cardinal features of fatigue, effort intolerance, edema, and clinical findings including pulmonary congestion and elevation of B-type natriuretic peptides [9]. When acutely decompensated heart failure is present, then a viscous cycle of worsened renal filtration function, venous and renal congestion, and further retention of salt and water can occur. This is commonly termed cardiorenal syndrome type 1 (Fig. 11.4) [10].

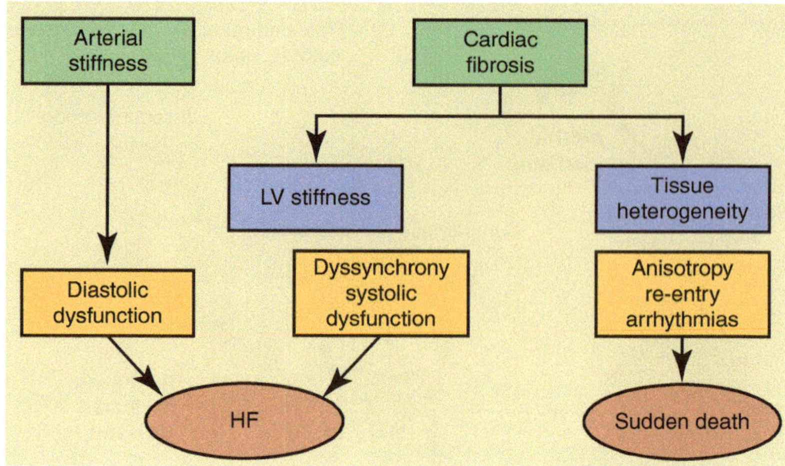

Fig. 11.5 Pathophysiologic pathways to heart failure and sudden arrhythmic death in patients with CKD and ESRD. *HF* heart failure (Reproduced from McCullough et al. [8])

11.5 Should I Hear a Murmur?

Accelerated aortic valvular and mitral annular calcification and fibrosis is common in patients with CKD and nearly universally present in patients with ESRD. The murmur of aortic valve sclerosis is found in the majority of patients, while the mitral annular disease is usually silent and detected only by echocardiography or other forms of imaging. The aortic valve sclerosis and calcification can progress to symptomatic aortic stenosis, while the mitral annular disease can result in very mild functional stenoses or regurgitation by Doppler but rarely requires surgical attention. Both valvular lesions can be the substrate for acute infective endocarditis in ESRD patients with temporary dialysis catheters and occur at a rate of 6–8 % per year. Staphylococcus aureus is the main cause (75 %) of vascular access-related bacteremia among patients receiving long-term hemodialysis [11]. When endocarditis occurs in this setting, the operative mortality rate can be in excess of 50 % [12]. Most patients with CKD should undergo echocardiography at some point in their care in order to evaluate not only for the extent of valve disease but also to assess left ventricular systolic and diastolic function.

11.6 Why Are There More Arrhythmias?

Patients with CKD have the myocardial and hemodynamic determinants of all forms of arrhythmias. In the United States Renal Data System database, 62 % of cardiac deaths (27 % of all deaths) are attributable to lethal arrhythmias [13]. Atrial fibrillation occurs at an elevated rate in patients with CKD and is associated with an increased risk of cardioembolic stroke compared to those with normal renal function. Because of accelerated myocardial fibrosis and the presence of macrovascular and microvascular disease, reentrant ventricular arrhythmias occur at increased rates and are believed to be the inciting event in sudden death (Fig. 11.5). Increased premature atrial and ventricular beats when seen on monitoring can be harbingers of atrial fibrillation and ventricular tachycardia, respectively. Electrolyte shifts and imbalance that occurs in CKD and is accentuated with forms of dialysis are also believed to play a role in ventricular arrhythmias and sudden death, most likely due to ventricular fibrillation. The roles of anticoagulation for stroke prevention in atrial fibrillation, atrial and ventricular antiarrhythmic medications, and the use of implantable cardio defibrillators are all controversial at the time of this writing [14]. Each guidelines-based approach in the population of patients with heart disease and normal kidney function is complicated by increased adverse events and even iatrogenic death in patients with CKD and ESRD [15]. Thus, therapy must be individualized and very frequent monitoring is required.

11.7 Summary

The connection between kidney and heart disease can be viewed in four domains: coronary atherosclerosis, myocardial disease, valvular abnormalities, and arrhythmias. Chronic kidney disease plays a role in the pathogenesis, presentation, outcomes, and management of each manifestation of CVD. Future research is needed to better understand the unique mechanisms at work in patients with CKD that promotes and worsens CVD outcomes. Practical strategies are needed to guide clinicians in the most appropriate management of this high-risk population.

Before You Finish: Practice Pearls for the Clinician

- Osteoblastic transformation of vascular smooth muscle cells is responsible for the calcification of atherosclerosis and the vascular media in patients with kidney disease.
- Both myocyte hypertrophy and increases in the interstitial matrix account for the phenotypic changes seen in the myocardium.
- Valvular thickening and calcification result in murmurs and risk for endocarditis, particularly in dialysis patients.
- Increased premature atrial contractions and premature ventricular beats can be harbingers for atrial fibrillation and ventricular tachycardia.
- Sudden death is the greatest cardiovascular concern among end-stage renal disease patients.

References

1. Ronco C, McCullough PA, Anker SD, Anand I, Aspromonte N, Bagshaw SM, et al. Cardiorenal syndromes: an executive summary from the consensus conference of the Acute Dialysis Quality Initiative (ADQI). Contrib Nephrol. 2010;165:54–67.
2. Levey AS, de Jong PE, Coresh J, El Nahas M, Astor BC, Matsushita K, et al. The definition, classification, and prognosis of chronic kidney disease: a KDIGO Controversies Conference report. Kidney Int. 2011; 80(1):17–28.
3. McCullough PA, Li S, Jurkovitz CT, Stevens LA, Wang C, Collins AJ, Kidney Early Evaluation Program Investigators, et al. CKD and cardiovascular disease in screened high-risk volunteer and general populations: the Kidney Early Evaluation Program (KEEP) and National Health and Nutrition Examination Survey (NHANES) 1999–2004. Am J Kidney Dis. 2008;51(4 Suppl 2):S38–45.
4. McCullough PA, Chinnaiyan KM, Agrawal V, Danielewicz E, Abela GS. Amplification of atherosclerotic calcification and Mönckeberg's sclerosis: a spectrum of the same disease process. Adv Chronic Kidney Dis. 2008;15(4):396–412.
5. McCullough PA, Agarwal M, Agrawal V. Review article: risks of coronary artery calcification in chronic kidney disease: do the same rules apply? Nephrology (Carlton). 2009;14(4):428–36.
6. Charytan DM, Kuntz RE, Garshick M, Candia S, Khan MF, Mauri L. Location of acute coronary artery thrombosis in patients with and without chronic kidney disease. Kidney Int. 2009;75(1):80–7.
7. Lubanski MS, McCullough PA. Kidney's role in hypertension. Minerva Cardioangiol. 2009;57(6): 743–59.
8. McCullough PA, Olobatoke A, Vanhecke TE. Galectin-3: a novel blood test for the evaluation and management of patients with heart failure. Rev Cardiovasc Med. 2011;12(4):200–10.
9. Hanson ID, McCullough PA. B-type natriuretic peptide: beyond diagnostic applications. In: Bakris GL, editor. The kidney in heart failure. New York: Springer; 2012. p. 67–77.
10. Ronco C, Cicoira M, McCullough PA. Cardiorenal syndrome type 1: pathophysiological crosstalk leading to combined heart and kidney dysfunction in the setting of acutely decompensated heart failure. J Am Coll Cardiol. 2012;60:1031–42.
11. Maraj S, Jacobs LE, Maraj R, Kotler MN. Bacteremia and infective endocarditis in patients on hemodialysis. Am J Med Sci. 2004;327:242–9.
12. Nucifora G, Badano LP, Viale P, Gianfagna P, Allocca G, Montanaro D, et al. Infective endocarditis in chronic haemodialysis patients: an increasing clinical challenge. Eur Heart J. 2007;28(19): 2307–12.

13. Herzog CA, Mangrum JM, Passman R. Sudden cardiac death and dialysis patients. Semin Dial. 2008; 21(4):300–7.
14. McCullough PA, Wase A. Do implantable cardioverter-defibrillators improve survival in dialysis patients after cardiac arrest? Nat Clin Pract Nephrol. 2006;2(2):70–1.
15. Dager WE, Kiser TH. Systemic anticoagulation considerations in chronic kidney disease. Adv Chronic Kidney Dis. 2010;17(5):420–7.

Screening and Diagnosing Cardiovascular Disease in Chronic Kidney Disease

12

Peter A. McCullough and Mohammad Nasser

Before You Start: Facts You Need to Know

- Cardiovascular disease is a leading cause of morbidity and mortality in patients with chronic kidney disease as determined by reduced estimated glomerular filtration rate and/or albuminuria.
- Atherosclerosis is both accelerated in development and in calcification in patients with chronic kidney disease.
- Heart failure is the most common symptomatic manifestation of cardiovascular disease requiring hospitalization in patients with chronic kidney disease.
- Blood B-type natriuretic peptide, N-terminal pro B-type natriuretic peptide, galectin-3, and soluble ST-2 are approved tests as these aid in the diagnosis, prognosis, and management of heart failure; however, caution should be exercised in the interpretation of these markers in the setting of chronic kidney disease.
- Aortic valve sclerosis and mitral annular calcification are common valve pathologies associated with chronic kidney disease.
- All forms of arrhythmias are more common in chronic kidney disease, especially sudden death which is markedly increased in risk in dialysis patients.

P.A. McCullough, MD, MPH
Department of Cardiovascular Medicine, Baylor Heart and Vascular Institute, Baylor University Medical Center, Baylor Jack and Jane Hamilton Heart and Vascular Hospital, Dallas, TX, USA

The Heart Hospital, Plano
e-mail: peteramccullough@gmail.com

M. Nasser, MD (✉)
Department of Internal Medicine, Providence Hospitals and Medical Centers, 16001 West Nine Mile Rd, Southfield, MI 48075, USA
e-mail: mnasser23@yahoo.com

12.1 What Are the Approaches to Screen for Coronary Artery Disease?

All adult patients including those with chronic kidney disease (CKD) should undergo an assessment for coronary artery disease (CAD) risk using a standard risk assessment such as that proposed by the Framingham investigators [1]. Variables in the Framingham risk calculation include age, total (or low-density lipoprotein [LDL-C]) cholesterol, high-density lipoprotein, smoking, and systolic blood pressure [2]. A 20 % 10-year risk (2 % annual risk) of nonfatal myocardial infarction or

M. Arici (ed.), *Management of Chronic Kidney Disease*,
DOI 10.1007/978-3-642-54637-2_12, © Springer-Verlag Berlin Heidelberg 2014

cardiovascular death is considered high risk and is a call for full prevention measures in the general population. Most patients with CKD (67 %) will be in Framingham moderate- or high-risk groups; however, as shown in Fig. 12.1, patients with Stages 3–5 CKD in these groups will have a 10–20 % annual risk of cardiovascular events (tenfold that of subjects in Framingham) [1]. Since the risk connoted by traditional risk factors is markedly amplified in CKD, it is reasonable to use exercise stress testing for exercise prescription and prognosis in high-risk individuals. Because of high rates of abnormal baseline electrocardiogram (ECG), left ventricular hypertrophy, and conduction abnormalities, exercise stress testing combined with either echocardiographic imaging or nuclear scintigraphy is reasonable. For those who cannot exercise, both dobutamine and dipyridamole/adenosine/regadenoson can be used as a pharmacological means of achieving myocardial perfusion imaging. Large areas of ischemia (>10 % of the left ventricular myocardium) usually call for invasive assessment of coronary lesions and consideration for revascularization. In the setting of diabetes and multivessel disease, coronary artery bypass surgery is the preferred method of revascularization [3]. Coronary computed tomographic angiography in patients with CKD is not advised given the very high rates of coronary calcification which causes "bloom" artifact which works to make lesion severity difficult to assess [4]. However, if vascular calcification is detected incidentally on computed tomography or roentgenography, it is indicative of advanced atherosclerosis, and attention should be paid to both atherosclerosis risk factors and the elements of CKD mineral and bone disorder (phosphate retention, hyperparathyroidism, and relative hypocalcemia) (Fig. 12.2) [5, 6].

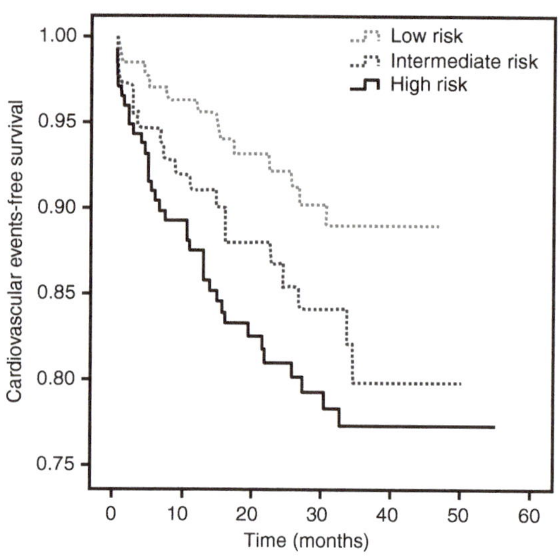

Fig. 12.1 Event-free survival from major cardiac events according to the Framingham risk score applied to a population of patients with chronic kidney disease

12.2 Should Patients with Chronic Kidney Disease Undergo Routine Echocardiography?

Because of the very high incidence of left ventricular hypertrophy, risk for Stage A and Stage B heart failure, and known associations between

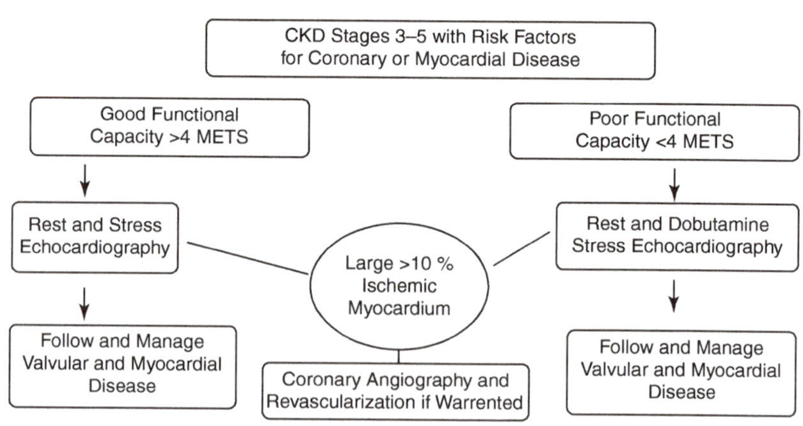

Fig. 12.2 Coronary artery disease screening algorithm (*METS* metabolic equivalents of functional capacity)

Box 12.1. Five Cardiorenal Syndromes and Their Common Clinical Scenarios

Cardiorenal Syndrome (CRS) General Definition

A pathophysiologic disorder of the heart and kidneys whereby acute or chronic dysfunction in one organ may induce acute or chronic dysfunction in the other organ

CRS Type I (Acute Cardiorenal Syndrome)

Abrupt worsening of cardiac function (e.g., acutely decompensated congestive heart failure) leading to acute kidney injury

CRS Type II (Chronic Cardiorenal Syndrome)

Chronic abnormalities in cardiac function (e.g., chronic congestive heart failure) causing progressive and permanent chronic kidney disease

CRS Type III (Acute Renocardiac Syndrome)

Abrupt worsening of renal function (e.g., acute kidney injury) causing acute cardiac disorder (acute heart failure)

CRS Type IV (Chronic Renocardiac Syndrome)

Chronic kidney disease (diabetic nephropathy) contributing to decreased cardiac function and cardiac hypertrophy and fibrosis and/or increased risk of adverse cardiovascular events

CRS Type V (Secondary Cardiorenal Syndrome)

Systemic condition (e.g., sepsis) causing both acute cardiac and renal injury and dysfunction

CKD and valvular heart disease, all patients with CKD should be considered for echocardiography at the time CKD is determined by the presence of reduced estimated glomerular filtration rate (eGFR) <59 ml/min/1.73 m^2 or evidence of kidney damage manifest by an increased urine albumin: creatinine ratio or imaging evidence of kidney disease such as polycystic kidneys by ultrasound [7]. Importantly, cardiovascular disease including coronary disease and heart failure occurs at much earlier ages than in the general population [8]. The presence of combined heart and kidney failure is now considered a "cardiorenal syndrome" and should be considered in the context of the more antecedent abnormality with respect to both diagnosis and management [9]. Five subtypes of cardiorenal syndromes are displayed in (Box 12.1). The current Kidney Disease Outcomes Quality Initiative (KDOQI) guidelines recommend echocardiograms for all CKD 5D patients 1–3 months after renal replacement therapy initiation and at 3-year intervals thereafter [10] (Boxes 12.2 and 12.3). Echocardiography with complete Doppler assessment reliably estimated left ventricular ejection fraction (normal 55–75 %), left ventricular hypertrophy (left ventricular mass index >115 and >95 g/m^2), and assesses both the morphology and flow characteristics of all four cardiac valves. Findings suggesting reduced ejection fraction, diastolic dysfunction, or regional wall motion abnormalities may prompt an evaluation for chronic cardiac ischemia as discussed above [11]. Diastolic dysfunction is ideally graded according to the European Association of Echocardiography/American Society of Echocardiography criteria as normal, Grade I (impaired relaxation), Grade II, and Grade III (most severe) with evidence of restriction and increased left atrial pressure. Echocardiographic evaluation of left ventricular diastolic dysfunction can be complicated. It consists of measuring E/è and E/A ratios to determine impaired relaxation as well as restrictive patterns and LV filling pressures. E and A represent velocities of the rapid early and late transmitral diastolic flow, while è is a measurement of mitral annulus recoil velocity. Chronic kidney disease is associated with a form of uremic or CKD cardiomyopathy as shown in Fig. 12.3. The cardiomyopathy associated with CKD is characterized by the presence of left ventricular hypertrophy, evidence of diastolic dysfunction, and, in more severe cases, superimposed systolic dysfunction with reduced ejection fraction.

A finding of significant valvular or pericardial disease warrants clinical correlation and

Box 12.2. What the Guidelines Say You Should Do

- Patients with chest pain should receive a complete history and physical examination to assess the probability of coronary disease before additional testing.
- A resting ECG is recommended in patients without an obvious, noncardiac cause of chest pain.
- Assessment of resting left ventricular function and evaluation for abnormalities of myocardium, heart valves, or pericardium are recommended with the use of Doppler echocardiography in patients with known or suspected coronary disease and a prior MI, pathological Q waves, symptoms or signs suggestive of heart failure, complex ventricular arrhythmias, or an undiagnosed heart murmur.
- Standard exercise stress testing is recommended for risk assessment in patients with stable coronary disease who have an interpretable ECG and no disabling comorbidity. Pharmacological stress with nuclear myocardial perfusion imaging or echocardiography is an alternative in those who are incapable of exercising to an accepted workload.
- Coronary computed tomography angiography is reasonable for patients with a low to intermediate pretest probability of ischemic heart disease who have a disabling comorbidity.

Source: Data from Refs. [16–18].

Box 12.3. Relevant Guidelines

1. *American Heart Association Guidelines*:
   - 2012 ACCF/AHA/ACP/AATS/PCNA/SCAI/STS guideline for the diagnosis and management of patients with stable ischemic heart disease: executive summary. A report of the American College of Cardiology Foundation/American Heart Association Task Force on Practice Guidelines, and the American College of Physicians, American Association for Thoracic Surgery, Preventive Cardiovascular Nurses Association, Society for Cardiovascular Angiography and Interventions, and Society of Thoracic Surgeons. Circulation. 2012;126:3097–137 [16].
   - 2011 ACCF/AHA/SCAI guideline for Percutaneous Coronary Intervention: executive summary. A Report of the American College of Cardiology Foundation/American Heart Association Task Force on Practice Guidelines and the Society for Cardiovascular Angiography and Interventions. Circulation. 2011;124:2574–609 [17].
2. *National Kidney Foundation Guidelines*:
   - National Kidney Foundation. K/DOQI clinical practice guidelines for cardiovascular disease in dialysis patients. Am J Kidney Dis. 2005;45 Suppl 3:S1–154 [18].

follow-up. Most patients with moderate or more aortic stenosis/regurgitation or mitral regurgitation will require annual echocardiography and cardiology consultation for surveillance. In general, severe symptomatic aortic stenosis (Fig. 12.4) and/or regurgitation is an indication for valve replacement [5].

Pericardial disease may develop in kidney failure as pericarditis, pericardial effusion, or chronic constrictive pericarditis. BUN elevations over 60 mg/dl may lead to inflammation in the pericardial membranes causing uremic pericarditis. Fluid overload can also lead to pericardial inflammation without uremia. Typical symptoms include fever and pleuritic chest pain that is relieved by sitting up or bending forward. Platelet function impairment may cause a hemorrhagic pericardial effusion and possibly tamponade depending on the

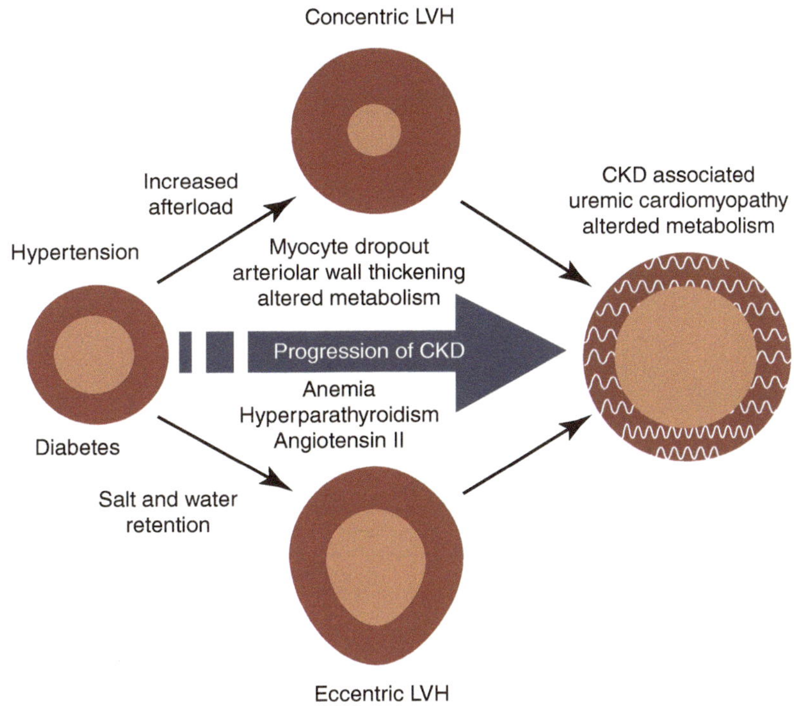

Fig. 12.3 Hypertension, diabetes mellitus, and the development of chronic kidney disease cardiomyopathy

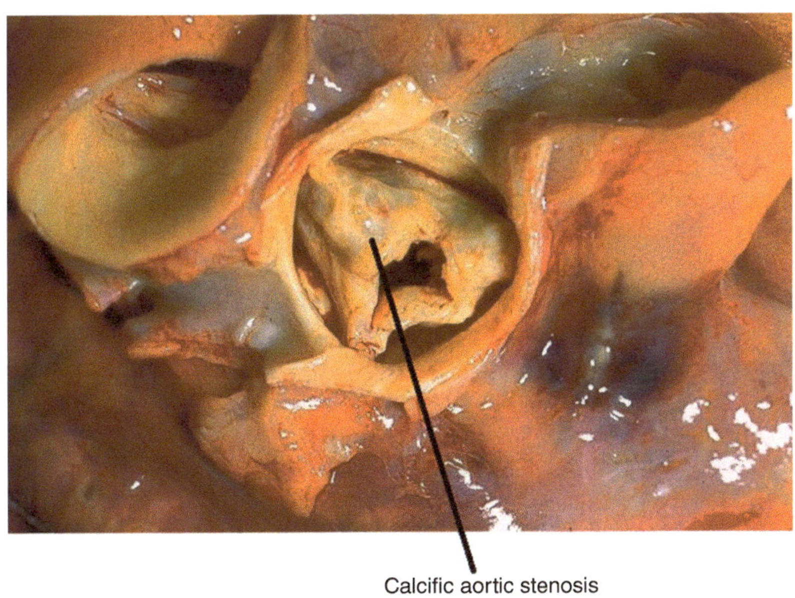

Fig. 12.4 Calcific aortic stenosis

rate of fluid accumulation. Typical diffuse ST elevations observed with acute pericarditis are generally not shown when uremia is the cause [12]. Echocardiography is able to exclude silent effusions and useful in determining associated myocarditis and altered ventricular function.

12.3 What Blood Biomarkers Are Useful in Heart Failure?

Both blood B-type natriuretic peptide (BNP) and N-terminal pro B-type natriuretic peptide (NT-proBNP) have been approved, guidelines

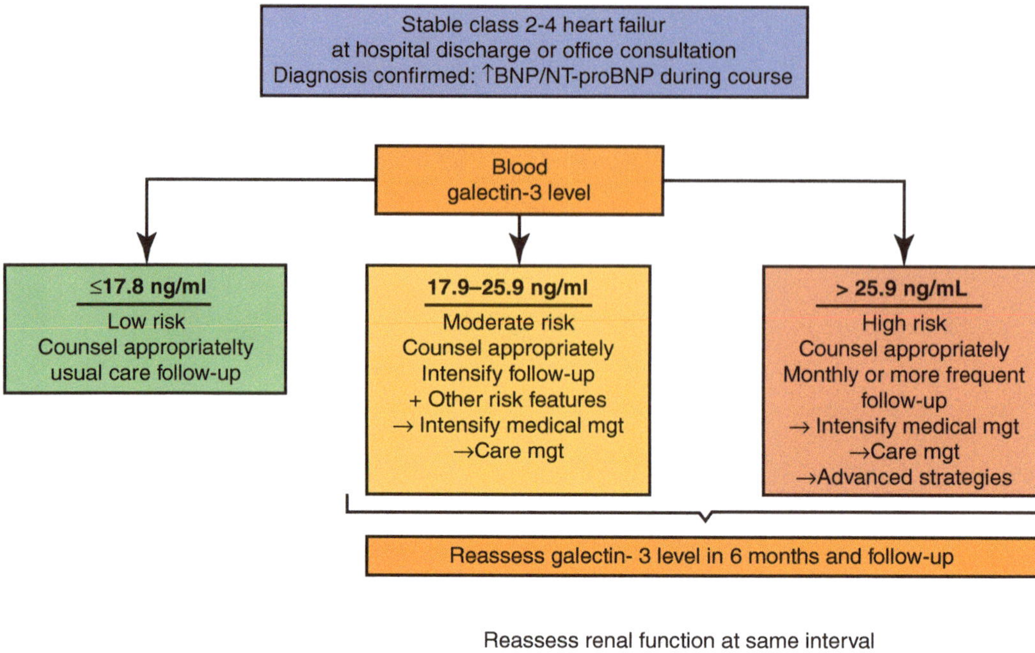

Fig. 12.5 Suggested algorithm for the management of heart failure patients using galectin-3 levels measured in blood

recommended, and are commercially available for several years. When measured in blood, they are indicated as diagnostic aids for the evaluation of patients with acute shortness of breath, prognostic indicators for death and heart failure hospitalization, and aids in the management of patients particularly with respect to the titration of chronic medications. In general, when BNP >200 pg/ml and NT-proBNP >2,000 pg/ml, there is increased myocardial production even in the presence of reduced clearance by the kidneys. The higher the levels, the greater the positive predictive value for heart failure and the worse the prognosis for hospitalization or death. Chronic use of angiotensin-converting enzyme inhibitors, angiotensin receptor antagonists, aldosterone receptor blockers, and beta-adrenergic receptor antagonists and use of biventricular pacing have been shown to reduce BNP/NT-proBNP over time. In approximately 25 % of patients with preserved renal function, natriuretic peptides can be normalized (BNP <100 pg/ml, NT-proBNP <150 pg/ml) with therapy for heart failure. In the setting of CKD, it is rare for natriuretic peptides to normalize; however, relatively lower levels (~50 % reduction from prior levels) are associated with a favorable prognosis. Conversely, a doubling of levels over a time frame of 6 weeks or more portends a high rate of future hospitalization and death, both from pump failure and arrhythmias.

Galectin-3 is a paracrine substance produced by macrophages that are participating in myocardial fibrosis. Increased levels of galectin-3 (>25.9 ng/ml) are strongly prognostic for short-term death and hospitalization in patients with either diastolic or systolic dysfunction. There have been no published studies evaluating the clinical value of galectin-3 in patients with CKD; however, many subjects in the heart failure studies where it was measured met the criteria for CKD according to an eGFR < 60 ml/min [13]. A suggested algorithm for the management of heart failure using galectin-3 is shown in Fig. 12.5.

Soluble ST2 (ST2) and interleukin-33 compete for the transmembrane protein ligand (ST2L) and induce production of T helper type 2 cytokines. In heart failure, serum ST2 is elevated and indicates increased abnormal immune cell signaling related to myocardial dysfunction. ST2 aids in prognostication in patients with acute and chronic heart failure, particularly when at very high levels (ST2 >36.3 ng/ml). However, an elevated concentration of serum sST2 is found in CKD patients and correlates with the severity of renal disease. Serum sST2 may be also associated

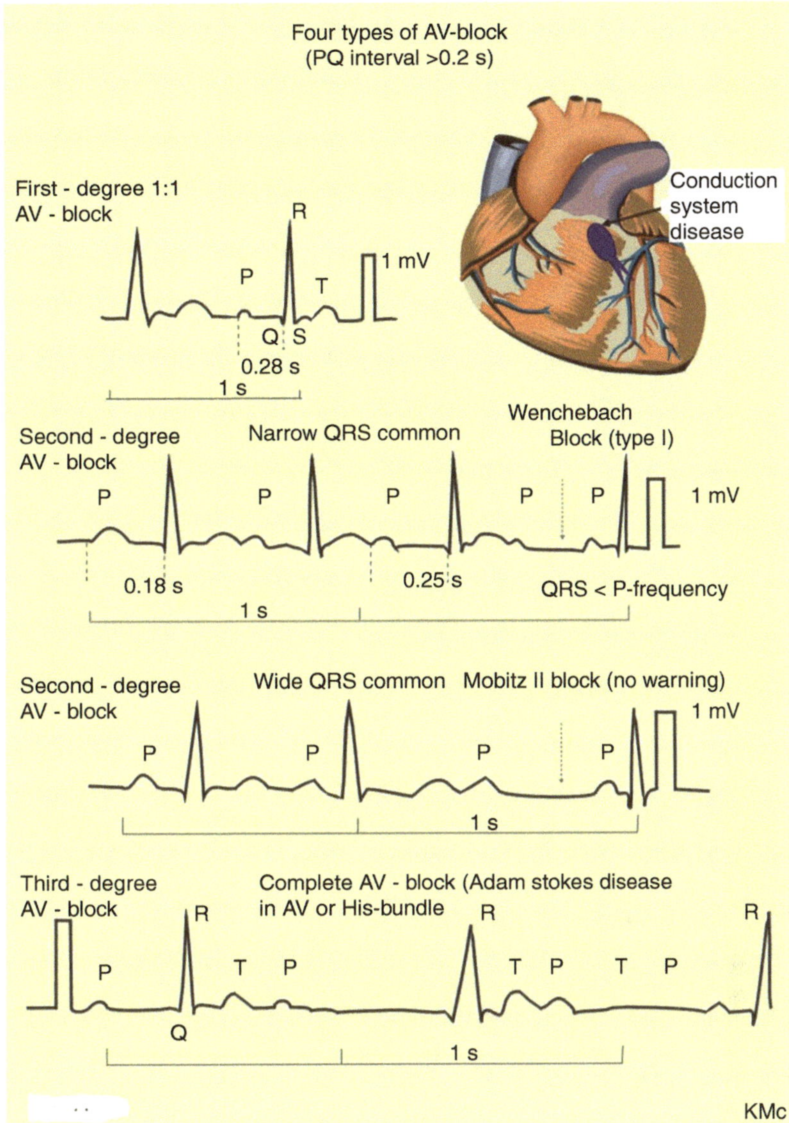

Fig. 12.6 Types of atrioventricular block as identified by electrocardiography

with secondary hyperparathyroidism. The sST2 may have an important role in the development of CKD or as a marker of disease severity, particularly in those with incipient heart failure. Future research in this area is warranted.

12.4 Should Patients with Renal Dysfunction Have Arrhythmia Surveillance?

Maintenance of normal sinus rhythm can become progressively more difficult in patients with CKD who develop left ventricular hypertrophy, left atrial dilatation, right ventricular strain and hypertrophy, and right atrial dilatation. With activation of factors that promote cardiac fibrosis, the conduction system of the heart can show signs of failure at all levels. Thus, at the minimum in an asymptomatic patient with CKD, a 12-lead electrocardiogram should be obtained on an annual basis and with any change in cardiac symptoms. Failure of conduction at the level of the sinus node can lead to sick sinus syndrome (episodes of sinus pauses and tachycardia), atrioventricular node block (Mobitz Type II second degree and complete heart block (Fig. 12.6), and bundle branch blocks. These lesions in symptomatic

Fig. 12.7 Atrial flutter

Atrial flutter: a right atrial macro re-entrant rhythm

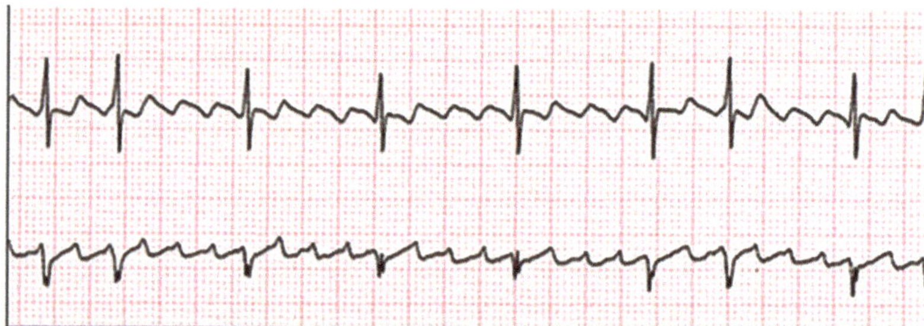

Heart Rate	Rhythm	P wave	PR interval (in seconds)	QRS (in seconds)
A: 220–430 bpm V: <300 bpm	Regualr or variable	Sawtoothed appearance	N/A	<.12 Winder if BBB

A=atrial, V=ventricular
BBB=bundle branch block

patients are indications for permanent pacemaker implantation.

Right atrial dilatation can create a macro reentrant circuit which facilitates atrial flutter. This rhythm is recognized by sawtooth atrial depolarization waves and ventricular conduction typically in a 2:1 or 3:1 ratio (Fig. 12.7). Atrial flutter is easily managed by radio-frequency ablation and deserves electrophysiology referral. Left atrial dilatation and left ventricular hypertrophy as well as advanced age and hypertension are strong determinants for the development of atrial fibrillation (AF). Atrial fibrillation is the most common dysrhythmia among the general and CKD populations. Because the disorganized rhythm leads to stasis of blood in the left atrial appendage, thrombi can form and be ejected into the left circulation resulting in stroke and systemic cardio-embolism (Fig. 12.8). Thus, AF presents multiple management dilemmas including rhythm versus rate control, anticoagulation, and heart failure prevention. Any patient who presents with palpitations, tachycardia, or stroke symptoms should be assessed for AF with inpatient monitoring, 24- or 48-h outpatient Holter monitoring, or patient-triggered event monitoring. For difficult cases, an implantable loop recorder can be placed subcutaneously in the infraclavicular region and give information about cardiac rhythm for several years using noninvasive computer interrogation. In the setting of cryptogenic stroke, use of intensive rhythm monitoring has shown that approximately one third of cases can have the stroke be attributable to paroxysmal AF that was previously unrecognized.

The leading cause of death in CKD and ESRD is sudden arrhythmic death. The details surrounding these cases are often difficult to pull together since many occur in the home and out of hospital. Presumably heart block, electromechanical dissociation, pump failure, or ventricular fibrillation is the terminal scenario. Patients with left ventricular ejection fractions <35 %, those with a history of a prior resuscitated cardiac arrest, and spontaneous sustained ventricular tachycardia on monitoring should all be considered for implantable cardio-defibrillators. These devices reduce cardiac mortality in the general population but have not definitively been shown to prolong survival in patients with CKD or ESRD. The two major therapies delivered by implantable cardio-defibrillators are anti-tachycardia pacing and defibrillation as shown in Fig. 12.9. Because of increased myocardial interstitial matrix in CKD and left ventricular hypertrophy, CKD and ESRD patients can be expected to have higher defibrillation thresholds and should undergo more frequent monitoring by the electrophysiologist using noninvasive programmed stimulation [14].

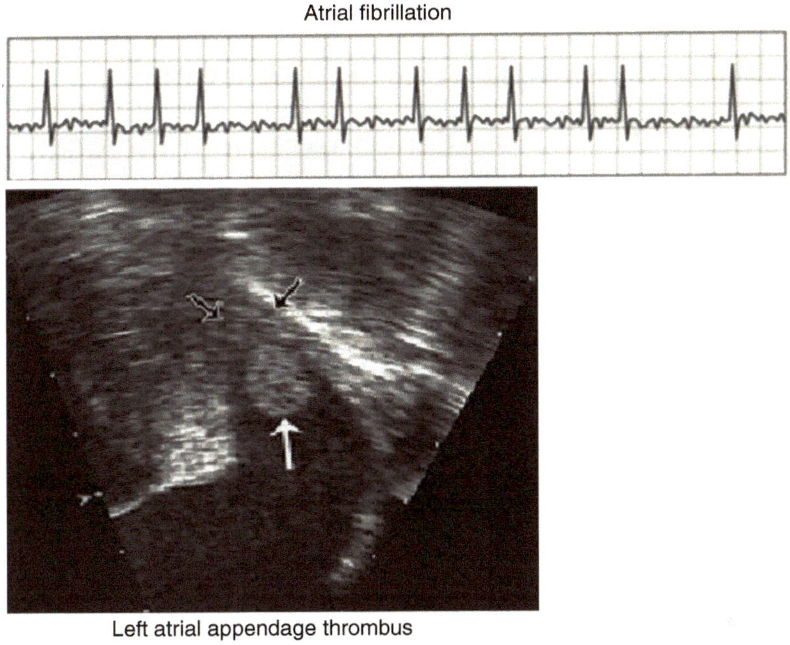

Fig. 12.8 Atrial fibrillation on electrocardiography and a left atrial appendage identified by transesophageal echocardiography

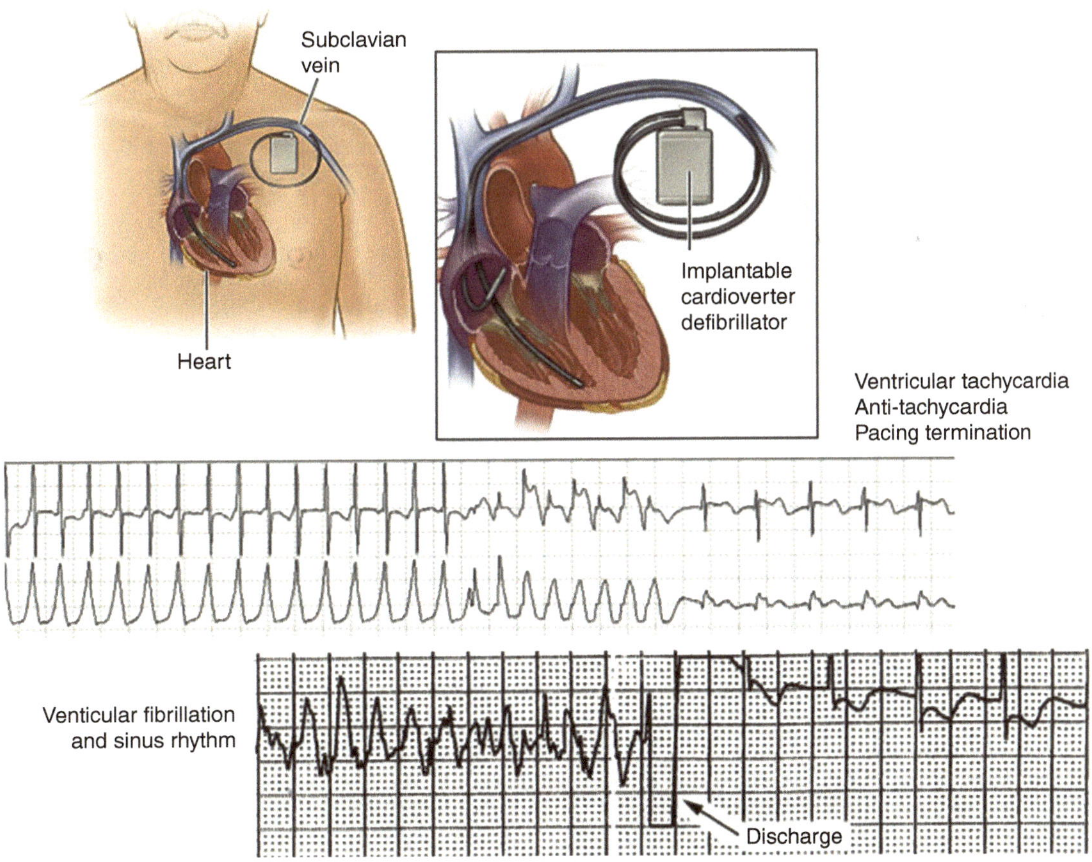

Fig. 12.9 Implantable cardio-defibrillator and demonstration of its two major forms of therapy: (1) anti-tachycardia pacing termination of ventricular tachycardia and (2) defibrillation for ventricular fibrillation

12.5 Summary

High rates of serious cardiovascular disease in patients with CKD and ESRD call for a more attentive approach to both routine and responsive testing in patients at risk or with potential cardiac symptoms [15]. The nephrologist needs a basic understanding of electrocardiographic interpretation both on routine single-lead monitoring and with 12-lead electrocardiography. Use of stress imaging, echocardiography, and continuous forms of rhythm monitoring provide an approach for the diagnosis and management of cardiovascular disease. Early detection and prompt management offer the hope for prevention of myocardial infarction, heart failure, valvular-induced structural damage, stroke, and fatal arrhythmias.

Before You Finish: Practice Pearls for the Clinician

- Assess atherosclerosis risk factors on all patients and work to manage them to optimal levels.
- Diagnose significant cardiac ischemia with stress imaging. Large amounts of ischemia (>10 % of the left ventricle) deserve coronary angiography and consideration of revascularization.
- Obtain routine 12-lead electrocardiography and have a low threshold to obtain more advanced forms of monitoring in patients with palpitations, near syncope, syncope, and stroke.
- Consider echocardiography for all patients with CKD and ESRD for assessment of myocardial function and valvular disease. Patients with considerable abnormalities need cardiology consultation and surveillance.
- In acute or chronic dyspnea, or when heart failure is suspected, elevated levels of BNP, NT-proBNP, galectin-3, and ST2 are supportive of the diagnosis of heart failure and can portend decompensation and death.
- Resuscitated sudden death is an indication for an implantable cardio-defibrillator.

References

1. Chen SC, Su HM, Tsai YC, Huang JC, Chang JM, Hwang SJ, et al. Framingham risk score with cardiovascular events in chronic kidney disease. PLoS One. 2013;8(3):e60008.
2. McCullough PA. Cardiovascular disease in chronic kidney disease from a cardiologist's perspective. Curr Opin Nephrol Hypertens. 2004;13(6):591–600.
3. Keeley EC, McCullough PA. Coronary revascularization in patients with coronary artery disease and chronic kidney disease. Adv Chronic Kidney Dis. 2004;11(3):254–60.
4. McCullough PA, Agrawal V, Danielewicz E, Abela GS. Accelerated atherosclerotic calcification and Mönckeberg's sclerosis: a continuum of advanced vascular pathology in chronic kidney disease. Clin J Am Soc Nephrol. 2008;3(6):1585–98.
5. McCullough PA, Agarwal M, Agrawal V. Review article: risks of coronary artery calcification in chronic kidney disease: do the same rules apply? Nephrology (Carlton). 2009;14(4):428–36.
6. KDIGO clinical practice guidelines for the diagnosis, evaluation, prevention, and treatment of chronic kidney disease-mineral and bone disorder (CKD-MBD). Kidney Int. 2009;76(113):S1–S130.
7. McCullough PA, Jurkovitz CT, Pergola PE, McGill JB, Brown WW, Collins AJ, KEEP Investigators, et al. Independent components of chronic kidney disease as a cardiovascular risk state: results from the kidney early evaluation program (KEEP). Arch Intern Med. 2007;167(11):1122–9.
8. McCullough PA, Li S, Jurkovitz CT, Stevens L, Collins AJ, Chen SC, KEEP Investigators, et al. Chronic kidney disease, prevalence of premature cardiovascular disease, and relationship to short-term mortality. Am Heart J. 2008;156(2):277–83.
9. Ronco C, McCullough PA, Anker SD, Anand I, Aspromonte N, Bagshaw SM, et al. Cardiorenal syndromes: an executive summary from the consensus conference of the acute dialysis quality initiative (ADQI). Contrib Nephrol. 2010;165:54–67.
10. National Kidney Foundation. K/DOQI clinical practice guidelines for cardiovascular disease in dialysis patients. Am J Kidney Dis. 2005;45:S1–153.
11. Vanhecke TE, Franklin BA, Soman P, Lahiri A, Mieres JH, Sias T, et al. Influence of myocardial ischemia on outcomes in patients with systolic versus non-systolic heart failure. Am J Cardiovasc Dis. 2011; 1(2):167–75.
12. Grunukula SR, Spodick DH. Pericardial disease in renal patients. Semin Nephrol. 2001;21:52.
13. McCullough PA, Olobatoke A, Vanhecke TE. Galectin-3: a novel blood test for the evaluation and management of patients with heart failure. Rev Cardiovasc Med. 2011;12(4):200–10.
14. Wase A, Basit A, Nazir R, Jamal A, Shah S, Khan T, et al. Impact of chronic kidney disease upon survival among implantable cardioverter-defibrillator recipients. J Interv Card Electrophysiol. 2004;11(3): 199–204.

15. Best PJ, Reddan DN, Berger PB, Szczech LA, McCullough PA, Califf RM. Cardiovascular disease and chronic kidney disease: insights and an update. Am Heart J. 2004;148(2):230–42.
16. Fihn SD, Gardin JM, Abrams J, Berra K, Blankenship JC, Dallas AP, Douglas PS, Foody JM, Gerber TC, Hinderliter AL, King 3rd SB, Kligfield PD, Krumholz HM, Kwong RY, Lim MJ, Linderbaum JA, Mack MJ, Munger MA, Prager RL, Sabik JF, Shaw LJ, Sikkema JD, Smith Jr CR, Smith Jr SC, Spertus JA, Williams SV, American College of Cardiology Foundation. 2012 ACCF/AHA/ACP/AATS/PCNA/SCAI/STS guideline for the diagnosis and management of patients with stable ischemic heart disease: executive summary. A report of the American College of Cardiology Foundation/American Heart Association Task Force on Practice Guidelines, and the American College of Physicians, American Association for Thoracic Surgery, Preventive Cardiovascular Nurses Association, Society for Cardiovascular Angiography and Interventions, and Society of Thoracic Surgeons. Circulation. 2012;126:3097–137.
17. Levine GN, Bates ER, Blankenship JC, Bailey SR, Bittl JA, Cercek B, Chambers CE, Ellis SG, Guyton RA, Hollenberg SM, Khot UN, Lange RA, Mauri L, Mehran R, Moussa ID, Mukherjee D, Nallamothu BK, Ting HH. 2011 ACCF/AHA/SCAI guideline for percutaneous coronary intervention: executive summary. A report of the American College of Cardiology Foundation/American Heart Association Task Force on Practice Guidelines and the Society for Cardiovascular Angiography and Interventions. Circulation. 2011;124:2574–609.
18. National Kidney Foundation. K/DOQI clinical practice guidelines for cardiovascular disease in dialysis patients. Am J Kidney Dis. 2005;45 Suppl 3:S1–154.

Management of Cardiovascular Disease in Chronic Kidney Disease

13

Mohammad Nasser and Peter A. McCullough

Before You Start: Facts You Need to Know

- Kidney patients should be assessed for signs and symptoms of coronary heart disease.
- Treating risk factors for atherosclerosis provides an amplified benefit for CKD patients.
- Management of heart failure is challenging in the context of CKD and may exacerbate kidney dysfunction.
- CKD predisposes patients to various arrhythmias, especially atrial fibrillation.
- Valvular heart disease commonly accompanies ESRD due to accelerated rate of calcification.

13.1 Coronary Atherosclerosis

Atherosclerosis begins with a fatty streak in young adult life. Lipoproteins then accumulate in the subendothelial space, thereby inducing inflammation by cytokines and oxidative stress. Macrophages attracted to the site promote foam cell formation by lipid phagocytosis. Vascular smooth muscle cells migrate and interact with the plaque as well as the vascular media taking on properties similar to osteoblasts. These cells respond to various lipid, inflammatory, and mineral stimuli to deposit calcium hydroxyapatite crystals in the plaque and vascular media. A fibrous plaque is gradually created by smooth muscle migration and proliferation. This process takes many years and is usually asymptomatic. When the lesion fills over 60 % of the arterial lumen, chronic stable heart disease evolves [1]. At this stage of atherosclerosis, virtually all lesions have histopathologic and x-ray evidence of calcification.

13.1.1 Dyslipidemia Management: Should Patients with Kidney Disease Receive Statins?

Chronic kidney disease (CKD) has been shown to be a risk factor for cardiovascular mortality. It is suggested to treat this disease as coronary heart disease (CHD) equivalent. Dyslipidemia, vascular stiffness, and elevated inflammatory markers are common findings in CKD patients and are

M. Nasser, MD (✉)
Department of Internal Medicine,
Providence Hospitals and Medical Centers,
16001 West Nine Mile Rd,
Southfield, MI 48075, USA
e-mail: mnasser23@yahoo.com

P.A. McCullough, MD, MPH
Department of Cardiovascular Medicine,
Baylor Heart and Vascular Institute,
Baylor University Medical Center,
Baylor Jack and Jane Hamilton Heart
and Vascular Hospital, Dallas, TX, USA

The Heart Hospital, Plano
e-mail: peteramccullough@gmail.com

M. Arici (ed.), *Management of Chronic Kidney Disease*,
DOI 10.1007/978-3-642-54637-2_13,

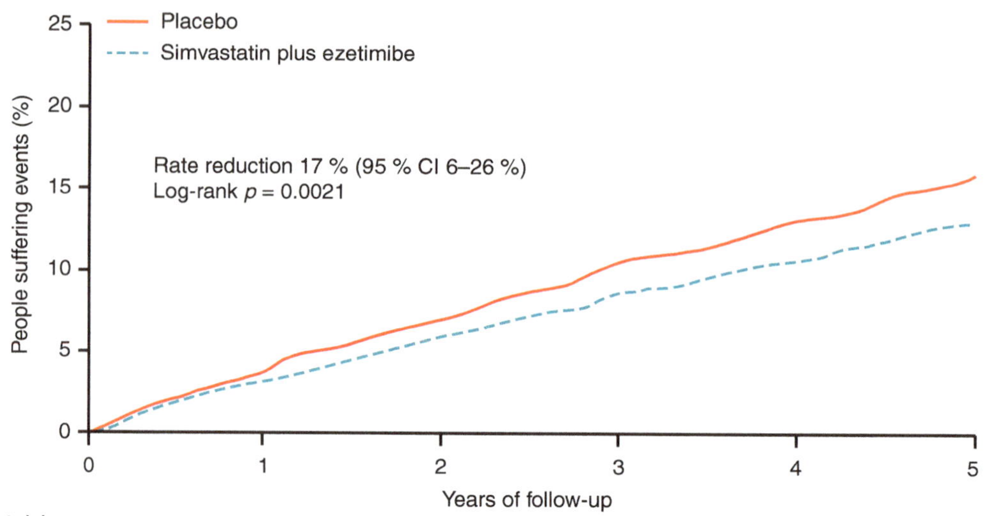

Number at risk

	0	1	2	3	4	5
Placebo	4,620	4,204	3,849	3,469	2,566	1,269
Simvastatin plus ezetimibe	4,650	4,271	3,939	3,546	2,655	1,265

Fig. 13.1 Primary results from the Study of Heart and Renal Protection (SHARP) trial testing simvastatin 20 mg plus ezetimibe 10 mg versus placebo in patients with pre-dialysis and dialysis requiring CKD (Reprinted from Baigent et al. [21], Copyright 2011, with permission from Elsevier)

associated with a faster decline in kidney function, especially if proteinuria is present. Dyslipidemia may accelerate proteinuria and progression of kidney disease. Statins are among the most potent cholesterol-lowering agents as they exhibit unique pleiotropic effects. They work by inhibiting HMG-CoA reductase, a rate-limiting enzyme involved in cholesterol formation, and have been studied in both pre-dialysis and dialysis patients. "The Study of Heart and Renal Protection (SHARP)" trial among other meta-analyses of randomized controlled trials demonstrated the benefit of lowering LDL levels in relation to cardiovascular mortality, myocardial infarction (MI), and stroke reduction (Fig. 13.1). Compared to patients without kidney dysfunction, high-dose statins further enhanced cardiovascular protection in the CKD population; therefore, they should be initiated if possible (Box 13.1).

In November of 2013 the AHA (American Heart Association) and ACC (American College of Cardiology) have collaborated with the NHLBI (National Heart, Lung, and Blood Institute) to develop guidelines for assessment and management of blood cholesterol and cardiovascular risk [2]. The recommendations were designed using data from randomized controlled trials to identify patients that will most likely benefit from statin therapy. Their updated strategy for managing high LDL levels is deviated from the common practice of lowering cholesterol levels to a certain target and the lower the better. The Expert Panel has failed to identify trials that examined titrating statin therapy to achieve a certain LDL goal. Instead, previous studies compared fixed doses of statins to placebo or compared higher and lower doses. Moreover, there is no evidence that nonstatin drugs or therapy to improve HDL has a positive impact on survival. Therefore, current guidelines focus on four groups in which benefit from statin use clearly exceeds risk. These groups include individuals with the following: (1) clinical cardiovascular disease – defined as history of MI, angina, arterial revascularization, stroke, TIA or peripheral vascular disease, (2) diabetics (age 40–75) with LDL levels 70–189 mg/dl and without clinical cardiovascular disease, (3) primary LDL levels of ≥190 mg/dl (secondary causes must be ruled

Box 13.1. What the Guidelines Say You Should Do

- Targeting LDL levels is no longer recommended. All CKD patients over 50 years of age should be on statin therapy. Younger patients should be treated when indicated.
- Lifestyle modification should be encouraged such as maintaining a healthy weight, lowering salt intake, and undertaking exercise programs.
- Statins are not indicated in dialysis-dependent patients due to lack of beneficial evidence.
- Lifestyle changes such as reduction of monosaccharide and disaccharide intake, reducing the total amount of dietary carbohydrates, and replacing long-chain triglycerides and fish oils are indicated in adults with CKD or dialysis with hypertriglyceridemia ≥500 mg/dl.
- Fibrates should be offered to patients with triglycerides ≥500 mg/dl and to patients with triglycerides ≥200 mg/dl and non-HDL level ≥130 mg/dl who are intolerant to statins.
- Antiplatelet agents should be offered in CKD patients unless contraindicated.
- When heart failure is present, acute clinical decompensation and addition or escalation in therapy should prompt close eGFR and potassium monitoring.

Source: Data from 2013 ACC/AHA Guideline on the Treatment of Blood Cholesterol to Reduce Atherosclerotic Cardiovascular Risk in Adults: A Report of the American College of Cardiology/American Heart Association Task Force on Practice Guidelines [2]; Kidney Disease: Improving Global Outcomes (KDIGO) Lipid Work Group [3]; Smith et al. [15]; and Yancy et al. [16].

out such as hypothyroidism, diabetes, drugs, diet, nephrotic syndrome, obesity, CKD, pregnancy, and biliary obstruction), or (4) without diabetes or clinical cardiovascular disease with LDL level of 70–189 mg/dl and an estimated 10-year risk of atherosclerotic cardiovascular disease (defined as nonfatal MI, CHF death, and fatal and nonfatal stroke) of ≥7.5 %. The Pooled Cohort Equations is used to estimate the 10-year cardiovascular risk (available at http://my.americanheart.org/cvrisk-calculator). This equation does not include CKD because data is uncertain about the net improvement in prediction after adding CKD; however, a typical kidney patient such as a 50-year-old African American male with a history of treated hypertension will have a 10-year risk >7.5 % even in the absence of smoking, LDL >189 mg/dl, and diabetes. Therefore, most CKD patients will be candidates for statin therapy.

Individuals with either clinical cardiovascular disease, diabetes plus a 10-year risk ≥7.5 %, or LDL level >189 mg/dl should be on high-intensity statin therapy if tolerated, defined as lowering LDL level by ≥50 % with atorvastatin 40–80 mg or rosuvastatin 20–40 mg. Diabetics with an estimated risk <7.5 % or those with a 10-year risk ≥7.5 % (without clinical cardiovascular disease or diabetes) should be started on moderate-intensity treatment. Atorvastatin 10–20 mg, rosuvastatin 5–10 mg, simvastatin 20–40 mg, or pravastatin 40–80 mg decreases LDL levels by 20–50 % and is considered moderate-intensity drugs. Primary prevention in individuals with no diabetes, LDL levels 40–189 mg/dl, <7.5 % 10-year cardiovascular risk, and ages <40 or >75 should be customized depending on several high-risk factors for coronary disease that include evidence of genetic hyperlipidemias, family history of a first-degree relative with premature coronary heart disease (age <55 for males and <65 for females), calcium score ≥300 Agatston units or ≥75 % of sex, age, and ethnicity, sensitivity-C-reactive protein ≥2 mg/dl, or Ankle Brachial Index <0.9.

The 2013 Kidney Disease: Improving Global Outcomes (KDIGO) guidelines agree with the AHA/ACC guidelines in many areas [3]. LDL values and titrating treatment to certain levels are no longer indicated. In fact, association between LDL and coronary heart disease gets weaker with the glomerular filtration rate (eGFR) potentially misleading clinicians since this population is still at very high risk. Although following LDL values is not currently the method of choice to direct treatment, lipid profile should still be evaluated in all CKD patients to assess those who will benefit from investigating secondary causes if triglyceride level is >1,000 mg/dl or LDL level is >190 mg/dl. Statins or statin/ezetimibe is the best pharmacologic approach. The cardiovascular risk in CKD patients is age dependent with a rate of cardiovascular death of >10 per 1,000 patient-years in individuals over 50. Therefore, statins are indicated in those ≥50 years with any eGFR but not dialysis dependent. Due to higher rates of toxicity, when eGFR is <60 ml/min/1.73 m^2, lower doses should be initiated and can be increased if patients tolerate because higher doses reduce events more than lower doses. In patients aged 18–49 with CKD but not dialysis dependent, statins are indicated when one or more of the following conditions are present: coronary heart disease, history of ischemic stroke, diabetes, and estimated 10-year risk >10 %. Those patients may also be considered for treatment according to the ACC/AHA guidelines. In this age group, therapy should be customized based on presence of aforementioned high-risk factors for coronary disease.

In contrast to CKD, it appears that hemodialysis (HD)-dependent patients may not benefit from statin therapy. Statins failed to add a significant mortality benefit in ESRD patients in the "German Diabetes and Dialysis Study" (4-D), "A Study to Evaluate the Use of Rosuvastatin in Subjects on Regular Hemodialysis (AURORA)," and SHARP trials. Unprofitable use of statins in this setting may be the result of other methods causing accelerated atherosclerosis. These methods include inflammation, oxidative stress, and accumulation of lipids and high oxidation potential molecules (e.g., intermediate-density lipoproteins). The 2013 ACC/AHA guidelines did not make any recommendation regarding statin therapy in individuals with class III and IV heart failure as well as patients on HD due to insufficient evidence. Similarly, due to lack of definite improvements in cardiovascular events in the ESRD population, KDIGO guidelines do not recommend initiating statins or statin/ezetimibe in HD patients. These drugs can, however, be continued if individuals were already taking them at the time dialysis was started. It may also be reasonable to treat diabetics on dialysis. It would be reassuring to see a large trial examining statin use in the face of ESRD.

Aside from lowering non-HDL cholesterol levels, statins have been proven to reduce inflammation, stabilize endothelial function, and decrease atherosclerotic burden. Therefore, it is not surprising that their use translates into cardiovascular and kidney stability. In some studies, statins reduced C-reactive protein (CRP) levels and improved vascular flow. Also, statins improved mortality in patients without hyperlipidemia but with elevated high-sensitivity CRP levels. Statin efficacy is similar in patients with and without albuminuria. However, their role in retarding CKD progression is still conflicting. Subgroup analysis of the "Cholesterol and Recurrent Events" (CARE) trial showed beneficial outcomes on eGFR in patients with moderate to severe kidney disease and baseline proteinuria. Higher doses seem to offer positive effects on progressive loss of kidney function – in particular atorvastatin. In contrast, other large studies failed to prove these favorable effects of statin therapy on kidney disease progression. Additionally, there are mixed data about statin activity against albumin excretion. While a series of trials described a significant reduction in proteinuria, other large trials found no further benefit when patients received angiotensin-converting enzyme inhibitors (ACEIs) and optimal blood pressure control.

Risk of statin toxicity is the same in CKD patients compared with the general population. Because hepatic failure associated with these drugs is rare, routine liver function monitoring is not necessary. It is sufficient to obtain a baseline transaminase levels prior to therapy initiation and to obtain a liver function test if symptoms of hepatotoxicity arise. Statins can be used in patients with chronic liver disease and baseline-elevated aminotransferase unless progressive liver failure is evident. Statin-related myopathies are more commonly encountered in clinical practices. Pravastatin, fluvastatin, and rosuvastatin appear to have a lower risk of myopathy and a safer use in kidney patients. Atorvastatin and fluvastatin are not required to be adjusted in CKD and offer convenience in this setting. Other statins are more dependent on the CYP3A4 enzyme; therefore, they accumulate in slow metabolizers or when CYP3A4 inhibitors are administered (Table 13.1). When muscle toxicity is an issue, patients should be evaluated for other conditions (hypothyroidism, worsening liver or kidney

Table 13.1 Lipid-lowering therapy for primary and secondary prevention in patients with CKD

Medication	Normal dose	CKD population	Pharmacology
Simvastatin	*Cardiovascular event protection*: 20 mg by mouth once daily combined with ezetimibe 10 mg by mouth once daily	Consider starting dose at 5 mg in the evening in patients with CKD	*Metabolism*: liver, CYP450
	Maximum dose: 40 mg by mouth given at hour of sleep	In SHARP, lipid lowering with statin + ezetimibe was beneficial in patients with CKD	*Excretion*: bile primarily, urine <2 %
Atorvastatin	*Cardiovascular event protection*: 10 mg by mouth once daily	No specific dose adjustments for patients with CKD	*Metabolism*: liver, CYP450
		Atorvastatin 10 mg in patients with CKD revealed a significantly lower risk of the primary end point (nonfatal MI or cardiac death) when compared with placebo	*Excretion*: bile primarily, urine <2 %
		With the TNT and GREACE studies, atorvastatin showed improvement in renal function in patients with CKD	
Fluvastatin	*Cardiovascular event protection*: 40 mg by mouth twice daily	No specific dose adjustments for patients with CKD	*Excretion*: feces 90 %, urine 5 %
	Extended release: 80 mg by mouth once daily	Caution for increased risk of rhabdomyolysis A multicentre, randomized, double blind, placebo-controlled trial of fluvastatin was conducted in kidney transplant recipients Fluvastatin reduced LDL cholesterol levels by 32 %. Although the primary end point did not achieve statistical significance, secondary analysis showed that the fluvastatin group experienced fewer cardiac deaths and nonfatal MI than did the placebo group. Coronary intervention procedures were not significantly different between the two groups	
Pravastatin	*Cardiovascular event protection Start*: 40 mg by mouth once daily, may adjust dose every 4 weeks	Start at 10 mg by mouth once daily in patients with CKD	*Excretion*: feces 70 %, urine 20 %
	Maximum dose: 80 mg by mouth once daily	A randomized trial of pravastatin versus placebo in patients with previous MI and CKD Secondary analysis showed coronary death or nonfatal MI was lower in patients receiving pravastatin, suggesting that pravastatin is effective for secondary prevention of cardiovascular events in patients with CKD	

Abbreviations: *ACS* acute coronary syndrome, *CKD* chronic kidney disease, *MI* myocardial infarction

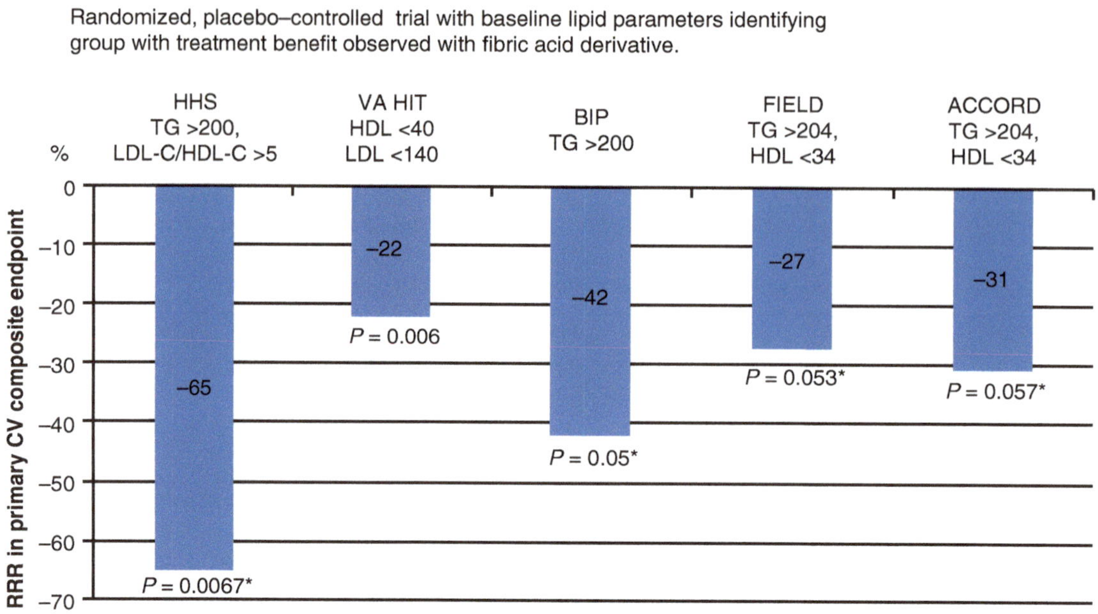

Fig. 13.2 Reductions in cardiovascular events with fibrates in patients with hypertriglyceridemia (From Goldfine et al. [22], Copyright © 2011 Massachusetts Medical Society. Reprinted with permission from Massachusetts Medical Society)

function, muscle disease, or rheumatologic conditions) after stopping statin therapy. When myopathy resolves, restart same therapy with lower doses. If myotoxicity still exists, patients may be switched to the safer statins mentioned above. Reducing the dose to every other day is also reasonable. Other remedies such as coenzyme Q10 and vitamin D have not been shown to be effective in preventing statin-induced myopathy and data is contradictory; therefore, they are not currently recommended. Also evaluating for new onset diabetes mellitus while on statin therapy is indicated by new guidelines. New-onset diabetics should be encouraged to follow a healthy diet and engage in an exercise program.

Hypertriglyceridemia is a prominent abnormality that often accompanies renal impairment. Diminished elimination of lipids and impaired lipoprotein lipase activity are the primary causes of hypertriglyceridemia. Fibrates are effective in decreasing triglyceride concentrations. In a recent meta-analysis of ten clinical trials, fibric acid therapy reduced the risk of cardiovascular events in patients with CKD, but had no effect on all-cause mortality. However, fibrates were observed to cause worsening in kidney function and increased risk of rhabdomyolysis among kidney patients [4]. For that reason, KDIGO guidelines do not currently recommend use of fibrates to reduce cardiovascular risk or pancreatitis in the CKD population. However, some clinicians believe that fibrates should be used in patients with a triglyceride level ≥200 mg/dl where subgroup analysis has shown consistent benefit or concomitantly with low- or moderate-dose statins if benefits of atherosclerotic heart disease risk reduction overweight risk. Kidney function should be assessed before fenofibrate initiation, 3 months later, and every 6 months thereafter (Fig. 13.2). Fenofibrate dose should not exceed 54 mg daily if eGFR is between 30 and 50 ml/min and should be discontinued if eGFR is below 30 ml/min. Gemfibrozil should not be used with statins due to risk of rhabdomyolysis.

Nicotinic acid is also used in treating hypertriglyceridemia. It is also effective in increasing high-density lipoprotein (HDL) levels. Despite these benefits, niacin does not improve cardiovascular events when added to statin therapy. Side effects include flushing, hyperglycemia, hyperuricemia, and hepatotoxicity. Flushing can be subsided with pretreatment with aspirin. Its use is not recommended by KDIGO guidelines.

13.1.2 Antiplatelet Therapy: Which Agents for What Syndromes?

Platelets play a cardinal role in the pathogenesis of acute coronary artery syndrome and atherosclerosis. Endothelial injury induces platelet activation, aggregation, and adherence to the exposed subendothelium. Antagonizing early phases of activation is the main mechanism of action of many antiplatelet agents such as aspirin and thienopyridines. Aspirin is the most widely utilized agent. It inhibits thromboxane A_2 by irreversible COX-1 acetylation, resulting in attenuation of platelet activation [1]. This drug exhibits a low potential for nephrotoxicity compared with other nonsteroidal anti-inflammatory drugs (NSAIDS) owing to the partial renal prostaglandin inhibition. Evidence strongly supports use of aspirin in secondary prevention of CHD. Aspirin therapy offers a 22 % reduction in the risk of subsequent cardiovascular events in patients with known coronary or vascular disease. Low doses are equal in effectiveness compared with high doses and therefore are recommended. In primary prevention, adverse reactions may exceed the benefit of preventing first MI in *low-risk* individuals. Therefore, benefit versus risk assessments should be conducted prior to aspirin initiation. Aspirin can induce various gastrointestinal (GI) adverse effects with peptic ulcer disease being the most serious. The risk of developing major GI bleeding is 1–3 percent/year. Patients who have a strong indication for aspirin therapy and a history of GI bleeding should be started on a proton pump inhibitor for gastric protection.

Thienopyridines also improve cardiovascular outcomes when used as monotherapy. They act by inhibiting ADP-induced platelet aggregation. These drugs are favored when aspirin allergy is present as well as in patients with severe vascular disease, previous myocardial infarction (MI), or stroke. Dual antiplatelet therapy did not enhance beneficial outcomes in patients with stable atherosclerotic disease and was associated with an increased risk of bleeding compared with monotherapy [5]. Addition of a thienopyridine to aspirin should be reserved for certain cases, such as acute ischemia or after stent implantation. In the setting of cryptogenic stroke, the escalating sequence of aspirin, then aspirin plus clopidogrel, and then warfarin is usually in response to repeated events where there is nonsurgical carotid or aortic arch disease in the absence of atrial fibrillation.

13.1.3 Angina Relief

The commonly used antianginal drugs include nitrates, beta-blockers, calcium channel blockers, and ranolazine. These agents display distinct properties and actions.

13.1.3.1 Nitrates

The antianginal efficacy associated with nitrates is a result of venodilation, decreased cardiac preload, and oxygen demand, as well as improvement of collateral coronary flow in a more relaxed myocardium. The sublingual preparations have the fastest onset of action; however, their effects only lasts 30–60 min. They are useful in the acute setting. On the contrary, isosorbide 5-mononitrate is a long-acting agent with effects lasting up to 12 h (Table 13.2). It is an active metabolite of the dinitrate form. This medication should be used once daily allowing a 12-h drug-free period, which helps avoid tolerance. Adverse effects of nitrates include flushing, headache, and hypotension. No dosing adjustment is needed in patients with CKD [1].

13.1.3.2 Beta-Blockers

Beta-blockers (B-blockers) should not be used as first-line therapy to treat hypertension. Recent evidence suggests that they do not offer any mortality benefit in hypertensive patients when compared with other antihypertensive therapy such as calcium channel blockers, diuretics, and ACEIs [6]. In healthy individuals, B-blockers diminish exercise endurance due to antagonizing the sympathetic nervous system. That is not the case in patients with coronary artery disease. B-blockers lead to an increase in exercise capacity in patients

Table 13.2 β-adrenergic receptor blockers for ACS in patients with CKD

Medication	Normal dose	CKD population	Pharmacology
Metoprolol	*Acute MI*	No specific dose adjustments for patients with CKD	*Dialysable: Yes.*
	Metoprolol tartrate: 2.5–5 mg rapid IV every 2–5 min, up to 15 mg over 10–15 min, then 15 min after last IV and receiving 15 mg IV or 50 mg by mouth every 6 h for 48 h, then 50–100 mg by mouth twice daily	Recommend close monitoring for adverse effects	*Metabolism*: hepatic CYP2D6
	Angina		*Metabolites*: inactive
	Metoprolol tartrate: initially 50 mg by mouth twice daily then titrated to 200 mg by mouth twice daily		*Excretion*: urine 95 %
	Metoprolol succinate: 100 mg by mouth once daily, no more than 400 mg per day		
Esmolol	*Immediate control*	No specific dose adjustments for patients with CKD	*Metabolism*: extensively metabolized by esterase in cytosol of red blood cells
	For intraoperative treatment give an 80 mg (approximately 1 mg/kg) bolus dose over 30 s followed by a 150 μg/kg per min *infusion, if needed*		*Metabolites*: major acid metabolite (ASL8123), methanol (inactive)
	Maximum infusion rate: 300 μg/kg per min		
	Gradual control		*Excretion*: urine <1–2 %
	For postoperative treatment, give loading dosage infusion of 500 μg/kg per min over 1 min followed by a 4 min infusion of 50 μg/kg per min		
	If no effect within 5 min, repeat loading dose and follow with infusion increased to 100 μg/kg per min		
Carvedilol	*Hypertension and post-MI protection*:	No specific dose adjustments for patients with CKD	*Elimination*: mainly biliary
	6.25–25 mg by mouth twice daily Start at 6.25 mg by mouth twice daily, then increase every 3–14 days to 12.5 mg by mouth twice daily, then 25 mg by mouth twice daily	In a small study of patients on dialysis with dilated cardiomyopathies, carvedilol improved left ventricular function and decreased hospitalization, cardiovascular deaths and total mortality	*Excretion*: primarily via feces

Hemodialysis reduces blood levels of atenolol, acebutolol, and nadolol; by contrast, levels of carvedilol and labetalol do not change significantly. Abbreviations: *ACS* acute coronary syndromes, *CKD* chronic kidney disease, *IV* intravenous, *MI* myocardial infarction

with angina. Anginal relief with beta-blockade is owed to increased diastolic duration and oxygen requirement reduction (Fig. 13.3). In contrast to patients with no prior MI, B-blockers reduce mortality when used after an acute event, which makes this piece of evidence the reason ACC/AHA committee recommends B-blockers as first-line therapy for chronic stable angina. Beattie and coworkers demonstrated that beta-blockade in patients with CKD and acute myocardial infarction may have enhanced benefit over the general population. This therapy should

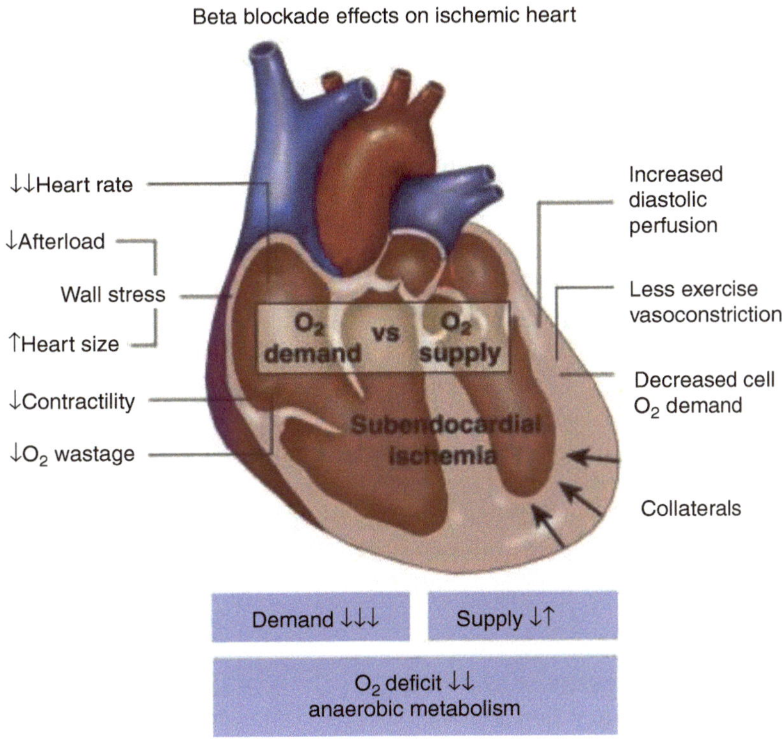

Fig. 13.3 Physiological effects of beta-adrenergic receptor blockade on the myocardium. Effects of beta-blockade on the ischemic heart. Beta-blockade has beneficial effects on the ischemic myocardium unless (1) the preload rises substantially, as in left-sided heart failure or (2) vasospastic angina is present, in which case spasm may be promoted in some patients. Note the suggestion that beta-blockade diminishes exercise-induced vasoconstriction (Adapted from Morrow and Boden [23], with permission from Elsevier)

be customized for every patient and requires careful monitoring. A reduced heart rate to 50–60 beats/min and exercise tolerance determine efficacy. Adverse effects include bronchoconstriction, weight gain, insulin resistance (with the exception of carvedilol), bradycardia, hypotension, sexual dysfunction, and fatigue. These agents have no effect on kidney function. Water-soluble B-blockers (e.g., atenolol, nadolol, and sotalol) are not well metabolized by the liver and are usually excreted unchanged in the urine. Hydrophobic agents (e.g., propranolol, metoprolol) are tolerated well in the setting of kidney disease [1] (Table 13.2).

13.1.3.3 Calcium Channel Blockers

Calcium channel blockers (CCBs) work by antagonizing calcium channels on vascular smooth muscle cells and myocytes, thereby reducing the cytoplasmic calcium influx. The net effect is vasodilation, improved coronary blood flow, and reduced contractility. When combined with B-blockers, CCBs are more effective in treating angina than either drug alone. They are categorized into three classes: dihydropyridines (e.g., nifedipine, amlodipine), benzothiazepines (e.g., diltiazem), and phenylalkylamines (e.g., verapamil) [1].

Several studies have shown that short-acting nifedipine may exacerbate ischemia and worsen heart failure, making its use a major concern. Longer-acting dihydropyridines appear to be safer and better tolerated. Amlodipine reduced cardiovascular events in clinical trials. It is eliminated by the liver allowing safe use in CKD patients. On the contrary, the non-dihydropyridines have a greater potency in reducing contractility with less profound vasodilatory effects. Verapamil has more cardiodepressive actions and therefore more adverse effects than diltiazem. Caution should be taken in patients with atrioventricular nodal disease and heart failure in the face of negative ionotropic actions of the non-dihydropyridines. Given the safety and efficacy of amlodipine compared with B-blockers regarding the end points of death, myocardial infarction, and frequency of angina, it should be tried first in the setting of hypertension.

13.1.3.4 Ranolazine

Ranolazine works by inhibiting the late inward sodium channels, thereby reducing calcium concentration and diastolic tension. It is contraindicated in patients with preexisting QT interval prolongation, hepatic disease, or taking medications that prolong the QT interval. It also produces a 0.1 mg/dl elevation in creatinine regardless of previous renal function. However, this effect is reversible upon discontinuation of the drug. Ranolazine does not appear to cause progressive renal dysfunction with long-term therapy. It is suggested to decrease the dose to 500 mg twice daily in patients with CKD [7].

13.1.4 Management of Acute Coronary Syndrome

End-stage renal disease and CKD patients appear to display silent ischemia more frequently. Acute coronary syndrome (ACS) suspicion should be high when ECG changes and abnormal cardiac enzyme levels are present. Standard ACS pharmacotherapy provides an amplified benefit in renal patients. Treatment includes dual antiplatelet therapy, statins, B-blockers, ACEIs, low molecular weight heparin, and glycoprotein IIb/IIa antagonists. Dose adjustment of these agents is recommended (Tables 13.3, 13.4, and 13.5). ACEIs offer a survival benefit after an acute event and should be continued thereafter. Although several studies have demonstrated superiority of early intravenous B-blocker use in acute MI, other trials have not been consistent with such benefit. In the "Global Utilization of Streptokinase and Tissue Plasminogen Activator for Occluded Coronary Arteries" (GUSTO) and "Clopidogrel and Metoprolol in Myocardial Infarction" (COMMIT) trials, early beta-blockade resulted in increased risk of cardiogenic shock and even death. Therefore, it is wise to be cautious with initiating early B-blockers in acute ST elevation MI during hemodynamic instability. High loading doses of clopidogrel lead to a reduction in death, MI, and stroke compared with low doses. Duration of dual antiplatelet therapy should be tailored to every patient. Trials have continued therapy for at least 9 months. It is reasonable to continue aspirin plus clopidogrel beyond a year for patients with severe vascular disease [8].

13.1.5 Revascularization Therapy

There is a paucity of data examining outcomes with percutaneous coronary intervention (PCI) versus coronary artery bypass grafting (CABG) in kidney patients. Physicians should base their choice upon patient characteristics. Kidney disease appears to be a predictor of worsened prognosis whether PCI or CABG is utilized.

13.1.5.1 PCI

PCI can be selected as a method of revascularization for patients who are suitable candidates. It does not prolong life compared with medical therapy. It is indicated in treating symptomatic single or double vessel disease. There is mixed data about association of CKD with increased restenosis rates. Patients with chronic total occlusion of an infarct-related artery should not undergo PCI due to excess risk of reinfarction and no clinical benefit with respect to death or heart failure. Drug-eluting stents (DES) are known to hold lower rates of in-stent restenosis than bare metal stents (BMS). Post-PCI pharmacotherapy should include dual antiplatelet targeting with aspirin and a thienopyridine. Prasugrel provides a greater inhibition of platelet aggregation with a more rapid onset of action than clopidogrel. When compared with clopidogrel in post-PCI patients, prasugrel was more effective in lowering the incidence of cardiovascular death, MI, stroke, and stent thrombosis. However, these advantages were balanced against higher rates of life-threatening and fatal bleeding with prasugrel. The risk of bleeding was particularly higher in patients with a history of transient ischemic attacks and strokes and in older patients. Prasugrel is therefore contraindicated in these patients. Duration of treatment is recommended to last for at least a year post-intracoronary stent implantation [9].

Table 13.3 Acute and chronic treatments for ACS in patients with CKD

Medication	Normal dose	CKD population	Pharmacology
Antiplatelets			
Aspirin	*Acute MI*: 160–325 mg by mouth as soon as possible	No specific dosing adjustments in patients with CKD	*Metabolism*: liver, microsomal enzyme system
	MI prophylaxis: 81–162 mg by mouth once daily	Meta-analysis involving patients on dialysis demonstrated a benefit of aspirin therapy on cardiovascular outcomes	*Renal clearance*: 80–100 % 24–72 h
	PCT: 325 mg by mouth 2 h pre-surgery, then 160–325 mg by mouth maintenance		*Excretion*: principally in urine (80–100 %). sweat, saliva, and feces
	UA: 75–162 mg by mouth once daily		
Antiplatelets (ADP receptor antagonists)			
Clopidogrel	*UA/NSTEMI*: 300–600 mg initial loading dose, followed by 75 mg by mouth once daily with aspirin	No specific dosing adjustments in patients with CKD	*Metabolism*: CYP3A4, CYP2C19 (predominantly) and others to generate active metabolite; also by esterase to an inactive metabolite
	STEMI: 75 mg by mouth once daily with aspirin 75–162 mg per day		*Excretion*: urine and feces
	Recent MI: 75 mg by mouth once daily		
Prasugrel	*ACS*: Loading dose- 60 mg by mouth once Maintenance dose: 10 mg by mouth once daily with aspirin 81–325 my per day; bleeding risk may increase if weight <60 kg, consider 5 mg by mouth once daily (efficacy/safety not established)	No specific dose adjustments in patients with CKD	*Metabolism*: liver; CYP450, CYP2B6, CYP2C9/ CYP2C19 (minor). CYP3A4 substrate; CYP2B6 (weak) inhibitor
			Excretion: urine (68 %) and. feces (27 %)
Ticagrelor	*ACS with PCI and stent*:	No specific dose adjustments in patients with CKD	*Metabolism*: hepatic CYP450
	Starting dose: 180 mg by mouth once		
	Maintenance dose: 90 mg by month twice daily		*Excretion*: bile primarily, urine <1 %
	To be given for 1 year with aspirin as an alternative option for dual antiplatelet therapy		
ACE inhibitors			
Captopril, zofenopril, enalapril, ramipril, quinapril, perindopril, lisinopril, benazepril, imidapril, trandolapril, fosinopril	Indicated for the treatment of hypertension, prevention of cardiovascular events including heart failure in those at risk, reduction in the progression of type 1 diabetic nephropathy, and reduction in cardiovascular events in patients post MI with left ventricular dysfunction or heart failure	The dosing schedules may need to be individualized for each dialysis session in order to avoid intradialytic hypotension	*Elimination*: mainly renal with an elimination half-life of 12.6 h in healthy individuals
	Also indicated for the treatment of heart failure		In patients with impaired renal function (CrCl ≤30 ml/min) a longer half-life and accumulation have been observed without clinical consequences

(continued)

Table 13.3 (continued)

Medication	Normal dose	CKD population	Pharmacology
ARBs			
Losartan, irbesartan, olmesartan, candesartan, valsartan, telmisartan	Indicated for treatment of hypertension, to reduce the progression of type 2 diabetic nephropathy, and reduce cardiovascular events in patients post-MI with left ventricular dysfunction or heart failure	As first-line treatment in the majority of patients with CKD, we recommend the use of ACE inhibitors or ARBs; both have been shown to reduce LVH in patients on hemodialysis	Losartan has 88 % hepatic and 12 % renal clearance
	Indicated for heart failure in those intolerant to ACE inhibitors	Levels of ARBs do not change significantly during hemodialysis	
CCBs			
Dihydropyridines; Amlodipine, nimodipine, nitrendipine; Non-dihyrdropyridines: e.g., diltiazem, verapamil, felodipine, nicardipine, nifedipine,	In UA/NSTEMT, if B-blockers are contraindicated, a non-dihydropyridine CCB should be chosen in the absence of clinically significant left ventricular dysfunction or other contraindications	No specific dose adjustments for patients with CKD	Amlodipine has renal elimination as the major route of excretion with about 60 % cleared in the urine
		The management of chronic CAD in patients on dialysis should follow that of the general population and use of CCBs as indicated	Diltiazem undergoes primary liver metabolism
		The hemodynamic and electrophysiological effects of CCBs are markedly different from each other and should be evaluated when selecting a suitable therapy	
Nitrates			
Nitroglycerin	*2 % ointment*	No specific dose adjustments for patients with CKD	*Metabolism*: mainly in liver, extrahepatic sites such as vascular wall, red blood cells
	Angina: 0.5–2 in. applied in morning and 6 h later to truncal skin	Care must he used to avoid hypotension in low volume states such as dialysis sessions	*Excretion*: urine
	Heart failure: 1.5 in., increase by 0.5–1 in. up to 4 in., every 4 h		
	Sublingual: 0.4 mg for relief of chest pain in ACS every 5 min		
	Maximum: 3 doses within 15 min		
Antianginal			
Ranolazine	500–1.000 my by mouth twice daily	No specific dose adjustments for patients with CKD Prolongs QTc interval Recommend close monitoring	Excretion: urine 73–75 %, feces 25 %
	Max: 2,000 mg per day		

Abbreviations: *ACE* angiotensin-converting enzyme, *ACS* acute coronary syndromes, *ADP* adenosine diphosphate, *ARB* angiotensin receptor blocker, *CAD* coronary artery disease, *CCB* calcium-channel blocker, *CKD* chronic kidney disease, *CrCl* creatinine clearance, *LVH* left ventricular hypertrophy, *MI* myocardial infarction, *NSTHM1* ruth-ST-elevation myocardial infarction: *PCI* percutaneous coronary intervention, *STEMI* ST elevation myocardial infarction, *UA* unstable angina

Table 13.4 Intravenous glycoprotein IIb/IIIa inhibitors for unstable angina/NSTEMI and STEMI

Agent	Normal dose	CKD population[a]	Pharmacology
Abciximab	*Adjunct to PCI*: 0.25 mg/kg IV bolus over at least 1 min, 10–60 min before start of PCI, then 0.125 μg/kg per min (not to exceed 10 μg per min) continuous IV infusion for 12 h	No specific dose adjustments for patients with CKD	*Metabolism*: unknown, but likely by the reticuloendothelial system
	Unstable angina with PCI planned within 24 h: 0.25 mg/kg IV bolus over at least 1 min, then 0.125 μg/kg per min (not to exceed 10 μg per min) IV infusion for 18–24 h concluding 1 h after PCI	Abciximab should also be considered as adjunctive therapy in patients with ACS on dialysis In CKD, safety of abciximab has been shown for creatinine levels >152.5 μmol/1	*Excretion*: urine
		Although increased bleeding with abciximab in patients with CKD has been reported, other studies have shown no increase in bleeding for CKD versus no CKD for abciximab in PCI	
Eptifibatidc	*ACS*: 180 μg/kg IV bolus, then 2 μg/kg per min IV for up to 72 h	*Creatinine clearance <50 ml/min and ACS*: 180 μg/kg IV, then continuous infusion 1 μg/kg per min Safety and use during hemodialysis is not established	*Metabolism*: other, minimal
	PCI: 180 μg/kg IV, then a continuous infusion at 2 μg/kg per min with another 180 μg/kg IV bolus 10 min after first bolus		*Excretion*: urine 50 %
	Continue infusion for at least 12 h		
Tirofiban	In patients undergoing PCI, tirofiban is not recommended as an alternative to abciximab	*Creatinine clearance <30 ml/min and ACS*: reduce dose to 50 % of normal rate	*Excretion*: urine 65 % (primarily unchanged), feces 25 % (primarily unchanged)
	ACS: 0.4 μg/kg per min IV for 30 min, then 0.1 μg/kg per min IV for 48–108 h	Safety and use during hemodialysis not established	
	PCI: Continue 0.1 μg/kg per min IV through procedure and for 12–24 h after		

[a]When a glycoprotein IIb/IIIa antagonist is used, abciximab and tirofiban should be considered preferred agents, as no dosing changes are required for abciximab, and dialysis-specific dosing recommendations are available for tirofiban. Increased bleeding but reduced in-hospital mortality in CKD patients with ACS treated with glycoprotein IIb/IIIa antagonists has also been shown. Abbreviations: *ACS* acute coronary syndromes, *CKD* chronic kidney disease, *IV* intravenous, *NSTEMI* non-ST-elevation myocardial infarction, *PCI* percutaneous coronary intervention, *STEMI* ST elevation myocardial infarction

13.1.5.2 CABG

There is increasing evidence demonstrating that CABG is associated with lower rates of long-term adverse outcomes and revascularization in HD patients. CABG is superior to PCI in diabetic patients with multivessel disease in terms of reducing rates of death and MI. This method is supported as the treatment of choice in HD patients with severe CHD. CKD patients with a creatinine greater than 2.5 mg/dl bear a risk of requiring dialysis post surgery. Larger trials are required to further elucidate the role of PCI versus CABG in this patient population.

13.2 Heart Failure

Heart failure (HF) is diagnosed in approximately 20 % of kidney patients approaching HD. Concomitant kidney dysfunction makes HF management challenging and complex. Restoration of hemodynamic abnormalities remains the aim

Table 13.5 Antithrombotic agents for unstable angina/NSTEMI and STEMI

Agent	Normal dose	CKD population	Pharmacology
Indirect factor Xa inhibitors			
Unfractionated heparin	Recommended dosage and desired aPTT values as per institutional protocol	In patients with CKD. suggested starting dose of heparin is 50 IU/kg bolus, then 1S IU/kg per h	*Metabolism*: liver (partial)
	PCI: 60–100 units/kg IV given once	Monitor aPTT level and adjust accordingly as per institutional protocol	Metabolites; none
	Target ACT 250–350 s		*Excretion*: urine
	In patients receiving glycoprotein IIb/IIIa inhibitor. give 50–70 units/kg IV to target ACT 200 s		
	STEMI, adjunct treatment, streptokinase use:		
	800 units/h when <80 kg body weight or 1,000 units per h when >80 kg body weight		
	Start: 5,000 units IV, adjust dose to target aPTT 50–75 s		
	NSTEMI: 1,215 units/kg per h IV		
	Start: 60–70 units/kg IV; Max 5,000 units bolus, max rate 1,000 units per h		
	Adjust dose to target aPTT 50–75 s		
Low-molecular-weight heparin (e.g., enoxaparin)	*Unstable angina, nonQ-wave myocardial infarction*: 1 mg/kg subcutaneously twice daily	*CrCl <30 ml/min*	*Excretion*: urine 40 %
	STEMI, aged <75 years: 30 nig IV bolus plus 1 mg/kg subcutaneously, then 1 mg/kg subcutaneously every 12 h	*STEMI, aged <75 years*: 30 mg IV bolus plus 1 mg/kg subcutaneously. then 1 mg/kg subcutaneously once a day	
	PCI: additional 0.3 mg/kg IV bolus it last subcutaneous administration given >8 h before balloon inflation	*STEMI, aged >75 years*: 1 mg/kg subcutaneously once a day	
	STEMI, aged >75 years: 0.75 mg/kg subcutaneously every 12 h (no IV bolus)		
Direct factor Xa inhibitor			
Fondaparinux	*Unstable angina/NSTEMI*	*CrCl 30–50 ml/min*: use with caution	*Excretion*: urine (primarily unchanged)
	Conservative strategy: 2.5 mg subcutaneously once daily	*CrCl <30 ml/min*: not indicated	
	During PCI: add unfractionated heparin 50–60 units/kg IV bolus for prophylaxis of catheter thrombosis		
Direct thrombin inhibitors			
Bivalirudin	Intended for use with aspirin 300–325 mg per day 0.75 mg/kg TV bolus initially, followed by continuous infusion at rate of 1.75 mg/kg per h for duration of procedure	*CrCl 10–29 ml/min*: usual bolus dose, then initial infusion of 1 mg/kg per h IV up to 4 h	*Dialysable*: with 25 % reduction in levels
	Perform ACT 5 min after bolus dose	*Hemodialysis*: usual bolus dose, then initial infusion of 0.25 mg/kg per h IV up to 4 h	*Excretion*: urine
	Administer additional 0.3 mg/kg bolus if necessary	Bivalirudin is a direct thrombin inhibitor with specific dosing adjustments for patients on dialysis and should be preferentially considered	
	May continue infusion following PCI beyond 4 h (optional post-PCI, at discretion of treating healthcare provider) initiated at rate of 0.2 mg/kg per h for up to 20 h as needed		

Table 13.5 (continued)

Agent	Normal dose	CKD population	Pharmacology
Dabigatran	Indicated for prevention of stroke and thromboembolism associated with nonvalvular atrial fibrillation	*CrCl 15–30 ml/min*: 75 mg by mouth twice daily	*Excretion*: urine 7 %, feces 86 %
	CrCl > 30 ml/min: 150 mg by mouth twice daily	*CrCl <15 ml/min or hemodialysis*: not indicated	
		For patients currently taking dabigatran, wait 12 h (CrCl ≥30 ml/min) or 24 h (CrCl <30 ml/min) after the last dose of dabigatran before initiating treatment with a parenteral anticoagulant	
		If possible, discontinue dabigatran 1–2 days (CrCl ≥50 ml/min) or 3–5 days (CrCl <50 ml/min) before invasive or surgical procedures because of increased risk of bleeding	
Rivaroxaban	Indicated for prevention of stroke and thromboembolism associated with nonvalvular atrial fibrillation	*CrCl 15–50 ml/min*: 15 mg by mouth at hour of sleep	*Metabolism*: liver CYP450
	CrCl >50 ml/min: 20 mg by mouth at hour of sleep	*CrCl <15 ml/min*: not indicated	*Excretion*: urine 66 %, feces 28 %
			Half life: 5–9 h or 11–13 h in elderly

Abbreviations: *ACT* activated clotting time, *aPTT* activated partial thromboplastin time, *CKD* chronic kidney disease, *CrCl* creatinine clearance, *IV* intravenous, *NSTEMI* non-ST elevation myocardial infarction, *PCI* percutaneous coronary intervention, *STEMI* ST elevation myocardial infarction

of HF therapy. Reversible causes and precipitating factors should be identified and targeted.

13.2.1 Management of Acute Decompensated Heart Failure

When treating HF, we should keep in mind that the traditional pharmacotherapy used to improve the hemodynamic profile might also aggravate kidney function. Fluctuating creatinine during HF management is associated with a worse prognosis. Acute decompensated heart failure (ADHF) treatment includes diuretics, vasodilators, and inotropes.

13.2.1.1 Diuretics

Diuretic therapy is an essential element in volume status restoration and symptom relief. The array of diuretics, location and mechanism of action, and physiological consequences are shown in Fig. 13.4. Intravenous diuretics should be initiated given their potency and efficacy compared with oral treatment. In addition, edema of the gastrointestinal tract may retard oral drug absorption. Loop diuretics are used as first-line therapy and can be given as either intravenous infusion or boluses. "The Diuretic Optimization Strategies Evaluation" (DOSE) trial compared both strategies and showed similar efficacies in relieving symptoms and change in serum creatinine [10]. In diuretic naïve patients, intravenous furosemide can be initiated at a dose of 20–40 mg. In chronic users, the initial dose should be at least double of their daily dose. Thiazides work synergically with loop diuretics and can be added for more effective diuresis. Higher furosemide doses are linked with greater dyspnea relief, net fluid loss, and weight loss compared with low doses. These favorable findings, however, are at the expense of more frequent transient creatinine elevations due to further activation of the renal angiotensin and sympathetic nervous systems (Fig. 13.5).

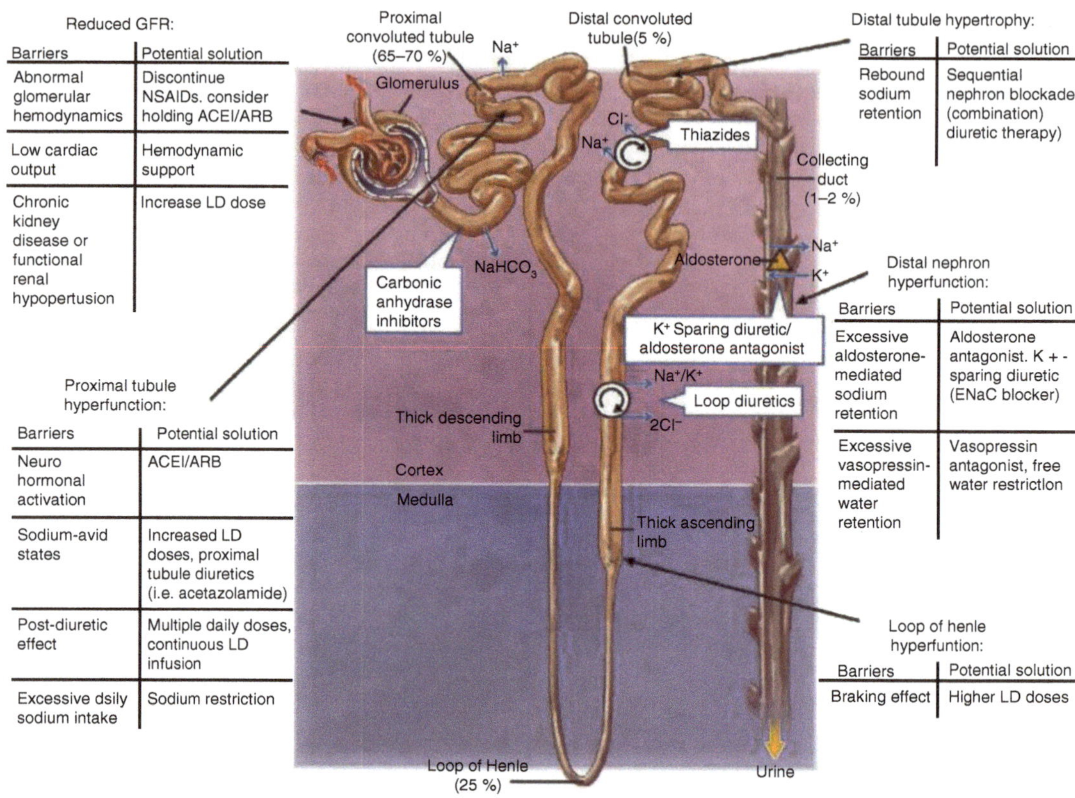

Fig. 13.4 Location, mechanism of action, and physiological effects of commonly used diuretics in cardiovascular patients with CKD (Reprinted from Jentzer et al. [24], Copyright 2010, with permission from Elsevier)

Changes in creatinine during diuretic therapy depend on the degree of both cardiac and kidney dysfunction counterbalanced by diuresis. Renal venous pressure reduction and cardiac output improvement with diuretics may help maintain or improve GFR. Nonetheless, excessive intravascular depletion may cause acute kidney injury, particularly in patients with a low left ventricular ejection fraction (LVEF). The initial manifestation of renal perfusion deprivation is a rise in BUN. In stable patients with mild congestive symptoms and elevation in BUN, diuresis should be downgraded to avoid kidney injury. If symptoms are persistent and severe diuresis should be continued, inotropes can be added as adjunctive therapy.

A decline in kidney function in ADHF treatment is associated with a worse prognosis and should be avoided if possible. However, in severe volume overload cases, kidney injury may be inevitable. These negative findings are compensated for by mortality improvement associated with lower intracardiac filling pressures [1].

13.2.1.2 Vasodilators

Nitrates, sodium nitroprusside, and nesiritide are among the vasodilators used in treating hypertensive ADHF patients. In combination with diuretics, careful blood pressure monitoring should be established. Sodisum nitroprusside should be used with caution in kidney patients due to the increased risk of cyanide toxicity. It may also cause coronary steal syndrome exacerbating MI [1].

Nesiritide was evaluated in the "Vasodilation in the Management of Acute Congestive Heart Failure" (VMAC) trial. It did not make an impact on improving dyspnea when compared with nitroglycerin. Additionally, there was evidence of worsening kidney function and

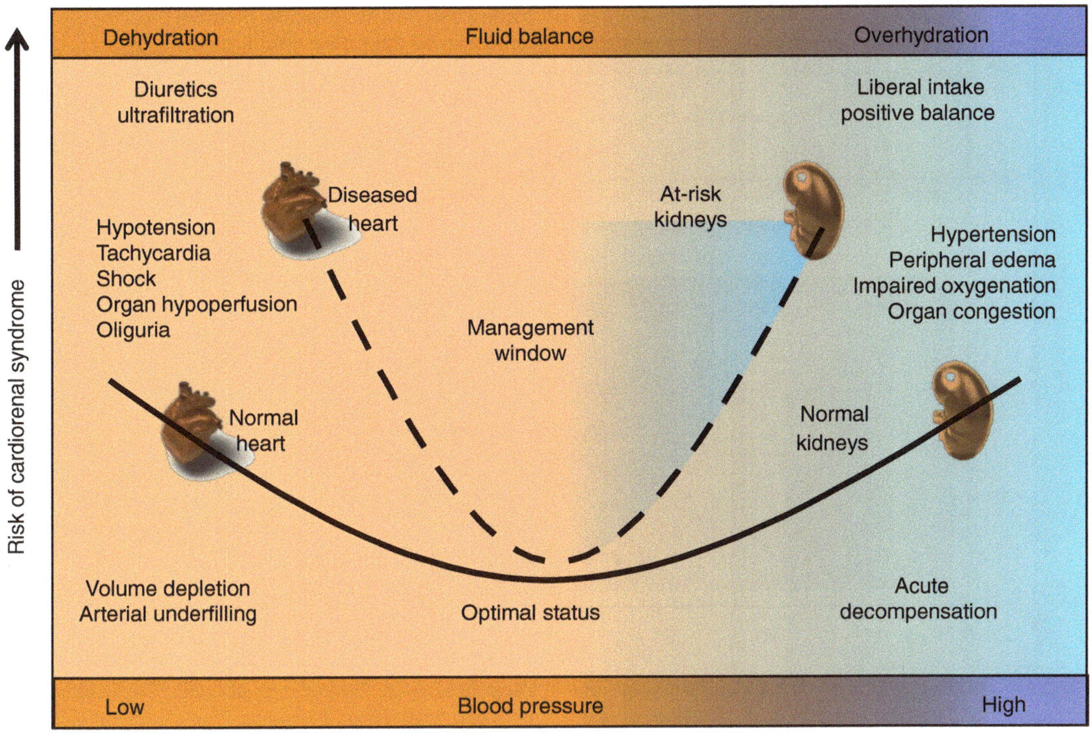

Fig. 13.5 Narrow therapeutic window between elevations in blood pressure and volume and dehydration with overaggressive diuresis in heart failure patients at risk for cardiorenal syndromes (Reprinted from Ronco et al. [25], Copyright 2012, with permission from Elsevier)

increasing mortality. This drug was subsequently investigated in the "Acute Study of Clinical Effectiveness of Nesiritide in Decompensated Heart Failure" (ASCEND-HF) trial. This study suggested that nesiritide has no effect on mortality or kidney function. Nesiritide can be used in selected patients resistant to other therapies given its longer half-life and persistence of side effects.

13.2.1.3 Inotropes

Inotropic agents improve cardiac output and decrease pulmonary capillary wedge pressure (PCWP). Dobutamine, milrinone, and dopamine are among the inotropes used in ADHF treatment. It is well established that these drugs adversely impact survival during their short-term use. They should only be used if poor tissue perfusion is resulting in resistance to diuretic therapy. These agents also increase the risk of atrial and ventricular arrhythmias and should be avoided in patients at risk [1].

13.2.2 Ultrafiltration

Previous trials have shown greater fluid removal with ultrafiltration compared with diuretics. Ultrafiltration or dialysis can be used as alternative treatment in patients with progressive worsening in kidney function; however, clinical trials are not concordant. The multicenter UNLOAD trial (Fig. 13.6) demonstrated that the use of ultrafiltration before the development of AKI improved decongestion and reduced hospitalization with no impact on kidney function. In the more recent "Cardiorenal Rescue Study in Acute Decompensated Heart Failure" (CARESS-HF) trial, ultrafiltration started once AKI development was associated with a rise in creatinine and more adverse events (Fig. 13.7). Thus, this method is a reasonable choice in selected patients with persistent symptoms despite medical therapy [11].

If sleep apnea syndrome is present, it should be treated in the hospital to minimize

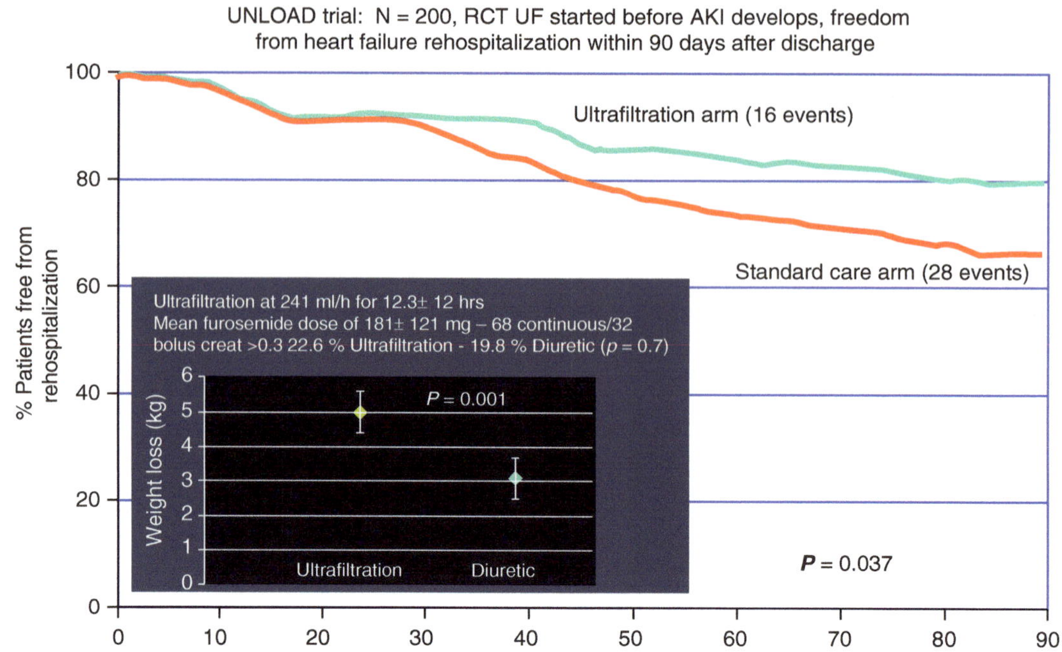

Fig. 13.6 Primary results of the randomized ultrafiltration versus IV diuretics for patients hospitalized for acute decompensated congestive heart failure (UNLOAD) trial (Reprinted from Costanzo et al. [26], Copyright 2007, with permission from Elsevier)

apneic-hypoxic events. This will lower activity of the renin-angiotensin system and along with selected treatments for ADHF shown in, lead to the most favorable outcomes with the least risk for developing cardiorenal syndrome.

13.2.3 Management of Chronic Heart Failure

Congestive heart failure frequently overlaps with kidney dysfunction. Therapeutic measures should be directed toward blood pressure and hyperglycemia control, as well as volume equilibrium. Early recognition of decompensation is vital. Clinicians should look for and target any imbalances such as excessive salt or water intake, anemia, and worsening ventricular or kidney function. Agents that have demonstrated a positive impact on survival include diuretics, aldosterone antagonists, ACEIs, B-blockers, and hydralazine plus nitrates.

13.2.3.1 Diuretics

Diuretic therapy is a cardinal component in maintaining sodium balance in chronic HF management. They are known to improve dyspnea, cardiac function, and exercise tolerance. They are capable of decreasing cardiac filling pressures and pulmonary congestion. There are limited data available on the long-term mortality benefit associated with these agents. The CKD population is predisposed to diuretic resistance and is more likely to achieve fluid balance with higher doses. This is in part due to decreased elimination of sodium. In addition, diminished cardiac output and diuretic secretion into renal tubules decrease drug delivery to the kidney.

Loop diuretics have been adopted as the preferred agents for HF treatment. Low doses should be started initially, then titrated upward to achieve target diuresis. Increasing frequency may be necessary in certain individuals. In cases of worsening kidney function, diuresis may be slowed until euvolemia is achieved. These agents enhance the RAAS (renin-angiotensin-aldosterone system), which acts to counterbalance sodium loss. The hemodynamic response to the RAAS is arterial vasoconstriction. This leads to an increase in afterload, which may result in reducing cardiac output. The potential detrimental effects of the

Baseline characteristics

Creatinine–mg/dl‡		
Median	2.09	1.90
Interquartile range	1.71–2.65	1.57–2.37
Qualifying increase creatinine–mg/dl§		
Median	0.46	0.43
Interquartile range	0.37–0.70	
NT-proBNP–pg/ml¶		
Median	4,007	5,013
Interquartile range	1,128–8,534	2,310–10,381

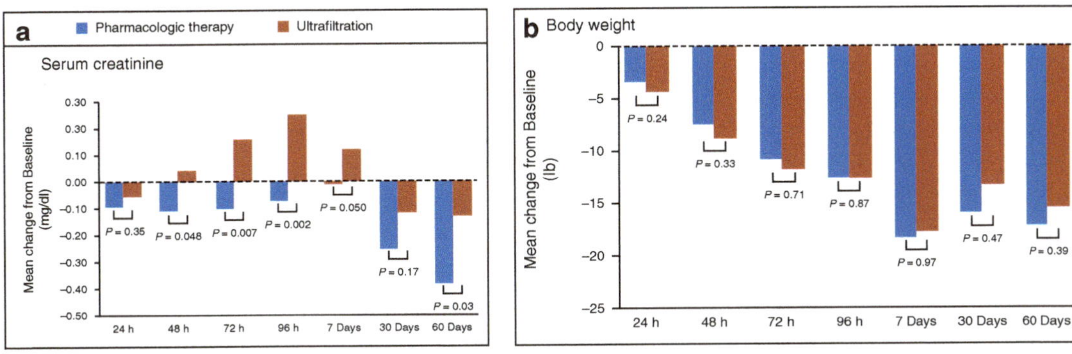

Clinical outcomes

Death – no. (%)	13 (14)	16 (17)	0.55
Hospitalization – no./total no. (%)			
For heart failure	27/93 (26)	23/90 (26)	0.97
For any cause	37/93 (40)	46/90 (51)	0.12
Unscheduled emergency department or clinic visit – no./total no. (%)	13/93 (14)	19/90 (21)	0.21

Fig. 13.7 Primary results of the Cardiorenal Rescue Study in Acute Decompensated Heart Failure (CARESS-HF) trial (From Bart et al. [27], Copyright 2010 Massachusetts Medical Society. Reprinted with permission from Massachusetts Medical Society)

RAAS on the cardiovascular system reinforce the importance of antagonizing this neurohormonal axis with either ACEIs or angiotensin receptor blockers (ARBs) [18].

Patients with diuretic resistance should be reevaluated for worsening cardiorenal function. All drugs that exacerbate volume overload should be terminated. Coadministering a thiazide diuretic is effective particularly when eGFR is over 40 ml/min/1.73 m [2]. Furosemide can also be substituted with other loop diuretics (e.g., torsemide, bumetanide) that have higher bioavailabilities [1].

13.2.3.2 Aldosterone Antagonists

Plasma aldosterone levels are markedly elevated in patients with heart failure. Aldosterone has several detrimental consequences on the failing heart such as myocardial hypertrophy, fibrosis, and endothelial dysfunction. Aldosterone may also be produced by endothelial and vascular smooth muscle, which explains why ACEIs (only inhibit aldosterone produced by adrenal glands) do not effectively lower aldosterone levels. Therefore, aldosterone antagonists have a greatly appreciated impact in heart failure and should be included as part of therapy. Furthermore, aldosterone antagonists reduce proteinuria and may retard progression of kidney disease in patients with CKD and diabetes. Published data on aldosterone antagonists have described their favorable effects on long-term cardiovascular morbidity, mortality, and frequency of hospitalization. These agents impede cardiac fibrosis, a principal determinant of pathologic remodeling. They work in synergism with ACEIs and ARBs. Aldosterone blockade is indicated in patients with class III to IV HF and an LVEF <35 %, or in patients who suffered a myocardial infarction with an LVEF <40 % plus HF symptoms. Spironolactone is generally contraindicated when eGFR is below 30 ml/min/1.73 m^2 or when potassium is above 5 mEq/l. This is because risk of developing hyperkalemia is higher.

13.2.3.3 ACEIs

Heart failure-induced organ hypoperfusion stimulates the renin-angiotensin-aldosterone system to maintain hemodynamic stability. However, angiotensin II produces deleterious effects on myocytes. It induces hypertrophy, apoptosis, and fibrosis. Therefore, the use of ACEIs is a vital component in the management of HF. These agents slow down and even reverse ventricular remodeling, enhance survival, and improve symptoms. ARBs are used when ACEIs are not well tolerated in certain patients and are as effective in prolonging life. A number of studies suggest that dual targeting with an ACEI and an ARB translates into an amplified clinical benefit although impact on mortality is nonsignificant. This is explained by antagonizing alternative pathways involved in angiotensin II production. Nonetheless, other studies have shown that this dual therapy poses an increased risk of adverse effects, complications, and mortality. Thus, routine administration of this combination therapy is not suggested unless compelling benefit is evident. Current guidelines recommend ARB therapy to be initiated in patients intolerant to ACEIs. Addition of an ARB may be considered in patients with persistent heart failure who are on a BB and an ACEI but intolerant to aldosterone antagonists [18].

Efficacy of ACEIs was apparent in multiple studies. In trials like "Studies of Left Ventricular Dysfunction" (SOLVD), "Survival and Ventricular Enlargement" (SAVE), and "Trandolapril Cardiac Evaluation" (TRACE), patients with asymptomatic LV dysfunction treated with ACEIs had a reduced rate of rehospitalization and development of symptomatic disease. Other trials such as "Cooperative North Scandinavian Enalapril Survival Study" (CONSENSUS I) have examined use of these agents in symptomatic stage IV HF. Enalapril reduced the 6-month and 12-month mortality by 40 and 31 %. Data suggests that correlation between disease severity and mortality exists. Effects of higher doses were elucidated by the "Assessment of Treatment with Lisinopril and Survival" (ATLAS) trial. High-dose lisinopril was associated with a reduced mortality and hospitalization rate. Importantly, it should be stressed that patients with creatinine levels >2.5 mg/ml have generally been excluded from these trials; therefore, the efficacy of ACEIs in this patient population is less well known. Further studies should be conducted to delineate ACEI efficacy in patients with impaired kidney function.

13.2.3.4 B-Blockers

In HF, the sympathetic nervous system is stimulated to preserve hemodynamics. It results in systemic and renal vasoconstriction, renal sodium retention, increased heart rate, and enhanced contractility. Unfortunately, chronic induction of the sympathetic tone causes consequences that far outweigh the benefits. Catecholamines decrease cardiac perfusion, increase myocardial oxygen deficit, induce hypertrophy, and promote apoptosis of myocytes leading to less pronounced contractility overtime. Metoprolol succinate, carvedilol, and bisoprolol have demonstrated enhanced survival as well as symptomatic benefit in a number of trials. In addition to ACEIs, diuretics, salt restriction, and aldosterone antagonists, B-blockers should be part of the pharmacotherapy when the LVEF is below 40 %. Patients should not be in decompensated HF when this regimen is started. Carvedilol may be preferred in hypertensive patients given its vasodilatory activity. The American Heart Association recommends targeting blood pressure to a level below 120/80 mmHg for those with HF plus an LVEF below 40 %. It should be emphasized to uptitrate the dose of B-blockers over weeks to avoid worsening volume overload [1].

13.2.3.5 Hydralazine Plus Nitrates

Combined hydralazine and nitrate therapy prolonged survival in blacks with class III to IV HF when evaluated in the "Vasodilator-Heart Failure" trials (V-HeFT). Mortality reduction is more pronounced when added to standard HF therapy including ACEIs, B-blockers, and spironolactone. The combination of hydralazine and a nitrate is recommended in patients with depressed

LV function and intolerant of ACEIs/ARBs or optimized on HF therapy [18].

13.2.3.6 Digitalis

Digitalis works by inhibiting the Na-K-ATPase pump, thereby increasing intracellular calcium and contractility. In addition, it enhances the vagal tone, which antagonizes the sympathetic pathway. It is indicated in HF patients with atrial fibrillation. Symptomatic and functional benefit seen with this drug is offset by an increase in mortality observed in females and patients with trough levels over 1.0 ng/ml [12]. Target serum levels should fall between 0.5 and 0.8 ng/ml. It is usually combined with a B-blocker or CCB to control the ventricular rate in atrial fibrillation. Digitalis is cleared by the kidneys making patients with low eGFR susceptible to its toxic effects. Electrolyte abnormalities, in particular hypokalemia, are common in patients on diuretics, which may also precipitate acute digitalis toxicity. This drug is eliminated unchanged in urine; therefore, the loading and maintenance doses must be reduced in CKD. Dose should be decreased 50 % when eGFR is below 60 ml/min/1.73 m^2 and 75 % when eGFR is below 30 ml/min/1.73 m^2. Patients must be aware of early signs of high digitalis levels such as nausea, vomiting, and confusion. Both digitalis and its antidote digoxin-specific antibody have a prolonged elimination in kidney failure. Hemodialysis has not been shown to be effective in this setting and recurrence of symptoms is common [18].

13.3 Arrhythmias

Cardiovascular complications of CKD can also be manifested as arrhythmias. Renal patients are predisposed to having a higher incidence of almost all arrhythmias. Adjusting antiarrhythmic dosing according to creatinine clearance is a caveat clinicians have to confront (Table 13.6). Atrial fibrillation is exceptionally prevalent among dialysis patients. Age, left atrial dilation, and duration of dialysis are identified as precipitating factors for this arrhythmia. The "Atrial Fibrillation Follow-up Investigation of Rhythm Management" (AFFIRM) and "Rate Control Versus Electrical Cardioversion for Persistent Atrial Fibrillation "(RACE) trials revealed no improvement in cardiovascular morbidity and mortality and quality of life when rate control strategy was compared to rhythm control. In elderly patients without severe symptoms, rate control is the preferred strategy.

All patients with atrial fibrillation are at risk of having an embolic event. Kidney failure further increases the risk of developing an embolic stroke attributable to higher levels of blood stasis. Antithrombotic therapy is an accepted treatment to decrease risk of embolization. At the same time, this patient population is prone to bleeding complications associated with antithrombotics. Patients should be carefully assessed before applying thromboprophylaxis, and benefits versus risks should be weighed. The CHAD-VASC scoring system is used to stratify clotting risk.

Table 13.6 Antiarrhythmic agents

Agent	Normal dose	CKD population	Pharmacology
Flecainide	100 mg BID. Maximum of 400 mg/day	*CrCl <50 ml/min*: Decrease dose by 50 %. Monitor serum levels	*Half-life*: 11–12 h
			Excretion: 80–90 % in urine.
Procainamide	*IV*: Loading dose of 15–18 mg/Kg.	*CrCl <50 ml/min*: Administer BID	*Half-life*: 2.5–4.7 h
	Maintenance dose of 1–4 mg/min	*HD*: Administer QD	*Excretion*: Urine
	Oral: 50 mg/Kg/24 h QID		
Dofetilide	*Oral*: 500 mcg BID	*CrCl 40–60 ml/min*: 250 meg BID	*Half-life*: 10 h
		CrCl 20–39 ml/min: 125 meg BID	*Excretion*: Urine
		CrCl <20 ml/min: Contraindicated	
Amiodarone	*Oral*: 200–400 mg/day	No dosage adjustment. Not dialyzable	*Half-life*: 40–55 days
	IV: Loading dose of 150 mg, then 1 mg/min for 6 h, followed by 0.5 mg/min infusion		*Excretion*: Feces

Box 13.2. CHAD-VASC Scoring System

Condition		Score
C	Congestive heart failure or left ventricular dysfunction	1
H	Hypertension	1
A_2	Age ≥75	2
D	Diabetes mellitus	1
S_2	Prior stroke or TIA	2
V	Vascular disease (e.g., peripheral artery disease, myocardial infarction, aortic disease)	1
A	Age 65–74	1
SC	Sex category (female gender)	1

Source: EHRA/EACT/ESC Committee for Practice Guidelines [17]

A score of 2 or greater is considered high risk and such patients require antithrombotic therapy (Box 13.2). Rivaroxaban, apixaban, and dabigatran are among the newer antithrombotic medications (Table 13.5). Subgroup analyses of a number of trials addressing stroke prevention in CKD stage 3 proved these drugs to be noninferior to warfarin. Apixaban exhibits a favorable adverse effect profile when compared with warfarin.

ESRD patients encounter electrolyte imbalances often during dialysis sessions, which predispose them to higher rates of ventricular arrhythmias. Implantable cardiac defibrillator (ICD) is indicated in HD patients who have suffered a life-threatening ventricular arrhythmia or sudden cardiac arrest (Box 13.3). However, increased defibrillation thresholds and higher rates of infections add weight to the challenge as they can cause ICD failure [13]. Clinical trials addressing the role of prophylactic ICDs in this patient population are underway.

Box 13.3. Class I Indications for ICD Implantation

- Left ventricular dysfunction (EF ≤35 %) preceded by a myocardial infarction at least 40 days ago and who are in NYHA functional Class II or III
- Nonischemic cardiomyopathy (EF ≤35 %) that is persistent 3 months post-optimal medical therapy and who are in NYHA functional class II or III
- Ischemic cardiomyopathy (EF ≤35 %) that is persistent 3 months post revascularization
- Survivors of ventricular tachycardia (VT) or ventricular fibrillation (VF) with an unidentified reversible cause (this excludes patients who experience an acute MI within 48 h)
- Spontaneous sustained VT in the presence of known structural heart disease
- Syncope in the presence of sustained VT or VF induced at electrophysiologic study
- Myocardial infarction causing nonsustained VT with EF ≤40 % and induced at electrophysiologic study

Source: Tracy et al. [18]

13.4 Valvular and Pericardial Heart Disease

ESRD is associated with increased prevalence of valvular heart disease, particularly aortic valve sclerosis and mitral annular calcification. Predisposing factors include older age, hyperphosphatemia, hypercalcemia, secondary

Box 13.4. Prevention of Infective Endocarditis

Prophylactic antimicrobial therapy is now limited to those considered high risk of developing infective endocarditis. Dental procedures are considered to be high risk for causing bacteremia especially if gingival manipulation is involved. Genitourinary and gastrointestinal tract procedures do not generally cause significant bacteremia, and AHA does not recommend the use of prophylactic therapy in high-risk patients undergoing such procedures. However, it is still recommended to use infective endocarditis prophylaxis prior to invasive respiratory tract procedures that involve incision of the respiratory mucosa. High-risk patients are identified as those who have one of the following:

- Prosthetic heart valve (bioprosthetic or homograft valve)
- Prosthetic material used for valve repair
- Previous history of infective endocarditis
- Persistently cyanotic congenital heart disease
- Completely/incompletely repaired congenital heart disease with prosthetic material
- Cardiac valve leaflet pathology or regurgitation in cardiac transplant recipients

Source: Data from Nishimura et al. [19]; and Habib et al. [20]

hyperparathyroidism, and duration of dialysis. It is estimated that 80 % of HD patients have the murmur of aortic sclerosis. Preventive measures should be focused on maintaining proper calcium and phosphorous levels, as well as hyperparathyroidism management. Regarding valve replacement surgery, this patient population is at risk for endocarditis whether a bioprosthetic or a mechanical valve is used, which increases surgical mortality. The most important preventive technique is maintaining good oral health. Both tissue and mechanical valves carry the same survival in patients who receive surgical intervention for valve failure following endocarditis [14]. Current recommendations for endocarditis prophylaxis are presented in Boxes 13.4 and 13.5. Mechanical valves are more resistant to calcification and last longer; however, tissue valves are favored when anticoagulation therapy is contraindicated and in ESRD patients where survival is shortened due to factors besides valvular heart disease.

Many patients with kidney disease are high risk for cardiac surgery (open or limited thoracotomy) and could be considered for transcatheter aortic valve replacement (TAVR). This procedure can be done using a femoral, aortic arch, or direct left ventricular percutaneous catheter insertion approach and a porcine valve loaded on a balloon-expandable stent. Severe symptomatic mitral regurgitation and asymptomatic severe mitral regurgitation with left ventricular dilatation/reduced ejection fraction are both indications for mitral valve repair or replacement. Both procedures require a thoracotomy at this time.

As discussed in Chap. 12, kidney failure is associated with either uremic or fluid overload pericarditis. Development of this disease is usually caused by inadequate or missed dialysis. With that being said, dialysis is the principal treatment of these two forms of pericarditis. Dialysis may also help decrease effusion size if present. Uremic patients may respond quicker to therapy. Systemic anticoagulation may increase risk of

Box 13.5. Relevant Guidelines

1. *Kidney Disease: Improving Global Outcomes Guidelines*
   Kidney Disease: Improving Global Outcomes (KDIGO) Lipid Work Group. KDIGO clinical practice guideline for lipid management in chronic kidney disease. Kidney Int Suppl. 2013;3:259–305.
2. *American Heart Association Guidelines*
   - 2013 ACC/AHA guideline on the treatment of blood cholesterol to reduce atherosclerotic cardiovascular risk in adults: a report of the American College of Cardiology/American Heart Association Task Force on Practice Guidelines. Circulation. 2013.10.1161 [2]
   - ACCF secondary prevention and risk reduction therapy for patients with coronary and other atherosclerotic vascular disease: 2011 update: a guideline from the American Heart Association and American College of Cardiology Foundation. Circulation. 2011;124:2458–73.
   - 2012 ACCF/AHA/HRS focused update of the 2008 guidelines for device-based therapy of cardiac rhythm abnormalities: a report of the American College of Cardiology Foundation/American Heart Association Task Force on Practice Guidelines and the Heart Rhythm Society. Circulation. 2012;126:1784–800.
   - ACC/AHA 2008 guideline update on valvular heart disease: focused update on infective endocarditis: a report of the American College of Cardiology/American Heart Association Task Force on Practice Guidelines: endorsed by the Society of Cardiovascular Anesthesiologists, Society for Cardiovascular Angiography and interventions, And Society of Thoracic Surgeons. Circulation. 2008;118(8):887.
   - 2013 ACCF/AHA Guideline for the Management of Heart Failure: Executive Summary. A Report of the American College of Cardiology Foundation/American Heart Association Task Force on Practice Guidelines. Circulation 2013;128:1810–52.
3. *European Society of Cardiology Guideline*
   - EHRA/EACT/ESC Committee for Practice Guidelines. Guidelines for the management of atrial fibrillation: the Task Force for the Management of Atrial Fibrillation of the European Society of Cardiology (ESC). Europace. 2010;12(10):1360–420. doi: 10.1093/europace/euq350.
   - Guidelines on the prevention, diagnosis, and treatment of infective endocarditis (new version 2009): the Task Force on the Prevention, Diagnosis, and Treatment of Infective Endocarditis of the European Society of Cardiology (ESC). Endorsed by the European Society of Clinical Microbiology and Infectious Diseases (ESCMID) and the International Society of Chemotherapy (ISC) for infection and Cancer. Eur Heart J. 2009;30(19):2369.

developing hemorrhagic effusions especially when uremia is present and should be avoided if possible. Ineffective dialysis may lead to large effusions, which may cause hemodynamic instability or diastolic compromise. Pericardiocentesis is recommended in these high-risk patients. Anti-inflammatory drugs may be also be used in resistant cases. Colchicine is associated with lowest rates of recurrences. Surgical pericardiectomy is preserved for persistent or recurrent effusions.

Before You Finish: Practice Pearls for the Clinician

- Statin therapy is proven to be the most effective treatment of hypercholesterolemia. Adverse effect profile is the same in kidney patients as in the general population.
- HD and CKD patients display silent ischemia more frequently, which may disguise ACS. Treatment includes dual antiplatelet therapy, statins, B-blockers, ACEIs, low molecular weight heparin, and glycoprotein IIb/IIa antagonists.
- Clinicians should assess fluid balance and target any imbalances that may lead to decompensated heart failure.
- Heart failure therapy should include a diuretic, an ACEI, a B-blocker, and an aldosterone antagonist if possible due to the survival benefit they provide.
- Maintaining excellent oral hygiene is pivotal in preventing infective endocarditis.

References

1. Libby P, Braunwald E. Braunwald's Heart disease: a textbook of cardiovascular medicine. 9th ed. Philadelphia: Elsevier Inc; 2012.
2. 2013 ACC/AHA guideline on the treatment of blood cholesterol to reduce atherosclerotic cardiovascular risk in adults: A report of the American College of Cardiology/American Heart Association Task Force on Practice Guidelines. Circulation. 2013. doi:10.1161.
3. Kidney Disease: Improving Global Outcomes (KDIGO) Lipid Work Group. KDIGO clinical practice guideline for lipid management in chronic kidney disease. Kidney Int Suppl. 2013;3:259–305.
4. Keech A, Simes RJ, Barter P, et al. Effects of long-term fenofibrate therapy on cardiovascular events in 9795 people with type 2 diabetes mellitus (the FIELD study): Randomized controlled trial. Lancet. 2005; 366:1849.
5. Bhatt D, Fox KA, Hacke W, et al. Clopidogrel and aspirin versus aspirin alone for the prevention of atherothrombotic events. N Engl J Med. 2006;354:1706.
6. Bangalore S, Messerli F, Kostis J, Pepine C. Cardiovascular protection using beta-blockers. J Am Coll Cardiol. 2007;50:563–72.
7. Vadnais DS, Wenger NK. Emerging clinical role of ranolazine in the management of angina. Dovepress. 2010;6:517–30.
8. McCullough PA. Acute coronary syndromes in patients with renal failure. Curr Cardiol Rep. 2003;5:266.
9. Szczeh LA, Reddan DN, Owen NF, et al. Differential survival after coronary revascularization procedures among patients with renal insufficiency. Kidney Int. 2001;60:292.
10. Brater DC. Update in diuretic therapy: clinical pharmacology. Semin Nephrol. 2011;31:483.
11. Bart BA, Goldsmith SR, Lee KL, et al. Ultrafiltration in decompensated heart failure with cardiorenal syndrome. N Engl J Med. 2012;367:2296.
12. Rathore SS, Wang Y, Krumholz HM. Sex-based differences in the effect of digoxin for the treatment of heart failure. N Engl J Med. 2002;347:1403–11.
13. Wase A, Basit A, Nazir R, et al. Impact of chronic kidney disease upon survival among implantable cardioverter-defibrillator recipients. J Interv Card Electrophysiol. 2004;11:199–2014.
14. Manian FA. Vascular and cardiac infections in end-stage renal disease. Am J Med Sci. 2003;325:243.
15. Smith Jr SC, Benjamin EJ, Bonow RO, Braun LT, Creager MA, Franklin BA, Gibbons RJ, Grundy SM, Hiratzka LF, Jones DW, Lloyd-Jones DM, Minissian M, Mosca L, Peterson ED, Sacco RL, Spertus J, Stein JH, Taubert KA, World Heart Federation and the Preventive Cardiovascular Nurses Association. AHA/ACCF secondary prevention and risk reduction therapy for patients with coronary and other atherosclerotic vascular disease: 2011 update: a guideline from the American Heart Association and American College of Cardiology Foundation. Circulation. 2011;124:2458–73.
16. Yancy CW, Jessup M, Bozkurt B, Butler J, Casey Jr DE, Drazner MH, Fonarow GC, Geraci SA, Horwich T, Januzzi JL, Johnson MR, Kasper EK, Levy WC, Masoudi FA, McBride PE, McMurray JJ, Mitchell JE, Peterson PN, Riegel B, Sam F, Stevenson LW, Tang WH, Tsai EJ, Wilkoff BL. 2013 ACCF/AHA guideline for the management of heart failure: executive summary. A report of the American College of Cardiology Foundation/American Heart Association Task Force on Practice Guidelines. Circulation. 2013;128:1810–52.
17. EHRA/EACT/ESC Committee for Practice Guidelines. Guidelines for the management of atrial fibrillation: the Task Force for the Management of Atrial Fibrillation of the European Society of Cardiology (ESC). Europace. 2010;12(10):1360–420. doi:10.1093/europace/euq350.

18. Tracy CM, Epstein AE, Darbar D, DiMarco JP, Dunbar SB, Estes 3rd NA, Ferguson Jr TB, Hammill SC, Karasik PE, Link MS, Marine JE, Schoenfeld MH, Shanker AJ, Silka MJ, Stevenson LW, Stevenson WG, Varosy PD, Ellenbogen KA, Freedman RA, Gettes LS, Gillinov AM, Gregoratos G, Hayes DL, Page RL, Stevenson LW, Sweeney MO, American College of Cardiology Foundation; American Heart Association Task Force on Practice Guidelines; Heart Rhythm Society. 2012 ACCF/AHA/HRS focused update of the 2008 guidelines for device-based therapy of cardiac rhythm abnormalities: a report of the American College of Cardiology Foundation/ American Heart Association Task Force on Practice Guidelines and the Heart Rhythm Society. Circulation. 2012;126:1784–800.
19. Nishimura RA, Carabello BA, Faxon DP, Freed MD, Lytle BW, O'Gara PT, O'Rourke RA, Shah PM, Bonow RO, Carabello BA, Chatterjee K, de Leon Jr AC, Faxon DP, Freed MD, Gaasch WH, Lytle BW, Nishimura RA, O'Gara PT, O'Rourke RA, Otto CM, Shah PM, Shanewise JS, Smith Jr SC, Jacobs AK, Buller CE, Creager MA, Ettinger SM, Krumholz HM, Kushner FG, Lytle BW, Nishimura RA, Page RL, Tarkington LG, Yancy Jr CW, American College of Cardiology/American Heart Association Task Force. ACC/AHA 2008 guideline update on valvular heart disease: focused update on infective endocarditis: a report of the American College of Cardiology/ American Heart Association Task Force on Practice Guidelines: endorsed by the Society of Cardiovascular Anesthesiologists, Society for Cardiovascular Angiography and interventions, And Society of Thoracic Surgeons. Circulation. 2008;118(8):887.
20. Habib G, Hoen B, Tornos P, Thuny F, Prendergast B, Vilacosta I, Moreillon P, de Jesus Antunes M, Thilen U, Lekakis J, Lengyel M, Müller L, Naber CK, Nihoyannopoulos P, Moritz A, Zamorano JL, ESC Committee for Practice Guidelines. Guidelines on the prevention, diagnosis, and treatment of infective endocarditis (new version 2009): the Task Force on the Prevention, Diagnosis, and Treatment of Infective Endocarditis of the European Society of Cardiology (ESC). Endorsed by the European Society of Clinical Microbiology and Infectious Diseases (ESCMID) and the International Society of Chemotherapy (ISC) for infection and Cancer. Eur Heart J. 2009;30(19): 2369.
21. Baigent C, Landray M, Reith C. The effects of lowering LDL cholesterol with simvastatin plus ezetimibe in patients with chronic kidney disease (Study of Heart and Renal Protection): a randomized placebo-controlled trial. Lancet. 2011;377:2181–92.
22. Goldfine AB, Kaul S, Hiatt WR. Fibrates in the treatment of dyslipidemias-time for a reassessment. N Engl J Med. 2011;365:481–4.
23. Morrow DA, Boden WE. Chapter 57: Stable ischemic heart disease. In: Bonow RO, Mann DL, Zipes DP, Libby P, editors. Braunwald's heart disease: A textbook of cardiovascular medicine. 9th ed. Philadelphia: Elsevier; 2011.
24. Jentzer JC, Dewald TA, Hernandez AF. Combination of loop diuretics with thiazide-type diuretics in heart. J Am Coll Cardiol. 2010;56(19):1527–34.
25. Ronco C, Cicoira M, McCullough PA. Cardiorenal syndrome type 1: Pathophysiological crosstalk leading to combined heart and kidney dysfunction in the setting of acutely decompensated heart failure. J Am Coll Cardiol. 2012;0735:1097.
26. Costanzo MR, Guglin ME, Saltzberg MT, et al. Ultrafiltration versus intravenous diuretics for patients hospitalized for acute decompensated heart failure. J Am Coll Cardiol. 2007;49(6):675–83.
27. Bart BA, Goldsmith SR, Lee KL, et al. Ultrafiltration in decompensated heart failure with cardiorenal syndrome. N Engl J Med. 2012;367(24):2296–304.

14 Cerebrovascular Disease and Chronic Kidney Disease

Semih Giray and Zülfikar Arlier

Before You Start: Facts You Need to Know

- Patients with low glomerular filtration rate (GFR) and/or albuminuria are at risk for both thrombotic and hemorrhagic events.
- In cases of CKD, endothelial dysfunction in brain arterioles, atherosclerotic changes of the large vessels, blood pressure elevation due to the activation of the renin-angiotensin system, and coagulation abnormalities probably underlie both hemorrhagic and ischemic stroke.
- Hypertension is the primary, manageable risk factor for both hemorrhagic and ischemic stroke.
- Hemorrhagic infarction is a major concern after thrombolytic therapy in CKD patients, because hemorrhagic transformation or cerebral microbleeds are more prevalent in these patients.
- Although CT is the gold standard for diagnosis of intracerebral hemorrhage, MRI (magnetic resonance imaging) gradient-echo sequences are also an effective way to delineate small or large hemorrhagic foci.

S. Giray, MD • Z. Arlier, MD (✉)
Neurology Department, Baskent University Medical Faculty, Adana Teaching and Research Hospital, Adana, Turkey
e-mail: sgiray72@hotmail.com; zarlier@gmail.com

14.1 Introduction

Several misconceptions exist about stroke. Stroke is not only a pure cerebral event (CVE) but also it is a primary or secondary devastating disease of the blood vessels of the brain. There is a presumed reason or cause for every stroke. Stroke is not one illness but it involves several diseases that lead to occlusion of arteries that deprive blood supply to certain parts of the brain or that predispose to bleeding into or around the brain. In the United States, nearly three fourths of a million individuals have a stroke, and 150,000 people die from stroke each year. In China, approximately 1.5 million people die each year because of stroke. Someone in the United States has a stroke every 45 sec., and every 3.1 min, someone dies of stroke. Stroke affects three times as many women as breast cancer and yet receives much less public attention. For a long time, stroke has been the third leading cause of death in most countries in the world, surpassed as a killer only by heart disease and cancer. Strokes are an even more important cause of prolonged disability.

Stroke is anything but a homogeneous entity. Disorders as different as rupture of a large blood vessel that causes flooding of the brain with blood and occlusion of a tiny artery with softening in a small but strategic brain site both qualify as strokes. These two pathologic caricatures of stroke subtypes are as divergent as grapes and watermelons, two very different substances that fit in the general category of fruit. Stroke refers

M. Arici (ed.), *Management of Chronic Kidney Disease*,
DOI 10.1007/978-3-642-54637-2_14, © Springer-Verlag Berlin Heidelberg 2014

to any damage to the brain or the spinal cord caused by an abnormality of the blood supply. The term stroke is typically used when the symptoms begin abruptly, whereas cerebrovascular disease is a more general term that carries no connotation as to the tempo of brain injury. Of course, many patients with severely diseased blood vessels have no injury to the brain tissue. A blood or cardiovascular abnormality precedes and subsequently leads to the brain injury. Recognition of the cardiac or cerebrovascular lesion or hematologic disorder before the brain becomes damaged offers clinicians a window of opportunity during which brain damage can be prevented. At times, even when brain injury has occurred, the patient is unaware of any symptoms, and neurologists may not be able to detect any abnormality on neurologic examination. Sophisticated neuroimaging techniques have taught clinicians that such "silent strokes" are common.

Diagnosis and treatment of stroke patients require a basic understanding of the anatomy, physiology, and pathology of the major structures involved—the brain and spinal cord, the heart and blood vessels that supply blood to these structures, and the blood itself. To be effective, clinicians caring for stroke patients must be intimately familiar with the appearance of the normal brain and the usual locations and course of arteries supplying the brain and spinal cord and veins that drain blood from these regions.

14.2 Mechanisms of Cerebrovascular Damage to Brain Tissue

There are two major categories of brain damage in stroke patients, namely, ischemia and hemorrhage. Bleeding damages the brain by cutting off connecting pathways and by causing localized or generalized pressure injury to brain tissue; biochemical substances released during and after hemorrhage also may adversely affect nearby vascular and brain tissues [1].

14.2.1 Ischemia

Ischemia can be further subdivided into three different mechanisms: thrombosis, embolism, and decreased systemic perfusion.

14.2.2 Thrombosis

The most common type of vascular pathology is atherosclerosis, in which fibrous and muscular tissues overgrow in the subintima, and fatty materials form plaques that can encroach on the lumen. Next, platelets adhere to plaque crevices and form clumps that serve as nidi for the deposition of fibrin, thrombin, and clot. Atherosclerosis affects chiefly the larger extracranial and intracranial arteries. Occasionally, a clot forms within the lumen because of a primary hematologic problem, such as polycythemia, thrombocytosis, or a systemic hypercoagulable state. The smaller, penetrating intracranial arteries and arterioles are more often damaged by hypertension than by atherosclerotic processes. Less common vascular pathologies leading to obstruction include (1) fibromuscular dysplasia, an overgrowth of medial and intimal elements that compromises vessel contractility and luminal size; (2) arteritis, especially of the Takayasu or giant-cell type; (3) dissection of the vessel wall, often with a luminal or extraluminal clot temporarily obstructing the vessel; and (4) hemorrhage into a plaque, leading to acute or chronic luminal compromise. At times, the focal vascular abnormality is a functional change in the contractility of blood vessels. Intense focal vasoconstriction can lead to decreased blood flow and thrombosis. Dilatation of blood vessels also alters local blood flow and clots often form in dilated segments.

14.2.3 Embolism

In embolism, material formed elsewhere within the vascular system lodges in an artery and blocks blood flow. Blockage can be transient or may persist for hours or days before moving distally. In contrast to thrombosis, embolic luminal blockage is not caused by a localized process originating within the blocked artery. The material arises proximally, most commonly from the heart; from major arteries such as the aorta, carotid, and vertebral arteries; and from systemic veins. Cardiac sources of embolism include the heart valves and clots or tumors within the atrial or ventricular cavities. Artery-to-artery emboli are composed of clots, platelet clumps, or fragments of plaques that break off from the proximal vessels. Clots originating in systemic veins travel to the brain through cardiac defects such as an atrial septal defect or a patent foramen ovale, a process termed paradoxical embolism. Also, occasionally air, fat, plaque material, participate matter from injected drugs, bacteria, foreign bodies, and tumor cells enter the vascular system and embolize to brain arteries.

14.2.4 Decreased Systemic Perfusion

In decreased systemic perfusion, diminished flow to brain tissue is caused by low systemic perfusion pressure. The most common causes are cardiac pump failure (most often due to myocardial infarction or arrhythmia) and systemic hypotension (due to blood loss or hypovolemia). In such cases, the lack of perfusion is more generalized than in localized thrombosis or embolism and affects the brain diffusely and bilaterally. Poor perfusion is most critical in border zone or so-called watershed regions at the periphery of the major vascular supply territories.

14.2.5 Damage Caused by Ischemia

The three mechanisms of brain ischemia may lead to temporary or permanent tissue injury. Permanent injury is termed infarction. Capillaries or other vessels within the ischemic tissue may also be injured, so that reperfusion can lead to leakage of blood into the ischemic tissue, resulting in a hemorrhagic infarction. The extent of brain damage depends on the location and duration of the poor perfusion and the ability of collateral vessels to perfuse the tissues at risk. The systemic blood pressure, blood volume, and blood viscosity also affect blood flow to the ischemic areas.

14.2.6 Hemorrhage

Hemorrhage can be further subdivided into four subtypes: subarachnoid, intracerebral, subdural, and epidural. These subtypes have different causes, pose different clinical problems, and have different managements.

14.2.7 Subarachnoid Hemorrhage

In subarachnoid hemorrhage, blood leaks out of the vascular bed onto the brain's surface and is disseminated quickly via the spinal fluid pathways into the spaces around the brain. Bleeding most often originates from aneurysms or arteriovenous malformations, but bleeding diatheses or trauma can also cause subarachnoid bleeding. The blood within the subarachnoid space often contains substances that promote vasoconstriction of the basal arteries that are bathed in cerebrospinal fluid.

14.2.8 Intracerebral Hemorrhage

The cause is most often hypertension, with leakage of blood from small intracerebral arterioles damaged by the elevated blood pressure. Bleeding diatheses, especially from the iatrogenic prescription of anticoagulants or from trauma, drugs, vascular malformations, and vasculopathies (such as cerebral amyloid angiopathy), can also cause bleeding into the brain. The degree of damage depends on the location, rapidity, volume, and pressure of the bleeding.

14.2.9 Subdural and Epidural Hemorrhages

These hemorrhages are almost always caused by head trauma. Subdural hemorrhages arise from injured veins that are located between the dura mater and the arachnoid membranes. The bleeding is most often slow and accumulates during days, weeks, and even a few months. When a large vein is lacerated, bleeding can develop more rapidly over hours to days. Epidural hemorrhages are caused by tearing of meningeal arteries, most often the middle meningeal artery. Blood accumulates rapidly over minutes to hours between the skull and the dura mater. Both subdural and epidural hemorrhages cause symptoms and signs by compressing brain tissue and increasing intracranial pressure.

14.3 General Measures to Prevent Stroke

Prevention is the most effective way to avoid death or suffering from stroke. Successful preventive strategies are cost-effective because they eliminate the expenses of acute hospital care and rehabilitation. Prevention of stroke involves two different tactics. One consists of interventions applied to large segments of the population and includes health promotion and identification and treatment of common factors that increase the risk of either hemorrhagic or ischemic stroke (Box 14.1). These measures (e.g., control of hypertension) may have limited benefit for individual persons, but their aggregate effects are substantial when prescribed to large populations. The second approach involves the use of more expensive and potentially more dangerous therapies given to smaller groups of persons judged to be at the highest risk. *Primary prevention* includes therapies to forestall ischemic vascular events, including stroke, in either large populations or small high-risk groups of asymptomatic people. *Secondary prevention* implies the use of treatments to prevent stroke or other ischemic vascular event in persons who already have had symptoms. Secondary prevention of stroke can include treatment of a spectrum of people to include those without neurological symptoms. The symptomatic high-risk groups especially include those patients who have evidence of atherosclerosis, such as:

- Myocardial infarction
- Angina pectoris
- Claudication
- Amaurosis fugax
- Transient ischemic attack (TIA)
- Ischemic stroke

Box 14.1. Factors Associated with an Increased Risk of Stroke

Epidemiologic

Age—(Elderly > middle-aged or young adults > children)

Gender—(Men > women in each age group)

Race—(Blacks > Asians or Hispanics > Whites)

Geographic region—(Eastern Europe > Western Europe; Asia > Europe or North America)

Family history—(Stroke or heart disease < aged 60)

Other, potentially modifiable, factors:

- Diastolic or isolated systolic hypertension
- Diabetes mellitus, type 1 or type 2
- Hyperlipidemia (hypercholesterolemia)
- Elevated low-density lipoprotein (LDL) cholesterol or low high-density lipoprotein (HDL) cholesterol
- Hyperhomocysteinemia
- Smoking
- Alcohol abuse
- Drug abuse
- Oral contraceptive use
- Pregnancy
- Migraine headaches

14.3.1 Risk Factors for Stroke

The conditions or factors that predispose to or increase the risk of a cerebrovascular event are diverse (Table 14.1 and Boxes 14.2, 14.3, and 14.4). While some conditions that lay the groundwork for ischemic stroke also lead to brain hemorrhage, additional factors may promote intracranial bleeding. Some conditions that predispose to stroke are not modifiable. Advancing age is the single most common factor that predicts a high risk for stroke. Although stroke is much more common in

Table 14.1 Nonatherosclerotic vasculopathies causing ischemic stroke

Noninflammatory causes	Inflammatory causes	Infectious causes
Dissection	PAN	Syphilis
Fibromuscular dysplasia	Wegener granulomatosis	Herpes zoster
Moyamoya disease	SLE	Cysticercosis
Ehlers-Danlos syndrome tip4	RA	AIDS
Fabry disease	Scleroderma	Bacterial meningitis
Hyperhomocysteinemia	Sjögren syndrome	
Marfan syndrome	Takayasu syndrome	
Menkes disease	Temporal arteritis	
Amyloid angiopathy	Behçet disease	
	Ulcerative colitis	
	Sarcoidosis	
	Cogan syndrome	
	Kawasaki syndrome	
	Polymyositis	
	Dermatomyositis	

PAN polyarteritis nodosa, *SLE* systemic lupus erythematosus, *RA* rheumatoid arthritis, *AIDS* acquired immunodeficiency syndrome

elderly people than in children or young adults, it also is an important disease in these latter groups. Approximately 3 % of ischemic strokes occur among people under the age of 45. The ratio of hemorrhagic stroke to ischemic stroke is higher in younger people than in the elderly. The causes of stroke also vary by age. Atherosclerosis and cardioembolism secondary to atrial fibrillation are the leading causes of ischemic stroke in the elderly, while the differential diagnosis of ischemic stroke etiologies is much broader in younger people. Similarly, cerebral amyloid angiopathy and chronic hypertension are leading causes of intracerebral hemorrhage in older persons, while vascular malformations and aneurysms are more common causes in younger adults [2].

Box14.2. Cardiac Causes of Embolization to the Brain

Atrial Fibrillation

Left Ventricle or Intraventricular Lesions

- Dilated cardiomyopathy
- Recent myocardial infarction (MI), anterior in particular
- Ventricular aneurysm (post-MI)
- Akinetic segment (post-MI)
- Mural or intraventricular thrombus

Left Atrium, Intra-atrial, or Interatrial Lesions

- Atrial septal aneurysm
- Atrial septal defect
- Patent foramen ovale
- Atrial turbulence
- Atrial thrombus
- Myxoma

Valvular Lesions

- Mechanical or bioprosthetic valve
- Congenital valvular abnormality
- Rheumatic mitral stenosis
- Mitral valve prolapse
- Infective endocarditis
- Nonbacterial thrombotic endocarditis (marantic)
- Libman-Sacks endocarditis
- Mitral annulus calcification
- Calcific aortic stenosis
- *Cardiac Procedures*
- Coronary artery bypass surgery
- Cardiac catheterization
- Percutaneous transluminal coronary angioplasty
- Percutaneous transluminal valvuloplasty
- Intra-aortic balloon pump procedure

Box 14.3. Atherosclerotic Causes of Ischemic Stroke

- Atherosclerosis of the aortic arch
- Extracranial large-artery atherosclerosis:
  - Origin of the internal carotid artery
  - Origin of the vertebral artery
  - Subclavian artery
- Intracranial larger-artery atherosclerosis:
  - Distal portion of internal carotid artery
  - Proximal portion of middle cerebral artery
  - Distal portion of vertebral artery
  - Middle portion of the basilar artery
  - Disseminated atherosclerosis
- Fusiform aneurysm:
  - Basilar artery
  - Internal carotid artery
- Small-artery disease (lipohyalinosis/microatheroma)

Box14.4. Hematologic or Coagulation Disorders Causing Ischemic Stroke

- Polycythemia rubra vera
- Sickle-cell disease
- Essential thrombocytosis
- Thrombotic thrombocytopenic purpura
- Heparin-induced thrombocytopenia
- Antithrombin III deficiency
- Protein C or S deficiency
- Deficiency of factors V, VII, XII, or XIII
- Heparin cofactor II deficiency
- Dysfibrinogenemias
- Antiphospholipid/anticardiolipin antibodies
- Nephrotic syndrome
- Malignancy
- Pregnancy
- Oral contraceptives
- Dehydration

14.3.2 Modifiable Risk Factors

Some of the interventions to prevent stroke are aimed primarily at slowing the course of atherosclerosis, preventing fracture of an atherosclerotic plaque, or stabilizing the arterial endothelium. Many therapies are aimed at controlling risk factors or conditions that promote development of advanced atherosclerotic conditions. Attention to these risk factors is critical when making decisions about the primary or secondary prevention of stroke.

14.3.2.1 Hypertension

Hypertension is the primary manageable risk factor for both hemorrhagic and ischemic stroke. Regardless of age, the presence of diastolic arterial hypertension greatly increases the likelihood of stroke. Among older persons, isolated systolic hypertension also promotes stroke. The relationship between hypertension and stroke is much closer than the association between an elevated blood pressure and coronary artery disease. Hemorrhagic stroke also complicates chronic hypertension and acute hypertensive crises, including eclampsia. A number of antihypertensive agents are available. The selection of medications is made on a case-by-case basis and involves consideration of factors such as concomitant diseases.

In most cases, β-blockers or oral diuretic agents are prescribed initially. Patients with concomitant symptomatic heart disease often are treated with β-blockers or calcium channel blocking medications. Recent evidence suggests that some of the newer angiotensin-converting enzyme (ACE) inhibitors may have additional potential benefits for stroke prevention. These agents may have some efficacy in stabilizing the vascular endothelium, which in turn might lower the risk of thromboembolism. In one trial, the ACE inhibitor ramipril was found to reduce the risk of stroke in asymptomatic high-risk patients, especially those with diabetes mellitus. The medication was given in conjunction with other measures to prevent stroke. Patients with hypertension secondary to renal artery stenosis usually are not treated with an ACE inhibitor.

14.3.2.2 Diabetes Mellitus

Diabetes mellitus promotes both atherosclerotic large-artery and small-artery disease of the brain. Stroke is a common complication in both younger, insulin-dependent diabetic patients and older persons with type 2 diabetes. Diabetic patients may have more severe strokes, and hyperglycemia also may exacerbate the severity of the neurologic impairments. Current recommendations advise careful control of diabetes mellitus and elevated blood glucose concentrations.

14.3.2.3 Hypercholesterolemia

Hyperlipidemia encourages early development of atherosclerosis. Hyperlipidemia is a likely important factor for stroke secondary to atherosclerosis, especially in middle-aged adults. Patients with ischemic stroke should be evaluated for the presence of hyperlipidemia. If the blood levels cannot be assayed within the first 24–48 h after stroke, the test should be delayed until the patient is convalescent. The cholesterol levels might be falsely low during the acute stage of stroke.

14.3.2.4 Smoking

Cessation of smoking probably is the single most cost-effective strategy to lower the risk of either hemorrhagic or ischemic stroke. Smokers have an increased risk of atherosclerosis. Even passive exposure to smoking has been implicated. Smoking also potentiates the use of oral contraceptives in young women. In addition, smoking adds to the risk of intracranial bleeding, including rupture of saccular aneurysms.

14.3.2.5 Other Potential Risk Factors

Other potential risk factors for stroke include:

- Migraine
- Use of oral contraceptives
- Obesity
- Excessive alcohol consumption
- Drug abuse
- Sleep disorders (including sleep apnea)

Excessive consumption of alcohol has been associated with an increased risk of intracranial bleeding. Elevated blood levels of homocysteine may augment the development of atherosclerosis and associated thrombosis. Supplementing the diet with folic acid, vitamin B12, and pyridoxine will lower homocysteine levels and might be helpful in preventing ischemic events. Inflammation also may play a role in the course of atherosclerosis.

14.3.3 Patients at Highest Risk

Persons with the following conditions are at the highest risk for ischemic stroke:

- Atrial fibrillation (AF)
- Asymptomatic stenosis of the carotid artery
- Amaurosis fugax
- TIA
- Previous ischemic stroke

14.3.3.1 Atrial Fibrillation

Atrial fibrillation (AF) is the primary cardiac abnormality associated with ischemic stroke. It is the most important risk factor for stroke in persons older than 75, especially in women. AF complicates a number of cardiac diseases and the presence of the arrhythmia is associated with an increased risk of cardioembolism. The most common cardiac diseases complicated by AF are:

- Coronary artery disease
- Hypertensive heart disease
- Cardiomyopathies
- Rheumatic heart disease
- Prosthetic cardiac valves

Persons younger than 60 years old who have AF and no other cardiac disorder (lone AF) appear to have a relatively low risk for stroke. Thus, the importance of AF is as an abetting factor leading to the formation of intra-atrial thrombi in a patient with another heart disease. Both people with chronic, sustained AF and those with an intermittent arrhythmia are at risk, and embolization can complicate intermittent or new-onset AF. The risk of embolization is relatively low during the first 2–3 days after the start of AF. Many patients do not have symptoms corresponding to the onset of the arrhythmia and the time the AF began becomes inferential. Thus, determining the onset of AF is problematic. Either electrical or pharmacologic cardioversion can be associated with embolization, and therefore, anticoagulation is prescribed for several weeks before and after correction of the arrhythmia. Several factors identify those persons with AF who are at greatest risk for embolization:

- Prior stroke or TIA
- Aged >75 years, especially women
- History of hypertension or systolic blood pressure >160 mmHg

- Diabetes mellitus
- Coronary artery disease
- Congestive heart failure
- Left ventricular dysfunction

14.3.3.2 Asymptomatic Cervical Stenosis or Bruit

Severe asymptomatic stenosis of the extracranial portion of the internal carotid artery can be detected after a physician auscultates a cervical bruit. Besides being a marker for a high risk for stroke, an asymptomatic carotid stenosis also forecasts an increased risk of myocardial infarction or vascular death. The risk of ipsilateral stroke in patients with narrowing >60 % appears to be approximately 2 % per year. The chance of stroke probably correlates with the severity of the arterial narrowing; patients with high-grade stenosis are assumed to be at the greatest risk. Doing carotid endarterectomy to treat an asymptomatic lesion at the same time as a major cardiovascular operation is not recommended because the chances for serious complications are excessively high.

14.3.3.3 Transient Ischemic Attack/ Amaurosis Fugax

Patients with ischemic symptoms of the brain or eye have the greatest risk of ischemic stroke. In general, the risk is highest among patients with a previous stroke, higher among patients with a TIA, and high in patients with amaurosis fugax. Amaurosis fugax (transient monocular blindness) is an episode of painless visual loss in one eye that is secondary to retinal ischemia. Amaurosis fugax usually is associated with atherosclerotic disease of the ipsilateral internal carotid artery. Global symptoms, including confusion, wooziness, light-headedness, and loss of consciousness, usually are not due to a TIA. The symptoms of a TIA usually involve weakness, numbness, or incoordination and represent a loss of normal neurologic activity. Positive neurologic symptoms, such as scintillating visual phenomena, seizure activity, or involuntary movements, rarely are due to transient brain ischemia. A migration or march of symptoms from one body part to another is uncommon with a TIA. The pattern of symptoms of a TIA in the vertebrobasilar circulation (binocular visual loss, diplopia, vertigo, unilateral or bilateral weakness, numbness, heaviness or clumsiness, ataxia, dysarthria, dysphagia, hearing loss, drop attack) differs from the pattern of symptoms in the carotid territory (ipsilateral monocular visual loss-amaurosis fugax, contralateral weakness, numbness, heaviness, or clumsiness, dysarthria, aphasia) [3].

14.4 Immediate Evaluation of Patients with Suspected Stroke

Early differentiation of ischemic stroke from hemorrhagic stroke is especially important because it influences acute treatment and subsequent care. A limited number of rapidly performed diagnostic tests are required, while extensive testing to determine the cause of stroke can be done after admission to the hospital. These diagnostic tests should be performed on an urgent basis because timing is critical (Box 14.5).

Box 14.5. Emergent Diagnostic Tests for Evaluation of a Patient with Suspected Stroke

- Computed tomography (CT) of the brain without contrast
- Electrocardiogram (ECG)
- Chest x-ray (if hypoxia or acute lung disease suspected)
- Complete blood count and platelet count
- Prothrombin time/international normalized ratio (INR)
- Activated partial thromboplastin time (aPTT)
- Blood glucose
- Serum chemistries, including electrolytes
- Cervical spine x-ray (if the patient is unresponsive and trauma is possible)
- Arterial blood gases (if hypoxia is suspected)
- Cerebrospinal fluid (CSF) examination (if subarachnoid hemorrhage is suspected but no blood or mass effect is seen on CT)

Brain imaging (computed tomography [CT]) is the most important diagnostic test because it is the most reliable way to differentiate hemorrhagic stroke from ischemic stroke (Box 14.6). Clinical presentations of the two types of cerebrovascular disease are sufficiently similar to make the diagnosis of brain hemorrhage or infarction problematic when using only the history and physical examination. Patients should not be treated with anticoagulants or thrombolytic agents until CT has helped exclude the presence of intracranial hemorrhage.

Because of the strong relationship between heart disease and stroke and because of the critical nature of early cardiopulmonary complications and their effect on emergent management and outcomes, an electrocardiogram (ECG) and chest x-ray are important as initial diagnostic tests. The coagulation tests also screen for the presence of an underlying hematologic (coagulation) disorder that could lead to either ischemic or hemorrhagic stroke. The tests also can influence decisions about use of thrombolytic agents to treat acute ischemic stroke. Examination of the cerebrospinal fluid (CSF) is an important study to search for bleeding if the patient's clinical findings suggest SAH. A lumbar puncture is not necessary if the CT has demonstrated hemorrhage.

Box 14.6. Sequence of Vascular Imaging Tests with Acute Stroke

- Imaging of the brain should be performed first (CT or MRI)
- Consider vascular imaging if:
  - Results would alter acute management
  - Patient has unexplained symptoms suggesting brain stem dysfunction
  - Acute intra-arterial intervention is planned
  - Patient has SAH or unexplained intraparenchymal hemorrhage
- Sequence:
  - If available, do CTA after CT
  - If MRI is performed, do MRA
  - If available, consider ultrasonography
  - DSA can be done if other tests are unavailable or if they give inconclusive results

Abbreviations: CT, computed tomography; CTA, computed tomographic angiography; DSA, digital subtraction angiography; MRA, magnetic resonance angiography; MRI, magnetic resonance imaging; SAH, subarachnoid hemorrhage

14.4.1 Subsequent Diagnostic Evaluation

Magnetic resonance imaging (MRI) is more sensitive than CT in detecting small ischemic lesions, particularly in the posterior fossa. MRI also can be used to assess the presence of an underlying arterial or venous occlusion. In addition, advances in MRI technology allow evaluation of perfusion, diffusion, and metabolic studies of the brain. The role of MRI in emergent evaluation will likely increase. In particular, mismatches between perfusion and other imaging sequences might become a key early diagnostic finding in determining eligibility for emergent stroke care. The recent development of gradient-echo T2-weighted magnetic resonance imaging (MRI) has enabled the highly accurate detection of prior cerebral microbleeds (CMBs), which might indicate a higher risk of future intracerebral hemorrhage (ICH) and be a marker of cerebral small-vessel disease in the general population. The cerebral vasculature can be examined by several diagnostic tests (Table 14.2). Arteriography (digital subtraction angiography [DSA]) is the preferred method for evaluation of patients with intracranial hemorrhage. Because early surgery often is recommended for those with ruptured aneurysms, DSA is performed as an emergent procedure for persons with SAH. Imaging of the heart usually is recommended because of the high prevalence of cardiac disease that can be the source of emboli in people with ischemic stroke. Transthoracic and transesophageal echocardiography (TTE and TEE) are the two most commonly ordered cardiac tests. If another likely cause for stroke, such as a carotid artery dissection, is found or if the results of cardiac imaging are not likely to alter

Table 14.2 What can be imaged in patients with acute stroke?

Imaging test	Imaging results
CT	Brain tissue, CSF space, skull, brain tissue perfusion
MRI	Brain tissue, CSF space, brain tissue proton diffusion and perfusion, brain function
CTA	Blood vessels in neck or brain (arteries and veins)
MRA	Same as CTA
DSA	Same as CTA
US	Same as CTA
TDU	Same as CTA
SPECT	Brain tissue perfusion
PET	Brain tissue perfusion, brain metabolism
MRS	Brain metabolism

Abbreviations: *CSF* cerebrospinal fluid, *CT* computed tomography, *CTA* computed tomographic angiography, *DSA* digital subtraction angiography, *MRA* magnetic resonance angiography, *MRI* magnetic resonance imaging, *MRS* magnetic resonance spectroscopy, *PET* positron emission tomography, *SPECT* single photon emission computed tomography, *TDU* transcranial Doppler ultrasound, *US* duplex ultrasound

management, these tests could be avoided. On the other hand, echocardiography can be informative in young people with ischemic symptoms or those who have other evidence suggesting a cardiac source for embolization. In general, TTE has a low yield in detecting cardiac abnormalities; it is most likely to find abnormalities in the left ventricle. The test should be ordered if a mural thrombus following a myocardial infarction or a left ventricular aneurysm or an akinetic left ventricular segment is suspected.

14.5 Emergent Medical Management

Acute cardiovascular and cerebrovascular events have several similarities. These life-threatening conditions usually are of arterial origin and accompanied by complications that add to morbidity and mortality. Complications of stroke can occur at any time during the acute illness, but they are most common during the first 24–48 h. Both acute coronary artery occlusion and acute occlusion of an artery to the brain can be treated with emergent administration of thrombolytic agents. Both conditions can be treated successfully and outcomes can be improved. Like management of those persons with acute heart disease, modern stroke care requires urgent treatment.

14.5.1 Fever

Fever is uncommon during the first day after stroke. It can result from complications, such as aspiration pneumonia, or be a marker of an infectious cause of stroke, such as endocarditis. People with intracranial bleeding often have an elevated temperature secondary to disturbances of the thermoregulatory center in the hypothalamus. An elevated temperature can be found in patients with intracranial hemorrhage, and its presence is a poor prognostic sign. An elevated temperature can potentiate the effects of acute ischemia. Measures to lower the temperature in febrile patients are encouraged.

14.5.2 Cardiac Complications

While heart disease is a leading cause of stroke, cardiac disorders are important, potentially life-threatening complications of cerebrovascular events. Myocardial ischemia, cardiac failure, and pulmonary edema are potential complications of intracranial hemorrhage. Acute myocardial injury and secondary arrhythmias are potential causes of sudden death in patients with major strokes. Cardiac monitoring to detect abnormal rhythms should be part of the initial observation of all patients with possible stroke. If serious arrhythmias are detected, medications should be prescribed using the rules of advanced cardiac life support.

14.5.3 Arterial Hypertension

During the first hours after stroke, most patients have an elevated blood pressure. Both acutely elevated and low blood pressures are associated with poor outcomes after stroke. The degree of hypertension is associated with the severity of neurological impairments; in general, blood pressures are highest among those patients with the most severe strokes. The high blood pressure can also be a compensatory mechanism to maintain adequate perfusion to the brain. Cerebrovascular autoregulation is lost in the ischemic bed and blood flow becomes pressure dependent. The brain may need an elevated blood pressure to limit the scope of the ischemic injury, and sudden lowering of the blood pressure might result in worsening of the neurologic signs. Information is lacking about what level of blood pressure is too high in the setting of acute stroke or about the best response to the finding of arterial hypertension. The best approach lies in not lowering the blood pressure too steeply or too rapidly. Rather, the blood pressure should be measured at frequent intervals and treatment responses should be based on sustained elevations of arterial hypertension.

For patients with ischemic stroke, the values that should lead to treatment are systolic >220 mmHg or mean >130 mmHg. The aim is to cautiously lower the blood pressure by approximately 15 % during the first 24 h after stroke. Parenteral agents can be given to rapidly lower arterial pressures in more urgent situations (Table 14.3). The current guidelines for the use of thrombolytic agents for treatment of acute ischemic stroke recommend that the medications not be used when a patient's systolic blood pressure is >185 mmHg or diastolic blood pressure is >110 mmHg. Lowering the blood pressure can be attempted so that recombinant tissue-plasminogen activator (rt-PA) can be administered. Given the

Table 14.3 Approach to elevated blood pressure in acute ischemic stroke

Blood pressure level (mmHg)	Treatment
Not eligible for thrombolytic therapy	
Systolic <220 or diastolic <120	Observe unless other end-organ involvement, e.g., aortic dissection, acute myocardial infarction, pulmonary edema, and hypertensive encephalopathy. Treat other symptoms of stroke such as headache, pain, agitation, nausea, and vomiting. Treat other acute complications of stroke, including hypoxia, increased intracranial pressure, seizures, or hypoglycemia
Systolic >220 or diastolic 121–140	Labetalol 10–20 mg IV over 1–2 min. May repeat or double every 10 min (maximum dose 300 mg) or nicardipine 5 mg/h IV infusion as initial dose; titrate to desired effect by 2.5 mg/h every 5 min to maximum of 15 mg/h, aim for a 10–15 % reduction of blood pressure
Diastolic >140	Nitroprusside 0.5 ug/kg/min IV infusion as initial dose with continuous blood pressure monitoring, aim for a 10–15 % reduction of blood pressure
Eligible for thrombolytic therapy	
Pretreatment	
Systolic >185 or diastolic >110	Labetalol 10–20 mg IV over 1–2 min. May repeat x 1 or nitropaste 1 –2 in.
	If blood pressure is not reduced and maintained at desired levels (systolic <185 and diastolic <110), do not administer rt-PA
During and after treatment	
1. Monitor BP	Check BP every 15 min for 2 h, then every 30 min for 6 h, and then every hour for 16 h
2. Diastolic >140	Sodium nitroprusside 0.5 ug/kg/min IV infusion as initial dose and titrate to desired blood pressure
3. Systolic >230 or diastolic 121–140	Labetalol 10 mg IV over 1–2 min, may repeat or double labetalol every 10 min to a maximum dose of 300 mg or give the initial labetalol bolus and then start a labetalol drip at 2–8 mg/min or nicardipine 5 mg/h IV infusion as initial dose; titrate to desired effect by increasing 2.5 mg/h every 5 min to maximum of 15 mg/h. If BP is not controlled by labetalol, consider sodium nitroprusside
4. Systolic 180–230 or diastolic 105–120	Labetalol 10 mg IV over 1–2 min. May repeat or double labetalol every 10–20 min to a maximum dose of 300 mg or give the initial labetalol bolus and then start a labetalol drip at 2–8 mg/min

Source: Adams et al. [18]

current relatively short window of time for the safe and effective use of rt-PA, management of arterial hypertension becomes problematic in the setting of acute stroke. In most instances, time will not be sufficient to determine if the blood pressure is stabilized at acceptable levels before rt-PA is given. The potential risks of exacerbating brain ischemia by lowering the blood pressure also may counteract any benefits from treating with rt-PA. The possibility of an elevated blood pressure increasing the risk of hemorrhagic transformation of the infarction after rt-PA treatment requires that monitoring and control of the blood pressure be aggressive during and following the use of the agent (Box 14.7).

Box 14.7. Treatment of Increased Intracranial Pressure Following Acute Stroke

General Prophylaxis

- Control fever, agitation, nausea and vomiting, hypoxia, hypercarbia
- Modest fluid restriction (approximately 1.5–2.0 l/day)
- Avoid potentially hypo-osmolar intravenous fluids (5 % dextrose/water)
- Elevate the head of the bed to augment venous drainage

Acute Interventions

- Intubation to protect the airway and to permit hyperventilation
- Goal to lower pCO2 to approximately 30 mmHg
- Mannitol 0.5 g/kg given in a 20 % solution over approximately 20–30 min:
  - Can repeat 0.25 g/kg every 6 h as needed
  - Usual maximal daily dose is 2 g/kg
  - Replace lost fluids
- Furosemide, 20–40 mg given intravenously
- Monitor intracranial pressure
- Drainage of CSF via a ventricular catheter
- Corticosteroids (dexamethasone or methylprednisolone) are not recommended

Surgical Procedures

- Evacuation of a hematoma
- Resection of infarcted brain
- Craniectomy with removal of a large section of skull

Abbreviations: *CSF* cerebrospinal fluid, *pCO2* partial pressure of carbon dioxide

14.5.4 Hypoglycemia and Hyperglycemia

Approximately one third of patients with stroke have hyperglycemia detected upon admission. Persistent hyperglycemia during the first 24 h predicts expansion of stroke and poor outcomes. The hyperglycemia may be a manifestation of underlying diabetes or it may be a secondary stress reaction. Treatment of hyperglycemia should be a component of emergent management.

14.5.5 Seizures

Seizures complicate approximately 5 % of strokes but status epilepticus is uncommon. Frequent seizures can intensify the brain injury from stroke, and they are a neurologic emergency in their own right. Seizures are most numerous in patients with subarachnoid hemorrhage (SAH) or cortical infarctions secondary to embolism. Phenytoin is the most commonly prescribed agent. Short-acting benzodiazepines can be given to patients who are having active seizures. Prophylactic administration of anticonvulsants to those patients who have had a recent stroke, but who have not had a seizure, is not recommended.

14.5.6 Increased Intracranial Pressure (ICP)

Patients with multilobar infarction or large hemorrhages of the cerebral hemisphere are at high risk for severely elevated ICP. A high ICP can worsen brain ischemia by reducing cerebral blood flow and cerebral perfusion pressure. In addition, pressure gradients between compartments within the cranial vault can lead to herniation and secondary brain injury. Elevations of ICP usually result from brain edema of the mass effect of the vascular lesion. In addition, large strokes in the posterior fossa or hemorrhages with ventricular or SAH can be complicated by acute hydrocephalus. The mass effects of the brain hematoma or acute hydrocephalus secondary to blockage of CSF pathways by clots mean that marked rises in ICP during the first hours after stroke are largely a problem in patients with hemorrhagic stroke. Usually, the course of brain edema and increased ICP is slower in patients with ischemic stroke; the symptoms evolve over the first 2–4 days in people with large hemispheric infarctions. Those with large hematomas or infarctions in the cerebellum or brain stem can develop signs of increased ICP rapidly. In this situation, the mass effects of the vascular lesion can cause both hydrocephalus and brain stem compression. Signs of herniation, such as unilateral oculomotor nerve (III) palsy, appear late in the course. Management of increased ICP after stroke includes both prophylactic and urgent treatment (Box 14.7). Osmotic therapy (saline, mannitol, or glycerol) is given to patients with signs of clinically significant brain edema and elevated ICP following stroke. Mannitol is administered intravenously over a 20-min period in a dose of 0.5 g/kg. Subsequent doses can be given every 4–6 h. The usual maximal daily dose is 2 g/kg. The ICP usually drops within 20 min of starting the infusion and effects will persist for approximately 4–6 h. A hyperosmolar state is a potential complication of repeated use of mannitol. In order to lessen the risk of this side effect, intravenous fluids can be administered to compensate for losses that are occurring. The level of monitored ICP can be used to time subsequent doses of mannitol. In patients with secondary hydrocephalus, drainage of CSF can be achieved via an intraventricular catheter. Removal of a small amount of fluid often can lower ICP dramatically. Continuous CSF drainage can be done, especially in patients with SAH. Repeated lumbar punctures can be performed if a patient does not have a mass; the only likely situation is severe SAH without a focal hematoma. Hypothermia also has been used to treat increased ICP following stroke.

14.6 Characteristics of Stroke in CKD Patients

14.6.1 Stroke Subtypes

CKD is an independent risk factor for ischemic, as well as hemorrhagic, stroke. In a population-based cohort study, the relative risk for ischemic stroke was 4.3–10.1 and that for hemorrhagic stroke was 4.1–6.7, respectively, in dialysis patients [4]. Even in the patients with a mild level of glomerular dysfunction, the risk for stroke appears to be increased. Recently, our group also demonstrated that CKD is associated with recurrent ischemia but not with hemorrhagic transformation in acute stroke patients [5]. A recent study with 20,386 participants without previous stroke has revealed that the incidence of stroke symptoms increased in patients with a lower estimated GFR (eGFR) and a higher level of albuminuria [6]. The impact of CKD on the stroke subtype may be different depending on gender. In 539,287 Swedish men and women free of previous stroke, the hazard ratios of renal dysfunction for ischemic stroke were 1.09, 1.24, and 2.27 for those with a mildly, moderately, and severely decreased GFR, respectively. This trend was observed in both genders. In contrast, hemorrhagic stroke was only related to renal dysfunction in females: 1.39, 1.70, and 3.46 for a mildly, moderately, and severely decreased GFR [7]. In a study of 12,222 Japanese men and women living in four communities, CKD increased the risk of hemorrhagic stroke, especially for males, but that of ischemic stroke for females. In that study, it was concluded that the gender difference was due to the differences in the prevalence of alcohol drinkers [8]. Therefore, CKD may have a gender-specific association with ischemic and hemorrhagic stroke, but this may differ according to the presence of other risk factors or in different ethnic groups.

14.6.2 Subtypes of Ischemic Stroke

Atherosclerosis is progressive in CKD patients. The prevalence of intracranial artery calcification was shown to be high in acute ischemic stroke patients with a reduced GFR [9]. Another study reported that proteinuria was an independent risk factor for ischemic stroke due to thrombotic arterial occlusion in patients with non-insulin-dependent diabetes mellitus [10]. A reduced GFR and increased excretion of albumin are factors closely associated with increased permeability or vulnerability of the small vessels, independent of other risk factors. These changes are causative of white matter lesions, cerebral microbleeds, and lacunar infarction. Recent studies showed that patients with a reduced GFR had more frequent lacunar strokes, as assessed by MRI. Cerebral microbleeds were also shown to be associated with proteinuria and with the level of microalbuminuria. The prevalence of atrial fibrillation is high in patients with late-stage CKD, ranging from 7 to 27 % in various studies. The hypercoagulable state deteriorates in parallel with the severity of renal dysfunction. Go et al. [11] reported that in patients with atrial fibrillation, proteinuria and a lower eGFR increased the risk of thromboembolism, independent of other known risk factors. Albuminuria or proteinuria is a surrogate for an increased permeability of the brain vasculature and thus implies an increased susceptibility to hemorrhagic transformation after infarction. A recent study showed that albuminuria was an independent predictor for hemorrhagic transformation following acute ischemic stroke, even after adjustment for possible confounding factors. Albuminuria was shown to be associated with parenchymal hemorrhage [12].

14.7 Clinical Outcomes in Stroke Patients with CKD

14.7.1 Functional Outcomes

CKD is associated with the functional outcomes in patients with acute stoke. Ovbiagele et al. [13] investigated the association between proteinuria or a low eGFR and functional activities in patients with an acute ischemic stroke without known CKD. They found that the clinical outcomes were poorer in relation to proteinuria, but not to a low GFR. It has been shown that in patients with lacunar stroke, the progression of neurological symptoms occurred more often in those with albuminuria. Albuminuria was an independent predictor of the neurological progression in patients with a lacunar stroke, and the progression was associated with a worse outcome at 90 days. Recent studies showed that patients with microalbuminuria showed a more severe neurological deficit and presented more decreased levels of consciousness. In cases of hemorrhagic stroke, moderate-to-severe CKD was associated with a larger hematoma volume. However, another study showed that, in patients with intracerebral hemorrhage, proteinuria and a low eGFR were not linked to the patient being discharged directly to home [14].

14.7.2 Mortality

A recent study showed that CKD was also significantly associated with in-hospital mortality after stroke, regardless of the stroke subtypes, ischemic stroke, intracerebral hemorrhage, and subarachnoid hemorrhage. This association was more pronounced in patients with a younger age and in females. A low GFR or proteinuria, or both, have been suggested to be involved in the short-term mortality after stroke. In patients with ischemic stroke, both proteinuria and a lower eGFR were predictive factors for the 30-day mortality. The mechanism by which CKD is associated with poor outcomes after stroke is unknown. In patients with ischemic stroke, acute kidney injury tended to occur in those with a reduced GFR after acute stroke and was associated with short-term survival. Since baseline kidney function was an independent predictor for acute kidney injury, poor functional outcomes may be partially mediated by acute kidney injury [11–14].

14.8 Management of Acute Stroke in CKD Patients

14.8.1 Tissue-Plasminogen Activator

It still remains controversial as to whether tissue-plasminogen activator is beneficial or detrimental to the clinical outcomes after ischemic stroke complicated by CKD. Hemorrhagic infarction is a major concern after thrombolytic therapy in CKD patients, because hemorrhagic transformation or cerebral microbleeds are more prevalent in these patients. Agrawal et al. [15] reported that an eGFR <60 ml/min/1.73 m^2 was not associated with an increased risk of symptomatic intracranial hemorrhage, poor functional outcomes, or in-hospital death in patients receiving thrombolytic therapy. They concluded that the clinical outcomes after the use of thrombolytic therapy were similar between those with and without CKD. However, another recent study has shown contradictory results, thus suggesting that a reduced eGFR was associated with early intracerebral hemorrhage and poor outcomes after 3 months in patients treated with tissue-plasminogen activator [16].

14.8.2 Anticoagulation Therapy

In patients with CKD, a variety of factors, including the treatments being administered, affects the coagulation and fibrinolytic states, leading to thrombosis and/or hemorrhage. The use of warfarin is associated with an improved survival in dialysis patients with atrial fibrillation. In high-risk patients with stage 3 CKD, an adjusted dose of warfarin was suggested to be effective to reduce the risk of ischemic stroke and systemic embolism. Anticoagulation therapy with warfarin targeting an INR between 2.0 and 3.0 is probably effective in CKD patients with atrial fibrillation to reduce the risk of thromboembolic stroke without increasing major bleeding. However, the efficacy and optimal intensity of anticoagulation to prevent early recurrence after cardioembolic stroke in CKD patients with atrial fibrillation are currently unknown.

14.9 Management of Symptomatic Carotid Stenosis in CKD Patients

CKD carries an increased risk for cardiovascular disease (CVD) including cerebrovascular events (CVE). There are multiple etiologies for CVE, and among them extracranial carotid artery disease accounts for approximately 25 % of ischemic strokes. It has been shown that carotid revascularization by carotid endarterectomy and carotid artery angioplasty and stenting can decrease the risk of CVE in appropriately selected population with carotid artery disease. Both these techniques of carotid revascularization have been shown to be safe and clinically effective in many large multicentered randomized clinical trials. However, most of these large trials have predominately excluded the patients with kidney failure. Most of the evidence for the management of carotid disease in CKD is based on small clinical trials and expert opinions. There is an urgent need to conduct large clinical trials in patients with CKD to enable better understanding and to improve techniques of various carotid revascularization therapies in CKD patients. A recent study showed that *individuals who have symptomatic moderate- to high-grade carotid stenosis and also have CKD benefit from and tolerate carotid endarterectomy. How this compares with the use of carotid stenting or with the use of maximal medical therapy in an era of statin use and good BP management is still unclear and warrants further study.*

14.10 Secondary Prevention

Secondary prevention includes the treatment of patients who have had ischemic symptoms, including prior ischemic stroke, transient ischemic attack (TIA), or amaurosis fugax. These persons have a much higher risk of stroke than any other population, and of these groups, those patients with previous ischemic stroke have the highest risk. Because persons with ischemic cerebrovascular disease also are at high risk for symptomatic coronary artery disease, prophylactic measures should include interventions to prevent or treat any ischemic heart disease. Fortunately, most medications that are effective in lowering the risk of ischemic stroke also lower the risk of myocardial infarction and vascular death. Still, one must remember that none of the measures to prevent stroke or other serious ischemic events will be uniformly successful. Rather, these therapies lower risks.

14.11 Medications to Prevent Thromboembolism

Several therapies that prevent thromboembolism are of proven usefulness in preventing stroke in high-risk patients (Box 14.8). Decisions about the prescription of medications to prevent thromboembolism are based on several factors including:

- Presumed vascular territory
- Likely cause of the ischemic symptoms
- Previous use of medications or prior surgery
- Contraindications for any specific intervention
- Wishes of the patient

14.11.1 Oral Anticoagulants

Warfarin or one of its derivatives is the usual oral anticoagulant that is prescribed for long-term stroke prophylaxis. As antagonists of vitamin K, these agents reduce plasma levels of the active factors II, VII, IX, and X and proteins C and S. Oral anticoagulants are of established utility for treatment of deep-vein thrombosis and for prevention of cardioembolic stroke. Patients with cardiac diseases associated with a high risk for thromboembolism should receive long-term anticoagulant therapy unless a specific contraindication exists. Hemorrhage is the most frequent adverse experience resulting from the use of oral anticoagulants; the leading fatal complication is intracranial hemorrhage [17].

Box 14.8. Therapies That Prevent Thromboembolic Stroke

Anticoagulants
- Warfarin

Antiplatelet-Aggregating Agents
- Aspirin
- Aspirin and dipyridamole
- Clopidogrel
- Ticlopidine

Surgical Interventions
- Carotid endarterectomy
- Other reconstructive operations
- Endovascular procedures

14.11.2 Antiplatelet Agents

14.11.2.1 Aspirin

Aspirin interferes with platelet function and thromboxane A2 production by irreversible acetylation and inactivation of cyclooxygenase. It has little effect on platelet adhesion or aggregation at high sheer stress. Aspirin is the most commonly prescribed medication for the primary or secondary prevention of ischemic stroke in patients with arterial diseases. Meta-analyses show that aspirin is effective in preventing stroke, myocardial infarction, and vascular death in high-risk men and women regardless of age. Presence of hypertension or diabetes mellitus does not affect responses to treatment. Aspirin also is used as an alternative to oral anticoagulants for those persons with cardiac sources of thromboembolism, such as AF, who cannot take warfarin. Aspirin can be started safely within the first days after stroke. Aspirin is recommended for the prevention of stroke for most high-risk patients with arterial diseases. It is the usual choice for the medical prevention of arterial thromboembolism for patients with symptoms in either the carotid or vertebrobasilar circulation. Aspirin alone, in a daily dose of 325 mg, is effective in preventing thromboembolism in people with AF, and it is recommended for treatment of those patients who cannot tolerate oral anticoagulants.

14.11.2.2 Dipyridamole and Aspirin/Dipyridamole

Dipyridamole has reversible effects on platelet aggregation through its inhibition of phosphodiesterase. In addition, the medication causes vasodilation. Dipyridamole has few side effects, with headache being the most bothersome complaint. Some patients with unstable angina pectoris might not tolerate the medication. Bleeding complications are few. No trial has directly compared the efficacy of clopidogrel or the combination of aspirin and extended-release dipyridamole in preventing stroke among high-risk patients. The combination of low-dose aspirin plus extended-release dipyridamole is an important option for management when a patient has a TIA or stroke.

14.11.2.3 Clopidogrel

Clopidogrel is a potent antiplatelet agent that blocks adenosine diphosphate (ADP)-induced platelet aggregation. Its usual daily dose is 75 mg. Some groups have used a "loading dose" of approximately 300 mg of clopidogrel to start treatment in order to rapidly achieve maximal effects on platelet aggregation. The need for this tactic when treating patients with stroke is not clear. Because it is pharmacologically similar to ticlopidine, it can also be associated with gastrointestinal symptoms and allergic reactions. However, unlike ticlopidine, the risk of neutropenia is relatively low. In addition, patients undergoing cerebrovascular angioplasty and stenting often are prescribed the medication for a period that usually lasts 6–8 weeks after the procedure. Clopidogrel can be considered a treatment alternative in a patient who has recurrent symptoms despite use of aspirin or in a patient in which treatment with aspirin is contraindicated.

14.12 Surgical Procedures

Several surgical procedures are available to treat patients with extensive intracranial or extracranial cerebrovascular disease. The goals of these operations are to either remove a source for thromboembolism or to improve flow to a vulnerable area of the brain. Carotid endarterectomy (CEA) is the most widely performed operation for prevention of stroke [17].

14.12.1 Carotid Endarterectomy

Carotid endarterectomy is of proven utility for prevention of stroke in patients with symptomatic high-grade stenosis (>50 %) of the origin of the internal carotid artery. The role of the operation for prevention of stroke in patients with an asymptomatic stenosis >60 % is more controversial than its use in patients who have had an ipsilateral TIA or ischemic stroke, but recent evidence suggests that CEA can be recommended for carefully selected patients. The advantage of surgical treatment increases in patients with marked narrowing of the carotid artery (>70 % stenosis). The benefit of surgery in patients with very severe narrowing (99+% stenosis) is not as clear. The presence of severe ulceration in addition to a high-grade stenosis increases the potential advantage to be derived from CEA. Patients with occlusion of the internal carotid artery and those with an intraluminal thrombus usually are not treated with operation.

14.12.1.1 Extracranial-Intracranial Arterial Anastomoses and Other Operations

Superficial temporal artery-middle cerebral artery anastomosis (extracranial-intracranial [EC/IC] bypass) was tested in a large clinical trial. Patients with occlusion of the internal carotid artery and stenoses of the middle cerebral artery were treated. Although operatively treated patients did very well, their outcomes were not superior to those of patients who were treated medically. As the result, EC/IC bypass has been abandoned other than for exceptional cases, such as those people who have moyamoya disease [17].

14.12.1.2 Angioplasty and Placement of Arterial Stents

Angioplasty, with or without stent placement, is being used to treat patients with stenotic lesions in the intracranial or extracranial arteries. The use of this procedure is controversial. In particular, the utility of angioplasty and stenting as an alternative to CEA is not known. While preliminary studies suggest that angioplasty and stenting are a feasible way to manage stenotic lesions of the arteries perfusing the brain, there are concerns about the safety and long-term efficacy of these procedures. One trial demonstrated that endarterectomy and angioplasty were roughly equal in safety, although recurrent stenosis was more common with the endovascular procedure. Most of the patients did not have stents. Additional studies currently are under way.

Before You Finish: Practice Pearls for the Clinication

- Individuals who have symptomatic moderate- to high-grade carotid stenosis and also have CKD benefit from and tolerate carotid endarterectomy.
- In high-risk patients with stage 3 CKD, an adjusted dose of warfarin was suggested to be effective to reduce the risk of ischemic stroke and systemic embolism.
- CKD has significantly associated with in-hospital mortality after stroke, regardless of the stroke subtypes, ischemic stroke, intracerebral hemorrhage, and subarachnoid hemorrhage.

References

1. Adams Jr HP, Brott TG, Crowell RM, Furlan AJ, Gomez CR, Grotta J, Helgason CM, et al. Guidelines for the management of patients with acute ischemic stroke. A statement for healthcare professionals from a special writing group of the Stroke Council, American Heart Association. Circulation. 1994;90(3):1588–601.
2. Hill MD, Hackinski V. Stroke treatment: time is brain. Lancet. 1998;352(Suppl 3):SIII10–4.
3. Hacke W, Kaste M, Olsen TS, Orgogozo JM, Bogousslavsky J. European stroke initiative: recommendations for stroke management. Organisation of stroke care. J Neurol. 2000;247:732–48.
4. Seliger SL, Gillen DL, Longstreth Jr WT, Kestenbaum B, Stehman-Breen CO. Elevated risk of stroke among patients with end-stage renal disease. Kidney Int. 2003;64:603–9.
5. Micozkadioglu H, Ozelsancak R, Giray S, Arlier Z. CKD is associated with recurrent ischemia but not with hemorrhagic transformation in acute ischemic stroke patients. Ren Fail. 2013;35(11):1512–8.
6. Muntner P, Judd SE, McClellan W, Meschia JF, Warnock DG, Howard VJ. Incidence of stroke symptoms among adults with chronic kidney disease: results from the REasons for Geographic And Racial Differences in Stroke (REGARDS) study. Nephrol Dial Transplant. 2012;27:166–73.
7. Holzmann MJ, Aastveit A, Hammar N, Jung-ner I, Walldius G, Holme I. Renal dysfunction increases the risk of ischemic and hemorrhagic stroke in the general population. Ann Med. 2012;44:607–15.
8. Shimizu Y, Maeda K, Imano H, Ohira T, Kitamura A, Kiyama M, Okada T, Ishikawa Y, Shimamoto T, Yamagishi K, Tanigawa T, Iso H. Chronic kidney disease and drinking status in relation to risks of stroke and its subtypes. The Circulatory Risk in Communities Study (CIRCS). Stroke. 2011;42:2531–7.
9. Bugnicourt JM, Chillon JM, Massy ZA, Canaple S, Lamy C, Deramond H, Godefroy O. High prevalence of intracranial artery calcification in stroke patients with CKD: a retro-spective study. Clin J Am Soc Nephrol. 2009;4:284–90.
10. Guerrero-Romero F, Rodriguez-Moran M. Proteinuria is an independent risk factor for ischemic stroke in non-insulin-dependent diabetes mellitus. Stroke. 1999;30:1787–91.
11. Go AS, Fang MC, Udaltsova N, Chang Y, Pomernacki NK, Borowsky L, Singer DE. Impact of proteinuria and glomerular filtration rate on risk of thromboembolism in atrial fibrillation: the anticoagulation and risk factors in atrial fibrillation (ATRIA) study. Circulation. 2009;119:1363–9.
12. Rodriguez-Yanez M, Castellanos M, Blanco M, Millan M, Nombela F, Sobrino T, Liza-soain I, Leira R, Serena J, Davalos A, Castillo J. Micro- and macroalbuminuria predict hemorrhagic transformation in acute ischemic stroke. Neurology. 2006;67:1172–7.
13. Ovbiagele B, Liebeskind DS, Pineda S, Saver JL. Strong independent correlation of proteinuria with cerebral microbleeds in patients with stroke and transient ischemic attack. Arch Neurol. 2010;67:45–50.
14. Ovbiagele B, Pineda S, Saver JL. Renal dysfunction and discharge destination in patients with intracerebral hemorrhage. J Stroke Cerebrovasc Dis. 2011;20:145–9.
15. Agrawal V, Rai B, Fellows J, McCullough PA. In-hospital outcomes with thrombolytic therapy in patients with renal dysfunction presenting with acute ischaemic stroke. Nephrol Dial Transplant. 2010;25:1150–7.
16. Naganuma M, Koga M, Shiokawa Y, Nakaga-wara J, Furui E, Kimura K, Yamagami H, Okada Y, Hasegawa Y, Kario K, Okuda S, Nishiyama K, Minematsu K,

Toyoda K. Reduced estimated glomerular filtration rate is associated with stroke outcome after intravenous rt-PA. The Stroke Acute Management with Urgent Risk-Factor Assessment and Improvement (SAMURAI) rt-PA registry. Cerebrovasc Dis. 2011;31:123–9.
17. Adams Jr HP, del Zoppo GJ, von Kummer R. Management of stroke. A practical guide for the prevention, evaluation and treatment of acute stroke. 2nd ed. Caddo: Professional Communications Inc.; 2002. ISBN 1-884735-517.
18. Adams Jr HP, et al. Guidelines for the early management of patients with ischemic stroke: a scientific statement from the Stroke Council of the American Stroke Association. Stroke. 2003;34:1056–83.

Part IV

Chronic Kidney Disease Complications: Assessment and Management

15 Anemia and Disorders of Hemostasis in Chronic Kidney Disease

Joshua S. Hundert and Ajay K. Singh

Before You Start: Facts You Need to Know

- Anemia, defined as a blood hemoglobin (Hb) level less than 13.0 g/dL for men and 12.0 g/dL for women, is a frequently occurring comorbidity of chronic kidney disease (CKD), and its prevalence jumps from 5 % in patients with estimated glomerular filtration rate (eGFR) greater than 60 mL/min/1.73 m^2 to 40 % in those with eGFR <30 mL/min/1.73 m^2.
- In general, anemia in CKD can be caused by both iron deficiency and decreased erythropoietin (EPO) production, though in later stages hyporesponsiveness to EPO may further contribute to low blood counts.
- In patients with CKD, concurrent anemia is associated with a higher risk of hospitalization, mortality from cardiac and other causes, progression to end-stage renal disease (ESRD), and an overall decrease in quality of life.
- Specific evidence-based guidelines have been published by several organizations for both screening for and treatment of anemia in CKD; these guidelines provide algorithms for the appropriate use of oral and intravenous iron preparations as well as use of erythropoiesis-stimulating agents (ESAs).
- Patients with chronic kidney disease also experience both endothelial dysfunction and abnormal coagulation activation, both of which increase risk of cardiovascular events.

Abbreviations

CKD	Chronic Kidney Disease
CERA	Continuous Erythropoiesis Receptor Activators
dDAVP	Desmopressin
eGFR	Estimated Glomerular Filtration Rate
EPO	Erythropoietin
EPO-R	Erythropoietin receptor
ESA	Erythropoiesis-stimulating agents
ESRD	End-Stage Renal Disease
GI	Gastrointestinal
Hb	Hemoglobin

J.S. Hundert, MD
Renal Division, Department of Medicine, Brigham and Women's Hospital, 1620 Tremont Street, OBC 3rd Floor, Boston, MA 02130, USA
e-mail: jhundert@partners.org, jhundert@gmail.com

A.K. Singh, MBBS, MBA (✉)
Renal Division, Brigham and Women's Hospital, 75 Francis Street, MRB 4th Floor, Boston, MA 02115, USA
e-mail: asingh@partners.org

M. Arici (ed.), *Management of Chronic Kidney Disease*,
DOI 10.1007/978-3-642-54637-2_15, © Springer-Verlag Berlin Heidelberg 2014

HIV	Human Immunodeficiency Virus
K/DOQI	Kidney Disease Outcomes Quality Initiative
KDIGO	Kidney Disease: Improving Global Outcomes
KDQOL	Kidney Disease Quality of Life
LVH	Left Ventricular Hypertrophy
MI	Myocardial Infarction
NKF	National Kidney Foundation
pRBC	Packed Red Blood Cells
PRCA	Pure Red Cell Aplasia
QoL	Quality of Life
RAAS	Renin-Angiotensin-Aldosterone System
rHuEpo	Recombinant Human Erythropoietin
SF-36	Medical Outcomes Study Short Form-36 (SF-36) or the
SFLC	Serum-Free Light Chains
SIFE	Serum Immunofixation Electrophoresis
SPEP	Serum Protein Electrophoresis
TIBC	Total Iron-Binding Capacity
TRALI	Transfusion-Related Acute Lung Injury
TSAT	Transferrin Saturation
vWF	von Willebrand Factor

15.1 Anemia in CKD

The link between chronic kidney disease and anemia is well known to internists and nephrologists alike, and patients with these conditions require careful management once diagnosed. In patients with early CKD, anemia may be mild and asymptomatic and thus often goes undiagnosed or untreated. Despite having slightly low or even normal Hb concentrations, patients with CKD may suffer from iron deficiency, and this will go undetected if iron studies are not drawn. It is important for clinicians to rule out other cause of anemia aside from iron deficiency, including but not limited to B12 and folate deficiencies, hypothyroidism, anemia of other chronic disease, and bone marrow disorders (Table 15.1). Practitioners must also exclude sources of active bleeding, such as from the gastrointestinal (GI) tract, prior to treating patients with iron supplementation, so that treatment does not mask further undiagnosed blood loss.

Table 15.1 Differential diagnosis of anemia in CKD

Common causes of anemia in patients with CKD	Other causes of anemia to consider
Iron deficiency	B12 deficiency
Functional iron deficiency – iron is present in the bone marrow at sufficient levels but it cannot be incorporated into RBC production	Folate deficiency
Absolute iron deficiency – iron stores are depleted, and bone marrow staining does not reveal iron	Anemia of another chronic disease
ACE inhibitor use	Hypothyroidism
Inflammation	Hemoglobinopathies
Infection Hyperparathyroidism Occult blood loss Bone marrow suppression Multiple myeloma	Other types of anemia if they correspond with the clinical picture

Recent studies of the pathophysiology of iron deficiency in CKD have focused on hepcidin, a peptide hormone that regulates iron absorption and homeostasis [1]. Hepatocytes, macrophages, and enterocytes take in iron through ferroportin channels present on the cell membrane. When stimulated by sufficient levels of iron in the body, hepcidin that is made by the liver binds to ferroportin channels, stimulating them to internalize and then undergo degradation, which in turn causes the downstream effects of sequestration of iron in the liver and decreased iron absorption in the GI tract. In the setting of infection, upregulation of hepcidin is a protective mechanism meant to decrease iron available to pathogens, but hepcidin levels also rise in inflammatory states, such is in CKD; in this case, high hepcidin limits the availability of iron for red cell production. Studies have shown that as eGFR worsens, hepcidin levels rise, and treatments with either iron or an ESA in patients with CKD have both been shown to lower hepcidin level in addition to their primary purpose of raising Hb levels [2].

Another hormone that becomes dysregulated in CKD is erythropoietin (EPO). EPO is produced by the peritubular cells of the kidney, but as CKD progresses these cells decrease in number and function. Secreted EPO binds to the EPO receptor (EPO-R) on erythroid progenitor cells in the bone marrow, and this binding stimulates red cell production via activation of the JAK2 pathway. In 1989, recombinant human erythropoietin (sometimes abbreviated rHuEpo) was approved to treat anemia in patients with ESRD [3], but since then its use has been widely expanded, and it is now frequently prescribed to patients with CKD and anemia who are not on dialysis. For two decades, ESAs were used to push Hb levels to normal levels in patients with both CKD and ESRD, but in recent years, an abundance of evidence suggests that ESAs used at a high dose are associated with increased adverse events and overall mortality. In 2010, with the introduction of the bundling program for dialysis reimbursement, ESA injections were no longer reimbursed separately from dialysis, and this has led to further reduction in their usage.

Though not as common in patients with CKD, patients with ESRD may have worsening anemia due to increased incidence of major bleeding events. These events partly arise as a result of multiple mechanisms of platelet dysfunction that occur in the setting of uremia. In uremic conditions, platelet binding to fibrinogen is impaired, glycoprotein IIb-IIIa receptors are dysfunctional, and levels of von Willebrand factor (vWF), a necessary component of platelet aggregation, are reduced [4]. Further blood loss can occur in patients undergoing hemodialysis due to routine complications of the procedure, such as clotting within the dialysis tubing, though this aspect has improved in recent years.

15.2 Diagnosis and Evaluation of Anemia in CKD

15.2.1 Screening and Diagnosis

In 1997, National Kidney Foundation (NKF) published the first set of guidelines for detection and management of CKD. The NKF expanded upon their original work and in 2002 published the Kidney Disease Outcomes Quality Initiative (K/DOQI) clinical practice guidelines. In these first standardized guidelines, the recommendations to physicians regarding anemia were as follows: evaluate all patients with CKD (GFR <60 mL/min/1.73 m^2) for anemia by drawing a complete blood count and other appropriate diagnostic studies as indicated, follow serial Hb concentrations over time, and prescribe treatment appropriate to the etiology of the anemia. In 2006, K/DOQI published an updated set of guidelines that focused more on treatment recommendations, which were not a part of the 2002 report, and there were few significant changes to screening recommendations for anemia in patients with CKD [5]. In 2012, an international board similarly under the direction of the NKF called Kidney Disease: Improving Global Outcomes (KDIGO) published the most recent set of guidelines to date, which are well researched, are evidenced based, and provide a good framework for screening and diagnosis as well as treatment of anemia in patients with CKD [6]. In a commentary published in 2013 in the American Journal of Kidney Disease, the K/DOQI panel weighed in and agreed with the majority of the newly proposed 2012 KDIGO recommendations, making these guidelines the present standard of care for patients with CKD and anemia [7].

The KDIGO guidelines from 2012 now suggest that physicians measure a Hb concentration at least once a year in all patients with CKD Stage 3 (eGFR between 30 and 60 mL/min/1.73 m^2), twice per year for patients with

Table 15.2 Diagnostic workup of anemia in patients with CKD

Signs and symptoms	Recommended baseline laboratories	Extended laboratories
Fatigue	Complete blood count, including:	Serum protein electrophoresis (SPEP)
Tachycardia	Hemoglobin (Hb)	Serum immunofixation electrophoresis (SIFE)
Pallor	Red cell indices	Serum-free light chains (SFLC)
Chest pain	White blood count and differential	Spot urine protein/creatinine ratio
Dyspnea	Absolute reticulocyte count	Urine Bence-Jones protein (UBJP, also known as urine immunofixation electrophoresis, or UIFE)[a]
Depression	Serum ferritin	TSH
Cold intolerance	Serum iron	Hemoglobin electrophoresis
	Total iron-binding capacity (TIBC)	Hemolysis labs (if indicated)

[a]It is useful to check a urine protein/creatinine ratio prior to sending a UBJP as it is an expensive test that does not need to be ordered on a urine specimen that contains no protein

CKD Stage 4 and pre-dialysis CKD Stage 5 (eGFR between 15 and 30 mL/min/1.73 m^2 and eGFR <15 mL/min/1.73 m^2, respectively), and every 3 months for patients on dialysis. For patients with CKD that receive ESA therapy, it is recommended that patients with eGFR <30 have a Hb level checked at least every 3 months and patients on dialysis have a Hb checked monthly. KDIGO recommended that clinicians check the following laboratory tests as part of the initial evaluation of anemia: a complete blood count, including red cell indices, a white blood cell count and differential, and a platelet count; an absolute reticulocyte count; a serum ferritin level and a serum transferrin saturation; and serum folate and vitamin B12 levels (Table 15.2) [6].

Aside from the recommended routine panel of labs, other laboratory tests may be effective in unveiling the etiology of anemia associated with CKD. For example, multiple myeloma is a common condition that causes CKD and may present with the infamous triad of kidney failure, anemia, and bone pain; in patients who present with these or similar symptoms – or even in those with CKD, anemia, and advanced age – a clinician should consider ordering a serum protein electrophoresis (SPEP), a serum immunofixation electrophoresis (SIFE), as well as a serum-free light-chain (SFLC) assay to assess for a plasma cell dyscrasia, such as myeloma, or other abnormalities of the bone marrow. In certain cases, referral to a hematologist for a bone marrow aspirate and biopsy may be indicated. Additionally, hemoglobinopathies can be associated with kidney disease, and a Hb electrophoresis may be considered if clinically indicated. Presently there are no evidence-based guidelines for performing these extended laboratory tests, but KDIGO does recommend against drawing serum EPO levels, since these titers have been shown to have little clinical utility.

Despite the multitude of labs that can be drawn to diagnose and characterize anemia, a comprehensive history and physical exam are of critical importance in detecting other underlying medical conditions that may be caused by or associated with anemia. It is the responsibility of both the primary caretaker as well as the nephrologist to ensure that patients are offered – and preferably undergo – all age-appropriate cancer screenings, particularly those for colon cancer, a common cause of iron deficiency and anemia in older patients. Clinicians must be mindful that other types of anemia may exist in patients with kidney disease, such as hemolytic anemia in the setting of a thrombotic microangiopathy, and these should be diagnosed and treated expectantly. Screening for the signs and symptoms of anemia, which include fatigue, tachycardia, pallor, chest pain, dyspnea, depression, and cold intolerance, among many others, should be performed at each visit in patients with CKD, since symptomatology plays a role in both the KDIGO and K/DOQI guidelines for treatment of anemia in patients with CKD (Boxes 15.1 and 15.2).

Box 15.1. What the Guidelines Say You Should Do

Use of Iron to Treat Anemia in CKD

A trial of IV iron (or alternatively a 1–3 month trial of oral iron) should be given to patients with CKD when:

- An increase in Hb concentration without starting ESA treatment is desired.
- An increase in Hb concentration or a decrease in ESA dose is desired for those already on an ESA.
- TSAT is ≤30 % and ferritin is ≤500 ng/mL (≤500 mg/L).

Use of ESAs and Other Agents to Treat Anemia in CKD

- Weigh the potential benefits of reducing blood transfusions and anemia-related symptoms against the risks of harm in individual patients (e.g., stroke, vascular access loss, hypertension) prior to starting ESA therapy.
- For patients with CKD not on dialysis:
  - Do not start ESAs for Hb concentration ≥10.0 g/dL (≥100 g/L) unless patients have symptomatic anemia despite sufficient iron stores or therapy.
  - In general, ESAs should not be used to maintain Hb concentration above 11.5 g/dL (115 g/L).
- ESA dose should be chosen using the patient's Hb concentration, body weight, and clinical circumstances.
- Choice of ESA should be based on pharmacodynamics, safety information, clinical outcome data, costs, and availability.

Red Cell Transfusion to Treat Anemia in CKD

- When managing chronic anemia, we recommend avoiding, when possible, red cell transfusions to minimize the general risks related to their use, especially in potential transplant recipients to minimize the risk of allosensitization.
- When managing chronic anemia, we suggest that the benefits of red cell transfusions may outweigh the risks in patients in whom:
  - ESA therapy is ineffective (e.g., hemoglobinopathies, bone marrow failure, ESA resistance).
  - The risks of ESA therapy may outweigh its benefits (e.g., previous or current malignancy, previous stroke).

Source: Data from KDIGO [6]

Box 15.2. Relevant Guidelines

1. *KDIGO Guidelines*
   Kidney Disease: Improving Global Outcomes (KDIGO) Anemia Work Group. KDIGO clinical practice guideline for anemia in chronic kidney disease. Kidney Int Suppl. 2012;2: 279–335.
   http://kdigo.org/home/guidelines/anemia-in-ckd
2. *CARI Guidelines*
   Biochemical and Haematological Targets: Haemoglobin Levels in Patients Using Erythropoiesis Stimulating Agents. May 2011.
   http://www.cari.org.au/DIALYSIS_bht_published/KHA_CARI_Anaemia_guidelines_November_ 2011.pdf
3. *NICE Guidelines*
   Anaemia management in people with chronic kidney disease. February 2011.
   http://www.nice.org.uk/nicemedia/live/13329/52853/52853.pdf
4. *NKF/KDOQI Guidelines*
   KDOQI clinical practice guideline and clinical practice recommendations for anemia in chronic kidney disease: 2007 update of hemoglobin target. Am J Kidney Dis. 2007;50(3):471–530.
   http://www.kidney.org/PROFESSIONALS/kdoqi/guidelines_anemiaUP/index.htm
   KDOQI clinical practice guidelines and clinical practice recommendations for anemia in chronic kidney disease: 2006. Am J Kidney Dis. 2006;47(5 Suppl 3):S11–145.http://www.kidney.org/Professionals/kdoqi/guidelines_anemia/index.htm

15.2.2 Iron Indices

Iron indices, also known as iron status tests or iron studies, include a serum ferritin concentration and a transferrin saturation, usually abbreviated as TSAT (calculated by serum iron divided by the total iron-binding capacity, or TIBC). These tests give information about the total stores of iron in the body, but the presence of systemic illness or inflammation can alter these values. As previously mentioned, patients with CKD have decreased ability to absorb iron because of the abnormal upregulation of hepcidin; over time this leads to depletion of body iron stores that are necessary for normal erythropoiesis. The first recommendations to monitor iron indices in patients with CKD came in the 2006 K/DOQI guidelines, which suggested that iron status tests be drawn during the initial workup of anemia but should be also checked every 3 months in patients receiving an ESA. For patients with CKD and anemia that were not on an ESA, no recommendations were made for rechecking iron studies after the initial diagnosis was made. For patients with CKD on an ESA, K/DOQI 2006 recommended that iron be given after exclusion of other causes of blood loss for patients whose serum ferritin level was less than 200 ng/mL and whose TSAT was less than 20 %. These 2006 K/DOQI guidelines were based on several randomized trials that stratified patients with CKD and anemia receiving an ESA to two treatment groups, one with a goal of achieving high iron indices with supplementation and the other with a goal of attaining normal iron parameters; the patients with higher iron indices after treatment with iron supplementation required lower doses of ESAs to reach K/DOQI target Hb than those with normal iron indices, and many subsequent studies have reinforced these original conclusions [5].

In the 2012 KDIGO guidelines, much more attention was paid to patients with CKD and anemia who did not require ESAs than in the previous 2006 K/DOQI guidelines. The most significant change in these guidelines was a redefinition of iron deficiency as a TSAT less than 30 % and a ferritin level less than 500 ng/mL, a substantial increase from the K/DOQI 2006 values of 20 % and 200 ng/mL, respectively. KDIGO agreed with the earlier suggestion that all patients have iron studies drawn early in the course of CKD, but the group went further and also recommended that follow-up iron studies be checked in all patients at the discretion of the clinician; still, KDIGO made no formal recommendations for frequency of monitoring iron studies in patients receiving either oral or intravenous therapies [7]. Though complete evidence is lacking, it is generally agreed that iron studies should not be rechecked until after 3 months of treatment with iron supplementation have commenced in order to determine whether or not the treatment was effective.

15.3 Management of Anemia in CKD

15.3.1 Risks and Benefits of Anemia and Treatment

In the past decade, the risks of anemia in patients with CKD, and the risks and benefits of its treatment with iron supplementation and/or ESA therapy, have been highly debated and publicized in both the scientific literature and popular media. A number of studies have shown a direct relationship between the severity of anemia and mortality rates in patients with CKD, with the focus being predominantly on the occurrence cardiovascular events, the leading causes of death for patients with CKD and ESRD. One popular theory to explain this phenomenon is that anemia, regardless of etiology, causes an increase in cardiac output as a compensatory mechanism meant to preserve oxygen delivery to tissues in the setting of low red cell mass. Over time, this is believed to lead to left ventricular hypertrophy, a well-known and independent prognostic marker of poor outcomes in patients with CKD [8]. Anemia is not the only cause of LVH in patients with CKD, and unfortunately, large randomized controlled studies have failed to demonstrate that LVH improves with elevation of the Hb concentration. Anemia itself has also been correlated with worsening kidney function; it is believed that in the setting of anemia, tubulointerstitial cells of the kidney can become hypoxic, and their death leads to further progression of kidney failure and decreased renal mass. Several small, randomized studies have suggested that anemia correction with either iron or ESA therapy may slow the progression of CKD, but this has yet to be demonstrated in a large randomized controlled trial. Finally, treatment of anemia in patients with CKD leads to decreased use of red blood cell transfusions, which themselves are associated with antibody sensitization, transfusion reactions, and a variety of infectious complications.

Treating anemia in patients with chronic kidney disease may have other benefits that are harder to quantify, the most important and frequently assessed being the improvement in quality-of-life (QoL) scores, typically measured by a standardized assessment tool such as the Medical Outcomes Study Short Form-36 (SF-36) or the Kidney Disease Quality of Life (KDQOL) Instrument. Patients with CKD often complain of profound fatigue, pain, depression, and many other subjective symptoms that may be directly caused or influenced by anemia. Many studies have shown that in both patients with and without CKD, those with a lower Hb concentration are more likely to report an overall poorer quality of life than those with normal Hb concentrations.

Trials of ESA use in patients with CKD since their introduction have for the most part been run by pharmaceutical companies, and these studies have examined the effects of different preparations and doses of ESAs on QoL scores. In addition to being run by the makers of the drug, many of these trials were open label and did not contain a placebo arm, making it difficult to prove that increased QoL scores were indeed due to drug effect. In recent years, however, independent investigators have conducted several trials that examined the medical risks and benefits as well as impact on QOL scores of ESA treatment in patients with CKD, and the results of these investigations have significantly changed clinical practice patterns (Table 15.3).

Both published in 2006, the Cardiovascular Risk Reduction by Early Anemia Treatment with Epoetin Beta (CREATE) [9] trial and the Correction of Hemoglobin and Outcomes in Renal Insufficiency (CHOIR) [10] trial were parallel-group treatment studies of ESAs in patients with CKD. In CREATE, 603 patients with eGFR between 15 and 35 mL/min/1.73 m^2 with Hb levels between 11.0 and 12.5 g/dL were randomized to either the high or low target Hb groups; in the high target group, epoetin beta (NeoRecormon, Roche, only available in Europe) was prescribed and titrated to achieve a Hb value between 13.0 and 15.0 g/dL, and in the low Hb target group, epoetin beta was only given if Hb concentration fell below 10.5 g/dL, with the Hb goal for this cohort ranging from 10.5 to 11.5 g/dL. The study followed patients for 3 years, and the primary outcome was time to any one of these cardiovascular events: sudden cardiac death, myocardial infarction (MI), acute heart failure, stroke or transient ischemic attack, unstable angina, cardiac arrhythmia, or a peripheral vascular disease complication. Secondary outcomes assessed included death from any cause, hospitalization, changes in LV mass by echocardiography, initiation of renal replacement therapy (RRT, either hemodialysis or peritoneal dialysis), changes in body-mass index, changes in serum albumin, and changes in quality of life using the SF-36 assessment tool.

As for the primary outcome, CREATE found that the rates of cardiovascular events were the same in both the high target Hb and low target Hb groups, showing the lack of cardiovascular benefit with normalization of Hb levels; perhaps even more significant was the finding that all-cause mortality was higher in the high Hb target group. Almost 40 % of patients in this study started dialysis before the end of the 3-year study period, with similar rates in both treatment groups, but patients in the high Hb target group had a significantly shorter time to initiation of RRT. Interestingly, approximately 60 % of patients in both groups received oral iron therapy and similar percentages of each group received intravenous iron or at least one red blood cell transfusion. The CREATE investigators did find a significant improvement in QoL for patients in the high Hb target group, with improvements in the areas of general health, mental health, physical functioning, social function, and vitality. The main conclusion of the study authors was that complete correction of anemia to normal Hb concentrations in patients with CKD did not lead to improved

Table 15.3 Landmark clinical trials anemia in patients with CKD

Study (year)	US normal hematocrit study [17] (1998)	Scandinavian normal hematocrit study [18] (2003)	Early correction of anemia on progression of CKD (ECAP) [19] (2006)	Cardiovascular risk reduction by early anemia treatment with epoetin beta (CREATE) [9] (2006)	Correction of hemoglobin and outcomes in renal insufficiency (CHOIR) [10] (2006)	Trial to reduce cardiovascular events with Aranesp therapy (TREAT) [11] (2009)
Patient type (*N*)	Dialysis with CAD or CHF (N=1,233)	HD, PD, CKD Excluded heart disease (N=416)	Stage 3–4 CKD (N=241)	CKD patients, eGFR 15–35 mL/min/1.73 m^2 (N=603)	CKD patients, eGFR 15–50 mL/min/1.73 m^2 (N=1,432)	CKD patients with DM eGFR 20–60 m/min/1.73 m^2 (N=4,038)
Low target	HCT 30 %	9–12 g/dL	11–12 g/dL	10.5–11.5 g/dL	11.3 g/dL	>9 g/dL
High target	HCT 42 %	13.5–16 g/dL	13–15 g/dL	13.0–15.0 g/dL	13.5 g/dL	13.0 g/dL
1° endpoint	Death + MI	6-min walking test	Delay in CKD progression	Composite endpoint: angina, heart failure, arrhythmias, stroke, sudden death, TIA, PVD	Composite endpoint: death, MI, stroke, CHF, hospitalization	Composite endpoint: cardiovascular event, death from CV cause, death from any cause
Results	High target arm worse, relative risk for 10 endpoints was 1.3 (0.9, 1.9). Total deaths: High arm: 183 Low arm: 150	High arm insignificantly worse	No statistically significant difference Cardiovascular adverse events: High arm: 25 %, Low arm: 18 %	No statistically significant difference Primary events: High arm: 58 Low arm: 47	Target Hb 13.5 worse than Hb 11.3, HR for composite endpoint: 1.337, p=0.03 Total deaths: High arm: 52 Low arm: 36	No statistically significant differences between the groups for time to first cardiac event, or mortality from cardiac or any other cause
Comment	Terminated early due to high arm losing	Unable to measure 1° outcome	–	Excluded patients with rapid progression of CKD	Median follow-up was only 14 months as the trial was terminated early	Randomized, blinded trial comparing ESA to placebo Twofold increase in the rate of both fatal and nonfatal stroke in the treatment group

medical outcomes – and may in fact be harmful – but it did confer a significant QoL benefit.

The CHOIR study design was similar to that of the CREATE study, though the drug used was a different ESA, epoetin alfa (Procrit®, Johnson and Johnson; also available as Epogen®, Amgen); additionally, enrollment criteria were slightly different, as patients needed a Hb concentration <11 g/dL and an eGFR between 15 and 50 mL/min/1.73 m^2. In CHOIR, 1,432 patients were randomly assigned to one of two groups, the first with a high Hb goal of 13.5 g/dL, and the other with a low Hb goal of 11.3 g/dL. Though it enrolled more patients than CREATE and was supposed to also last 3 years, the CHOIR study was terminated early with all patients completing 16 months and only 46 % completing the whole 36 months. The study was stopped because at an interim analysis, investigators determined that there was a <5 % chance that there would be a significant benefit for the high-hemoglobin group with respect to reducing cardiovascular events. Full analysis revealed that patients in the high target Hb group had not only an increased risk of cardiovascular events, but they also had higher rates of progression to ESRD and there was no difference between the performance of either group on the SF-36 QoL assessment.

In 2009, the Trial to Reduce Cardiovascular Events with Aranesp Therapy (TREAT) investigators published results of their randomized controlled trial, which was a study of darbepoetin alfa (Aranesp®, Amgen) versus placebo [11]. This study was much larger than both CREATE and CHOIR and enrolled 4038 patients with a diagnosis of type 2 diabetes, an eGFR between 20 and 60 mL/min/1.73 m^2, a Hb concentration <11 g/dL, and a TSAT >15 %. Prior to this trial, there were no specific data from a randomized controlled trial regarding use of ESAs in patients with diabetes, a condition that itself confers a great deal of cardiovascular risk. For patients in the treatment group, a third party monitored Hb, and the appropriate dose of darbepoetin was automatically and blindly selected to get patients to a goal Hb of 13.0 g/dL. Patients in the placebo group could receive darbepoetin if their Hb level fell below 9 g/dL, and this was discontinued as soon as their Hb stabilized above 9 g/dL. Patients were followed for 48 months, and once again, primary endpoints were cardiac events and mortality, as well as all-cause mortality. In this study, the high target Hb group achieved an average Hb of 12.5 g/dL, and the low target group had an average Hb of 10.6 g/dL. There were no significant differences between the groups for time to first cardiac event or mortality from cardiac or any other cause, but there was a twofold increase in the rate of both fatal and nonfatal stroke in the treatment group compared with that of the placebo group (5 % versus 2.6 %, respectively). There was no difference in rate of progression to ESRD between the groups. In terms of QoL benefit, the TREAT study used the Functional Assessment of Cancer Therapy – Fatigue (FACT-Fatigue) Instrument in addition to the SF-36; while patients in the treatment group had statistically significant improvement in fatigue as measured by the FACT-fatigue score, there were no differences in the SF-36 scores between the treatment and placebo groups.

In light of the number of studies and guidelines that have been published on this topic, particularly in the last 10 years, it can be confusing for clinicians to determine the appropriate Hb target for patient with CKD, whether to initiate treatment with an ESA, and what dose to choose. High Hb concentrations were once thought to be beneficial for patients, and there was a financial advantage to physicians who prescribed ESAs, especially at high dose, but the pendulum has swung widely on both of these issues. The evidence from the CHOIR and CREATE studies, among other randomized controlled trials and meta-analyses, forced K/DOQI to revise their 2006 guidelines just 1 year after publication and release a special statement; in 2007, K/DOQI made the recommendation that Hb levels above 13 g/dL in patients with CKD should be avoided as they are associated with increased cardiovascular events and mortality and the goal Hb target for patients receiving an ESA should be in the range of 11.0–12.0 g/dL [12]. In 2012, KDIGO made even stricter guidelines regarding the use of ESAs and therefore lowered goal Hb targets for patients with CKD, suggesting that ESA therapy not be initiated in patients with Hb concentration greater than 10 g/dL unless benefits and risks are evaluated and symptomatic anemia is present and recommending that ESAs not be used to raise Hb concentration above 11.5 g/dL except in only the most extreme situations.

15.3.2 Iron Treatment

15.3.2.1 When and How to Use Iron for Treatment of Anemia in CKD

In general, the 2012 KDIGO guidelines recommend initiating iron therapy in patients when an increase in Hb concentration or decrease in ESA dose is sought, and when TSAT is ≤30 % and the ferritin is ≤500 ng/mL. Iron supplementation can be given either orally or intravenously, and many studies to date have compared these two treatment modalities. Though oral iron is inexpensive and has few significant adverse effects, it frequently causes nausea and constipation, and compliance to three times daily dosing, which aims to provide a total daily dose 200 mg of elemental iron (one 325 mg tablet of ferrous sulfate contains 65 mg of elemental iron), is often poor (Table 15.4). Intravenous iron has been shown to be only slightly more effective at raising Hb levels than oral forms, likely because GI absorption of iron is poor in patients with CKD, but is associated with infusion reactions and other risks, including placement of a parenteral line that can damage blood vessels which may be needed for future dialysis-access placement [6]. The consensus reached by the KDIGO 2012 group was that there was no significant advantage to using intravenous iron over oral iron in patients with CKD and oral iron therapy should be tried first except when not feasible due to patient intolerance, impairment of absorption due to GI disease (including celiac disease, Whipple's disease, chronic GI bleeding, and bacterial overgrown syndromes), prior lack of response, or when severity of anemia necessitates rapid treatment with intravenous iron. Intravenous iron can be given to patients in the hospital, but more commonly it is administered in an infusion clinic, private nephrology office or clinical practice, or at a dialysis unit for patients with ESRD.

Table 15.4 Oral iron preparation overview

Preparation	# Of pills required to provide 200 mg of elemental iron	Tablet size (mg)	Amount of elemental iron (mg)/pill
Ferrous sulfate	3	325	65
Ferrous gluconate	6	325	35
Ferrous fumarate	2	325	108
Iron polysaccharide	2	150	150

15.3.2.2 Intravenous Iron Preparations and Dosing

Once the decision is made to treat with intravenous iron, a clinician is then faced with choosing the appropriate agent. Not all agents may be available due to pharmacy and formulary restrictions, but it is important understand the differences between the different preparations that are currently available. For each of these agents, a full course contains of about 1,000 mg of elemental iron, but each preparation has different dosing schedules (Table 15.5).

- *Iron Dextran*
  Iron dextran is the oldest preparation and has largely fallen out of favor in recent years due to its side effect profile. Both high molecular weight and low molecular weight iron dextran preparations are associated with anaphylactic reactions, and a test dose given prior to the full infusion is required. Unlike the newer agents, an entire 1,000 mg of elemental iron may be given in one dose of iron dextran. Due to safety concerns, iron dextran was deleted from the World Health Organization List of Essential Medications in 2004.
- *Iron Gluconate (Ferrlecit®, Sanofi-Aventis) and Iron Sucrose (Venofer®, American Regent)*
  Unlike iron dextran, iron gluconate (also known as sodium ferric gluconate) and iron sucrose are newer preparations of intravenous iron that carry a significantly lower – if any –

Table 15.5 Intravenous iron preparation overview

Preparation	Test dose required	Typical dosing regimen	Total dose	Risk of anaphylaxis
Iron dextran High molecular weight (Dexferrum®) Low molecular weight (INFeD®)	Yes – 0.5 mL	Dose (mL) = 0.0442 (desired Hgb – observed Hgb) × LBW + (0.26 × LBW) Desired hemoglobin: usually 14.8 g/dL LBW = lean body weight in kg	One dose can complete course Concentration of iron dextran is 50 mg of elemental iron/mL	US box warning: IV iron preparations carry risk of anaphylaxis, HMW Fe > LWM Fe Anaphylaxis can occur even after a patient tolerates test dose
Iron sucrose (Venofer)	No	HD: 100 mg IV on 10 consecutive HD sessions CKD: 200 mg × 5 doses within 14 days	1,000 mg of elemental iron	Low risk of anaphylaxis
Iron gluconate (Ferrlecit)	No	HD patients: 125 mg IV on 8 consecutive HD sessions	1,000 mg of elemental iron	Low risk of anaphylaxis
Ferumoxytol (Feraheme)	No	510 mg	1,020 mg of elemental iron	Low risk of anaphylaxis

risk of anaphylaxis; as a result, these agents do not require a test dose. Randomized controlled trials comparing these agents do not show differences in rates of efficacy or occurrence of adverse events [13]. For patients with CKD, iron sucrose is generally given 5 times over 14 days at a dose of 200 mg for each infusion, or at a 100 mg dose for 10 doses in patients on hemodialysis. Iron gluconate is generally only given to patients on hemodialysis at a dose of 125 mg for 8 sequential infusions but can be given to patients with CKD as well.

- *Ferumoxytol (Feraheme®, AMAG Pharmaceuticals)*
  The newest and perhaps best parenteral agent for treating iron deficiency in CKD is ferumoxytol. Ferumoxytol is composed of small iron oxide particles coated by low molecular weight synthetic carbohydrates, and the safety profile is similar to that of both iron sucrose and iron gluconate. This agent also does not require a test dose, and in fact a full course of ferumoxytol consists of two 510 mg injections administered over 15 min, each 3–8 days apart. Because only two infusions are needed for a full course, this agent spares patients from placement of multiple intravenous lines, helping to preserve vascular access in patients with CKD [6].

15.3.2.3 Risks of Iron Treatment and Special Considerations

Though new preparations of parental iron have made the infusion itself safer, intravenous iron use is still associated with some significant risks and adverse events. Intravenous iron may be overused, and hemosiderosis, or deposition of iron in different body tissues, has been observed in hemodialysis patients and less frequently in patients with CKD. Parenteral iron infusion may also cause a flare of arthritis in patients with certain rheumatic diseases. Based primarily on animal models, intravenous iron is not recommended for use by KDIGO when patients have an active systemic infection as iron is needed for replication of bacteria, viruses, fungi, parasites, and helminthes, but there is little published clinical evidence to support these conclusions. Finally, in patients with hepatitis, particularly in those with chronic hepatitis C infection and already high serum ferritin levels, increased iron levels may accelerate fibrosis of the liver and iron supplementation should be used with caution.

15.3.3 ESA Treatment

15.3.3.1 When and How to Administer ESA for Treating Anemia in CKD

It is widely agreed and also recommended by KDIGO that iron deficiency be treated sufficiently prior to initiating therapy with ESAs for patients with anemia and CKD. As previously mentioned in this chapter, ESAs should not be given to asymptomatic patients with Hb greater than 10 g/dL. For patients with Hb <10 g/dL, KDIGO reinforces in its 2012 guidelines statement, "the decision whether to initiate ESA therapy be individualized based on the rate of fall of Hb concentration, prior response to iron therapy, the risk of needing a transfusion, the risks related to ESA therapy and the, presence of symptoms attributable to anemia," ultimately providing flexibility to physicians and simultaneously acknowledging that the decision to initiate an ESA is a complex one.

As for the route of administration of ESAs, they may be given either intravenously, which KDIGO recommends for patients on hemodialysis, or subcutaneously, recommended for patients with CKD. As with parenteral iron administration, it is important to minimize repeated peripheral vascular trauma for patients who may 1 day need vascular access for dialysis, and studies have demonstrated that subcutaneous dosing of ESAs in patients can be more effective at raising Hb values at lower doses than intravenous administration [6]. ESAs are often given in the office setting, but subcutaneous forms can be taken by patients at home, and this requires training and monitoring of patient compliance.

15.3.3.2 ESA Preparations and Dosing

Two main ESAs are used in the USA – epoetin alfa and darbepoetin – while epoetin beta is available and used widely outside the USA. Epoetin alfa and epoetin beta are made by different manufacturing processes and though they have the same amino acid sequence, they are coated with different carbohydrate moieties; epoetin beta has been shown to have a longer half-life than epoetin alfa for both the subcutaneous and intravenous administration routes, and this may lead to a more potent effect of the beta subtype of this drug. KDIGO only currently considers epoetin alfa and darbepoetin in its recommendations, however, and both drugs are effective and neither is superior for treating anemia in patients with CKD. Physicians should choose the appropriate ESA based on pharmacokinetics, cost, and availability [6]. Darbepoetin should be initially given once every 4 weeks, but some patients are unable to achieve goal Hb or symptomatic benefit at this frequency and require biweekly dosing. Epoetin should be initiated at a frequency of three times per week. Recently, trials of the third-generation ESAs, known as continuous erythropoiesis receptor activators (or CERAs) (methoxy polyethylene glycol-epoetin beta, brand name Mircera®, Roche), were carried out in the USA and abroad. This pegylated ESA was effective at reducing doses of other ESAs used when the two drugs were given in combination in patients with either CKD or ESRD, but due to patent issues arising in 2008, the drug can no longer be sold in the USA (Table 15.6).

15.3.3.3 Malignancy Risks Associated with ESA Treatment

ESAs are associated with risks other than cardiovascular complications as already described. ESA use is generally contraindicated in the setting of malignancy, as tumors may have EPO receptors and stimulation with ESAs may result in tumor growth; this was supported by secondary findings of the TREAT trial, which showed that patients who had a history of malignancy were significantly more likely to die of cancer if they received darbepoetin than if they received placebo [11]. While in general ESAs are avoided for patients with solid tumors, ESAs can be considered in patients with hematologic malignancies, as they are often used for supportive care in patients with leukemia or lymphoma on chemotherapy; however, use in multiple myeloma, a hematologic malignancy frequently associated with CKD and anemia, remains controversial.

Table 15.6 ESA preparation overview

Class	Drugs	Dosing recommendations and comments
1st generation	Epoetin alfa (Epogen/Procrit)	Initial dose: 50–100 units/kg injected subcutaneously 3 times per week Increase dose by 25 % if hemoglobin does not increase by >1 g/dL after 4 weeks If hemoglobin increases >1 g/dL in any 2-week period, reduce dose by ≥25 % Avoid frequent dose adjustments, and increase no more than once every 4 weeks When given subcutaneously in non-dialysis patients, half-life ranges from 5 to 24 h
	Epoetin beta (NeoRecormon)	Not currently available for use in the USA. According to National Institute for Health and Clinical Excellence (NICE, UK, 2011 guidelines), initial dosage is recommended at 450 IU/kg subcutaneously weekly
2nd generation	Darbepoetin alfa (Aranesp)	Initial dose: 0.45 mcg/kg injected subcutaneously every 4 weeks Increase dose by 25 % if hemoglobin does not increase by >1 g/dL after 4 weeks. May also increase frequency If hemoglobin increases >1 g/dL in any 2-week period, reduce dose by ≥25 % Do not increase dose more frequently than every 4 weeks (dose decreases may occur more frequently) When given subcutaneously in non-dialysis patients, half-life is 70 h (range 35–139 h)
3rd generation	Methoxy polyethylene glycol-epoetin beta (Mircera)	This drug class is called continuous erythropoietin receptor activators (CERAs). Not currently available in the USA due to patent issues but is widely used in other countries to decrease epoetin or darbepoetin doses or for insufficient response to these agents In the PROTOS study (Poland), Mircera was given subcutaneously to patients either once or twice monthly, and starting dose was based on the dose of epoetin that the patient was already receiving (between 60 and 180 mcg twice weekly or 120 and 360 mcg once weekly). Doses were titrated to achieve a Hb goal of 10–12 g/dL The European Medical Association recommends dosing Mircera as a monthly subcutaneous injection at doses of 120–360 mcg, based on the dose of epoetin or darbepoetin already used (2007 guidelines) Mircera should not be used to increase Hb to >12 g/dL

15.3.3.4 ESA Hyporesponsiveness and Pure Red Cell Aplasia

According to KDIGO, patients are classified as having initial ESA hyporesponsiveness if after 1 month of ESA treatment with appropriate weight-based dosing they experience no increase in Hb concentration. For these patients, it is acceptable to increase ESA dose but it should go no higher than double the original weight-based dose. ESA hyporesponsiveness more commonly develops over time in patients who were once on a stable dose of an ESA. Once again KDIGO recommends individualization of therapy to treat patients with this particular condition. The presence of ESA hyporesponsiveness has been shown to be a very poor and independent prognosticator in patients with anemia and CKD, and there is growing evidence that high doses of ESAs themselves can be toxic to patients [14]. The pathophysiology of ESA hyporesponsiveness is complex and not entirely understood, but it is thought to be multifactorial (Fig. 15.1).

In the catastrophic condition known as pure red cell aplasia (PRCA), ESA use leads to the production of anti-EPO antibodies that bind to both exogenous and endogenous EPO, which in turn leads to sudden and severe transfusion-dependent anemia; this anemia can be so severe that Hb concentration can drop by 4 g/dL 1 month after disease onset. Though this condition is rare,

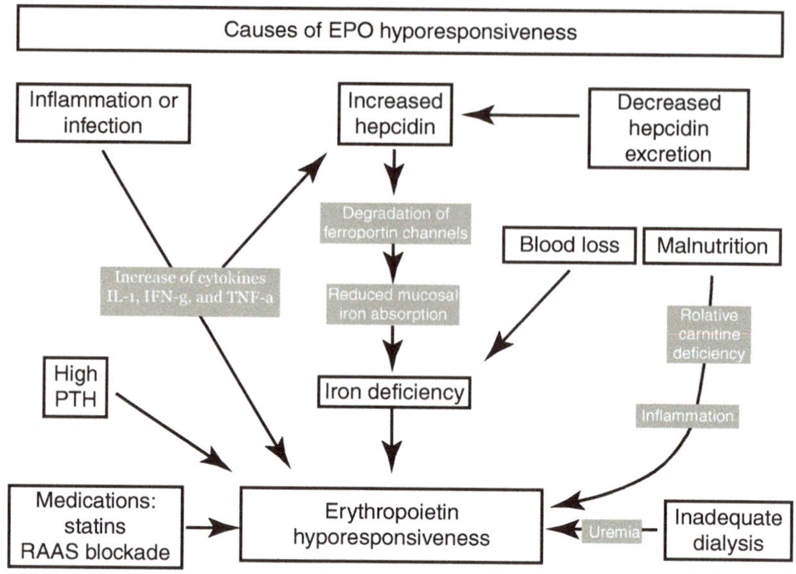

Fig. 15.1 Causes of ESA hyporesponsiveness

occurring in an estimated 5 cases/100,000 patient-years, it generally occurs in patients who receive subcutaneous rather than intravenous ESAs. Diagnosis of this condition can involve a very low peripheral reticulocyte count or bone marrow biopsy revealing few or no erythroblasts but most importantly is based upon the presence of serologic anti-EPO antibodies alongside the appropriate clinical scenario [6]. The mainstay of treatment for this condition is unfortunately regular red blood cell transfusions.

15.3.4 Red Cell Transfusions

Packed red blood cell (pRBC) transfusions can be lifesaving in patients with active hemorrhage or critical anemia that results in tissue hypoperfusion and hypoxia, but 2012 KDIGO guidelines recommend avoiding use of red cell transfusions whenever possible. KDIGO also states that there is no specific Hb threshold at which use of a red cell transfusion is indicated, and the signs and symptoms of anemia should guide clinicians in their prescribing practices [6].

Prior to ESA introduction in the late 1980s, pRBC transfusions were the most frequently used therapy for anemia, and data gathered since then by the US Renal Data System, which analyzes patients with ESRD, has consistently shown that patients who have received transfusions become HLA sensitized and are 2.4 times more likely to have a positive panel-reactive antibody than patients who have never had a transfusion. Sensitization caused by pRBC transfusion can cause patients to have longer wait times for an appropriate allograft, or in fact may make an allograft match impossible; additionally, HLA-mismatch caused by prior pRBC transfusion is correlated with early allograft loss [6]. Aside from risk of antibody-generation that will decrease potential for and later success of a kidney transplant, pRBC transfusions carry the risk of infections, but in the USA, all units of pRBCs are tested for presence of the hepatitis B and C viruses as well as for HIV. With each transfusion given, there is the risk of a transfusion reaction such as acute lung injury (TRALI), hypothermia, coagulopathy, hemolysis, or volume overload. Also of note, units of pRBCs contain citrate, which functions as an anticoagulant, and when several transfusions are given consecutively, citrate toxicity can lead to metabolic alkalosis and hypocalcemia; in this situation, physicians should monitor chemistries and ionized calcium values.

15.3.5 Other Treatments

15.3.5.1 Peginesatide

Peginesatide (Omontys®, formerly Hematide®, Takeda) is a synthetic peptide attached to polyethylene glycol that has been shown to activate the EPO receptor, thereby increasing erythropoiesis. Peginesatide is structurally distinct from EPO and therefore does not bind to antibodies to EPO, making it a useful agent with these antibodies or EPO resistance. In both the EMERALD study (in patients on hemodialysis) and the PEARL study (in patients with CKD), peginesatide was shown to be non-inferior to ESAs at raising Hb levels, but in early 2013, peginesatide was temporarily withdrawn from the market due to a high incidence of serious and possibly fatal hypersensitivity and anaphylactic reactions resulting from its use, with further investigation ongoing [15].

15.3.5.2 Androgens

In male patients with CKD, testosterone deficiency is common and increases this risk of patients developing anemia as well as its severity. Studies have demonstrated that patients with low testosterone levels required higher doses of ESAs to reach target Hb. Testosterone use has been in several studies to raise Hb levels in patients on dialysis, but KDIGO recommends against using androgen therapy as an adjuvant to ESAs for the purpose of treating anemia in CKD due to the side effects, including worsening cardiovascular risk and metabolic complications [6].

15.4 Disorders of Hemostasis

CKD is generally thought to be a hypercoagulable state, supported by observation of high plasma levels of fibrinogen, C-reactive protein, and interleukin-6, among many other proinflammatory cytokines in both human and animal studies to date. Activation of the renin-angiotensin-aldosterone system (RAAS), a common feature of CKD, also increases hypercoagulability, as does CKD-induced vascular endothelial dysfunction and clotting factor abnormalities. Also, patients with CKD have a higher prevalence of hypercoagulable risk factors than the general population, including smoking, type 2 diabetes, and obesity. All of these mechanisms and more are responsible for increased thrombosis in patients with CKD, which likely contributes to high incidence of cardiovascular events in these patients (Table 15.7). Primary prevention of thrombosis in patients with CKD is aimed at reducing cardiovascular risk factors by using RAAS blockade and statin use. No randomized controlled trials have shown a definitive benefit of aspirin therapy or other platelet inhibition in patients with CKD at reducing thrombotic events, but most patients with CKD are prescribed aspirin or similar agents given their baseline cardiovascular comorbidities; of note, it is well known that patients with CKD exhibit decreased responsiveness to clopidogrel.

As CKD progresses, platelets begin to function improperly from a variety of mechanisms [16]. Additionally, in the uremic state, toxic metabolites such as guanidinosuccinic acid and methyl guanidine build up, and these stimulate nitric oxide release that further inhibits platelets. Patients with qualitative platelet dysfunction exhibit the same signs and symptoms as those with thrombocytopenia, which usually starts with mucosal bleeding, but bleeding events in these patients can be severe. In these situations, administration of desmopressin (DDAVP), which increases levels of vWF and factor VIII, can improve platelet function. Cryoprecipitate is also rich in vWF and factor VIII and can also be given. Treatment of anemia with ESAs may also help bleeding in patients with CKD and uremia as increases in red cell mass are thought to decrease platelet contact with the endothelium, allowing them to aggregate when needed to stop bleeding. There are many other reasons for bleeding in late-stage CKD aside from those just described (Table 15.7). The primary and most effective treatment for bleeding in the uremic patient is use of renal replacement therapy to resolve uremia, as removal of causes of platelet dysfunction will hopefully help to restore normal hemostasis.

Table 15.7 Abnormalities of hemostasis in patients with CKD

Factors that may cause bleeding	Factors that may cause thrombosis
Endothelial dysfunction	Coagulation abnormalities
Decreased production of the largest multimers of von Willebrand factor	Increased tissue factor
Enhanced nitric oxide production	Increased von Willebrand factor
Enhanced prostacyclin production	Increased factor XIIa
Platelet dysfunction	Increased factor VIIa
Defective activation of glycoprotein IIb-IIIa receptors	Increased activated protein C
Defective cyclooxygenase activity (reduced ability to generate thromboxane A2)	Increased fibrinogen
High levels of cyclic adenosine monophosphate	Reduced tissue plasminogen activator
Low levels of serotonin and adenosine diphosphate	Increased plasminogen activator inhibitor 1
Uremic toxins (such as guanidinosuccinic acid, phenol, phenolic acid, urea)	Other hypercoagulable risk factors Diabetes Hypertension Smoking Obesity Activation of renin-angiotensin-aldosterone system (RAAS) Nephrotic syndrome

Before You Finish: Practice Pearls for the Clinician

- Both primary care practitioners and nephrologists play a role in the diagnosis and management of the anemia associated with CKD.
- Current KDIGO and K/DOQI recommend screening for anemia in any patient with eGFR <60.
- Prior to treatment with an ESA, it is imperative to ensure that deficient iron stores have been treated appropriately.
- If iron deficiency is diagnosed, careful consideration should be given by the primary caretaker to exclude other causes prior to initiation of iron supplementation.
- ESA dose should be minimized as much as possible while providing maximum and safe quality-of-life benefit. Red cell transfusions should be used as sparingly as possible, especially in potential transplant recipients.

Disclosures Joshua Hundert, MD, has no financial disclosures.
Ajay Singh, MB Bs, MBA, has financial disclosures with IHS Dialysis, Rockwell Medical, Keryx Biopharmaceuticals, and Sandoz-Novartis.

References

1. Nurko S. Anemia in chronic kidney disease: causes, diagnosis, and treatment. Cleve Clin J Med. 2006; 73(3):289–97.
2. Goldfarb S, et al. Chronic kidney disease and progression. NephSAP. 2011;10(5):496–501.
3. Eschbach JW. The anemia of chronic renal failure: pathophysiology and the effects of recombinant erythropoietin. Kidney Int. 1989;35:134–48.
4. Jalaj DI, Chonchol M, Targher G. Disorders of hemostasis associated with chronic kidney disease. Semin Thromb Hemost. 2010;36(1):34–40.
5. KDOQI; National Kidney Foundation. KDOQI clinical practice guidelines and clinical practice recommendations for anemia in chronic kidney disease: 2006. Am J Kidney Dis. 2006;47(5 Suppl 3):S11–145.
6. Kidney Disease: Improving Global Outcomes (KDIGO) Anemia Work Group. KDIGO clinical practice guideline for anemia in chronic kidney disease. Kidney Int Suppl. 2012;2:279–335.
7. Kliger AS, Foley RN. KDOQI US commentary on the 2012 KDIGO clinical practice guidelines for anemia

in CKD. Am J Kidney Dis. 2013;65:849–59. pii: S0272-6386(13)00978-5.
8. Locatelli F, Del Vecchio L, Pozzoni P. Anemia and cardiovascular risk: the lesson of the CREATE trial. J Am Soc Nephrol. 2006;17(12 Suppl 3): S262–6.
9. Drueke TB, Locatelli F, et al. Normalization of hemoglobin levels in patients with chronic kidney disease and anemia. N Engl J Med. 2006;355(20): 2071–84.
10. Singh AK, Szczech L, Tang KL, et al. Correction of anemia with epoetin alfa in chronic kidney disease. N Engl J Med. 2006;355:2085.
11. Pfeffer MA, Burdmann EA, et al. A trial of darbepoetin alfa in type 2 diabetes and chronic kidney disease. N Engl J Med. 2009;361:2019–32.
12. KDOQI. KDOQI clinical practice guideline and clinical practice recommendations for anemia in chronic kidney disease: 2007 update of hemoglobin target. Am J Kidney Dis. 2007;50(3):471–530.
13. Kosch M, Bahner U, Bettger H, et al. A randomized, controlled parallel-group trial on efficacy and safety of iron sucrose (Venofer) vs iron gluconate (Ferrlecit) in haemodialysis patients treated with rHuEpo. Nephrol Dial Transplant. 2001;16(6):1239–44.
14. Icardi A, Paoletti E, et al. Renal anaemia and EPO hyporesponsiveness associated with vitamin D deficiency: the potential role of inflammation. Nephrol Dial Transplant. 2013;28:1672–9.
15. Macdougal IC, Provenzano R, et al. Peginesatide for anemia in patients with chronic kidney disease not receiving dialysis. N Engl J Med. 2013;368(4):320–32.
16. Boccardo P, Remuzzi G, Galbusera M. Platelet dysfunction in renal failure. Semin Thromb Hemost. 2004;30(5):579–89.
17. Besarab A, et al. The effects of normal as compared with low hematocrit values in patients with cardiac disease who are receiving hemodialysis and epoetin. N Engl J Med. 1998;339:584–90.
18. Furuland H, et al. A randomized controlled trial of haemoglobin normalization with epoetin alfa in pre-dialysis and dialysis patients. Nephrol Dial Transplant. 2003;18:353–61.
19. Rossert J, et al. Effect of early correction of anemia on the progression of CKD. Am J Kidney Dis. 2006; 47:738–50.

Mineral and Bone Disorders in Chronic Kidney Disease

16

Jorge B. Cannata-Andía, Natalia Carrillo-López, Minerva Rodriguez-García, and José-Vicente Torregrosa

Before You Start: Facts You Need to Know

- After 60 years of use, the term "renal osteodystrophy" was changed to "chronic kidney disease–mineral and bone disorders" (CKD–MBD).
- CKD–MBD group is a complex clinical syndrome including biochemical parameters and other surrogated markers.
- "Renal osteodystrophy" is reserved to describe the bone histological lesions.
- The key regulators of CKD–MBD are calcium, phosphorus, PTH, FGF23, and the vitamin D hormonal system.
- The prevention and treatment of CKD–MBD needs to be done integrating all the components of the syndrome.

J.B. Cannata-Andía, MD, PhD (✉)
N. Carrillo-López, PhD
Bone and Mineral Research Unit,
Hospital Universitario Central de Asturias, Instituto Reina Sofía de Investigación (REDinREN-ISCIII),
Julián Clavería, s/n, Oviedo 33006, Spain
e-mail: cannata@hca.es; natalia@hca.es

M. Rodriguez-García, MD, PhD
Department of Nephrology,
Hospital Universitario Central de Asturias REDinREN,
Calle Celestino Villamil s/n, Oviedo 33006, Spain
e-mail: minrodgar@hotmail.com

J.-V. Torregrosa, MD
Nephrology and Renal Transplant,
Hospital Clinic REDinREN, University of Barcelona,
Villarroel, 170, Barcelona, Spain
e-mail: vtorre@clinic.ub.es

16.1 Mineral and Bone Disorders in CKD

16.1.1 General Aspects, Epidemiology, and Pathophysiology

In healthy individuals, kidneys regulate calcium and phosphorus homeostasis modifying their tubular resorption. Patients with CKD experience a progressive compromise of the homeostatic mechanisms, giving rise to different adaptive changes in calcium, phosphorus, parathyroid hormone (PTH), vitamin D, and fibroblast growth factor 23 (FGF23) levels. These elements and hormones exert their effects on several tissues, but they act mainly on their principal targets: the bone, kidney, and intestine.

For six decades, the mineral and bone abnormalities of CKD patients were known as "renal osteodystrophy." However, in 2006, the new term "chronic kidney disease–mineral and bone disorders" (CKD–MBD) was proposed by KDIGO guidelines (Box 16.1) to group and describe a more ample and complex clinical syndrome which includes not only biochemical and bone histological abnormalities but also other bone and cardiovascular complications such as fractures and cardiovascular abnormalities occurring in CKD patients. The term "renal osteodystrophy" was reserved to describe the bone abnormalities associated with CKD which require a bone biopsy for the diagnosis. For the latter, a new classification system was proposed based on parameters of bone turnover, mineralization, and volume (TMV) [1].

M. Arici (ed.), *Management of Chronic Kidney Disease*,
DOI 10.1007/978-3-642-54637-2_16, © Springer-Verlag Berlin Heidelberg 2014

Box 16.1. Relevant Guidelines

1. *KDIGO Guidelines*
   - KDIGO clinical practice guideline for the diagnosis, evaluation, prevention, and treatment of chronic kidney disease-mineral and bone disorder (CKD-MBD). Kidney Int Suppl. 2009; 76(113):S1–130 [1].
   - KDIGO 2012 clinical practice guideline for the evaluation and management of chronic kidney disease. Kidney Int Suppl. 2013;3(1):S1–150 [12].
2. *KDOQI Guidelines*
   - K/DOQI clinical practice guidelines for chronic kidney disease: evaluation, classification, and stratification. Am J Kidney Dis. 2002;39(2 Suppl 1): S1–266 [13].
3. *Spanish Society of Nephrology Guidelines*
   - Spanish Society of Nephrology recommendations for controlling mineral and bone disorder in chronic kidney disease patients (S.E.N.-M.B.D.). Nefrologia. 2011;31 Suppl 1:3–32 [14].

The mineral and endocrine functions disrupted in CKD are critically important in the regulation of bone modeling during growth and bone remodeling during adulthood. These CKD–MBD are found almost universally in patients requiring dialysis but also in the majority of patients in CKD stages 3–5. In recent years, there has been an increased concern with the nonskeletal calcification which increases early in the course of CKD, due to the deranged mineral and bone metabolism, but it might also occur as a result of therapies used to correct the CKD–MBD themselves. Numerous cohort studies have shown associations between several CKD–MBD, such as bone fractures, vascular calcification, and cardiovascular disease with increased mortality.

As mentioned, the key regulators of bone and mineral metabolism are calcium, phosphorus, PTH, FGF23, and the vitamin D hormonal system. Even though there is still some debate concerning the chronology of changes, it is currently accepted that the increments in FGF23 and the reduction of kidney mass are possibly the earliest events in the pathogenesis of CKD–MBD; both factors favor the reduction of 1-alpha-hydroxylase in the kidney, which in turn results in low levels of the active form of vitamin D (1,25-dihydroxyvitamin D_3-[1,25$(OH)_2D_3$] or calcitriol), impairing calcium absorption in the intestine favoring the reduction in serum calcium. The decrease in serum calcium stimulates PTH synthesis and release, which in turn increases bone turnover, increases bone resorption, and stimulates 1-alpha-hydroxylase (see Fig. 16.1). All these mechanisms lead to compensatory increases in serum calcium [2].

In addition, in non-advanced phases of CKD, the increments of FGF23 and PTH increase urinary phosphorus excretion in order to avoid phosphorus accumulation [2]. Despite FGF23 and PTH featuring synergic effects to increase phosphorus excretion, both have opposite effects on calcitriol synthesis: FGF23 inhibits 1-alpha-hydroxylase, decreasing calcitriol synthesis, whereas PTH stimulates 1-alpha-hydroxylase production, thus increasing calcitriol synthesis (see Fig. 16.1). FGF23 exerts its tubular effect binding the FGFR-1 and FGFR-3 receptors with their co-receptor Klotho and PTH with the PTH receptor. Both increase phosphate excretion by reducing apical abundance of sodium-coupled cotransporters NaPi2a and NaPi2c via both PKA- and PKC-dependent pathways.

Both calcium and calcitriol act on the parathyroid cells through their specific receptors, the calcium-sensing receptor (CaSR) and the vitamin D receptor (VDR), respectively (see Fig. 16.1). While CaSR is a cell membrane receptor member of the G protein-coupled receptor family, VDR is a nuclear receptor that, when bound to vitamin D, acts as a transcription factor. The differences in the nature of the two ligands and their receptors lead to two different mechanisms of action with complementary functions on the parathyroid cells.

On one hand, small decreases in extracellular calcium concentrations are rapidly sensed by the CaSR, triggering within seconds or minutes increments

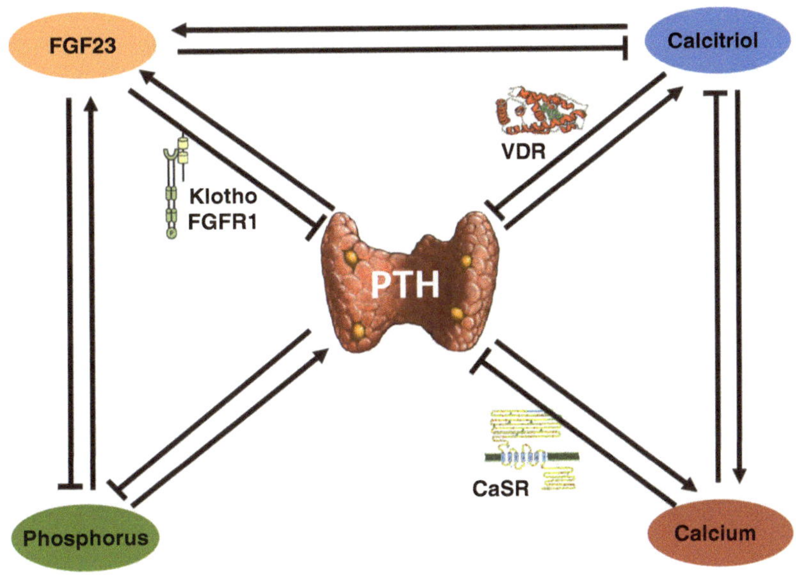

Fig. 16.1 Interrelationships between calcium and phosphorus and their hormones, PTH, FGF23, and calcitriol. The calcium ability to increase FGF23 and the low and high phosphorus to increase and, respectively, decrease serum calcitriol are not shown

in PTH release. Small increases in calcium are also sensed by the CaSR, yielding opposite results. If the stimulus persists for longer periods (hours, days), calcium is able to regulate PTH synthesis posttranscriptionally by modifying the mRNA stability through differences in binding of the parathyroid proteins to an element in its 3′-untranslated region. As a result, the decreases in serum calcium reduce mRNA degradation by increasing its stability and the half-life of mRNA PTH. On the contrary, the active form of vitamin D (calcitriol) acts at the transcriptional level and inhibits PTH gene transcription resulting in a reduction of PTH synthesis [2].

When kidney function decreases, all these complex and tightly interrelated mechanisms fail to adequately control the mineral metabolism. As a result, a progressive trend to reduce serum levels of calcitriol and increase phosphorus and calcium retention begins, ending at later stages of CKD, despite the permanent and progressive parathyroid hormone stimulation, in a manifest incapacity to control the mineral metabolism. As a result, in advanced stages of CKD–MBD, patients show severe forms of secondary hyperparathyroidism with diffuse and nodular hyperplasia and a significant reduction in CaSR, VDR, and FGFR/Klotho expression with a poor response of the parathyroid glands to the effect of calcium, VDR activators (VDRAs), and FGF23 (see Fig. 16.2) [3].

Cross-sectional studies have shown the pattern of abnormalities in serum calcium, phosphorus, PTH, 25(OH)D_3 (calcidiol), and calcitriol at different stages of CKD. As Fig. 16.3 shows, serum calcium and phosphorus values did not become abnormal until the glomerular filtration rate (GFR) fell below 40 mL/min and were relatively stable until GFR fell below 20 mL/min. By contrast, calcitriol started decreasing early in the course of CKD (GFR between 80 and 70 mL/min) and PTH increased a bit later (GFR between 70 and 60 and 40 mL/min) (see Fig. 16.3) [4].

Even though all the above discussed changes lead to the stimulation of the parathyroid gland and high bone turnover, the latter is not the most frequent histological finding of renal osteodystrophy in CKD patients. Due to several other important factors, such as aging, diabetes, and the medical management of CKD–MBD (calcium overload, high dose of VDRAs, aluminum salts), throughout the recent decades, the more frequent pattern of bone lesions has changed from high to low bone turnover forms of renal osteodystrophy (see Table 16.1). Despite high and low bone turnover being quite different and also opposite extremes of the CKD bone abnormalities, they have been associated with similar

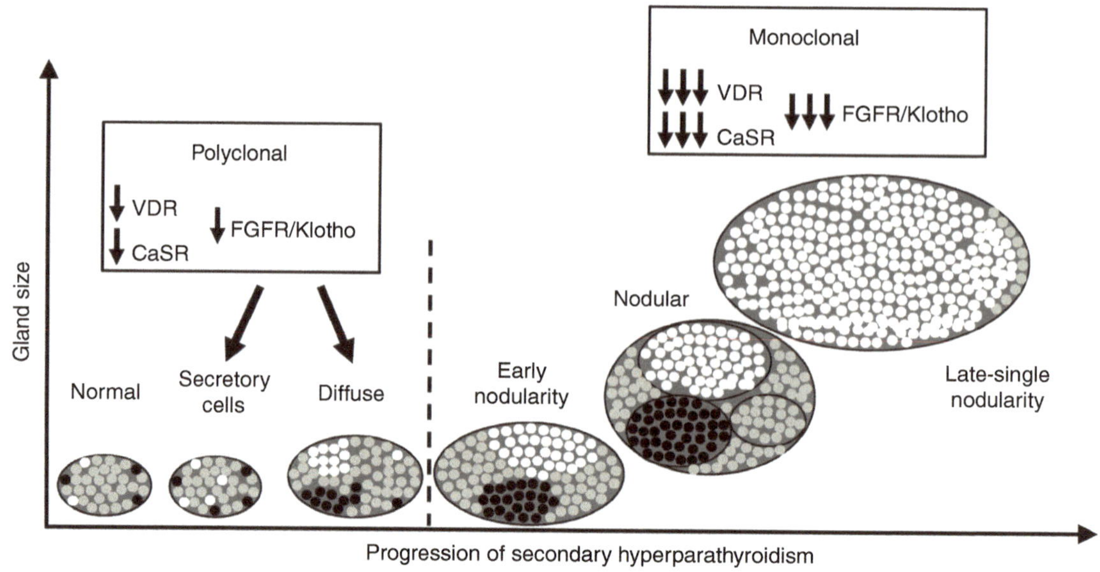

Fig. 16.2 Progression of secondary hyperparathyroidism: Initially, the parathyroid glands respond by increasing the number of secretory cells; this results in diffuse hyperplasia of the gland where cell growth is polyclonal and is accompanied by downregulation of CaSR, VDR, and FGFR/Klotho. As CKD progresses to end-stage renal disease (CKD stage 5), parathyroid hyperplasia evolves even further; monoclonal abnormalities lead to nodular hyperplasia of the glands associated with significant under-expression of CaSR, VDR, and FGFR/Klotho (Modified from Tominaga et al. [3], with permission from John Wiley and Sons)

clinical outcomes, such as a higher prevalence of vascular calcification and bone fragility fractures leading to a higher mortality risk.

16.2 Diagnosis of CKD–MBD

16.2.1 Biochemical Abnormalities

The changes in the biochemical parameters of CKD–MBD currently begin in CKD stage 3, but the rate of change and the severity of abnormalities vary greatly among patients. Therefore, assessment should begin at this stage, and the frequency of assessments, the type and duration of the identified abnormalities, the degree and rate of change of GFR, and the concomitant therapy need to be taken into account.

The diagnosis of CKD–MBD includes the use of laboratory testing of calcium, phosphorus, and PTH. In addition, the measurement of calcidiol, alkaline phosphatase (ALP) (total or bone specific), and bicarbonate may help in the diagnosis. The recommended frequency of assessment of these biochemical markers is detailed in Table 16.2 [1]. One important limitation of the biochemical markers used to diagnose, treat, and monitor CKD–MBD is the inter-assay variability and other variations as well (postprandial, diurnal, seasonal). The interpretation of values calls for the careful analysis of the type and precision of the assay used in order to avoid overemphasizing the role of minimal or inconsistent laboratory changes in the clinical decision-making process. *The importance of one single abnormal value of any one bone and mineral serum biochemical markers should not be determinant. By contrast, the diagnosis and the management of CKD–MBD should be based mainly on the trend of changes; this aspect is even more relevant in the interpretation of serum PTH and ALP values.*

In the last two decades, there has been a debate to better define the normal or acceptable upper and lower limits of these biochemical markers and thus inform managerial and therapeutical decisions. The

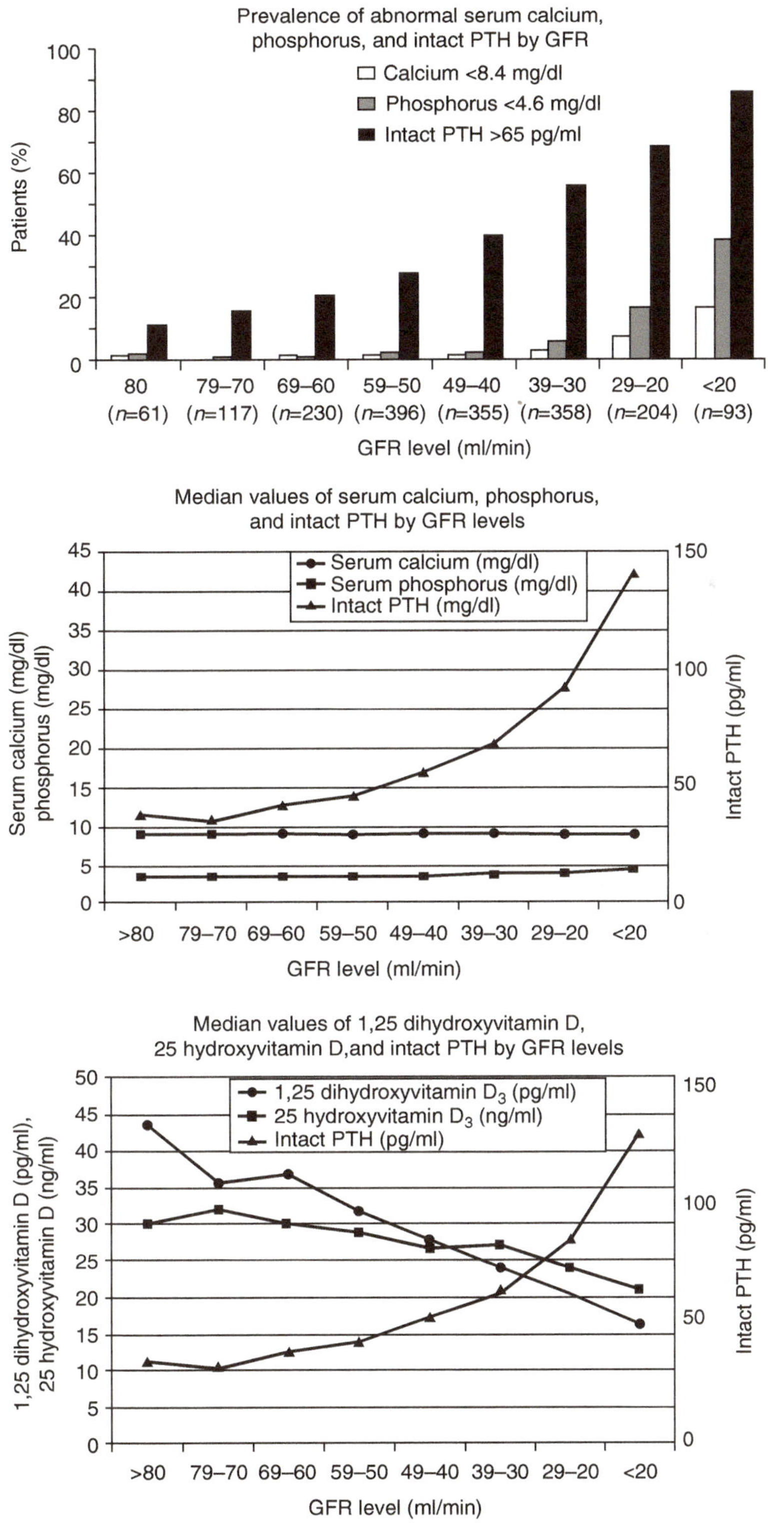

Fig. 16.3 Prevalence of abnormal mineral metabolism in CKD. (**a**) The prevalence of hyperparathyroidism, hypocalcemia, and hyperphosphoremia by GFR levels at 10 mL/min per 1.73 m^2 intervals. (**b**) Median values of calcium, phosphorus, and intact PTH by GFR levels. (**c**) Median values of 1,25(OH)$_2$D$_3$, 25(OH)D$_3$, and intact PTH by GFR levels (Republished by permission from MacMillan Publishers Ltd: Levin et al. [4], Copyright © 2007)

KDOQI (Box 16.1), the European, and more recently the KDIGO and national guidelines have established different cutoff levels [1, 12–14]. Table 16.3, which considers mainly the 2009 KDIGO recommendations, summarizes what we should consider as adequate or acceptable values of the main serum bone and mineral markers according to the degree of CKD [1]. Most of the recommendations are backed by a reasonable scientific rationale, but, unfortunately, the degree of evidence based on randomized clinical trials is very low. At present, most of the best available evidence comes from population-based or cohort-based prevalence studies.

Table 16.1 Change in the pattern of renal osteodystrophy throughout the recent decades from high to low bone turnover forms

	High bone turnover (%)	Low bone turnover (%)
Lorenzo et al. [5] (Spain)	71	25
Moriniere et al. [6] (France)	76	24
Sherrard et al. [7] (USA)	48	37
Hercz et al. [8] (USA)	50	50
Torres et al. [9] (Spain)	52	45
Ferreira et al. [10] (Portugal)	32	63
Asci et al. [11] (Turkey)	23	73

16.2.2 Bone Abnormalities

Bone tissue has an excellent biomechanical properties: it possesses a great mechanical tension to tensile stress, which is lower than that of iron, but it is at least three times lighter and ten times more flexible than iron. This outstanding property of bone explains why during long periods of life, only a reduced number of bone fractures occur despite the remarkable number of falls suffered by many people. Bone has such clinically relevant biomechanical properties thanks to the activity of the bone remodeling units, which during the young adult life allow for the renewal of a mean of 5–10 % of the skeleton per year. However, the capacity to renew bone tissue progressively decreases after age 50. Apart from the changes due to aging and gender differences, two bone disorders, osteoporosis and renal osteodystrophy,

Table 16.2 What the guidelines say you should do? Serum calcium, phosphorus, and PTH measurement frequencies according to CKD stages

	Progressive CKD stage 3	CKD stage 4	CKD stages 5 and SD
Calcium and phosphorus	6–12 months	3–6 months	1–3 months
PTH and alkaline phosphatases	Baseline	6–12 months	3–6 months
Calcidiol	Baseline	Baseline	Baseline

Source: Republished by permission from MacMillan Publishers Ltd: Kidney Disease: Improving Global Outcomes (KDIGO) CKD-MBD Work Group [1], Copyright © 2009

Table 16.3 What the guidelines say you should do? Recommended values from KDIGO [1] for the main serum bone and mineral markers according to the degree of CKD

	CKD stages 3–5	CKD stage 5
Serum phosphorus	Maintains serum phosphorus within the normal range	Lowers elevated serum P levels toward the normal range
Serum calcium	Maintains serum calcium within the normal range	Maintains serum Ca within the normal range
Serum PTH	Maintains serum PTH within the normal range	Maintains serum PTH within the range of 2–9 times more than normal for the assay
Serum calcidiol	Maintains serum calcidiol within the safe and biologically optimal range (20–40 pg/mL)	Maintains serum calcidiol within the safe and biologically optimal range (20–40 pg/mL)

greatly influence bone turnover, since they exert an important impact on bone mass and bone quality.

The rate of bone turnover impacts both cancellous (trabecular) and compact (cortical) bone, and it depends on the activity of the bone remodeling units which are regulated by several factors; among them, PTH plays a key role. Cortical bone is the most abundant type (85 % of the skeleton), but the most metabolically active is trabecular bone. Trabecular bone decreases in CKD patients, but due to the quantity of cortical bone and also the sustained major effect of PTH on the latter, in the current long-term evolution of the CKD–MBD, there is a predominant loss of cortical bone, which after several years of CKD leads to a generalized thin cortex with trabecular aspects due to insidious bone cortical erosions.

High serum PTH levels are associated with hyperdynamic bone. PTH stimulates bone cell proliferation and activity but also bone turnover. In secondary hyperparathyroidism, the cycles of the bone remodeling units are more rapid and active, but also more bone remodeling units are activated; as a result of these two mechanisms, an abnormal, immature, non-lamellar bone matrix is formed. At the end, a woven and less resistant bone is produced, which yields an increased fracture risk. Very high serum PTH levels (>450 pg/mL) have a good predictive value for high bone turnover, but moderately high serum PTH values (300–450 pg/mL) do not exhibit a good correlation with bone turnover; in fact, normal or low bone turnover can be found within these ranges of serum PTH values.

Low PTH levels are associated with adynamic bone, low bone cellular activity, and bone turnover [15]. Consequently, the inadequate renewal of bone increases its fragility. In practice, adynamic bone is currently suspected when serum PTH levels are below the normal values. PTH levels lower than 150 pg/mL have a good predictive value for low bone turnover and adynamic bone, but PTH between 150 and 450 pg/mL, currently considered normal or adequate serum PTH values, can be associated with adynamic bone. Then, despite the measurement of serum PTH levels in CKD patients being the current noninvasive method to assess bone turnover, its specificity within the previous mentioned ranges is limited. Overall, the clinical consequences of low bone turnover observed in adynamic bone are similar to those observed in osteoporosis, with a higher prevalence of bone fractures and more frequent and severe vascular calcification compared with patients in whom bone turnover remains close to normal [15].

For the precise diagnosis of high or low bone turnover (mainly for the latter), it is necessary to perform a bone biopsy. An increased number of osteoclasts and osteoblasts, a non-laminar osteoid, woven bone, high bone formation rate with high activation frequency, normal or high mineralization rate (double tetracycline labeling), and increased marrow fibrosis are typically found in high bone turnover states. By contrast, the reduction or absence of osteoblasts and osteoclasts, a decreased or null osteoid formation, and low or no bone mineralization rate (low or absent tetracycline labeling) with low activation frequency are found in adynamic bone [15]. Another histological diagnosis associated with low bone turnover is osteomalacia, which was the most common form of low bone turnover in the 1970s and 1980s and is currently associated with aluminum overload. The proper control of the sources of aluminum exposure (aluminum in dialysis fluids and the reduction of the massive use of aluminum-containing phosphate binders) has drastically reduced the incidence of osteomalacia in CKD patients.

A decrease in BMD and changes in the bone microarchitecture occur early in CKD and worsen as the disease progresses. As a result, CKD patients present flaws in the quantity and quality of bone, resulting in a higher risk of bone fracture, mainly of non-vertebral bone fractures (see Fig. 16.4) [1, 15]. The measurement of bone mass as bone mineral density (BMD) using dual-energy X-ray absorptiometry (DXA) is the best noninvasive marker to predict bone fractures in the general population, but this is not the case in CKD patients. Fracture rates and fracture-related mortality are elevated in CKD, but BMD measurement does not reliably predict fracture, neither the risk nor the type of renal osteodystrophy in patients in CKD stages 3B–5D [1].

Bone strength is determined by the density and quality of the bone, but the BMD measured using DXA is not able to capture bone quality (cortical and trabecular microarchitecture). Changes in

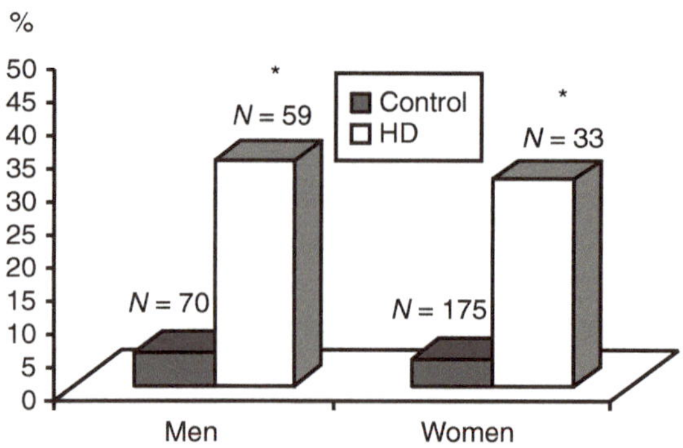

Fig. 16.4 Percentage of hemodialysis patients (*HD*) having non-vertebral fractures compared to a randomly selected general population of the same age and region (Asturias, Spain) (control). $p<0.001$ HD patients ($N=92$) compared to general population ($N=245$) (Adapted with permission of Società Italiana di Nefrologia, from Rodriguez Garcia et al. [16] permission conveyed through Copyright Clearance Center, Inc.)

quality are better studied using high-resolution peripheral quantitative computed tomography (HR-pQCT). Currently, neither technique is predictive of bone fracture in CKD patients. Thus, except in specific and particular cases, it is not recommended to follow the BMD or HR-pQCT measurement routine in patients in CKD stages 3B–5D as such techniques can lead to equivocal CKD–MBD diagnosis and management.

16.2.3 Diagnosis and Type of Vascular Calcification

The diagnosis of CKD–MBD includes the detection of cardiovascular calcification. The predisposition of patients with CKD toward developing vascular calcification was already mentioned in the nineteenth century; since then, this aspect has been a life-threatening complication of CKD but only recently has it awoken great interest in nephrology. Despite the debate still rages somewhat, it has been suggested that a lateral abdominal X-ray and an echocardiogram, both simple and inexpensive procedures, can be effectively used to detect vascular and valvular calcification, respectively.

Most studies examining calcification have been performed using CT-based techniques (electron beam tomography and multi-slice computed tomography, EBCT and MSCT, respectively), which are quite sensitive methods for the detection of and quantification of calcium in the vessels. However, these more precise techniques are not widespread available. The localization and extension of vascular calcification can be scored in a reproducible manner using X-ray. Several available methods such as the Kaupila, Adragao, and others are able to quantify and score vascular calcification, featuring a good correlation with the CT-based gold standard techniques and also with outcomes such as mortality. In addition, valvular calcification detected by echocardiography is a good predictor of coronary artery calcium. The information provided by these studies should help not only to evaluate risk and prognosis but also to guide the therapeutic management of CKD patients [16–18].

There are three types of arteries which differ according to their size and structure: elastic or large-caliber arteries, muscular or medium-caliber arteries, and small-caliber arteries.

The elastic or large-caliber arteries are responsible of conducting the blood to the distribution arteries; they show a relatively thin wall in proportion to their diameter and a rather thick tunica media containing more elastic fibers than smooth muscle with a fairly thin adventitia. The aorta, the subclavia, and the common carotid arteries belong to this group. The muscular or medium-caliber arteries are capable of withstanding further vasodilatation and vasoconstriction to adjust the volume of blood to the perfusion requirements; they have a tunica media which contains a high proportion of smooth muscle. The axillary, brachial, radial, coronary, femoral, and tibial arteries are included in this group. Finally, the small-caliber arteries are responsible for regulating the local blood flow and perfusion pressure through luminal size variations caused by vasoconstriction and vasodilatation; they are less than 2-mm thick, and their tunica media contains only smooth muscle. This group includes, among others, the palmar arch and the digital arteries [16].

Vascular calcification can occur in the intima and the media layers. Intimal calcification begins and progresses throughout lifetime mainly under the influence of genetic and lifestyle circumstances. Intimal calcification is associated with atherosclerosis including endothelial dysfunction, intimal edema, lipid cell formation, and blood cell migration that may cause a plaque rupture, leading to the formation of a thrombus. It is currently associated with chronic arterial

Table 16.4 Traditional and nontraditional uremia-related risk factors for vascular calcification in CKD patients

Traditional risk factors	Nontraditional risk factors (uremia related)
Hypertension	Time in dialysis
Diabetes mellitus	Hyperphosphoremia
Tobacco	High calcium–phosphorus product
Genetic	Hyperparathyroidism and hypoparathyroidism
Age	High dosage of vitamin D metabolites
Dyslipidemia	Low fetuin-A
History of premature coronary heart disease	Poor nutrition (low albumin)
Vitamin K inhibitors (warfarin)	Chronic inflammation (high IL-1, IL-6, TNF-α) Hyperhomocysteinemia Advanced glycated end products

IL-1 Interleukin 1, *IL-6* Interleukin 6, *TNF*-α tumor necrosis factor-alpha

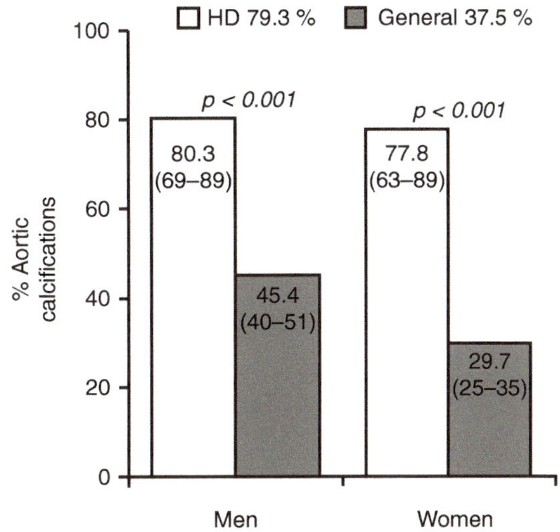

Fig. 16.5 Differences in the prevalence of aortic calcifications in hemodialysis (*HD*) patients and in a randomly selected general population of the same age and region (Asturias, Spain) (control). $p<0.001$ HD patients ($N=92$) compared to general population ($N=245$) (Adapted with permission of the American Society of Nephrology, from Cannata-Andia et al. [26] permission conveyed through Copyright Clearance Center, Inc.)

inflammation exacerbated by well-characterized risk factors, such as hypertension, diabetes, hypercholesterolemia, obesity, smoking, and a family history of heart disease.

Calcification of the media occurs in the elastic lamina of large-caliber and medium/small-sized arteries. It seems to be independent of atherosclerosis but can coexist with it. This type of calcification was known initially as "Monckeberg sclerosis," and it has been radiographically described as railroads. It affects the arteries that are less likely to develop atherosclerosis, such as visceral abdominal, thyroid, lung, limb, and femoral arteries, but it is also extremely common in the aorta. It is frequently observed in CKD patients and in other disorders with metabolic abnormalities such as diabetes and hypervitaminosis D. Table 16.4 summarizes the traditional and nontraditional uremia-related risk factors for vascular calcification in CKD patients.

16.2.4 Epidemiology and Pathophysiology of Vascular Calcification

CKD patients exhibit a very high prevalence of vascular calcifications exceeding the percentage observed in the general population of the same age, sex, and region (see Fig. 16.5), leading to cardiovascular disease, decreased life expectancy, and mortality, even in the early phases of CKD. Moreover, calcification of the cardiac valves involves a high risk of cardiovascular dysfunction. A recent study in patients in CKD stage 5D has shown that vascular calcifications are frequently localized in high-caliber arteries, such as the aorta (around 80 %); medium-caliber arteries, including coronary arteries (around 60–70 %); and small-caliber arteries (20–30 %), reflecting the heterogeneity of the three categories of arteries previously described [16]. Time on hemodialysis has been positively associated with vascular calcification, particularly in medium-caliber arteries. Each year on dialysis increased the risk of developing vascular calcifications by approximately 15 % [20].

The mechanisms by which vascular and valvular calcification are produced are complex. It is not a mere precipitation of calcium and phosphate; it involves active and modifiable processes. This regulated process involves several changes, such as a decrease of vascular calcification inhibitors, an increase of vascular calcification promoters, and the formation of calcification vesicles; the result is the induction of a cellular phenotypic change of vascular smooth muscle

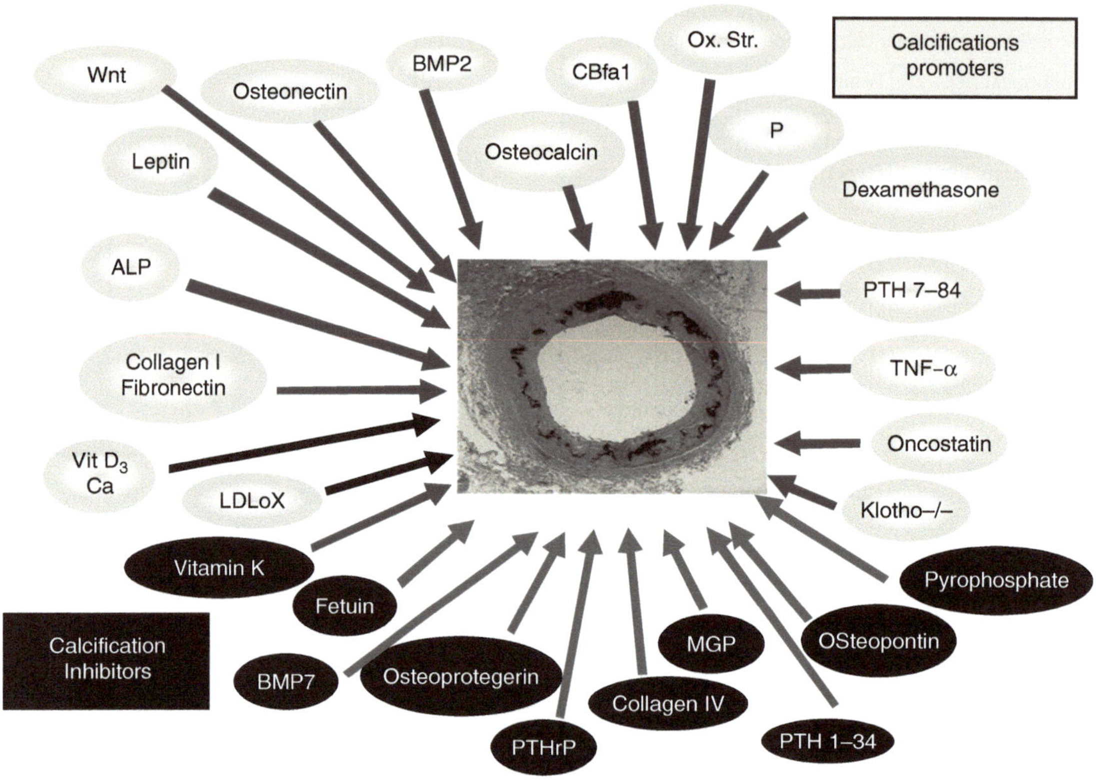

Fig. 16.6 Promoters and inhibitors of vascular calcification. *ALP* alkaline phosphatase, *Ca* calcium, *LDLox* oxidized low-density lipoprotein, *MGP* matrix GLA protein, *P* phosphorus, *PTHrP* parathyroid hormone-related protein, *TNF-a* tumor necrosis factor-alpha, *Vit* D_3 calcitriol (Republished with permission of Oxford University Press, from Cannata-Andia et al. [27])

cells which are turned into bone-like cells (see Fig. 16.6). The outcome is the formation of bone tissue inside the artery wall.

Among the promoters of vascular calcification, high serum phosphorus is considered the most important uremia-related, nontraditional risk factor associated to vascular calcification in CKD patients. Phosphorus is capable of acting as a secondary intracellular messenger, activating several molecular pathways related to bone formation. It reaches the intracellular space via a specific Na-dependent channel called Pit1 and exerts some important actions, such as the blockade of Pit1 which prevents vascular calcification. In vitro experiments have demonstrated that high intracellular phosphorus levels may directly increase Cbfa1, the bone-specific transcription factor, resulting in the activation of several osteogenic pathways and factors, including bone morphogenetic proteins (BMPs) which lead to the phenotypic changes of vascular smooth muscle cells into bone-like cells. Phosphorus also promotes the expression of osteocalcin and ALP in the vasculature.

Among the inhibitors of vascular calcification, pyrophosphates, fetuin-A, osteoprotegerin (OPG), and matrix Gla protein (MGP) are the most studied either in tissue or in serum. In the former, pyrophosphates are located in the vascular matrix to preserve the vascular smooth muscle cells phenotype inhibiting calcium phosphate crystal formation and the change of vascular smooth muscle cells into bone-like cells. In serum, the most abundant inhibitors of vascular calcification are fetuin-A, OPG, and MGP. Fetuin-A, a known inhibitor of osteogenesis, is capable of hampering vascular calcification. OPG holds back osteoclast differentiation, modulating bone resorption through its action as a decoy receptor of RANKL, but it may also act as inhibitor of vascular calcification. New players such as FGF23 and its co-receptor Klotho have been also related with vascular calcification. FGF23 and Klotho knockout mice showed low bone mass and accelerated aging with widespread tissue calcification. The mechanisms by which FGF23/Klotho affects bone health and vascular calcifications may involve phosphorus excretion, vitamin D synthesis, and also PTH regulation.

16.2.5 Vascular Calcification and Bone Health

Most of the previously discussed factors, either promoters or inhibitors of the vascular calcification process, have been related not only with vascular calcification but also with bone health, a fact which suggests there might be several links and common pathways between bone and vascular disorders. Vascular calcification, bone loss, and fragility fractures are very common disorders associated with aging, both in CKD patients and in the general population. In recent years, several studies have drawn attention to the fact that apart from aging there might be other common factors linking vascular calcification and bone health. Even though these factors are not still fully understood, in CKD patients and in animal models, there is evidence that the progression of vascular calcification is directly associated with the reduction of bone mass and an increased risk of fragility fractures. The more severe the vascular calcification, the greater the loss of bone mass [17].

16.2.6 Calciphylaxis

An infrequent but very severe form of medial calcification of small cutaneous arteries is calciphylaxis, also called "calcific uremic arteriolopathy" which is currently associated with a poor control of mineral metabolism, mainly PTH, calcium, and phosphorus. It is characterized by painful ischemic skin ulcerations which are frequently followed by superinfections. The pathogenesis of this form of severe vascular calcification is not yet fully understood, and apart from the uncontrolled mineral metabolism, dysregulation of some calcification inhibitors such as fetuin-A, MGP, and vitamin K have been implicated in its pathogenesis. This form of medial calcification is associated with high risk of mortality.

16.3 Management of CKD–MBD

16.3.1 Management of Biochemical Abnormalities

Even though for didactic reasons we shall describe individually the management of the main mineral and bone disorders, it is important to emphasize that in CKD–MBD, all the parameters need to be evaluated and put together in an integrated manner as they all are very tightly interrelated players.

In CKD stages 3–5, there is a clear trend to have a positive phosphate balance; thus, therapeutic strategies aim to avoid the accumulation of phosphorus. The rationale behind the importance of controlling serum phosphorus is based on epidemiological and solid experimental studies which have shown that hyperphosphoremia is an important risk factor, not only for secondary hyperparathyroidism but also for cardiovascular disease and mortality. In addition, despite the lack of evidence from randomized controlled trials that lowering serum phosphorus levels can improve clinical outcomes, most strategies aim to reduce serum phosphorus in CKD in patients with hyperphosphoremia. The approaches to achieve this goal include three levels of action: reduction of dietary phosphorus intake, use of phosphate binding agents, and increasing phosphorus removal by adding more hours of dialysis.

The control of serum phosphorus through dietary phosphorus restriction merits specific and important comments. The factors affecting gastrointestinal phosphorus absorption include vitamin D levels and phosphorus food content and bioavailability. Currently, the sources of dietary phosphorus are protein-rich foods, which in a nonvegetarian Western diet may represent around 60 % of the dietary phosphorus. Foods rich in phosphorus include dairy products, meat, fish, legumes, nuts, and chocolates. However, variable but not negligible amounts of phosphorus (e.g., inorganic phosphate) with a high bioavailability are found in food additives and preservatives. The phosphate content of plants is high in phosphorus, but its bioavailability and gastrointestinal absorption is low. The reduction of dietary phosphorus intake has a clear limitation: the need to ensure an adequate protein intake to avoid undernutrition. In fact, a restrictive prescription of dietary phosphorus has been associated with poorer indices of nutritional status, and a stepwise trend toward greater survival with more liberal phosphorus prescription has been postulated.

To obtain a higher removal of phosphorus, increasing the hours of dialysis, either by prescribing prolonged nocturnal dialysis or short daily dialysis, has become a useful approach to control hyperphosphoremia and to reduce serum PTH levels and the dose of phosphate binders prescription in CKD 5D patients. However, despite the progressive use of the two aforementioned useful strategies, still most patients in CKD stage 5D (between 80 and 90 %) need the use of phosphate binding agents to control hyperphosphoremia.

Although there is no evidence that lowering serum phosphorus to a specific level range would lead to improved clinical outcomes and despite all the available evidence is based on observational data, the recent guidelines suggest that serum phosphorus should be maintained within the normal range at all stages of CKD [1, 12]. The use of moderate phosphate-restricted diets in combination with phosphate-binding agents has become a reasonable approach to avoid phosphorus accumulation in patients in CKD stages 3–5D. This strategy allows a more liberal diet which leads to a better nutritional status which can positively impact survival, as it has been shown in recent large-scale epidemiological studies.

Several observational studies and clinical trials have shown that all available phosphate-binding agents are effective in reducing serum phosphorus, but to date, the available data do not support a strong superiority of the novel non-calcium-containing phosphate-binding agents on outcomes such as cardiovascular and mortality endpoints. In addition, the great differences in dietary phosphorus intake and availability of phosphate binders around the world, the different economic and social scenarios, and the individual clinical circumstances of each CKD patient are enough reasons to avoid making general and conclusive recommendations for the generalized use of one specific phosphate-binding agent (see Table 16.5) [22, 23].

However, based on the analyses of the individual circumstances of CKD patients, it is reasonable that the choice of the phosphate binder would take into account several aspects, such as the stage of CKD, the presence of other components of CKD–MBD, and any concomitant therapies. In CKD stages 3–5D patients with persistent or recurrent hypercalcemia, arterial calcification, adynamic bone disease, and persistent low serum PTH levels, the use and dose of calcium-based phosphate binders, calcitriol, or other less hypercalcemic and hyperphosphoremic VDRAs should be carefully and individually evaluated. It is recommended to avoid or restrict the long-term use of aluminum-containing phosphate binders to prevent aluminum overload.

Regarding calcium, apart from the limitations already discussed about the use of calcium-based phosphate agents and the need to individualize the therapy, the most appropriate approach for CKD stage 5D patients is to use a dialysate calcium concentration between 1.25 and 1.50 mmol/L (2.5 and 3.0 mEq/L). It is important to stress that the combined use of a high calcium concentration in the dialysate (>1.50 mmol/L) together with calcium-based phosphate binders should be avoided as they would increase the risk of calcium overload in CKD 5D patients.

In the case of CKD stages 3–5 patients not on dialysis, it is suggested that if PTH levels are above the upper normal limit of the assay, they should be first evaluated for hyperphosphoremia, hypocalcemia, and calcidiol deficiency and correct them if they are present. If serum PTH increases progressively and remains persistently above the upper limit despite having corrected the abovementioned factors, treatment with VDRAs can be initiated. There are several VDRAs in the market (see Table 16.6); all of them are effective in PTH suppression even though they may have a differential effect in calcium and phosphorus absorption [24].

Table 16.5 Comparison of advantages, disadvantages, benefits, and risks among the most currently used phosphate binders

	Aluminum hydroxide	Calcium salts	Sevelamer	Lanthanum carbonate
Years of use	>50	>40	>12	>6
Efficacy	++++	++	++	+++
Additional positive effects	Antacid	Antacid Control of acidosis	Improvement lipid profile and inflammation Pleiotropic effects?	Pleiotropic effects?
Short/medium-term adverse effects	–	Hypercalcemia	Digestive intolerance	Digestive intolerance
Long-term toxic effects	CNS, hematopoiesis, parathyroids and bone alterations	Vascular/valvular calcification	–	–
Accumulation	++++ tissues	++++ tissues ++++ vessels	No	+ tissues
Effect on bone turnover	Inhibition	Inhibition	No	No
Effect on vessels	?	Increase vascular calcification	Reduce progression of vascular calcification	Reduce progression of vascular calcification
Effect on survival	No advantage	Minor advantage	Advantage	Advantage

CNS central nervous system

Table 16.6 Comparisons between the different generations of VDRAs

	First generation	Second generation	Third generation
Generic name	Calcitriol (1α,25-dihydroxyvitamin D_3)	Alfacalcidol/doxercalciferol (1α-hydroxyvitamin D_3/D_2)	Paricalcitol (19-nor-1α, 25-dihydroxyvitamin D_2)
Characteristic	Mimics endogenous VDR hormone	Molecular modifications at the side chain	Molecular modifications at the side chain and A-ring
Comments	Active upon administration	Requires activation in the liver	Active upon administration
Well-established clinical indications	SHPT in CKD Osteoporosis	SHPT in CKD Osteoporosis	SHPT in CKD

SHPT secondary hyperparathyroidism, *CKD* chronic kidney disease

The approach is different for CKD stage 5D patients, for whom the KDIGO guidelines suggest to maintain serum PTH levels within the range of approximately two to nine times the upper normal limit for the assay [1]. Accordingly, changes in therapy should be based on the observed trends of changes, and therapy should be initiated or modified to avoid any progression to serum PTH levels outside this range in either direction. This recommendation makes it difficult to be implemented in clinical practice due to the wide range of PTH normality, then the KDOQI ranges (serum PTH levels between 150 and 300 pg/dL) and similar ranges from national guidelines are also currently used in practice [13, 14]. Despite the absence of definitive evidence, several large-scale observational studies released after the CKD–MBD KDIGO guidelines were published have confirmed that in CKD patients, the better outcomes are associated with serum PTH values around 150–300 pg/dL [19, 21].

To reduce PTH in CKD stage 5D patients, the suggested management is the use of VDRAs and/or calcimimetics. The selection of the initial drug for the treatment should be based on serum calcium and phosphorus levels and other aspects of CKD–MBD, such as the presence of vascular calcification. When using VDRAs, if either hyperphosphoremia or hypercalcemia is present, they should be reduced or stopped. Likewise, if hypocalcemia is present, the use of calcimimetics needs to be reduced or stopped. All changes in the therapy of secondary hyperparathyroidism should take into account other aspects, signs, symptoms, severity of the disorders, and concomitant medications.

If PTH levels fall and reach the range of low bone turnover, the use of VDRAs and/or calcimimetics should be reduced or stopped. In patients with severe hyperparathyroidism who did not respond with a clinically meaningful reduction of serum PTH levels after following the previous recommendations, parathyroidectomy should be considered. Even though there is no agreement regarding at which serum PTH level a parathyroidectomy should be indicated, the most current practice is to perform any type of parathyroidectomy when patients maintain PTH levels above 800 pg/mL despite an adequate medical treatment. Subtotal parathyroidectomy and total parathyroidectomy with parathyroid implants are the two techniques more currently used.

16.3.2 Osteoporosis

The CKD–MBD constellation also includes the study of bone fragility fractures, which can appear due to high and low bone turnover states but also due to osteoporosis, an age-dependent and highly prevalent bone disorder whose importance has greatly increased due to aging of our CKD population.

In osteoporosis there is a reduction in bone mass with no specific defect in bone formation. This occurs because the balance between bone formation and bone resorption is lost, favoring the latter. As a result, less new bone is formed to replace bone loss. The DXA definition of osteoporosis and the bone mass criteria followed for its diagnosis were adopted for the first time by the World Health Organization (WHO) in 1993. It stands as "a disease characterized by low bone mineral density and micro architectural deterioration leading to low bone strength and increased risk of fractures." Strictly speaking, the definition applied only to Caucasian postmenopausal women, and it was conceived to be used for diagnostic purposes, but not for treatment. However, its use progressively expanded to include men and also to help in the treatment decision process. The WHO definition of osteoporosis never included the CKD condition.

The T-score of the DXA measurement is used for the assessment of BMD and for the definition of osteoporosis. Each T-score difference in BMD represents 1 standard deviation (SD) from the peak bone mass. Values up to −1 SD BMD below the mean peak bone mass are considered normal; values between −1 SD and −2.5 SD BMD are indicative of osteopenia, and values below −2.5 SD BMD are indicative of osteoporosis (see Fig. 16.7) [15]. BMD measurement plays an important diagnostic, preventive, and managerial role in the general population, but as it has been already mentioned, in the case of CKD stages 3–5 patients, this technique has a rather limited utility which becomes worse the more advanced the CKD stages.

In addition to the aforementioned limitations in the interpretation of BMD, restrictions exist in the treatment of osteoporosis in CKD patients. Apart from the possibility of using calcium supplements and VDRAs (drugs which are also used in the management of osteoporosis), due to the complexity of CKD–MBD, the use of the currently available antiosteoporotic compounds also presents additional limitations. There are two main reasons for such limitations: the first is the fact that all large-scale, long-term clinical trials carried out to register active antiosteoporotic drugs have specifically excluded patients with low kidney function, particularly CKD stages 4–5; the second reason is the fact that kidneys play a key role in the clearance of some of these compounds (e.g., bisphosphonates and strontium ranelate). Thus, the available evidence comes from the post hoc analysis of the studies, selecting patients with reduced kidney function in whom the drug was administered. In some of these studies, there were enough CKD stage 3 patients, but that was not the case with CKD stages 4–5 patients. To fill that

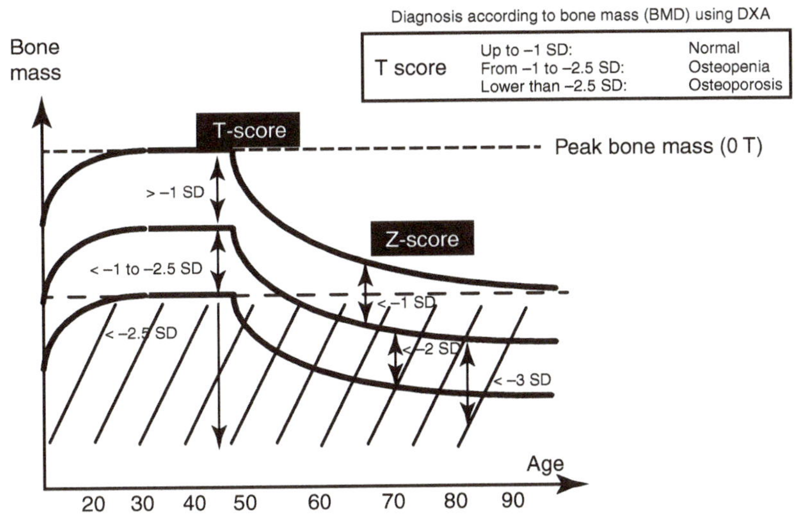

Fig. 16.7 The WHO osteoporosis diagnostic criteria: T-score values for normality, osteopenia, and osteoporosis using DXA (Adapted with permission of Società Italiana di Nefrologia, from Cannata-Andia et al. [15] permission conveyed through Copyright Clearance Center, Inc.)

gap, recent studies have started to address this issue such as a recent pilot single-dose study performed with denosumab in patients with different degrees of kidney impairment.

Despite the mentioned limitations, the KDIGO CKD–MBD 2009 guidelines [1], partly updated in 2013 [12], include the following advices: CKD stages 1–2 patients should be managed as the general population; CKD stage 3 patients should be individually evaluated taking into account other important biochemical parameters such as PTH values. In CKD stage 3B, since GFR is low (45–30 mL/min), it is necessary to carefully monitor the progression of kidney failure and the serum PTH levels. The prescription of bisphosphonates is not recommended in patients with GFR <30 mL/min without a strong clinical indication. In general, patients with biochemical anomalies, such as PTH or other serum bone parameter abnormalities, should be managed differently, and the treatment choices should take into account the magnitude and reversibility of those biochemical abnormalities as well as the progression of CKD. A bone biopsy should be always considered for this type of patients, and a greater caution needs to be taken when considering the use of antiresorptive agents when PTH levels are normal or low. In the latter, bisphosphonates cannot be used because the risk of further reducing bone turnover and bone fragility is very high.

16.3.3 Vascular Calcification

Another important aspect of CKD–MBD is to follow strategies to minimize or avoid the progression of vascular calcification. Any strategy designed to reduce the impact of vascular calcification needs to take into account primary prevention measures to control cardiovascular risk factors. It is crucial to promote a healthy lifestyle, a balanced diet, regular physical exercise, smoking cessation, and a low alcohol intake. Once vascular calcifications appear, secondary prevention must aim to reduce their complications, intensifying the measures and treatments previously described. Most strategies to reduce vascular calcifications focus on several risk factors such as hyperphosphoremia, hypercalcemia, secondary hyperparathyroidism, smoking, dyslipidemia, hypertension, diabetes, inflammation, and to stop the use of warfarin. Other strategies such as the use of bisphosphonates have shown to be effective, but they are still being researched and they cannot be used in clinical practice.

16.3.4 Calciphylaxis

Despite calciphylaxis is an infrequent form of vascular calcification, its management remains a challenge. As in the other forms of vascular calcification, the first step in the treatment of calciphylaxis is an effective control of serum phosphorus, calcium, and PTH using the most efficacious strategies, including parathyroidectomy if necessary. As the skin ulcerated lesions are frequently infected, antibiotic therapy is indicated.

On top of the abovementioned measure, there are new approaches that they can be successful, though still the evidence of its efficacy is based on case reports or short series. Among them, in patients receiving warfarin, the urgent withdrawal and switch to another anticoagulant is indicated. Sodium thiosulfate has been used due to its antioxidant effect and to its capacity to interfere with calcium and phosphate precipitation; however, its long-term potential side effects are unknown. Bisphosphonates have also been used based on the experimental available evidence of its capacity to reduce vascular calcification by decreasing bone resorption and calcium availability and due to its positive effect at the vascular cell level on MGP; the evidence of its beneficial effect is still based on short case series reports [25]. Finally, in an attempt to improve wound healing in the ischemic tissues, hyperbaric oxygen therapy and anti-inflammatory strategies have been successfully used in a small number of patients [18].

Before You Finish: Practice Pearls for the Clinician

- The changes in biochemical parameters of CKD–MBD currently begin in CKD stage 3, with important variations among patients. Assessment should start at this stage.
- The optimal or normal values for each of the serum biochemical markers of CKD–MBD have been obtained from population- or cohort-based studies. A single value can alert, but the diagnosis and management should be guided considering also the trend of changes.
- In CKD, both high and low bone turnover and osteoporosis are associated with vascular calcification, bone fractures, and increased mortality.
- Calcium overload should be avoided at all stages of CKD. Excess of calcium and phosphorus are two potent but avoidable promoters of vascular calcification with negative impact in outcomes.
- In CKD stages 3–5D, there is a clear trend to a positive phosphate balance that needs to be avoided using the available strategies but taking into account that aggressive dietary restriction of phosphorus may lead to undernutrition with possible negative effect on survival.

Acknowledgements The authors wish to thank the Fondo de Investigaciones Sanitarias (FIS), Fondo Europeo de Desarrollo Regional (FEDER), Redes Temáticas de Investigación Cooperativa en Salud (REDinREN; RD06/0016/1013, RD12/0021/1023), Instituto de Salud Carlos III (ISCIII), Fundación para el Fomento en Asturias de la Investigación Científica Aplicada y la Tecnología (FICYT), Instituto Reina Sofía de Investigación- Fundación Renal Iñigo Álvarez de Toledo (IRSIN-FRIAT), and University of Oviedo. The authors also would like to extend their appreciation to Marino Santirso for the language editing of this chapter.

References

1. Kidney Disease: Improving Global Outcomes (KDIGO) CKD-MBD Work Group. KDIGO clinical practice guideline for the diagnosis, evaluation, prevention, and treatment of chronic kidney disease-mineral and bone disorder (CKD-MBD). Kidney Int Suppl. 2009;76(113):S1–130.
2. Olgaard K, Salusky I, Silver J, editors. The spectrum of mineral and bone disorders in chronic kidney disease. Oxford: Oxford University Press; 2010. p. 61–136.
3. Tominaga Y, Tanaka Y, Sato K, Nagasaka T, Takagi H. Histopathology, pathophysiology, and indications for surgical treatment of renal hyperparathyroidism. Semin Surg Oncol. 1997;13(2):78–86.
4. Levin A, Bakris GL, Molitch M, Smulders M, Tian J, Williams LA, Andress DL. Prevalence of abnormal serum vitamin D, PTH, calcium, and phosphorus in patients with chronic kidney disease: results of the study to evaluate early kidney disease. Kidney Int. 2007;71(1):31–8.
5. Lorenzo V, Torres A, Gonzalez-Posada JM, Pestaña M, Rodriguez A, Diaz-florez L. Prevalencia de las distintas formas histológicas de osteodistrofia renal, con especial referencia a la osteomalacia. Nefrologia. 1986;VI(2):25–33.
6. Moriniere P, Cohen-Solal M, Belbrik S, Boudailliez B, Marie A, Westeel PF, Renaud H, Fievet P, Lalau JD, Sebert JL, et al. Disappearance of aluminic bone

disease in a long term asymptomatic dialysis population restricting A1(OH)3 intake: emergence of an idiopathic adynamic bone disease not related to aluminum. Nephron. 1989;53(2):93–101.
7. Sherrard DJ, Hercz G, Pei Y, Maloney NA, Greenwood C, Manuel A, Saiphoo C, Fenton SS, Segre GV. The spectrum of bone disease in end-stage renal failure–an evolving disorder. Kidney Int. 1993;43(2):436–42.
8. Hercz G, Pei Y, Greenwood C, Manuel A, Saiphoo C, Goodman WG, Segre GV, Fenton S, Sherrard DJ. Aplastic osteodystrophy without aluminum: the role of "suppressed" parathyroid function. Kidney Int. 1993;44(4):860–6.
9. Torres A, Lorenzo V, Hernandez D, Rodriguez JC, Concepcion MT, Rodriguez AP, Hernandez A, de Bonis E, Darias E, Gonzalez-Posada JM, et al. Bone disease in predialysis, hemodialysis, and CAPD patients: evidence of a better bone response to PTH. Kidney Int. 1995;47(5):1434–42.
10. Ferreira A, Frazao JM, Monier-Faugere MC, Gil C, Galvao J, Oliveira C, Baldaia J, Rodrigues I, Santos C, Ribeiro S, Hoenger RM, Duggal A, Malluche HH. Effects of sevelamer hydrochloride and calcium carbonate on renal osteodystrophy in hemodialysis patients. J Am Soc Nephrol. 2008;19(2):405–12.
11. Asci G, Ok E, Savas R, Ozkahya M, Duman S, Toz H, Kayikcioglu M, Branscum AJ, Monier-Faugere MC, Herberth J, Malluche HH. The link between bone and coronary calcifications in CKD-5 patients on haemodialysis. Nephrol Dial Transplant. 2011;26(3):1010–5.
12. Kidney Disease: Improving Global Outcomes (KDIGO) CKD-MBD Work Group 2012 clinical practice guideline for the evaluation and management of chronic kidney disease. Kidney Int Suppl. 2013;3(1): S1–150.
13. National Kidney Foundation. K/DOQI clinical practice guidelines for chronic kidney disease: evaluation, classification, and stratification. Am J Kidney Dis. 2002;39(2 Suppl 1):S1–266.
14. Torregrosa JV, Bover J, Cannata Andia J, Lorenzo V, de Francisco AL, Martinez I, Rodriguez Portillo M, Arenas L, Gonzalez Parra E, Caravaca F, Martin-Malo A, Fernandez Giraldez E, Torres A. Spanish Society of Nephrology recommendations for controlling mineral and bone disorder in chronic kidney disease patients (S.E.N.-M.B.D.). Nefrologia. 2011;31 Suppl 1: 3–32.
15. Cannata-Andia JB, Rodriguez Garcia M, Gomez Alonso C. Osteoporosis and adynamic bone in chronic kidney disease. J Nephrol. 2013;26(1):73–80.
16. Rodriguez Garcia M, Naves Diaz M, Cannata Andia JB. Bone metabolism, vascular calcifications and mortality: associations beyond mere coincidence. J Nephrol. 2005;18(4):458–63.
17. Roman-Garcia P, Rodriguez-Garcia M, Cabezas-Rodriguez I, Lopez-Ongil S, Diaz-Lopez B, Cannata-Andia JB. Vascular calcification in patients with chronic kidney disease: types, clinical impact and pathogenesis. Med Princ Pract. 2011;20(3):203–12.
18. Ketteler M, Floege J. Clinical management of vascular and soft tissue calcifications in chronic kidney disease patients. In: Olgaard K, Salusky I, Silver J, editors. The spectrum of mineral and bone disorders in chronic kidney disease. Oxford: Oxford University Press; 2010. p. 317–31.
19. Naves-Diaz M, Passlick-Deetjen J, Guinsburg A, Marelli C, Fernandez-Martin JL, Rodriguez-Puyol D, Cannata-Andia JB. Calcium, phosphorus, PTH and death rates in a large sample of dialysis patients from Latin America. The CORES study. Nephrol Dial Transplant. 2011;26(6):1938–47.
20. Rodriguez-Garcia M, Gomez-Alonso C, Naves-Diaz M, Diaz-Lopez JB, Diaz-Corte C, Cannata-Andia JB. Vascular calcifications, vertebral fractures and mortality in haemodialysis patients. Nephrol Dial Transplant. 2009;24(1):239–46.
21. Floege J, Kim J, Ireland E, Chazot C, Drueke T, de Francisco A, Kronenberg F, Marcelli D, Passlick-Deetjen J, Schernthaner G, Fouqueray B, Wheeler DC. Serum iPTH, calcium and phosphate, and the risk of mortality in a European haemodialysis population. Nephrol Dial Transplant. 2011;26(6):1948–55.
22. Jamal SA, Vandermeer B, Raggi P, Mendelssohn DC, Chatterley T, Dorgan M, Lok CE, Fitchett D, Tsuyuki RT. Effect of calcium-based versus non-calcium-based phosphate binders on mortality in patients with chronic kidney disease: an updated systematic review and meta-analysis. Lancet. 2013; 382(9900):1268–77.
23. Cannata-Andia JB, Fernandez-Martin JL, Locatelli F, London G, Gorriz JL, Floege J, Ketteler M, Ferreira A, Covic A, Rutkowski B, Memmos D, Bos WJ, Teplan V, Nagy J, Tielemans C, Verbeelen D, Goldsmith D, Kramar R, Martin PY, Wuthrich RP, Pavlovic D, Benedik M, Sanchez JE, Martinez-Camblor P, Naves-Diaz M, Carrero JJ, Zoccali C. Use of phosphate-binding agents is associated with a lower risk of mortality. Kidney Int. 2013;84(5): 998–1008.
24. Lund RJ, Andress DL, Amdahl M, Williams LA, Heaney RP. Differential effects of paricalcitol and calcitriol on intestinal calcium absorption in hemodialysis patients. Am J Nephrol. 2010;31(2):165–70.
25. Torregrosa JV, Duran CE, Barros X, Blasco M, Arias M, Cases A, Campistol JM. Successful treatment of calcific uraemic arteriolopathy with bisphosphonates. Nefrologia. 2012;32(3):329–34.
26. Cannata-Andia JB, Rodriguez-Garcia M, Carrillo-Lopez N, Diaz-Lopez B. Vascular calcifications: pathogenesis, management, and impact on clinical outcomes. J Am Soc Nephrol. 2006;17(12 Supp 3):S267–73.
27. Cannata-Andia JB, Roman-Garcia P, Hruska K. Connections between vascular calcification and bone health. Nephrol Dial Transplant. 2011;26(11):3429–36.

Protein–Energy Wasting and Nutritional Interventions in Chronic Kidney Disease

17

T. Alp Ikizler

Before You Start: Facts You Need to Know

- Protein–energy wasting is highly prevalent in CKD patients and is a significant predictor of their survival.
- Screening and assessment of nutritional status in CKD and ESRD patients are complicated due to a number of coexisting factors.
- The etiology of PEW in CKD and ESRD patients is multifactorial requiring a comprehensive approach.
- A number of preventive measures can be taken to avoid development of PEW.
- In patients where preventive measures cannot maintain adequate nutritional status, nutritional supplementation is shown to be effective in replenishing protein and energy stores.

17.1 Protein and Energy Wasting in CKD: Definition, Epidemiology, and Clinical Relevance

Among a number of complications of CKD, development of a state of metabolic and nutritional derangements, more aptly called protein–energy wasting (PEW) of chronic kidney disease, constitutes a major role [1]. In general terms, PEW is the state of decreased body stores of protein and energy fuels (i.e., body protein and fat masses) [2]. In CKD, protein or energy depletion can result from an inadequate diet (e.g., anorexia), nonspecific and specific inflammatory processes, factors related to renal replacement therapies, and metabolic and hormonal derangements. Regardless of the etiologic factors, the common physiological phenotype in PEW of CKD is the altered balance between protein synthesis and breakdown toward loss of lean body mass. The absolute or relative decreased lean body mass in turn predisposes the CKD patients to undesirable consequences such as increased risk for infections, development and progression of cardiovascular disease, and progressive sarcopenia and frailty, all of which are directly associated with increased risk of hospitalizations and death.

Virtually every study evaluating the nutritional status of patients with advanced CKD reports some degree of inadequate nutritional status in this population, particularly regarding protein and energy depletion. Due to the many

T.A. Ikizler, MD
Division of Nephrology, Department of Medicine, Vanderbilt University Medical Center, 1161 21st Avenue South, S-3223 Medical Center North, Nashville, TN 37232-2372, USA
e-mail: alp.ikizler@vanderbilt.edu

M. Arici (ed.), *Management of Chronic Kidney Disease*,
DOI 10.1007/978-3-642-54637-2_17,

different diagnostic tools utilized in separate studies, the prevalence of PEW in this patient population varies widely among different reports, ranging from 20 to 60 %. Once CKD patients are initiated on maintenance dialysis, the extent of PEW becomes more evident. Although there is evidence of improvement in nutritional parameters within 3–6 months following initiation of hemodialysis, PEW is still present in up to 40 % or more of the maintenance dialysis patients, and the prevalence seems to increase as the time on dialysis extends.

Most of the epidemiological reports on nutrition in CKD patients have been mainly based on serum albumin concentrations. In the baseline phase of the Hemodialysis (HEMO) Study, 29 % of the patients had albumin levels below 3.5 g/dL. Results from the Dialysis Outcomes and Practice Patterns Study (DOPPS) suggest a lower prevalence of hypoalbuminemia in countries other than the United States such that the lowest mean serum albumin level was observed in the United Kingdom for Europe, whereas the United States value was significantly lower than in all European countries (3.60 vs. 3.72 g/dL [36 vs. 37 g/L]). In a separate analysis, Japan had significantly higher albumin compared with the United States when adjusted for patient age, sex, and day of laboratory draw. In DOPPS II, 20.5 % of the US patients had a serum albumin level less than 3.5 g/dL (35 g/L). Results from the DOPPS also showed a prevalence ranging from 7.6 % (the United States) to 18 % (France) for moderately malnourished and 2.3 % (Italy) to 11 % (the United States) for severely malnourished maintenance hemodialysis (MHD) patients as diagnosed by subjective global assessment (SGA).

The clinical relevance of the aforementioned data is that practically every nutritional marker used in CKD patients has been associated with hospitalization and death risk. These observations are reproducible irrespective of patient demographics and geographical area. Recent epidemiological data also indicate a survival benefit with improvement in these markers over time. This alleged benefit has been observed for serum albumin and body mass index.

17.2 Screening and Assessment of Nutritional Status in CKD

A clinically meaningful assessment of nutritional status should be able to identify and risk-stratify patients with PEW, distinguishing the causes and consequences of both PEW and the underlying disease states, and determine whether there is potential benefit from nutritional interventions [3]. Therefore, no single nutritional marker is likely to adequately phenotype this comorbid state, and a comprehensive assessment of protein and energy nutritional status requires several different measurements. It is also important to apply the nutritional markers according to their appropriate use, i.e., for screening or assessment. Screening parameters are generally collected routinely in clinical practice, taking minimal to no training. They can be completed by any health professional and can provide a trigger to conduct more extensive assessment or to determine best course of treatment. Assessment, on the other hand, generally requires extensive training and provides comprehensive information to inform nutritional diagnosis, intervention, and monitoring plan. Table 17.1 provides a list of screening and assessment tools that can be used to both identify patients at risk and diagnose the ones with PEW.

A diagnosis of PEW necessitates confirmation by several tools and can be as strict as requirement of multiple findings as suggested by International Society of Renal Nutrition and Metabolism (ISRNM) criteria (Table 17.1) or could be less specific as suggested by others [4]. It is important that a number of considerations must be made on the unique situation of CKD patients for appropriate screening and assessment of their nutritional status (Box 17.1).

17.3 Etiology of Protein-Energy Wasting

The etiology of PEW in CKD is complex and multifactorial. As stated in a recent consensus statement by the ISRNM [1], although insufficient food intake (true undernutrition) due to

Table 17.1 Suggested strategies to screen and assess nutritional status in advanced CKD

Screening	*Threshold for detailed assessment*
Body weight	Continuous decline or <85 % IBW
Dietary nutrient intake	DEI <25 kcal/kg IBW/day DPI <0.8 g/kg IBW/day
Serum albumin	<4.0 g/dL
Serum creatinine	Relatively low value
MST	>2
Assessment	*Threshold for intervention*
Serum prealbumin	<28 mg/dL
hsCRP	>10 mg/dL
Anthropometrics	Deviation from norms
SGA	B or C (moderately or severely malnourished)
MIS	>5
Diagnosis (2 of the 4)[a]	*Threshold for intervention*
Serum chemistry	
Albumin	<3.8 g/dL
Prealbumin	<28 mg/dL[b]
Cholesterol	<100 mg/dL
Body mass	
BMI	<23 kg/m^2
Weight loss	>5 % over 3 months or 10 % over 6 months
Total body fat %	<10 %
Muscle mass	
Muscle wasting	>5 % over 3 months or 10 % over 6 months
Reduced MAMC	>10 % reduction compared to norms
Creatinine appearance	<1 g/kg/IBW
Dietary intake	
Low DPI	DPI <0.8 g/kg IBW/day
Low DEI	DEI <25 kcal/kg IBW/day

Source: Adapted from Ikizler [3], with permission of the American Society of Nephrology

IBW ideal body weight, *DEI* dietary energy intake, *DPI* dietary protein intake, *MST* malnutrition screening Tool, *hsCRP* high-sensitivity C-reactive protein, *SGA* subjective global assessment, *MIS* malnutrition inflammation score

[a]ISRNM criteria [2]

[b]Influenced by kidney function

poor appetite and dietary restrictions contributes, other highly prevalent factors are required for PEW to develop. These include alterations related to advanced CKD such as increased energy expenditure, persistent inflammation, metabolic acidosis, and multiple endocrine disorders that render a state of hypermetabolism leading to excess catabolism. In addition, comorbid conditions associated with CKD, poor physical activity, frailty, and the dialysis procedure per se further contribute to PEW. Figure 17.1 provides a conceptual model for etiology of PEW in CKD and its clinical consequences [5].

Box 17.1. Factors That Affect Interpretation of Nutritional Markers in CKD

- Fluid status: Altered body composition and biochemical markers.
- Systemic inflammation: Increased (hsCRP) or decreased (albumin, prealbumin, cholesterol) acute phase protein synthesis.
- Proteinuria: A major determinant of serum albumin levels.
- Residual renal function: Some biochemical markers such as prealbumin are cleared by the kidneys.

17.4 Prevention of PEW: A Cause-Specific Approach

Since a large number of factors affect nutritional and metabolic status in CKD patients leading to multiple adverse consequences [1], prevention and treatment of PEW of CKD should involve an integrated approach to reduce protein and energy depletion, in addition to therapies that will avoid further losses and replenish already wasted stores (Fig. 17.1).

17.4.1 Dietary Nutrient Intake in CKD Patients

A frequent and important cause of PEW in advanced CKD patients is inadequate dietary protein and energy intake relative to their needs, primarily due to uremic anorexia [1]. Anorexia has long been considered to be the hallmark of advanced CKD, and patients

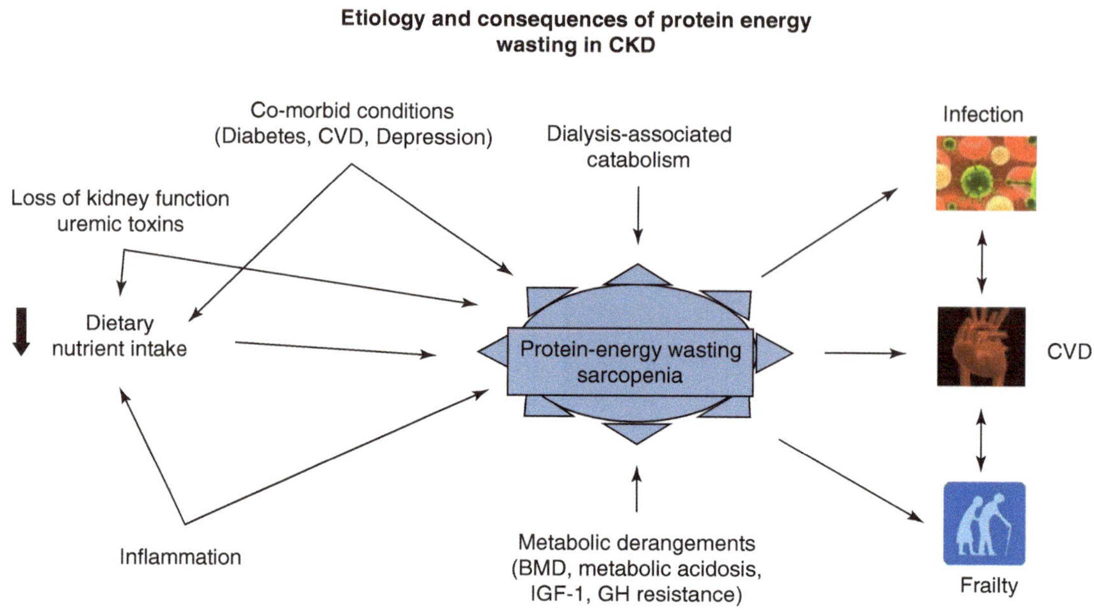

Fig. 17.1 The conceptual model for etiology and consequences of protein–energy wasting (PEW) in chronic kidney disease. *BMD* bone mineral disorders, *IR* insulin resistance, *HPT* hyperparathyroidism, *GH* growth hormone, *CVD* cardiovascular disease (Reprinted from Ikizler et al. [5])

spontaneously restrict their dietary protein intake often to levels less than 0.6 g/kg/day when estimated glomerular filtration rate (eGFR) falls below 15 mL/min. Anorexia in CKD may develop as a result of retention of uremic toxins, intercurrent illness, and inflammation. Inadequate nutrient intake may also be secondary to comorbid illness that affects gastrointestinal function, depression, and poor socioeconomic situation. In clinically stable stage 3–5 CKD patients not on dialysis, dietary protein and energy intakes of 0.6–0.8 g/kg of ideal body weight per day and 30–35 kcal/kg of ideal body weight per day, respectively, are sufficient to preserve their protein stores throughout the progression of kidney disease. However, these levels should be increased when hypermetabolic conditions such as acute illness and hospitalizations occur. Another important implication of anorexia in advanced CKD is its use as a relative indication for initiation of maintenance dialysis, especially when associated with other symptoms or findings such as significant weight loss.

17.4.2 Dietary Protein Restriction in CKD and the Use of Ketoacids

Dietary protein restriction, with or without supplementation of keto-analogs of certain amino acids, has long considered to be an attractive intervention to slow progression of kidney disease [6]. As suggested by a number of meta-analyses, this effect is real, albeit relatively small in the context of progressive kidney disease. Several smaller studies indicate that the favorable effects of dietary protein restriction extend beyond slowing the progression. These include amelioration of metabolic acidosis and insulin resistance, antioxidant effects, and decreasing dietary phosphorus load. The optimal range of dietary protein restriction to exert the most beneficial outcome is not established, and the applicability of dietary protein restriction is limited by compliance.

In addition to protein restriction alone, a number of studies have also examined the effects of keto or amino acid-supplemented low-protein diets [sLPD] or very-low-protein diets [sVLPD] on certain metabolic and renal outcome parameters. Several studies indicated that protein-restricted diets supplemented with keto/amino acids result in a significant decrease in urea production and a beneficial effect on insulin resistance and oxidative stress in humans. A recent consensus statement provided recommendations for obtaining maximum benefit from keto/amino acid-supplemented protein-restricted diets (Box 17.2) [7].

An important consideration regarding dietary protein restriction in CKD is the potential to adversely affect the nutritional status of patients. These concerns have been mostly defied by a number of studies showing that well-designed diets, planned by skilled dietitians and followed by motivated and compliant patients, are effective and do not have harmful effects on the nutritional condition. Long-term follow-up of several relatively large cohorts of CKD patients who received 0.47 g/kg/day protein with the keto acid supplementation showed no detrimental effect on the outcome of the patients after initiating any kind of renal replacement therapy. It was also demonstrated in a 5-year follow-up study that CKD patients treated with LPDs were found to rapidly increase their dietary protein intake with a gain in lean body mass index after beginning the renal replacement therapy with a low mortality and morbidity rate. Accordingly, one can conclude that prescribing low-protein diets with or without keto or amino acid supplementation with adequate caloric intake and close supervision does not seem to lead to protein–energy wasting.

Box 17.2. Considerations for Maximum Efficacy and Safety of Administration of Keto/Amino Acid-Supplemented Protein-Restricted Diets

- Patient selection: Motivation and ability to follow a protein-restricted diet
- Gradual implementation of intervention (i.e., progressive 0.2 g/kg/day steps)
- Support and educational tools along with regular dietary counseling (every 2–3 months initially)
- Involvement of dieticians

17.4.3 Renal Replacement Therapy as a Catabolic Stimulus

A minimum dose of dialysis is required to avoid uremic anorexia and maintain optimal dietary nutrient intake. Based on data from large randomized clinical trials, current guidelines for adequate dialysis are considered sufficient to preserve the nutritional status although HEMO study showed that MHD patients lose weight over time regardless of "adequate" dialysis dose. Increasing dialysis dose beyond current targets has not been shown to improve the nutritional status any further. There is suggestion that the use of high-flux dialysis membranes provides a nominally significant survival benefit in patients with baseline serum albumin levels <40 g/dL and with diabetes mellitus. The results of the frequent hemodialysis trial indicate no appreciable difference in nutritional markers between subjects randomized to 6×/week in-center HD versus standard 3×/week in-center HD.

In ESRD patients on maintenance dialysis, there are additional protein catabolic processes such as the unavoidable loss of amino acids (6–8 g per HD session and 1–2 g per day during PD) and albumin into the dialysate and the inflammatory stimulus associated with the dialysis procedure or other components of ESRD (i.e., hemodialysis catheters). This requires that dietary protein intake targets need to be adjusted once the patient is initiated on maintenance dialysis, which is provided in Table 17.2 [8]. Along with the protein intake, energy intake should be adjusted based on the physical activity levels as shown in Box 17.3. An important consideration regarding strategies to improve dietary protein intake in ESRD patients is the potential increase in the intake of several potentially harmful elements, especially phosphorus [11]. Dietary recommendations to improve protein intake should take into account the phosphorus content of the specific protein sources (i.e., vegetarian diet

Table 17.2 What the guidelines say you should do: protein intake recommendations in CKD

	Non-dialysis CKD	Hemodialysis	Peritoneal dialysis
National Kidney Foundation K/DOQI [8]	0.6–0.75 g/kgBW*/day	>1.2 g/kgBW/day	1.2–1.3 g/kgBW/day
British Dietetic Association [9]	N/A	>1.1 g/kgBW/day	>1/2 g/kgBW/day
ESPEN (Nutritional Support) [10]	0.6–0.8 g/kgBW/day	1.2–1/4 g/kgBW/day	1.2–1.5 g/kgBW/day
	Illness 1.0 g/kg	Illness >1/5 g/ideal body weight kg/day	

>50 % of high biological value (i.e., complete protein sources, containing the full spectrum of essential amino acids)
*BW = ideal body weight in nonobese patients. Use adjusted body weight in obese patients = ideal body weight + 0.25×(actual body weight − ideal body weight)

Box 17.3. What the Guidelines Say You Should Do: Energy Intake Recommendations in CKD

Sufficient energy (kcal) intake is critical to promote nitrogen balance.

Early and Predialysis CKD

Stages 1–2: Same as general population

Stages 3–5: 30–35 kcal/kg of ideal or adjusted body weight/day (age dependent)

Dialysis (*stage 5*): 30–35 kcal/kg of ideal or adjusted body weight (age dependent)

Decreased requirements	Increased requirements
Over ideal body weight	Maintenance dialysis
Age >60 years	Undernutrition
Limited activity	<60 years
Bed bound (no concurrent illness)	Routine or increased physical activity
	Acute illness, hypermetabolic state

Source: Data from NKF/KDOQI [8]

leading to lower serum phosphorus levels) and other phosphorus-containing nutrients especially the ones with additives/preservatives in processed food.

17.4.4 Systemic Inflammation

Systemic inflammation is a major contributor to PEW of CKD [12]. The elevated systemic concentrations of pro-inflammatory cytokines are thought to play an integral role in the muscle catabolism of ESRD patients. Interleukin-6 (IL-6) causes increased muscle proteolysis, which can be ameliorated by the administration of IL-6 receptor antibody and interleukin-1 (IL-1), and tumor necrosis factor-alpha (TNFα) can cause anorexia through their effects on the satiety center in the central nervous system.

There are a number of factors that can cause systemic inflammation in CKD and ESRD patients (Fig. 17.2). The most crucial step for treatment of systemic inflammation is elimination of etiologic factors such as the use of central hemodialysis catheters in MHD patients. As the dialysis procedure per se might stimulate the immune system, pro-inflammatory effects of dialysis membranes and fluids should also be taken into account in maintenance dialysis patients. Many uremic toxins are also known to be pro-inflammatory. Appropriate management of fluid status might improve systemic inflammation in ESRD patients since volume overload leads to immunoactivation and increased cytokine production via bacterial or endotoxin translocation.

17.4.5 Comorbidities in CKD

CKD patients often have other comorbid diseases that can adversely affect their nutritional status such as diabetes mellitus, cardiovascular disease, and depression. Diabetic CKD patients are likely to suffer protein depletion because of associated gastrointestinal disturbances (e.g., diabetic gastroparesis, nausea and vomiting, bacterial overgrowth in the gut and pancreatic insufficiency, impaired protein absorption in the gut) and increased protein breakdown secondary to insu-

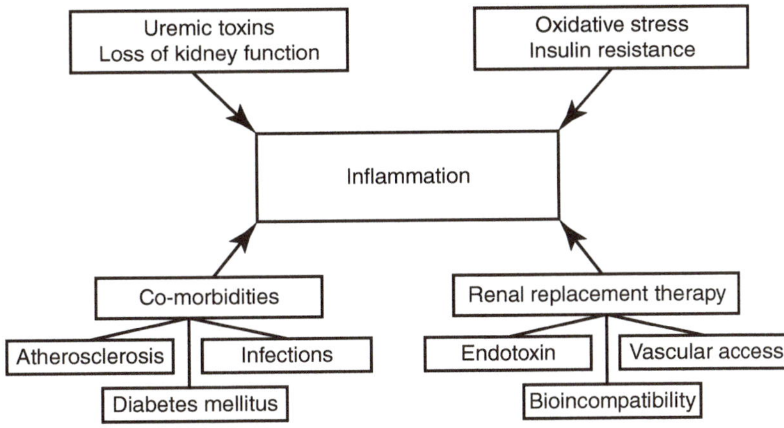

Fig. 17.2 A number of modifiable and non-modifiable factors lead to the chronic inflammatory state of chronic kidney disease (Reprinted from Ikizler [4])

lin resistance. Polypharmacy worsens these gastrointestinal complications. Uncontrolled hyperparathyroidism and cardiac cachexia are associated with systemic inflammation and increased energy expenditure. Depressive symptoms, which are common in CKD and ESRD patients, are linked to fatigue, lack of appetite, and weight loss. Early recognition and treatment are important components in the prevention of PEW.

17.4.6 Metabolic Acidosis

Metabolic acidosis is associated with increased muscle protein catabolism and promotes PEW in patients with advanced CKD. Metabolic acidosis stimulates the oxidation of essential amino acids and further raises protein requirements for patients on maintenance dialysis. Oral or intradialytic (specifically in PD patients) bicarbonate supplementation was associated with increased dietary protein and energy intake, improved mid-arm muscle circumference (MAMC), and improved serum albumin level, and progression of CKD was slowed in stage 3–4 CKD patients. A steady-state serum bicarbonate level should be greater than 24 mmol/L in CKD patients not yet on maintenance dialysis and PD patients. Based on epidemiological data, a target of predialysis serum bicarbonate level of 22–24 mmol/L is recommended in MHD patients.

17.5 Treatment of Protein–Energy Wasting

17.5.1 Oral and Enteral Nutritional Supplementation

In certain CKD and ESRD patients, the aforementioned standard preventive measures are unable to diminish loss of protein and energy stores [13]. In these circumstances, nutritional supplementation is a suitable next step with appropriate indications (Fig. 17.3).

The efficacy of oral supplementation has been studied in multiple settings (reviewed in detail by Ikizler et al. [5]). The beneficial nutritional effects of these supplements ranged from improvements in serum biomarkers such as albumin, prealbumin, and transferrin to gains in different body compartments such as weight and lean body mass and improvements in quality of life and physical functioning. The effects were evident as early as within a month and were sustained in most if not all studies. It is important to note that oral supplementation is the first choice for these patients. If it is not sufficient, enteral tube feeding should be instituted. For patients who are unable to tolerate nutritional supplementation by mouth, nasogastric tubes, percutaneous endoscopic gastroscopy, or jejunostomy tubes can be considered. Enteral tube feeding is most often used in conditions such as severe anorexia, swallowing troubles secondary to neurologic or head and neck diseases, perioperative periods, and stress. Hospitalized or institution-

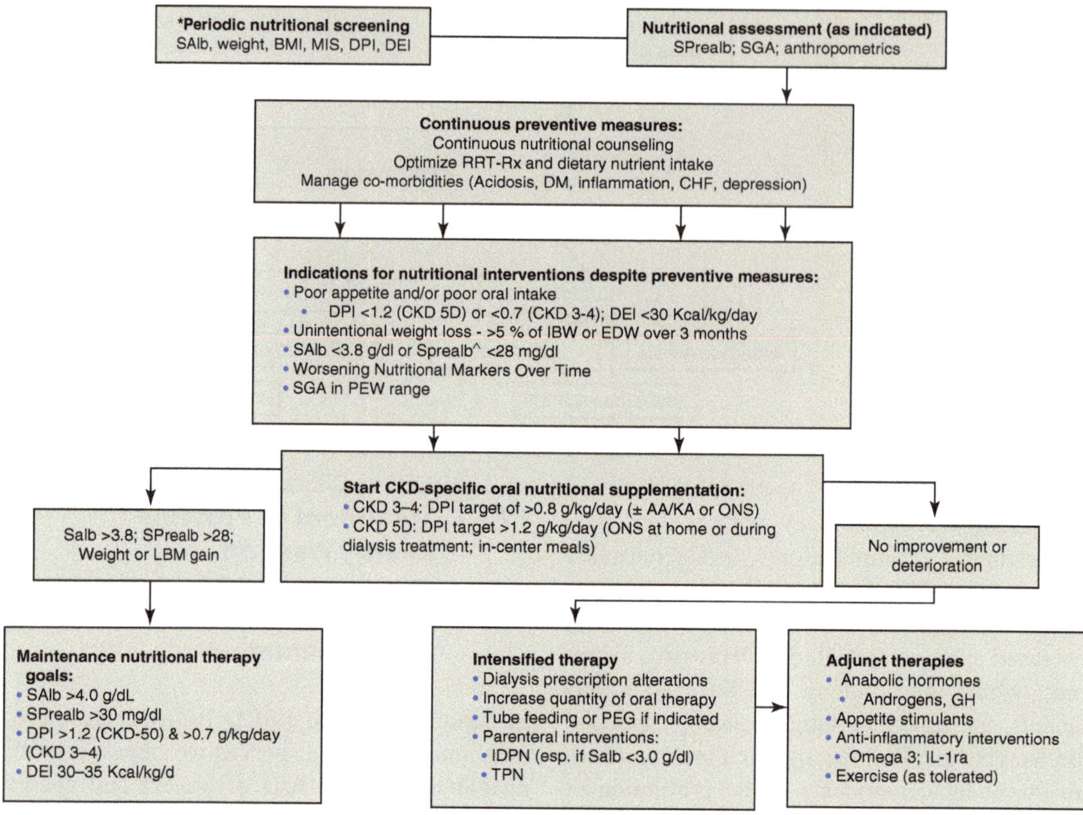

Fig. 17.3 Algorithm for nutritional management and support in patients with chronic kidney disease. *Minimum every 3 months, monthly screening recommended. ^ Only for ESRD patients without residual renal function. Abbreviations: *SAlb* serum albumin (measured by bromocresol green), *BMI* body mass index, MIS malnutrition–inflammation score, *DPI* dietary protein intake, *DEI* dietary energy intake, *SPrealb* serum prealbumin, *SGA* subjective global assessment, *RRT-Rx* renal replacement therapy prescription, *DM* diabetes mellitus, *CHF* congestive heart failure, *CKD* chronic kidney disease, *PEW* protein–energy wasting, *LBM* lean body mass, *ONS* oral nutritional supplement, *PEG* percutaneous endoscopic gastrostomy, *IDPN* intradialytic parenteral nutrition, *TPN* total parenteral nutrition, *GH* growth hormone, *IL-1ra* interleukin-1 receptor antagonist (Reprinted from Ikizler et al. [5])

alized CKD patients also often ingest even lower amounts of their usual protein and energy intake (as low as 66 and 50 %, respectively).

Oral supplementation should be given two to three times a day, preferably 1 h after main meals and/or during dialysis for MHD patients. Oral supplementation can provide an additional 7–10 kcal/kg per day of energy and 0.3–0.4 g/kg per day of protein. This requires a minimum spontaneous dietary intake of 20 kcal/kg per day of energy and 0.4–0.8 g/kg per day of protein in order to meet the recommended dietary energy intake (DEI) and dietary protein intake (DPI) targets. Oral nutritional supplements are typically multi-nutrient containing a mix of macronutrients (protein, carbohydrate, fat) and micronutrients (vitamins, minerals, trace elements). Most are liquid, but there are also puddings and bars available. Different flavors and components can be used to improve compliance and tolerability. Different formulations, including disease and stage (renal) specific, are also available [14].

Despite a large body of evidence indicating the nutritional efficacy of supplementation, there are a few studies that have carefully assessed their effects on hospitalization and mortality. Two recent large-scale observational studies reported significant survival benefit in favor of hypoalbuminemic MHD patients receiving nutritional supplementation versus similarly matched controls.

In these studies, oral nutritional supplement use was associated with higher serum albumin, lower hospitalization, and lower mortality. The limitations of these studies include their retrospective design, convenience sampling, and residual confounding from unmeasured variables. There are no prospective RCTs to examine the effects of oral nutritional supplementation on mortality and morbidity.

17.5.2 Intradialytic Parenteral Nutrition (IDPN)

Parenteral provision of nutrients, especially during the HD procedure (i.e., IDPN), has been shown to be a safe and convenient approach for individuals who cannot tolerate oral or enteral administration of nutrients. Parenteral nutrition is also administered in hospitalized patients with underlying CKD or newly developed acute kidney injury. The indications for parenteral nutrition in these patients are similar to any patients admitted to hospital. Box 17.4 outlines the additional guidelines that should be considered in ESRD patients (Box 17.5).

The efficacy of IDPN has been shown in several studies, albeit most of those are hampered by some design issues. In terms of comparison to oral supplementation, a large RCT showed that similar improvements in nutritional parameters are observed when adequate and comparable protein and energy are provided to the patients [15]. Other clinically relevant conclusions that can be driven from available RCTs using IDPN or ONS include the direct correlation between

Box 17.4. What the Guidelines Say You Should Do: Intradialytic Parenteral Nutrition (IDPN) in ESRD Patients

- In non-acutely ill malnourished HD patients, IDPN is infused through the venous line during dialysis with constant rate of infusion throughout the whole session.
- The rate should be progressively increased from 8 mL/kg during the first week to a maximum of 16 mL/kg.
- There should be controlled ultrafiltration to compensate fluid intake, and 75 mmol of Na should be added per liter of IDPN.

Box 17.5. Relevant Guidelines

1. Kopple JD. National kidney foundation K/DOQI clinical practice guidelines for nutrition in chronic renal failure. Am J Kidney Dis. 2001;37(1 Suppl 2): S66–70 [8].
2. Cano N, Fiaccadori E, Tesinsky P, Toigo G, Druml W; DGEM (German Society for Nutritional Medicine), et al. ESPEN guidelines on enteral nutrition: adult renal failure. Clin Nutr. 2006;25(2):295–310 [10].
3. Fouque D, Kalantar-Zadeh K, Kopple J, Cano N, Chauveau P, Cuppari L, et al. A proposed nomenclature and diagnostic criteria for protein-energy wasting in acute and chronic kidney disease. Kidney Int. 2008; 73(4):391–8 [2].
4. Cano NJ, Aparicio M, Brunori G, Carrero JJ, Cianciaruso B, Fiaccadori E, et al. ESPEN Guidelines on parenteral nutrition: adult renal failure. Clin Nutr. 2009;28(4):401–14 [16].
5. Ikizler TA, Cano NJ, Franch H, Fouque D, Himmelfarb J, Kalantar-Zadeh K, et al. Prevention and treatment of protein energy wasting in chronic kidney disease patients: a consensus statement by the International Society of Renal Nutrition and Metabolism. Kidney Int. 2013 [5].
6. Naylor HL, Jackson H, Walker GH, Macafee S, Magee K, Hooper L, et al. British Dietetic Association evidence-based guidelines for the protein requirements of adults undergoing maintenance haemodialysis or peritoneal dialysis. J Hum Nutr Diet. 2013;26(4):315–28 [9].

response to nutritional supplementation and the severity of PEW and the amount of nutrients received, diabetic patients showing a reduced response to nutritional support in terms of serum albumin and the observation that inflammatory status does not significantly affect the response to nutritional support. It should be noted that high cost of IDPN therapy and the regulatory concerns remain the greatest barriers for the use of IDPN, which should be reserved for patients where PO or enteral supplements are not feasible. Similar studies using amino acids in dialysate (AAD) as a nutritional intervention in PD patients with PEW have shown that AAD remains to be a viable option in PD patients with PEW who cannot tolerate or are not suitable for PO and other enteral supplements.

17.5.3 Adjunctive Therapies

17.5.3.1 Exercise

Abnormalities in muscle function such as reductions in oxidative capacity and type 1 fibers, exercise performance, and physical activity begin in the early stages of CKD and progress dramatically as ESRD develops [17]. A number of studies have shown the efficacy of cardiopulmonary fitness training in ESRD patients, whereas relatively few studies have examined the role of exercise training on stimulating the muscle growth. Collectively, the available data indicate that the presumed beneficial effects of exercise such as improvements in muscle quality and quantity, strength, and physical functioning are not consistently observed in ESRD patients. The possible explanations for the limited efficacy of exercise in CKD patients include the limitations of methods to assess body composition, inadequate intensity and/or duration of exercise, and the lack of understanding of the actual metabolic and morphologic abnormalities related to PEW in the setting of advanced CKD.

17.5.3.2 Anabolic Hormones

Recombinant human growth hormone (rhGH), an approved treatment of short stature in pediatric CKD patients, leads to improved growth, confirming that rhGH could overcome GH resistance associated with CKD. In adults with CKD, resistance to native GH may be responsible for the premature decline in body composition. In a large multicenter RCT, significant decreases were observed in C-reactive protein (CRP) and homocysteine levels along with increases in serum high-density lipoprotein (HDL) cholesterol and transferrin levels in hypoalbuminemic MHD patients. Unfortunately, this large RCT was prematurely terminated due to slow recruitment, without the ability to assess the effects of rhGH on hospitalization or death.

Testosterone deficiency is also very common in male MHD patients and is associated with increased mortality risk. Several RCTs performed in MHD patients showed significant benefits of nandrolone decanoate (ND) treatment in both anthropometric and biochemical parameters including body weight, body mass index, skinfold, MAMC, and serum levels of total protein, prealbumin, and transferrin. No consistent effect of ND was demonstrated on physical functioning in several studies, and high-dose ND (100 mg/week) was intolerable in females because of its virilizing effects. In clinical practice, anabolic steroids could be used for preventing sarcopenia, albeit under close supervision, and its use should be limited to 6 months.

17.5.3.3 Other Therapies for Treatment of PEW in CKD

Appetite stimulants have been long used for increasing nutrient intake in patients with chronic diseases and malnutrition. Examples of pharmacological agents that may stimulate appetite include megestrol acetate, dronabinol, cyproheptadine, melatonin, thalidomide, and ghrelin. Most of these drugs have not been studied systematically in CKD patients. In several small studies, megestrol acetate stimulated appetite and induced small increases in serum albumin and weight in maintenance dialysis patients, but large-scale prospective studies are needed to assess whether these drugs provide adjunctive nutritional therapy for CKD patients. Ghrelin is an orexigenic peptide released primarily from the stomach, which increases appetite and adjusts both short- and long-term energy balances making it a good candidate for treatment of anorexic ESRD patients. Several small studies in PD patients showed increased calorie intake with short-term ghrelin administration. When comorbidities and potential dialysis-related causes of inflammation have been evaluated and appropriately treated, other anti-inflammatory treatment strategies such as anti-oxidative and/or bioecological strategies or targeted anti-cytokine therapies could be considered in CKD patients who are persistently inflamed. There are no large-scale studies examining the effects of any of the targeted anti-inflammatory agents on nutritional markers in CKD patients.

17.5.4 Obesity in CKD

Insulin resistance (IR), glucose intolerance, prediabetes, and diabetes mellitus represent a continuum of abnormalities in glucose and insulin homeostasis, which are highly prevalent in CKD and ESRD patients. Obesity plays a central role in initiation and/or acceleration of these derangements [18]. Insulin resistance is an established risk factor for the development of cardiovascular and all-cause mortality in CKD patients, including those on dialysis. In addition, protein metabolism is dramatically affected by IR, leading to increased catabolism, to result in a higher incidence and prevalence of PEW. Insulin resistance can be caused by underlying metabolic acidosis, oxidative stress, inflammation, accumulation of uremic toxins, vitamin D deficiency, physical inactivity, and the accumulation of fat mass, in particular truncal fat mass, which is common in these patients [19]. Appropriate management of factors leading to or worsening IR is an important strategy to prevent or treat PEW in CKD patients.

Overweight and obesity are defined as abnormal or excessive fat accumulation that may impair health. Obesity increases the risk for CKD and its progression to ESRD in addition to carrying markedly increased risk for other comorbid complications, such as type 2 diabetes, cancer, hypertension, dyslipidemia, cardiovascular disease, Alzheimer's disease, and sleep apnea [18]. Obesity also leads to sarcopenia in CKD and ESRD patients. Obesity induced decrease in adipokine secretion combined with increased inflammation, and insulin resistance leads to muscle wasting and sarcopenia. Decreased physical activity and physical functioning in return further worsens obesity leading to the "sarcopenic obesity" phenotype which is characterized by a vicious cycle. Management of obesity in stage 1–5 CKD patients, not on maintenance dialysis and kidney transplant patients, is similar to general population. Specifically, lifestyle changes such as walking or cycling instead of driving, routine exercise such as 30 min 3×/week walking or running, and calorie restriction are key management strategies. Calorie restriction includes reduction by 500 kcal/day in the absence of physical activity, which could lead to weight loss of 1 lb/week.

Management of obesity of maintenance dialysis patients is more controversial. In the general population, a high BMI is associated with increased cardiovascular disease and all-cause mortality. However, the effect of overweight (BMI: 25–30) or obesity (BMI: >30) in ESRD patients is paradoxically in the opposite direction; i.e., a high BMI is associated with improved survival. It is suggested that residual confounding by protein–energy wasting, inflammation, and competing mortality risk factors explain this phenomenon. Despite overwhelming epidemiological data on this association, a generalization of this sort, i.e., increased BMI is always good in ESRD, would actually be inappropriate, and further consideration of certain phenotypic features is necessary for proper management of these patients. For example, additional data indicate that also differences in body composition, i.e., total fat mass versus muscle mass and visceral versus non-visceral fat mass, could be the underlying mechanism leading to differing morbidity and mortality risk in ESRD patients. Accordingly, certain ESRD patients may benefit from weight loss. These include candidates for kidney transplantation, diabetic ESRD patients with poor glycemic control, and patients with significant issues with physical activity due to morbid obesity. There are no pharmacological agents approved for weight loss. Bariatric surgery can be considered if above measures fail and if BMI >45 kg/m^2.

Before You Finish: Practice Pearls for the Clinician

- Screening and assessment of PEW require special consideration in CKD patients. Screening for patients at risk can be completed by any health professional and should provide a trigger to conduct more extensive assessment. Assessment should be performed by individuals with training and should guide intervention and monitoring plan.
- In CKD and ESRD patients, in whom a number of catabolic signals dominate, it is critical to maintain a dietary protein and energy intake relative to needs.
- Preemptive treatment of concurrent conditions that contribute to catabolism, such as metabolic acidosis, insulin resistance, and systemic inflammation, is of paramount importance for the prevention of PEW.
- Supplemental nutrition could be indicated in a significant number of CKD and ESRD patients, especially the ones with comorbid conditions and elderly.
- When prescribing oral nutritional support, physiological aspects of the patient and supplement, tolerability, nutritional efficacy, and availability should be taken to account. In general, oral or enteral nutrition are preferable to intradialytic or daily parenteral nutrition.
- Oral nutritional supplementation, especially when provided around the time of hemodialysis such as intradialytic administration, has been shown to exert both short- and long-term nutritional benefits in maintenance dialysis patients.
- Oral nutritional supplementation may improve clinical outcomes based on cohort studies. However, there are no large adequately powered randomized clinical trials that have tested the effectiveness of nutritional interventions on morbidity and mortality.

References

1. Carrero JJ, Stenvinkel P, Cuppari L, Ikizler TA, Kalantar-Zadeh K, Kaysen G, et al. Etiology of the protein-energy wasting syndrome in chronic kidney disease: a consensus statement from the International Society of Renal Nutrition and Metabolism (ISRNM). J Ren Nutr. 2013;23(2):77–90. Epub 2013/02/23.
2. Fouque D, Kalantar-Zadeh K, Kopple J, Cano N, Chauveau P, Cuppari L, et al. A proposed nomenclature and diagnostic criteria for protein-energy wasting in acute and chronic kidney disease. Kidney Int. 2008;73(4):391–8. Epub 2007/12/21.
3. Ikizler TA. A patient with CKD and poor nutritional status. Clin J Am Soc Nephrol. 2013;8(12): 2174–82.
4. Ikizler TA. Optimal nutrition in hemodialysis patients. Adv Chronic Kidney Dis. 2013;20(2):181–9. Epub 2013/02/27.
5. Ikizler TA, Cano NJ, Franch H, Fouque D, Himmelfarb J, Kalantar-Zadeh K, et al. Prevention and treatment of protein energy wasting in chronic kidney disease patients: a consensus statement by the International Society of Renal Nutrition and Metabolism. Kidney Int. 2013;84(6):1096–107.
6. Fouque D, Aparicio M. Eleven reasons to control the protein intake of patients with chronic kidney disease. Nat Clin Pract Nephrol. 2007;3(7):383–92. Epub 2007/06/27.
7. Aparicio M, Bellizzi V, Chauveau P, Cupisti A, Ecder T, Fouque D, et al. Keto acid therapy in predialysis chronic kidney disease patients: final consensus. J Ren Nutr. 2012;22(2):S22–4.
8. Kopple JD. National kidney foundation K/DOQI clinical practice guidelines for nutrition in chronic renal failure. Am J Kidney Dis. 2001;37(1 Suppl 2): S66–70.
9. Naylor HL, Jackson H, Walker GH, Macafee S, Magee K, Hooper L, et al. British Dietetic Association evidence-based guidelines for the protein requirements of adults undergoing maintenance haemodialysis or peritoneal dialysis. J Hum Nutr Diet. 2013; 26(4):315–28.
10. Cano N, Fiaccadori E, Tesinsky P, Toigo G, Druml W, Kuhlmann M, et al. ESPEN guidelines on enteral nutrition: adult renal failure. Clin Nutr. 2006; 25(2):295–310. Epub 2006/05/16.
11. Kovesdy CP, Shinaberger CS, Kalantar-Zadeh K. Epidemiology of dietary nutrient intake in ESRD. Semin Dial. 2010;23(4):353–8. Epub 2010/06/19.
12. Stenvinkel P. Can treating persistent inflammation limit protein energy wasting? Semin Dial. 2013;26(1): 16–9. Epub 2012/10/10.
13. Kalantar-Zadeh K, Ikizler TA. Let them eat during dialysis: an overlooked opportunity to improve outcomes in maintenance hemodialysis patients. J Ren Nutr. 2013;23(3):157–63. Epub 2013/01/15.

14. Rocco MV, Ikizler TA. Nutrition. In: Daugirdas J, Blake PG, Ing TS, editors. Handbook of dialysis. 4th ed. Philadelphia: Lippincott Williams & Wilkins; 2006. p. 462–81.
15. Cano NJ, Fouque D, Roth H, Aparicio M, Azar R, Canaud B, et al. Intradialytic parenteral nutrition does not improve survival in malnourished hemodialysis patients: a 2-year multicenter, prospective, randomized study. J Am Soc Nephrol. 2007;18(9):2583–91.
16. Cano NJ, Aparicio M, Brunori G, Carrero JJ, Cianciaruso B, Fiaccadori E, et al. ESPEN guidelines on parenteral nutrition: adult renal failure. Clin Nutr. 2009;28(4):401–14.
17. Ikizler TA. Exercise as an anabolic intervention in patients with end-stage renal disease. J Ren Nutr. 2011;21(1):52–6. Epub 2011/01/05.
18. Stenvinkel P, Zoccali C, Ikizler TA. Obesity in CKD–what should nephrologists know? J Am Soc Nephrol. 2013;24:1727–36.
19. Hung AM, Ikizler TA. Factors determining insulin resistance in chronic hemodialysis patients. Contrib Nephrol. 2011;171:127–34. Epub 2011/06/01.

18 Infectious Complications and Vaccination in Chronic Kidney Disease

Vivek Kumar and Vivekanand Jha

Before You Start: Things You Need to Know

- Infections are the second most common cause of morbidity and mortality in chronic kidney disease (CKD) patients.
- Infections increase the risk of adverse cardiovascular events in CKD.
- Uraemia-induced immune dysfunction, frequent visits to health-care facilities, frequent hospitalisation, need for vascular catheters and extracorporeal treatment increase infection risk.
- Preventing infections is of utmost importance both in pre-dialysis and dialysis-dependent CKD patients.

V. Kumar, MBBS, MD, DM
V. Jha, MD, DM, FRCP (✉)
Department of Nephrology, Postgraduate Institute of Medical Education and Research, Sector 12, Chandigarh 160 012, India
e-mail: enigma165@yahoo.co.in; vjha@pginephro.org

18.1 Infections and Chronic Kidney Disease

Chronic kidney disease (CKD) is recognised as an important global health-care concern. The National Chronic Kidney Disease Fact Sheet 2010 released by Centers for Disease Control and Prevention (CDC) estimates that >10 % of the US population aged 20 years or older have CKD. Besides being common, CKD affects the poor disproportionately and has major impact on the outcome of other major non-communicable diseases like diabetes and hypertension, 35 and 20 % of whom develop CKD [1].

Infection control remains a major public health goal worldwide. Over the last few decades, a complex interplay between infections and CKD has become evident. A number of infections can cause kidney disease, and CKD predisposes patients to various infections. Chronic infections with organisms like hepatitis C virus (HCV), hepatitis B virus (HBV) and human immunodeficiency virus (HIV) are responsible for a substantial proportion of CKD in some parts of the world. In addition, infection-related acute kidney injury may not recover completely and lead to CKD.

The high incidence of infections in CKD patients, including those on dialysis and after kidney transplantation, has been known for decades. Infections are the second most common cause of morbidity and mortality in these patients after cardiovascular disease [2]. A number of risk factors increase the risk for infections in patients

M. Arici (ed.), *Management of Chronic Kidney Disease*,
DOI 10.1007/978-3-642-54637-2_18, © Springer-Verlag Berlin Heidelberg 2014

with kidney disease (Box 18.1). These include alterations in specific functions of various components of innate and adaptive immune system (Box 18.2). These changes are also responsible for poor response to vaccinations and failure to maintain protective antibody titres in CKD.

Though infections and cardiovascular disease may appear to be distinct clinical problems, modulation of underlying inflammatory state may be a common denominator linking the two in CKD. Data from United States Renal Data System (USRDS) Wave 2 study showed that the presence of bacteremia or septicaemia was associated with increased risk of death [hazard ratio (HR) 2.33, 95 % confidence interval (CI) 1.38–2.28], myocardial infarction (HR 1.78, 95 % CI 1.38–2.28), heart failure (HR 1.64, 95 % CI 1.39–1.95), peripheral vascular disease (HR 1.64, 95 % CI 1.34–2.0) and stroke (HR 2.04, 95 % CI 1.27–3.28) [3]. Analysis of USRDS data revealed that the risk of cardiovascular events was increased by 25 and 18 % at 1 and 3 months after an episode of infection-related hospitalisation compared to control periods [4]. These observational studies lend support to the intriguing hypothesis that the superimposition of macro-inflammatory events like bacterial infections over the persistent micro-inflammatory state of CKD might increase cardiovascular disease risk, despite apparent recovery from the infectious episode.

Box 18.1. Risk Factors for Infections in Kidney Disease

1. Old age
2. Female sex
3. African American race
4. Presence of diabetes mellitus
5. Malnutrition
6. Hypoalbuminaemia
7. Impaired cutaneous defence
   (a) Severe oedema
   (b) Use of vascular access and peritoneal dialysis catheters
   (c) Needlestick injury for native arteriovenous fistulae or grafts
8. Therapy related
   (a) Use of immunosuppressive drugs for treatment of basic disease
   (b) RBC or blood products transfusion
   (c) Contaminated caregiver's hands or gloves, equipment, supplies and environmental surfaces
   (d) Use of iron preparations*
   (e) Bioincompatible dialysis*
9. Increased hospitalisation for non-infectious complications
10. Immunological dysfunction
11. Poor vaccine response

*Increase oxidative stress

Box 18.2. Immune System Alterations in CKD

1. *Polymorphonuclear leucocyte dysfunction*
   (a) Increased reactive oxygen species production
   (b) Increased apoptosis
   (c) Spontaneous activation and degranulation
   (d) Decreased phagocytosis
2. *Depletion of antigen presenting cells*
3. *Monocyte dysfunction*
   (a) Increased circulating monocytes (especially $CD14^{+}CD16^{+}$ monocytes)
   (b) Increased reactive oxygen species production
   (c) Increased basal integrin, toll-like receptor (TLR)-2 and TLR-4 expression
   (d) Increased cytokine production
   (e) Decreased phagocytosis
4. *T-cell dysfunction*
   (a) Decreased regulatory T (Treg) cells
   (b) Reduced CD4/CD8 T-cell ratio
   (c) Decreased memory T cells (both central and naïve)
5. *B-cell dysfunction*
   (a) Decreased B-cell number
   (b) Decreased antibody production

18.2 Epidemiology of Infections in CKD

For the purposes of discussion of infections, it is useful to divide the CKD population into two groups: pre-dialysis CKD and dialysis-dependent CKD. Besides becoming a defining moment for patient and treating physician as this change affects patient's daily lifestyle and management, initiation of dialysis also alters the risk and consequences of infection by repeatedly breaching the physical defences and altering immune functions.

Pre-dialysis CKD patients have 3 times more risk of developing infectious complications as compared to general population [5]. Based on the 2001 Medicare data, urinary tract infection (UTI), pneumonia and bacteraemia or sepsis were four times, three times and four times, respectively, more common in pre-dialysis CKD population in the USA compared to the general population [5]. Sepsis and pneumonia were encountered in end stage renal disease (ESRD) patients ten times and five times more commonly than general population [5]. Recent data from Cardiovascular Health Study (CHS) showed that after a median follow-up of 11.5 years, risk of all-cause hospitalisation secondary to infectious events increased 16, 37 and 64 % in participants over the age of 65 with estimated glomerular filtration rate (eGFR) of (calculated using serum cystatin C level) 60–89, 45–59 and 15–44 mL/min/1.73 m^2, respectively, as compared to those with eGFR ≥90 mL/min/1.73 m^2 [6]. The risks of UTI and pneumonia were 160 and 80 % more in patients with eGFR 15–44 mL/min/1.73 m^2 when compared to those with eGFR ≥90 mL/min/1.73 m^2 [6].

The USRDS 2012 Annual Data Report identified infections as an important consequence of declining GFR [2]. In this report, mortality rates due to infection in the US ESRD population on haemodialysis in 2010 were 40 and 21 per 1,000 patient-years at risk at 2 months and 12 months after initiation of dialysis, respectively, after adjustment for age, gender, race, Hispanic ethnicity and primary diagnosis [2]. Also, hospitalisation rates due to infection in CKD stages 4–5 were 50–72 % higher than the rates for lower stages of CKD. In 2010, hospitalisation rates in haemodialysis patients in the USA were 0.46 and 0.11 per patient per year for infections overall and vascular access-related infections, respectively [2]. Rehospitalisation rate during transition to dialysis was highest if the index hospitalisation was infection related. During the quarter before initiation of dialysis, 44 % of patients were readmitted within 30 days of discharge after an infection-associated hospitalisation [2]. In the quarter after dialysis initiation, 44 % of patients died or needed rehospitalisation within 30 days of discharge after infection-associated hospitalisation [2]. Therefore, it appears that infections not only lead to acute problems but may also identify patients at higher risk of repeated hospitalisations. Whether this risk is related to infections or is a marker of otherwise poor underlying state is not clear.

18.2.1 Urinary Tract Infections (UTI)

UTIs are more common in certain subpopulations with CKD. These include patients with vesicoureteric reflux; interference with the normal flow of urine, either due to structural lesions, stricture, renal stone disease or secondary to functional problems like neurogenic bladder and diabetic cystopathy; or specific abnormalities like polycystic kidney disease. In addition to the frequency, some conditions can lead to more severe and/or special forms of UTI such as acute pyelonephritis, renal abscesses, renal papillary necrosis, emphysematous and xanthogranulomatous pyelonephritis or renal mucormycosis.

Another important consideration is distinguishing colonisation from true UTI especially in patients with underlying risk factors. A diagnosis of UTI should be made only when a patient is symptomatic, urinalysis shows significant pyuria (>9 pus cells/hpf) and urine culture shows a significant growth. Asymptomatic bacteriuria is treated only in pregnant females and patients who have to undergo either surgery or instrumentation of the urinary tract which may involve mucosal breach.

Established UTI in patients with CKD is treated as in general population. However, certain important considerations apply in this situation.

First, if the basic disease leading to CKD is associated with any structural or functional alteration in the urinary tract, the initial treatment course is given for extended period (2–4 weeks depending on whether it is lower or upper UTI), and prophylaxis is given for 6–12 months if there are recurrent episodes of UTI. Second, the choice of antibiotics and their dosage may have to be changed in accordance with the degree of renal dysfunction. Nitrofurantoin which is commonly used for treatment and prophylaxis of UTI in general population is contraindicated in patients with eGFR <50 mL/min/1.73 m^2. Third, risk of other complications like hyperkalaemia in CKD patients especially those on angiotensin-converting enzyme inhibitors or angiotensin receptor blockers may forbid long-term use of drugs like trimethoprim-sulphamethoxazole which are commonly used in general population for prophylaxis. Fourth, cyst infection is a unique form of kidney infection seen in polycystic kidney disease patients which requires prolonged course of antibiotics (up to 6 weeks) and at times may be refractory and thus require surgical intervention. Whereas trimethoprim-sulphamethoxazole remains the first choice in acute, uncomplicated, lower UTI in patients with CKD stage 3a, either ciprofloxacin or extended spectrum penicillin like pivmecillinam (especially in European countries where it is available) are recommended in CKD stages 3b to 5. It is important to note that the duration of treatment of acute, uncomplicated, lower UTI in females and males without any predisposing factors is different at 3 and 7 days, respectively. It is very important that attempts at modifying risk factors for recurrent UTI (e.g. surgical relief of obstruction, clean intermittent self-catheterisation in large volume neurogenic bladder) are made early as treatment becomes increasingly difficult because of urinary tract colonisation with drug-resistant organisms.

18.2.2 Pneumonia

Community-acquired pneumonia is a common cause of hospitalisation in general population. The risk of pneumonia increases progressively with fall in GFR. This risk further translates into increased severity of disease at admission and higher mortality rates during admission and at 1 month after discharge. *Streptococcus pneumoniae* is the most common cause of community-acquired pneumonia in CKD patients [7]. Vaccination against pneumococcus has been shown to be beneficial in improving outcomes. CKD patients are also at increased risk of developing severe forms of influenza.

18.2.3 HIV Infection

The prevalence of CKD is increased in incident patients of HIV infection starting antiretroviral therapy. About one-third of patients with HIV infection have CKD. The spectrum of renal involvement in HIV infection ranges from asymptomatic proteinuria to nephrotic syndrome, acute kidney injury or progressive decrease in GFR. The majority of patients have HIV-associated nephropathy (HIVAN) which most frequently presents as nephrotic syndrome and is characterised histologically by collapsing glomerulopathy and variable tubulo-interstitial involvement. African American race, decreased CD4 counts and family history of kidney disease are risk factors for development of HIVAN. All patients with HIVAN should be given antiretroviral therapy irrespective of their eGFR. In CKD patients, the presence of HIV infection is considered a risk factor for accelerated decline in GFR. Conversely, presence of CKD is also a risk factor for progression of HIV infection. Drug interactions and drug-induced kidney injury are very important treatment considerations in patients with HIV and CKD. Calcium channel blockers are contraindicated in patients using protease inhibitors. The risk of lactic acidosis does not forbid the use of nucleoside analogues in patients with CKD, but careful monitoring is advisable. Ensuring adequate hydration (daily water intake >1.5 L) is of paramount importance in patients who take indinavir to prevent indinavir nephrolithiasis. Though annual screening for renal involvement by urine protein and eGFR estimation is recommended, this frequency should be increased to biannually in patients who take drugs like tenofovir and indinavir and are at risk of drug-induced kidney injury. Finally, as the life expectancy of HIV-infected population on therapy has progressively increased, unrelated risk factors for CKD, e.g. diabetes, hypertension, etc., have also become important now.

18.2.4 Vascular Access-Related Infections

Patients with CKD are at risk of potentially lethal vascular access-related infections later in the course of disease because attention is not paid to timely creation of appropriate access. As a result, large proportions of CKD patients start dialysis with central venous catheters. The risk is highest for non-tunnelled central venous catheters followed by tunnelled ones, arteriovenous grafts and native arteriovenous (AV) fistulae. Amongst 1846 participants in the HEMO study, of whom only 7.6 % were using catheters, first infection-related hospitalisation was due to non-access-related infection in 79 % patients [8]. However, in HD population using catheters for vascular access at a large centre in the USA, non-access-related infections accounted for just 12 % of all proven infectious episodes [9]. *Staphylococcus aureus*, coagulase-negative staphylococci and enterococci are the most common organisms responsible for access-related bloodstream infections and may become complicated by infective endocarditis or osteomyelitis. Of particular concern are infections with multidrug-resistant bacteria and nosocomial transmission to other patients. As a result of these problems, timely creation of AV fistulae, dubbed the 'Fistula First' initiative, is targeted at reducing catheter usage.

Despite decreasing vascular access and PD catheter-related infections, hospitalisation rates due to infection in 2010 in the US ESRD population were 31 % higher compared to 1994 [2]. The increase was more striking (43 %) in the HD population [2].

18.2.5 Blood-Borne Infections

Patients with CKD are at risk of acquiring blood-borne infections like hepatitis B and C due to repeated skin punctures, need of blood or blood products and sharing of contaminated machines, surfaces or supplies in hospitals. Better staff training, improved infection control practices, regular screening and universal vaccination of patients and staff have reduced the HBV prevalence and seroconversion rates [10]. However, HCV infection still remains an important problem with prevalence ranging from 0.7 to 18.1 % in Asia-Pacific countries and 2.7 to 20 % in Europe [10, 11]. The Kidney Disease: Improving Global Outcomes (KDIGO) guidelines recommend the use of nucleic acid-based testing to screen patients for these infections in areas with high prevalence so as to not miss occult infections (see Chap. 20). However, this recommendation is not universally followed. KDIGO also recommends strict infection control measures as the most important tool for preventing its spread.

18.2.6 Tuberculosis

Tuberculosis is an important infection in patients with CKD, with 10–15 times increased incidence in both endemic and non-endemic regions as compared to general population [12, 13]. The diagnosis is not straightforward as the disease is more commonly extra-pulmonary with variable nonspecific manifestations like fever, weight loss, malaise, etc., which frequently delay diagnosis. Therefore, a high index of suspicion is required. As definitive diagnosis by culture takes a long time and absence of acid-fast bacilli on staining does not rule out tuberculosis, treatment is often started empirically in a significant proportion of patients on the basis of strong clinical suspicion and suggestive investigations, e.g. granulomatous inflammation on histopathology [12]. There is controversy about the need and optimal method of screening for latent tuberculosis [12]. However, the utility of screening in endemic regions with high prevalence of this disease is not clear. Interferon gamma assays like QuantiFERON-TB Gold test have been shown to be better than tuberculin skin test for detecting latent tuberculosis [14]. Tuberculosis is treated as in non-CKD population, but drug dose modification for level of eGFR is recommended.

18.2.7 Other Infections

The incidences of dyspepsia and gastroduodenal disease are more in CKD patients as compared to general population. Though *Helicobacter pylori* infection has been found to be less prevalent in haemodialysis and peritoneal dialysis patients, whenever present, it is treated as in patients with normal renal function [15]. Similarly, infective endocarditis is also treated as in general population. Patients with CKD and risk factors for development of infective endocarditis (prosthetic heart valves, valvular heart disease, valvular calcification, etc.) should receive antibiotic prophylaxis (amoxicillin 2 g or clindamycin 600 mg) prior to invasive dental and periodontal procedures.

It has been shown that mortality after septic shock due to various reasons is significantly more in patients with reduced GFR. In fact, eGFR <60 mL/min/1.73 m^2 remains an independent predictor of early and late mortality in patients with septic shock even after correction for comorbidities like diabetes, hypertension and cardiovascular disease.

The treatment of essentially all infectious diseases is same as in general population. However, drug dose modification or choosing alternative drug may be required as per patient's eGFR.

18.3 Infection Control in CKD

Globally, infection control and prevention are one of the biggest goals of public health. According to the World Health Organization (WHO), the objective of infection prevention and control is to ensure protection of those who might be vulnerable to an infection either in general community or while utilising health-care facilities. WHO identifies hygiene as the basic principle of infection prevention and control.

Patients with CKD are treated in the same manner as in general non-CKD population for established infections. Important considerations in this population include the assessment of comorbidities and risk factors, antimicrobial dose adjustment for level of kidney function, consideration of drug interaction and preventing superimposed acute kidney injury due to infections and use of radiocontrast agents or drugs used to treat the infection.

18.3.1 Vaccination in CKD Patients

In addition to general measures, timely vaccination is important in infection control (Box 18.3). The impact of vaccination in preventing, eliminating and eventually eradicating the disease has been convincingly demonstrated throughout the world through the universal immunisation programmes. The Advisory Committee on Immunization Practices (ACIP) in the USA annually updates and recommends immunisation schedules for children and adults. Kidney disease patients are classified at having high infection risk. Although vaccination is effective in CKD, these patients mount an inferior response to vaccination and suffer relatively rapid decline in protective antibody titres as compared to general population.

It is important to assess and record immunisation history of every CKD patient at initial presentation. *Physician should be aware of differences between contraindications and precautions with respect to vaccination.* While a contraindication precludes vaccination because of significant risk of adverse events, a precaution either means slightly increased risk of adverse events or decreased immune response to vaccine.

Box 18.3. Measures Aimed at Reducing Infections in CKD Patients

1. Vaccination against vaccine-preventable diseases
2. Timely creation of dialysis access
3. Maximising use of native arteriovenous fistulae in prevalent and incident haemodialysis patients
4. Universal precautions to be followed at health-care facilities
5. Rationalising antibiotic use according to local antimicrobial resistance data
6. Practising hand hygiene by patient and care giver

Severe allergic reaction or anaphylactic response to a vaccine or its constituents (e.g. egg, gelatin, latex, adjuvants) is a contraindication. Usually, vaccines are not administered even in situations where precaution is advised. It is important to note that not all contraindications or precautions are permanent. Mild acute febrile illnesses, previous mild local reactions and breast-feeding are not contraindications to vaccination. Vaccination should be deferred for 4 weeks after recovery from acute febrile illnesses. Live virus vaccines (varicella, zoster and MMR) are contraindicated in pregnancy and states of severe immunosuppression, e.g. primary or acquired immunodeficiency, steroid dose equivalent of prednisolone dose ≥20 mg/day for ≥2 weeks, malignancies involving the bone marrow or lymphatic system, etc. Particular attention should be paid to storage conditions, vaccine diluents, dose, site and type of administration. Adult vaccines are usually administered by intramuscular route except varicella, zoster, MMR and inactivated meningococcal polysaccharide vaccine which are given by subcutaneous route. Multiple vaccines can be administered simultaneously, but sites should be separated by at least 1–2 in. However, if immune globulin is also administered, a different anatomic site should be used.

All HbsAg-negative and anti-HBs negative patients must be vaccinated against HBV at the time of initial diagnosis irrespective of the stage of CKD. Higher dose of 40 μg in a four-dose schedule (0–2 and 6 months) has been shown to achieve higher seroconversion rates [17]. Though seroconversion rates in pre-dialysis stages of CKD are better, they are still suboptimal as compared to general population. An anti-HBs titre of >10 IU/L is considered protective and titre below this level warrants booster dose. A number of strategies have been used to increase the immunogenicity: these include increasing dose and frequency of vaccination, intradermal route of administration, using pre-S2/S antigens, use of adjuvants like 3-0-desacyl-4′-monophosphoryl lipid A adsorbed on aluminium phosphate and immunostimulants like levamisole and granulocyte macrophage colony stimulating factor [18]. The data, however, is inconclusive because of small sample sizes, variable doses and schedules and conflicting results. The antibody titres should be monitored annually in all previously vaccinated patients to ensure maintenance of protective levels.

Annual vaccination against influenza decreases the risk of hospitalisation and death in CKD patients [17]. Only inactivated influenza vaccine is recommended. Pneumococcal vaccination is also recommended for all patients with renal failure. A recent, large retrospective analysis of about 37,000 patients on dialysis in the USA has shown that vaccination against influenza and pneumococcus was independently associated with survival [19]. As compared to no vaccination, adjusted odds ratio of all-cause mortality amongst patients vaccinated for influenza alone and both influenza and pneumococcal vaccination were 0.79 (95 % CI, 0.72–0.86) and 0.70 (95 % CI, 0.62–0.78), respectively [19]. The recent KDIGO clinical practice guidelines for management of CKD also recommend vaccination against influenza, pneumococcus and HBV. ACIP recommends that except for meningococcal and hepatitis A vaccines, all other recommended vaccines should be considered in adult patients with CKD if they have not received them (Table 18.1). Though not routinely recommended in CKD, *Haemophilus influenzae* type b vaccination elicits adequate immunological response in dialysis patients and should be given to eligible patients [20]. Vaccination against *Staphylococcus aureus* has not been found to be effective in preventing septicaemia in dialysis patients and is not recommended. Routine paediatric immunisation schedule should be followed in children with CKD. Only inactivated polio vaccine should be used in patients with renal failure. As previously stated, live influenza vaccine is contraindicated, and caution is required before use of other live vaccines in children with CKD.

All patients with advanced CKD should preferably be vaccinated before renal transplantation. The seroconversion rates come down drastically if vaccines are administered after transplantation. Live vaccines are contraindicated in renal transplant recipients, and it is preferable to postpone other vaccinations till 6 months after transplant.

Despite recommendations, vaccination rates remain low, varying from 26 to 65 % and 15 to

Table 18.1 Vaccine recommendations for adult patients (age ≥19 years) with chronic kidney disease

Vaccine	Dose	Frequency	Considerations
Hepatitis B[a]	3–4	Once. Revaccinate with booster dose if anti-HBs titres fall <10 mIU/L	Check anti-HBs titres
Inactivated influenza	Single	Annual	Intranasally administered live, attenuated influenza vaccine not recommended in renal failure patients
Tetanus, diphtheria, pertussis (Td/Tdap)[b]	Single	Every 10 years	None
Varicella	Two (4 weeks apart)	Once	None
Human papillomavirus female (HPV2/HPV4)[c]	Three doses	Once	Not recommended beyond 26 years of age
Human papillomavirus male (HPV4)	Three doses	Once	Not recommended beyond 21 years of age
Zoster	Single	Once	Recommended for all adults aged ≥60 years irrespective of past history of herpes zoster
Measles, mumps, rubella (MMR)	1–2[d]	Once	None
Pneumococcal polysaccharide (PPSV23)	1–2	Revaccinate once after 5 years till 64 years of age Revaccinate again at ≥65 years if ≥5 years have elapsed since last dose No revaccination if vaccinated ≥65 years of age	None
Pneumococcal 13-valent conjugate (PCV13)	1–2	Not previously received PCV13 or PPSV23: Give single dose of PCV13 followed by a dose of PPSV23 at least 8 weeks later Previously received one dose of PPSV23: PCV13 1 or more years after the PPSV23, repeat PPSV23 dose no sooner than 8 weeks after PCV13 and at least 5 years after the most recent dose of PPSV23 Previously received two doses of PPSV23: PCV13 1 or more years after the PPSV23	None
Meningococcal[e]	Two	Revaccinate every 5 years till risk factors present	Recommended only in adults with anatomic or functional asplenia or persistent complement component deficiencies, HIV infection or high risk, e.g. occupational exposure, dormitory residence
Hepatitis A	Two	Once	Recommended only in adults with risk factors, e.g. occupational exposure, gay men, chronic liver disease, travel to endemic areas

Source: Data from Advisory Committee on Immunization Practices (ACIP) [16]

All are recommended in CKD patients without documented previous vaccination or disease except meningococcal and hepatitis A vaccines which are recommended only in certain high-risk groups. Note that zoster vaccination is recommended irrespective of previous zoster infection

[a]40 μg/mL (Recombivax HB®) administered on a three-dose schedule at 0, 1 and 6 months or two doses of 20 μg/mL (Engerix-B®) administered simultaneously on a four-dose schedule at 0, 1, 2 and 6 months

Table 18.1 (continued)

[b]Substitute first dose of Tdap for Td booster, then boost with Td every 10 years; give primary vaccination if it is not received and no evidence of previous infection.
[c]HPV2: bivalent human papillomavirus vaccine, HPV4: quadrivalent human papillomavirus vaccine
[d]Two doses recommended for adults who are students in postsecondary educational institutions, work in a health-care facility or plan to travel internationally
[e]Meningococcal conjugate vaccine quadrivalent (MCV4) preferred in patients aged ≤55 years, meningococcal polysaccharide vaccine (MPSV4) preferred in patients aged ≥56 years. Administer in a two-dose schedule at either 0 and 6–12 months (Havrix) or 0 and 6–18 months (Vaqta)

46 % in dialysis and pre-dialysis CKD patients, respectively. Targeted interventions at educating health-care staff coupled with regular monitoring and review have been shown to improve vaccination rates.

Conclusion

Infections are common cause of morbidity and mortality in CKD patients. Increasing patient age, presence of multiple comorbidities, the underlying immunosuppressive uraemic milieu and the use of dialysis catheters contribute to the infection risk, complicate clinical presentation and make management complex. Prevention of infections requires institution and implementation of appropriate guidelines including vaccination (Boxes 18.4 and 18.5). Tuberculosis is an important infection in certain geographic areas and requires high degree of clinical suspicion for timely diagnosis.

Box 18.4. What the Guidelines Say You Should Do?

1. All general principles of infection control and management apply in CKD population.
2. Always consider drug dose modifications and try to prevent drug-induced nephrotoxicity in patients with CKD.
3. Trimethoprim-sulphamethoxazole is the drug of choice for acute, uncomplicated, lower UTI in patients with CKD stage 3a.
4. Ciprofloxacin or extended spectrum penicillin like pivmecillinam is the drug of choice for acute, uncomplicated, lower UTI in patients with CKD stage 3b to 5.
5. *Tuberculosis in CKD*
   (a) Tuberculin skin testing may be negative in CKD patients despite infection.
   (b) Patients with active tuberculosis should receive standard chemotherapeutic agents for standard duration with drug dose modifications for level of eGFR.
6. *HIV in CKD*
   (a) All patients with HIVAN should be given antiretroviral therapy irrespective of their eGFR.
   (b) Calcium channel blockers are contraindicated in patients using protease inhibitors.
   (c) Annual screening for renal involvement by urine protein and eGFR estimation is recommended. However, this frequency should be increased to biannually in patients who take drugs like tenofovir and indinavir.
   (d) Drug dose modification and interactions should be considered before prescribing drugs in CKD patients with HIV infection.
7. *Vaccination in CKD*
   (a) Consider individual's immune status and specific vaccine recommendations before using live vaccines in CKD patients.
   (b) All CKD patients should be vaccinated against hepatitis B virus, pneumococcus and influenza virus at diagnosis.
   (c) Revaccinate annually against influenza virus and every 5 years against pneumococcus.
   (d) Monitor anti-HB titres annually and revaccinate with booster dose if titres are below <10 IU/L.

Box 18.5. Relevant Guidelines

1. *KDIGO Clinical Practice Guideline for the Evaluation and Management of Chronic Kidney Disease*

   Chapter 4: Other complications of CKD: CVD, medication dosage, patient safety, infections, hospitalizations, and caveats for investigating complications of CKD. Kidney Int Suppl. 2013;3(1):91–111. http://www.nature.com/kisup/journal/v3/n1/full/kisup201267a.html
2. *Scottish Intercollegiate Guidelines Network*

   Management of suspected bacterial urinary tract infection in adults. Scottish Intercollegiate Guideline Network Guideline No.88 July 2012 (http://www.sign.ac.uk/pdf/sign88.pdf).
3. *Advisory Committee on Immunization Practices (ACIP) Guideline*

   Advisory Committee on Immunization Practices (ACIP) recommended immunization schedules for persons aged 0 through 18 years and adults aged 19 years and olde--nited States, 2013. MMWR. 2013;62(Suppl 1):1. (http://www.cdc.gov/mmwr/pdf/other/su6201.pdf)
4. *Infectious Diseases Society of America Guideline*

   Gupta SK, Eustace JA, Winston JA, Boydstun II, Ahuja TS, Rodriguez RA, et al. Guidelines for the management of chronic kidney disease in HIV-infected patients: recommendations of the HIV Medicine Association of the Infectious Diseases Society of America. Clin Infect Dis. 2005;40(11):1559–85. (http://cid.oxfordjournals.org/content/40/11/1559.long)
5. *British Thoracic Society Guideline*

   Milburn H, Ashman N, Davies P, Doffman S, Drobniewski F, Khoo S, et al. Guidelines for the prevention and management of Mycobacterium tuberculosis infection and disease in adult patients with chronic kidney disease. Thorax. 2010;65(6):557–70. (http://thorax.bmj.com/content/65/6/559.long)

Before You Finish: Practice Pearls for the Clinician

- Despite decrease in the rate of access-related and blood-borne infections, the overall rate of infections in dialysis patients remains high.
- Improving native arteriovenous fistula utilisation, reducing catheter use, timely vaccination and implementation of infection control guidelines are important for preventing access-related infections.
- CKD patients need to be vaccinated against hepatitis B virus, pneumococcus and influenza as early as possible.
- Vaccination response may be suboptimal and needs monitoring in subjects with CKD.
- Management considerations include measures to prevent acute kidney injury and drug toxicity.
- Tuberculosis is important in certain geographic areas and requires high degree of clinical suspicion for timely diagnosis.

References

1. Couser WG, Remuzzi G, Mendis S, Tonelli M. The contribution of chronic kidney disease to the global burden of major noncommunicable diseases. Kidney Int. 2011;80:1258–70.
2. U S Renal Data System, USRDS 2012 annual data report: atlas of chronic kidney disease and end-Stage renal disease in the United States. National Institutes of Health, National Institute of Diabetes and Digestive and Kidney Diseases. 2012. http://www.usrds.org/atlas.aspx. Accessed 25 Feb 2013.
3. Ishani A, Collins AJ, Herzog CA, Foley RN. Septicemia, access and cardiovascular disease in dialysis patients: the USRDS wave 2 study. Kidney Int. 2005;68:311–8.
4. Dalrymple LS, Mohammed SM, Mu Y, et al. Risk of cardiovascular events after infection-related hospitalizations in older patients on dialysis. Clin J Am Soc Nephrol. 2011;6:1708–13.
5. Naqvi SB, Collins AJ. Infectious complications in chronic kidney disease. Adv Chronic Kidney Dis. 2006;13:199–204.
6. Dalrymple LS, Katz R, Kestenbaum B, et al. The risk of infection-related hospitalization with decreased kidney function. Am J Kidney Dis. 2012;59:356–63.
7. Viasus D, Garcia-Vidal C, Cruzado JM, et al. Epidemiology, clinical features and outcomes of pneumonia in patients with chronic kidney disease. Nephrol Dial Transplant. 2011;26(9):2899–906.
8. Allon M, Depner TA, Radeva M, et al. Impact of dialysis dose and membrane on infection-related hospitalization and death: results of the HEMO study. J Am Soc Nephrol. 2003;14:1863–70.
9. Al-Solaiman Y, Estrada E, Allon M. The spectrum of infections in catheter-dependent hemodialysis patients. Clin J Am Soc Nephrol. 2011;6:2247–52.
10. Li PK, Chow KM. Infectious complications in dialysis–epidemiology and outcomes. Nat Rev Nephrol. 2012;8:77–88.
11. Johnson DW, Dent H, Yao Q, et al. Frequencies of hepatitis B and C infections among haemodialysis and peritoneal dialysis patients in Asia-pacific countries: analysis of registry data. Nephrol Dial Transplant. 2009;24:1598–603.
12. Richardson RM. The diagnosis of tuberculosis in dialysis patients. Semin Dial. 2012;25:419–22.
13. Malhotra KK, Parashar MK, Sharma RK, et al. Tuberculosis in maintenance haemodialysis patients. Study from an endemic area. Postgrad Med J. 1981;57:492–8.
14. Lee SS, Chou KJ, Dou HY, et al. High prevalence of latent tuberculosis infection in dialysis patients using the interferon-gamma release assay and tuberculin skin test. Clin J Am Soc Nephrol. 2010;5:1451–7.
15. Thomas R, Panackal C, John M, et al. Gastrointestinal complications in patients with chronic kidney disease–a 5-year retrospective study from a tertiary referral center. Ren Fail. 2013;35:49–55.
16. Advisory Committee on Immunization Practices (ACIP) recommended immunization schedules for persons aged 0 through 18 years and adults aged 19 years and olde--nited States, 2013. MMWR. 2013;62(Suppl 1):1. http://www.cdc.gov/mmwr/pdf/other/su6201.pdf.
17. Janus N, Vacher LV, Karie S, Ledneva E, Deray G. Vaccination and chronic kidney disease. Nephrol Dial Transplant. 2008;23:800–7.
18. Grzegorzewska AE. Hepatitis B, vaccination in chronic kidney disease: review of evidence in non-dialyzed patients. Hepat Mon. 2012;12:e7359.
19. Bond TC, Spaulding AC, Krisher J, McClellan W. Mortality of dialysis patients according to influenza and pneumococcal vaccination status. Am J Kidney Dis. 2012;60:959–65.
20. Hawdon N, Nix EB, Tsang RS, Ferroni G, McCready WG, Ulanova M. Immune response to Haemophilus influenzae type b vaccination in patients with chronic renal failure. Clin Vaccine Immunol. 2012;19:967–9.

Endocrine Disorders in Chronic Kidney Disease

19

Marcin Adamczak and Andrzej Więcek

Before You Start: Facts You Need to Know

- The kidney is the site of synthesis and degradation of several hormones.
- In CKD patients, deficiency of hormones like erythropoietin, calcitriol, insulin-like growth factor, and testosterone is present.
- In contrast, the accumulation of insulin, prolactin, aldosterone, and growth hormone occurred.

19.1 Introduction

Endocrine abnormalities in patients with chronic kidney disease (CKD) may arise from a number of different causes, which are summarized in Table 19.1. The kidney is the site of synthesis and degradation of several hormones. Moreover, different concomitant conditions like inflammation, malnutrition, and metabolic acidosis participate in the pathogenesis of endocrine alterations in these patients.

Table 19.1 Selected pathomechanisms leading to endocrine abnormalities in chronic kidney disease

Type of defect	Example
Abnormalities of hormone production	
Reduced hormone production by the kidney	Erythropoietin, $1,25(OH)_2D_3$
Reduced hormone production in endocrine organs	Testosterone, estrogen
Abnormal secretion pattern (pulsatility; circadian rhythm)	PTH, GH, LH
Reactive hypersecretion of hormone to reestablish homeostasis	Erythropoietin, PTH, FGF 23
Inappropriate hypersecretion due to disturbed feedback	LH, prolactin, corticotropin
Abnormalities of hormone catabolism	
Decreased metabolic clearance	PTH, insulin, gastrin, leptin, adiponectin
Abnormalities of hormone action	
Disturbed activation of prohormones	Proinsulin, thyroxin (T_4)
Increased isoforms with potentially less bioactivity (due to posttranscriptional modifications)	LH
Increased hormone-binding proteins in plasma reducing availability of free hormone	IGF
Decreased hormone-binding proteins increasing availability of free hormone	Leptin
Changed receptor number, structure, modification	Vitamin D receptor
Disturbed postreceptor cellular signaling	Insulin, GH

$1,25(OH)_2D_3$ 1,25-dihydroxyvitamin D_3, *PTH* parathyroid hormone, *GH* growth hormone, *LH* luteinizing hormone, *FGF 23* fibroblast growth factor 23, *IGF* insulin-like growth factor

M. Adamczak, MD, PhD (✉) • A. Więcek, MD, PhD, FRCP (Edin), FERA
Department of Nephrology, Endocrinology and Metabolic Diseases, Medical University of Silesia, Francuska Str. 20/24, Katowice 40-027, Poland
e-mail: madamczak1@op.pl; awiecek@spskm.katowice.pl

M. Arici (ed.), *Management of Chronic Kidney Disease*,
DOI 10.1007/978-3-642-54637-2_19, © Springer-Verlag Berlin Heidelberg 2014

The clinician is able to measure plasma concentration of different hormones, which may or may not be abnormal. However, such measurements have limitations in CKD patients. Estimation of plasma concentrations of different hormones per se failed to provide a proper assessment of the adequacy of the hormonal status (e.g., hormone concentrations may be inappropriate to the stimulating or suppressing signals, the test may detect inactive hormone isoforms, or the response of the target organ may be abnormal). It is therefore necessary in patients with CKD to interpret hormone concentrations in plasma within the appropriate underlying clinical context (e.g., insulin concentration in relation to glucose concentration, parathyroid hormone (PTH) concentration in relation to serum ionized calcium concentration).

19.2 Abnormalities in the Erythropoietin Secretion

In the adults, kidneys are producing ca. 85–90 % of circulating erythropoietin (EPO). The liver is the source of the rest 10–15 % of circulating EPO. Within the kidneys, EPO is synthesized by peritubular cells of the renal cortex. The main stimulus for EPO synthesis is renal hypoxia, which is caused by anemia or hypoxemia. Hypoxia stimulates hypoxia inducible factor (HIF), which activates a wide set of genes and among others also EPO gene. Besides hypoxia, angiotensin II stimulates EPO production. On the other hand, inflammatory proteins (interleukin-1 (IL-1) and tumor necrosis factor-α (TNF-α)) inhibit its secretion. The plasma EPO concentrations in anemic CKD patients are usually comparable to those obtained in non-anemic subjects with intact kidney function, but they are inappropriately low taking into account actual blood hemoglobin concentrations. Moreover in CKD patients the erythropoietin resistance also occurs [1]. Anemia is the direct clinical consequence of EPO deficiency in CKD patients. The measurement of plasma EPO concentration in CKD patients is not useful in clinical practice. Decisions concerning treatment with erythropoiesis-stimulating agents (ESAs) in CKD patients are based on blood hemoglobin concentration and entire clinical status, but not on plasma EPO concentration (see Chap. 15).

19.3 Abnormalities in the Vitamin D Metabolites

In the general population, vitamin D deficiency has been linked to increased prevalence of albuminuria, hypertension, cardiovascular diseases, metabolic syndrome, insulin resistance, and obesity. The prevalence of 25-vitamin D_3 deficiency increases with the progression of CKD and approaches 80 % in CKD stage 5 patients. Moreover, in patients with nephrotic syndrome, the $25(OH)D_3$ is lost with the urine and in CKD patients treated with peritoneal dialysis is lost with the peritoneal fluid. The repletion with ergocalciferol in CKD patients is considered safe. In patients with plasma $25(OH)D_3$ concentration below 30 ng/mL, such therapy is recommended.

$25(OH)D_3$ is transported to the kidneys for further hydroxylation, resulting in the production of the active metabolite $1,25(OH)_2D_3$. With worsening of kidney function, there is decline in the activity of 1α-hydroxylase, the enzyme converting $25(OH)D_3$ to 1,25-dihydroxyvitamin D_3 (calcitriol), and decline in the amount of $25(OH)D_3$ delivered to the kidney (via receptor-mediated mechanism involving megalin). Additionally increased plasma concentration of fibroblast growth factor 23 (FGF 23) may directly inhibit activation of $25(OH)D_3$ to $1,25(OH)_2D_3$. Therefore in CKD stage 5 patients, plasma $1,25(OH)_2D_3$ concentration is low. Moreover, CKD patients revealed organ resistance to the action of $1,25(OH)_2D_3$. There is a decrease in the density of $1,25(OH)_2D_3$ receptors (VDR) in these patients.

The $1,25(OH)_2D_3$ deficiency in CKD patients plays an important role in the genesis of secondary hyperparathyroidism, defective intestinal absorption of calcium, skeletal resistance to the calcemic action of PTH, defective mineralization of bone, growth retardation in children, and proximal myopathy. Clinical studies suggest that

$1,25(OH)_2D_3$ deficiency increases cardiovascular and general mortality in CKD patients. The results of the small interventional studies suggested that treatment with calcitriol or other VDR agonists may reduce the mortality among these patients. Recent studies showed that $1,25(OH)_2D_3$ deficiency increases proteinuria and paricalcitol treatment reduces proteinuria in CKD patients. However, these studies enrolled only low number of patients, and therefore more larger studies are needed in the abovementioned areas [2].

The other abnormalities in the endocrine regulation of calcium and phosphate metabolism (among others, PTH and fibroblast growth factor 23) in CKD are discussed in detail in Chap. 16.

19.4 Abnormalities in the Hormones of the Hypothalamic–Pituitary-Gonadal Axis in Male CKD Patients

Male CKD patients are characterized by a variety of derangements of the hypothalamic–pituitary–gonadal axis (Table 19.2). The most important abnormalities are related directly to the gonadal function.

19.4.1 Luteinizing Hormone

In CKD patients, the lack of appropriate cyclic release and decreased amplitudes of the secretory bursts of gonadotropin-releasing hormone (GnRH) by the hypothalamus leads to a loss of normal pulsatile luteinizing hormone (LH) release by the pituitary. The causes of impaired cyclic release of GnRH are hyperprolactinemia and high plasma GnRH and LH concentrations caused mainly by their reduced renal clearances [3].

In the majority of CKD patients, basal plasma LH concentrations are high. High plasma LH concentrations in CKD patients are due to a decreased rate of catabolism and lack of testosterone inhibition (due to low plasma testosterone concentration in CKD) of GnRH secretion and secondarily also LH secretion.

Table 19.2 Abnormalities in the hormones of hypothalamic–pituitary–gonadal axis in chronic kidney disease

	Male	Female
LH	↑	↑
FSH	↑	N
Prolactin	↑	↑
Testosterone	↓	–
Estradiol	–	↓
Progesterone	–	↓

FSH follicle-stimulating hormone, *LH* luteinizing hormone
N normal

19.4.2 Follicle-Stimulating Hormone

In CKD patients, plasma concentrations of follicle-stimulating hormone (FSH) are in the upper normal range or elevated. FSH is important for spermatogenesis. It stimulates testicular growth and increases the production of testosterone-binding protein by Sertoli cells. In CKD patients, spermatogenesis is impaired despite elevated blood levels of FSH. This is probably due to the resistance of the testis to the action of FSH occurred or due to primary testicular dysfunction [3].

19.4.3 Prolactin

Plasma prolactin concentrations are elevated in the majority of male hemodialysis patients. Apart from elevated basal prolactin concentrations, the circadian rhythm of prolactin secretion is also disturbed. Moreover, the sleep-induced secretory bursts are not observed, although episodic secretion occurs during the daytime. It seems that both diminished prolactin clearance and increased production rate (probably due to inadequate dopaminergic inhibition of prolactin release from pituitary) contribute to hyperprolactinemia in CKD patients [4]. Prolactin accumulation leads to inhibition of GnRH pulsatile secretion and testosterone synthesis which resulted among others with sexual dysfunction and infertility. It is of interest that in some CKD patients, correction of the hyperprolactinemia by bromocriptine caused improvement of sexual function. There is evidence, suggesting that hyperprolactinemia may participate in the endothelial dysfunction frequently observed in CKD patients. The association between hyperprolactinemia and negative cardiovascular outcome was found in CKD patients. In a small clinical study in patients with CKD, it was found that reduction of plasma prolactin concentration with bromocriptine reduced blood pressure and left ventricular hypertrophy [4].

19.4.4 Testicular Hormones

In most male hemodialysis patients, plasma testosterone concentrations are low. The normal circadian rhythm of plasma testosterone concentrations, with a peak at 4–8 a.m. and nadir at 8–12 p.m., is maintained in CKD patients. It is unknown whether decreased plasma testosterone concentrations are due to reduced synthesis, increased catabolism, or a combination of both. The response to 4 days administration of human gonadotropin is sluggish and delayed; no increase of testosterone concentration was seen after 8 h, but a two- to threefold increase was seen after 4 days. Malnutrition participates in the reduction of plasma testosterone concentration in CKD male patients. In CKD patients on a low-protein diet, essential amino acid and keto amino acid analog supplementation raised plasma testosterone concentration [3, 5].

With respect to the other androgens, decreased plasma concentration of androstenedione and dehydroepiandrosterone sulfate has been reported in CKD male patients.

Androgen deficiency in CKD males may cause changes in body composition: body fat increases while lean body mass (mainly muscles mass) is reduced. Androgen deficiency leads also to CKD-related bone disease and higher incidence of bone fractures, anemia and ESAs hyporesponsiveness (due to reduced growth of differentiated stem cells and decreased sensitivity of erythroid progenitors to EPO), depression, decreased libido, and impairment of sexual function. Finally, it was recently shown that low plasma testosterone concentrations were associated with worse outcomes in male hemodialysis patients [5].

Therapy with exogenous testosterone is not exempted from risks, and the evidence of clear benefits from large, clinical studies is necessary, before recommendation of such therapy in hypogonadal CKD males patients [4, 5].

19.5 Abnormalities in the Hormones of the Hypothalamic–Pituitary–Gonadal Axis in Female CKD Patients

Female CKD patients present a variety of derangements of the hypothalamic–pituitary–gonadal axis (Table 19.2). The consequences of these abnormalities are anovulatory menstrual cycles and infertility.

19.5.1 Luteinizing Hormone

Plasma LH concentration is elevated in most premenopausal CKD patients. In healthy premenopausal females, the secretion of LH is pulsatile. In females with CKD, the lack of appropriate cyclic release of GnRH by the hypothalamus leads to a loss of normal pulsatile LH release by the pituitary. In healthy females, estradiol lowers the amplitude of LH pulses. In females with CKD, estradiol fails to influence the LH surge, suggesting impaired feedback which results in impaired ovulation. The clinical consequence of the loss of normal pulsatile LH release by the pituitary in female CKD is infertility [6].

19.5.2 Follicle-Stimulating Hormone

In contrast to the abnormal plasma LH concentration, the plasma FSH concentration is normal in most premenopausal CKD female patients. Therefore the FSH/LH ratio is decreased. The decreased FSH/LH ratio argues against primary ovarian failure and suggests that hypothalamic–hypophyseal dysregulation occurred in CKD females [6].

19.5.3 Prolactin

Plasma prolactin concentrations are often elevated in female hemodialysis patients, and the increase of plasma prolactin after the administration of thyrotropin-releasing hormone (TRH) is blunted. In CKD females, amenorrhea is frequent in patients with high plasma prolactin concentrations [6].

19.5.4 Estrogens

In female CKD patients, plasma estradiol concentrations are normal or low and are consistently lower in CKD females with hyperprolactinemia. In the second half of the menstrual cycle, plasma progesterone concentrations are low because of defective luteinization of the follicles. The hormonal derangements of females with CKD are clearly the consequence of abnormal regulation at the level of the hypothalamus [6].

A major consequence of the low plasma estrogen concentration concerns bone disease [7]. Amenorrheic patients had not only lower plasma estrogen concentrations but also lower bone mineral density compared to normally menstruating female dialysis patients. Small clinical interventional studies suggest that treatment with transdermal estradiol and cyclic addition of norethisterone acetate or treatment with raloxifene, a selective estrogen receptor modulator (SERM), increased bone mineral density of the lumbar spine in hemodialysis postmenopausal females. In view of concern about the potential adverse cardiovascular effects of hormone replacement therapy, it must be emphasized that currently long-term studies safety of hormone replacement or SERM therapy in CKD females are not available.

19.6 Abnormalities in the Growth Hormone/Insulin-Like Growth Factor (Somatotropic) Axis

The somatotropic axis comprises growth hormone (GH), insulin-like growth factor 1 and 2 (IGF-1 and -2), six IGF-binding proteins (IGFBP-1 to -6), and the IGFBP proteases (BP-Pr). All are involved in the modulation of somatic growth, cellular proliferation, and metabolism. Several abnormalities (Box 19.1) in the somatotropic axis have been reported in children and adults with CKD [8, 9]. The clinical consequence of these abnormalities is slow growth and reduced final height in CKD children. It was also shown that growth failure in CKD patients is associated with increased morbidity and mortality [8, 9].

19.6.1 Growth Hormone

In children and adult CKD patients, plasma concentration of GH is usually elevated. The increased plasma GH concentration is caused by both a reduction of clearance rate by kidney failure and an increase of GH secretion. Hyperglycemia induced by glucose infusion suppresses GH secretion in normal individuals, but fails to do so in CKD patients. Moreover, in CKD patients, the response of GH secretion to the administration of GHRH is exaggerated.

In CKD patients, high plasma GH concentrations are counteracted by peripheral resistance to GH. The GH resistance appears to be both at the receptor and at the postreceptor level. Determination of the concentration of serum

Box 19.1. Abnormalities in the Growth Hormone/Insulin-Like Growth Factor Axis in Chronic Kidney Disease

Growth hormone
Increased plasma GH concentration
Peripheral resistance to GH due to defect in GH intracellular signal transduction
Insulin-like growth factor
Decreased IGF-1 plasma concentration
Reduced free IGF-1 plasma concentration
Increased IGFBPs (IGFBP-1, IGFBP-2, IGFBP-4, and IGFBP-6) plasma concentration
Presence of low molecular weight (1,000 Da) inhibitor of IGF-1 in plasma
Peripheral resistance to IGF-1 due to postreceptor defect in IGF-1 action

GH growth hormone, *IGF-1* and *IGF-2* insulin-like growth factor-1 and -2, *IGFBP* IGF-binding protein growth hormone-binding protein (GHBP), which is a cleaved product of the GH receptor, may be used to assess GH receptor density in tissues. GHBP plasma concentration is low in children and adults with CKD. Resistance to GH is also due to defective intracellular signal transduction. The impaired phosphorylation and nuclear translocation of GH-activated STAT protein was also found. Hyperparathyroidism, metabolic acidosis, and inflammation may participate in the pathogenesis of GH resistance in CKD [8, 9].

19.6.2 Insulin-Like Growth Factors

GH promotes linear growth partially by stimulating systemic and local concentrations of IGFs. IGF-1 and IGF-2 are produced locally by most tissues, including the growth plate, but the liver is the main source of circulating hormones. IGF-1 mediates most of the growth-promoting effects of GH. Plasma IGF-1 forms complexes with six IGF-binding proteins (IGFBP-1 to IGFBP-6).

In advanced CKD, the plasma concentration of IGF-1 is decreased and of IGF-2 is increased. In patients with advanced CKD, the resistance to the metabolic effects of recombinant human IGF-1 was found. Moreover the so-called somatomedin bioactivity in blood, an index of IGF activity measured by sulfate incorporation into porcine costal cartilage, is reduced in uremia. The discrepancy between normal or elevated total IGF plasma concentration and its low bioactivity in CKD may be explained by increased plasma concentration of IGFBPs, circulating IGF inhibitor and receptor or postreceptor defect.

Plasma concentrations of four of the six IGF-binding proteins (IGFBP-1, IGFBP-2, IGFBP-4, and IGFBP-6) are markedly higher in CKD patients. The increased binding capacity of IGF-1 decreases the concentration of free IGF-1. This imbalance between plasma IGF-1 and plasma IGFBP concentrations is relevant in the pathogenesis of growth failure in CKD.

A low molecular weight (1,000 Da) inhibitor of IGF-1 has been identified in the plasma of CKD patients, but molecular details have not yet been characterized.

Resistance to IGF-1 in CKD is also due to defective intracellular signal transduction (both autophosphorylation of the IGF-1 receptor tyrosine kinase and activity of the IGF-1R tyrosine kinase to the exogenous insulin receptor substrate 1) [8, 9].

19.6.3 Growth Hormone Therapy

Demonstration of the resistance to the action of GH and IGF-1 in CKD provides the rationale for the use of GH in the treatment of CKD children with retarded growth despite normal or elevated hormone concentrations. Administration of recombinant human GH in prepubertal children with CKD caused an increase in growth rate and in standardized height without undue advancement of bone age or significant side effects. In adults, recombinant human GH administration stimulates muscle mass gain and may be used in the treatment of protein energy wasting [8, 9].

19.7 Abnormalities in the Adrenocorticotropin–Cortisol Axis

The adrenocorticotropin–cortisol axis is only mildly affected in CKD. In CKD patients, plasma adrenocorticotropin (ACTH) and cortisol concentrations are normal or modestly elevated. The cortisol half-life is prolonged in CKD patients, and decreased catabolism may contribute to the mildly elevated plasma cortisol concentrations in CKD [10].

Clinical consequences of the abovementioned modest hormonal alterations are unclear, but hypercortisolemia may cause osteopenia, disturbed distribution of adipose tissue, and increased protein catabolism.

In CKD patients, ACTH secretion cannot be suppressed by standard oral doses of dexamethasone, but higher doses of dexamethasone suppress ACTH secretion. Therefore, when Cushing syndrome is suspected in CKD patients, a 2-day dexamethasone test is recommended.

19.8 Abnormalities in Vasopressin

In CKD patients, the plasma vasopressin (AVP) concentration is elevated. The major cause is decreased metabolic clearance rate. The main physiologic stimuli for AVP secretion are increased plasma osmolality and decreased cardiac output or arterial vasodilation. The osmotic and nonosmotic regulation of AVP secretion in CKD is intact. In hemodialysis patients, the plasma AVP concentration increases during ultrafiltration and plasma volume contraction and decreases during hypervolemia. The clinical significance of the elevated plasma AVP concentration in CKD is still uncertain. Experimental and observational human studies suggest that high plasma AVP concentration may participate in the CKD progression [11, 12].

Copeptin (CT-proAVP) is the C-terminal part of the vasopressin prohormone. CT-proAVP is secreted with AVP, and it is easier to estimate than AVP itself. In patients with diabetic nephropathy, high CT-proAVP copeptin plasma concentration predicts cardiovascular mortality [11, 12].

19.9 Abnormalities in the Thyroid Gland and Hypothalamic–Pituitary–Thyroid Axis

Abnormalities in the function of the thyroid gland and in the plasma concentrations of thyroid hormones are common in patients with CKD. A detailed profile of the indices of thyroid status in CKD as compared to primary hypothyroidism and chronic nonthyroid, nonkidney illness is presented in Table 19.3 [13].

Table 19.3 Abnormalities of hypothalamic–pituitary–thyroid axis in chronic kidney disease, chronic nonthyroidal, nonkidney illness and primary hypothyroidism

	T_4	T_3	rT_3	TSH
Chronic kidney disease	N, ↓	↓	N	N
Chronic nonthyroidal, nonkidney illness	N, ↓	↓	↑	N
Primary hypothyroidism	↓	↓	N	↑

N normal, *TSH* thyroid-stimulating hormone, T_4 thyroxin, T_3 triiodothyronine, rT_3 reverse triiodothyronine

19.9.1 Thyroid Hormones

The plasma concentrations of thyroxin (T_4) are normal and triiodothyronine (T_3) are normal or reduced in CKD patients. The reduced plasma T_3 concentration in CKD patients is the result of decreased peripheral conversion of T_4 to T_3 in several tissues. The impaired conversion of T_4 to T_3 in CKD may be the result of malnutrition or chronic metabolic acidosis.

Although T_3 is the most active thyroid hormone, CKD patients with low plasma T_3 concentrations appear usually clinically euthyroid. The expression of messenger RNA of c-erb-A α and β T_3 receptors by mononuclear cells is increased in CKD patients compared with normal subjects. This may help maintain a euthyroid state despite low T_3 concentrations.

In contrast to the other chronic nonthyroid diseases, rT_3 plasma concentration is normal in CKD patients.

In CKD, low thyroid hormone concentrations do not necessarily indicate a state of hypothyroidism, but are a reflection of the state of chronic illness and/or malnutrition. The low T_3 status of CKD can be traditionally viewed as being somehow protective, promoting the saving energy in response to uremic wasting. There is evidence, however, suggesting that low plasma T_3 concentration in CKD may lead to endothelial dysfunction, atherosclerosis, and cardiac abnormalities. In clinical studies low plasma T_3 was a predictor of total and cardiovascular mortality.

T_3 therapy is not exempted from risks (like negative protein balance), and the evidence from large, clinical studies in CKD patients is necessary before recommending its use in CKD patients [4, 13].

19.9.2 The Thyroid-Stimulating Hormone

Despite a tendency to low plasma concentrations of T_4 and T_3, the plasma concentration of thyroid-stimulating hormone (TSH) is usually normal in CKD patients. The normal plasma

TSH concentration despite low plasma concentrations of the thyroid hormones suggests an abnormal regulation of the hypothalamic–pituitary–thyroid axis. The TSH response to TRH is usually blunted. In CKD patients, the normal diurnal rhythm of TSH with a peak in the late evening or early morning is blunted, and the nocturnal TSH surge is reduced. The pattern of pulsatile TSH secretion is also altered [4, 13].

19.9.3 Primary Hypothyroidism and Hyperthyroidism

Primary hypothyroidism is two to three times more frequent in CKD patients than in the general population. It is difficult to make the clinical diagnosis of hypothyroidism in CKD patients. The signs and symptoms of hypothyroidism, such as pallor, hypothermia, and asthenia, are also found in patients with advanced CKD without hypothyroidism. The only reliable procedure to diagnose hypothyroidism in CKD is the finding of an elevated plasma TSH concentration and clearly low plasma T_4 concentrations. Heparin competes with T_4 at the binding site of the hormone-binding protein, causing an increase of plasma T_4 concentrations for at least 24 h. Therefore blood for the determination of thyroid hormones should be sampled before heparin administration at the beginning of a dialysis session. Clinical consequences of hypothyroidism in CKD are exacerbation of muscle wasting, anemia, and depression [4, 13].

The prevalence of hyperthyroidism in CKD is similar to that found in the general population.

19.10 Aldosterone

Plasma aldosterone concentrations are elevated in CKD patients when GFR is lower than 70 mL/min, and a correlation between plasma aldosterone concentration and the rate of CKD progression is found.

The results of the small interventional studies suggest that treatment with spironolactone reduced proteinuria in CKD patients. However, these studies are small, and more larger studies to define the safety and effectiveness of such treatment are needed [14].

Box 19.2. Insulin Metabolism in Chronic Kidney Disease

Fasting hyperinsulinemia with prolonged insulin half-life and elevated blood levels of proinsulin and C peptide
Usually decreased early, but exaggerated late-insulin response to hyperglycemia induced by oral or intravenous glucose administration
Decreased peripheral sensitivity to insulin action, but normal suppression of hepatic glucose production by insulin

19.11 Abnormalities in Insulin and Glucagon

In patients with chronic kidney disease (CKD), abnormalities in carbohydrate metabolism are encountered at different levels of the insulin–glucose cascade (Box 19.2) [15, 16].

19.11.1 Insulin Secretion and Clearance

Insulin secretion is impaired in CKD. Causes of this impairment are among others high PTH and low plasma $1{,}25[OH]_2D_3$ concentration.

The kidney plays an important role in insulin clearance. Insulin is filtered by the glomeruli and reabsorbed in the proximal tubule. In healthy subjects the renal clearance of insulin is about 200 mL/min. This value exceeds the glomerular filtration rate (GFR), indicating that, in addition, peritubular uptake of insulin takes place. It is estimated that 6–8 U of endogenous insulin are daily removed by the kidney, accounting for 25–40 % of the total removal of endogenous insulin. A decrease in the metabolic clearance rate of insulin is documented in patients with GFR <40 mL/min. In CKD patients, diminished insulin clearance accounts for fasting hyperinsulinemia. It also accounts for decreased insulin requirements in diabetic patients with impaired kidney function [15].

19.11.2 Insulin Resistance

Peripheral resistance to insulin is seen even in early CKD stages. The main sites of decreased insulin sensitivity are skeletal muscles. It was demonstrated that the defect is located not only at the level of the insulin receptor but presumably at the postreceptor level. Impairment of phosphatidyl-inositol 3-kinase activity (PI3-K) was documented in CKD patients. Higher plasma insulin concentrations are required to increase glucose uptake by skeletal muscle.

Peripheral resistance to insulin action is frequently found even in early stages of kidney disease and is found in the majority of patients with advanced CKD. The resistance to the peripheral action of insulin is markedly improved, however after several weeks of hemodialysis or peritoneal dialysis. Presumably, unidentified dialyzable uremic "toxins" are involved in the pathogenesis of deranged insulin action. Such compounds with a molecular weight of 1–2 kDa are specific for CKD, because they are not found in nonuremic patients with insulin resistance.

A number of other factors have been identified which are involved in the pathogenesis of insulin resistance in CKD patients and which are potential targets for intervention. In hemodialysis patients, insulin resistance is ameliorated by treatment with erythropoietin or $1,25(OH)_2D_3$. In predialysis patients it is ameliorated by dietary protein restriction.

Plasma concentrations of insulin antagonists glucagon and growth hormone are frequently elevated in CKD patients. It has been proposed that these two hormones contribute to insulin resistance. Metabolic acidosis, chronic inflammation, and increase of renin–angiotensin system activity may also participate in the pathogenesis of insulin resistance in CKD patients [16].

19.11.3 Clinical Consequences of Hyperglycemia and Insulin Resistance

Hyperglycemia and insulin resistance in CKD patients contribute to increased cardiovascular risk and CKD progression. Insulin resistance may also participate in the pathogenesis of the malnutrition often found in these patients. Insulin deficiency (or resistance) stimulates breakdown of muscle and activates a common proteolytic pathway via the ubiquitin–proteasome system. Insulin resistance also increases salt sensitivity through increased tubular sodium reabsorption and therefore contributes to hypertension [15, 16].

19.12 Abnormalities in the Cardiac Natriuretic Peptides

Plasma concentrations of ANP and BNP usually are elevated in CKD patients. Moreover, in these patients, the pulsatile secretion of ANP and BNP is characterized by abnormally high amplitude. The causes of high plasma concentrations of ANP and BNP in CKD are an increase in intravascular filling and atrial distension, concomitant heart failure, and diminished renal clearance. The removal of fluid by ultrafiltration during dialysis therapy is associated with a decrease in the plasma ANP and BNP concentrations.

The measurement of ANP and BNP plasma concentration was used as a biochemical marker of volume overload in CKD patients. The weight of evidence indicates that measurements of plasma ANP and BNP concentration add little to the clinical examination of these patients. However, high plasma concentrations of cardiac natriuretic peptides, particularly BNP, were strong predictors of cardiovascular mortality in CKD patients.

The estimation of plasma concentrations of cardiac natriuretic hormones (BNP and N-terminal proBNP) could be useful for a differential diagnosis of heart failure in general population. In CKD patients, most studies indicate that the upward adjustment of diagnostic cut points preserves the usefulness of BNP and N-terminal proBNP for the differential diagnosis of heart failure [17].

19.13 Abnormalities in Cardiotonic Steroids

Cardiotonic steroids (ouabain and marinobufagenin) act as physiological regulators of sodium pump activity and are implicated in regulation of natriuresis and vascular tone. In CKD patients, the plasma marinobufagenin but not ouabain concentration is elevated. Such an elevation seems to be of pathophysiological relevance because it was shown that in CKD patients erythrocyte Na/K-ATPase was inhibited, and plasma marinobufagenin concentration exhibited a negative correlation with this enzyme activity [18]. The clinical significance of the elevated plasma marinobufagenin concentration in CKD is uncertain. Results of experimental studies suggest that high plasma concentration may participate in the pathogenesis of hypertension, diastolic dysfunction, and both cardiac and renal fibrosis in CKD.

19.14 Abnormalities in Gastrointestinal Hormones

An elevated plasma gastrin concentration is found in CKD patients. The kidney is the main site of gastrin biodegradation; therefore, hypergastrinemia in uremic patients is mainly due to reduced renal degradation of this hormone. Hypergastrinemia in CKD patients is due predominantly to "big" gastrin (G34), but not "little" gastrin (G17) accumulation. G34 is biologically less active than G17. Postprandial gastrin secretion in CKD patients is similar to that in normal subjects, but the peak values were attained later and the response was more prolonged [19].

Elevated plasma ghrelin levels were observed in CKD. Increased ghrelin plasma concentration in CKD is due to the decreased degradation of ghrelin by the kidney. There are two forms of circulating ghrelin: acylated and des-acyl ghrelin. Acylated ghrelin promotes food intake, whereas des-acyl ghrelin induces negative energy balance. However, only plasma des-acyl ghrelin concentration was elevated in CKD. It is suggested that elevated des-acyl ghrelin plasma concentration may be involved in the pathogenesis of anorexia in CKD patients. The results of small interventional clinical studies suggest that ghrelin treatment in CKD patients enhanced food intake and may improve nutritional status [20].

The plasma concentrations of other gastrointestinal hormones, such as cholecystokinin, gastric inhibitory peptide, pancreatic polypeptide, secretin, gastrin releasing peptide, vasoactive intestinal polypeptide, and motilin, are elevated in CKD patients. The pathophysiological importance of these findings remains to be elucidated.

19.15 Abnormalities in the Hormones of Adipose Tissue

The adipose tissue is an important endocrine organ producing biologically active substances (adipokines). An elevated plasma concentration of different adipokines is found in CKD patients (Box 19.3). It was proved that some of them (such as leptin, adiponectin, resistin, and visfatin) are characterized by systemic actions [21].

Patients with CKD are characterized by increased plasma leptin concentration. The decreased leptin clearance by failed kidneys leads to its accumulation in the circulation. Leptin stimulates the proliferation and the differentiation of hematopoietic stem cells. It is likely that the effects of leptin and erythropoietin are synergistic. Apart from this, hyperleptinemia stimulates the activity of the sympathetic nervous system and therefore likely plays a pathophysiological role in the CKD progression, pathogenesis of hypertension, and cardiovascular diseases [21].

Patients with CKD are characterized by increased plasma adiponectin concentration. The increased plasma adiponectin concentration in CKD patients is owing to the disturbances of its biodegradation and elimination by the failed kidneys. Clinical consequences of increased plasma adiponectin concentration in CKD are not clear [21]. It seems however that in CKD patients

Box 19.3. Abnormalities in the Hormones of Adipose Tissue in Chronic Kidney Disease

Leptin	↑
Adiponectin	↑
Resistin	↑
Visfatin	↑

due to the receptor resistance, the unique anti-atherosclerotic actions of adiponectin are reduced.

Plasma concentration of resistin is increased in CKD patients. The main cause of high plasma resistin concentrations in CKD is its reduced renal clearance. Resistin, at concentrations seen in CKD patients inhibits neutrophil activity. Therefore, it may participate in the pathogenesis of the increased risk of infections in CKD patients. Resistin also appears to have a potential role in the pathogenesis of cardiovascular disease in CKD patients. Hemodialysis patients with the low serum resistin concentration had poor hospitalization-free survival [21].

The plasma concentration of visfatin gradually increases with the loss of kidney function and is related positively to endothelial dysfunction. This adipokine stimulates adhesion of monocytes to endothelial cells. Visfatin may also play a role in the pathogenesis of malnutrition in CKD. A high plasma visfatin concentration predicted mortality in CKD patients [21].

Box 19.4. What the Guidelines Say You Should Do [22]

- In patients with CKD stages 3–5D, 25(OH)D (calcidiol), levels might be measured; vitamin D deficiency and insufficiency be corrected using treatment strategies recommended for the general population.
- In children and adolescents with CKD stages 2–5D and related height deficits, treatment with recombinant human growth hormone when additional growth is desired, after first addressing malnutrition and biochemical abnormalities of CKD–MBD, is recommended.

Box 19.5. Relevant Guidelines

1. *KDIGO Guideline*: KDIGO clinical practice guideline for the diagnosis, evaluation, prevention, and treatment of Chronic Kidney Disease-Mineral and Bone Disorder. Kidney Int Suppl. 2009;113:S1–130. Available at: http://www.kdigo.org/clinical_practice_guidelines/pdf/CKD/KDIGO%20CKD-MBD%20GL%20KI%20Suppl%20113.pdf

Before You Finish: Practice Pearls for the Clinician

- The main clinical consequences of the endocrine abnormalities in CKD patients are anemia, bone disease, and infertility.
- Decisions concerning treatments with erythropoiesis-stimulating agents (ESAs) in these patients should be based on blood hemoglobin concentration and entire clinical status, but not on plasma EPO concentration.
- The repletion with ergocalciferol in CKD patients with plasma $25(OH)D_3$ concentration below 30 ng/mL is recommended.
- Therapy with testosterone is not exempted from risks, and the evidence of benefits from large, clinical studies is necessary, before recommendation of such therapy in hypogonadal CKD males.
- Similarly, in female CKD patients, there is no data from the large, clinical studies concerning the safety and efficiency of the estrogen therapy. The decision of hormone replacement therapy in female CKD patients should be individualized and made after discussion with gynecologist.
- The administration of recombinant human GH in prepubertal children with CKD caused an increase in growth rate without undue advancement of bone age or significant side effects.
- Blood samples for the determination of thyroid hormones should be taken before heparin administration at the beginning of a dialysis session.
- In CKD, low thyroid hormone concentrations do not necessarily indicate a state of hypothyroidism, but are a reflection of the state of chronic illness and/or malnutrition.

References

1. Fisher JW. Erythropoietin: physiology and pharmacology update. Exp Biol Med (Maywood). 2003;228:1–14.
2. Dusso A, González EA, Martin KJ. Vitamin D in chronic kidney disease. Best Pract Res Clin Endocrinol Metab. 2011;25:647–55.
3. Iglesias P, Carrero JJ, Díez JJ. Gonadal dysfunction in men with chronic kidney disease: clinical features, prognostic implications and therapeutic options. J Nephrol. 2012;25:31–42.
4. Ros S, Carrero JJ. Endocrine alterations and cardiovascular risk in CKD: is there a link? Nefrologia. 2013;33:181–7.
5. Carrero JJ, Stenvinkel P. The vulnerable man: impact of testosterone deficiency on the uraemic phenotype. Nephrol Dial Transplant. 2012;27:4030–41.
6. Holley JL. The hypothalamic-pituitary axis in men and women with chronic kidney disease. Adv Chronic Kidney Dis. 2004;11:337–41.
7. Sugiya N, Nakashima A, Takasugi N, Kawai A, Kiribayashi K, Tanaka J, et al. Endogenous estrogen may prevent bone loss in postmenopausal hemodialysis patients throughout life. Osteoporos Int. 2011;22:1573–9.
8. Mak RH, Cheung WW, Roberts Jr CT. The growth hormone-insulin-like growth factor-I axis in chronic kidney disease. Growth Horm IGF Res. 2008;18:17–25.
9. Gupta D, Gardner M, Whaley-Connell A. Role of growth hormone deficiency and treatment in chronic kidney disease. Cardiorenal Med. 2011;1:174–82.
10. Luger A, Lang I, Kovarik J, Stummvoll HK, Templ H. Abnormalities in the hypothalamic-pituitary-adrenocortical axis in patients with chronic renal failure. Am J Kidney Dis. 1987;9:51–4.
11. Meijer E, Boertien WE, Zietse R, Gansevoort RT. Potential deleterious effects of vasopressin in chronic kidney disease and particularly autosomal dominant polycystic kidney disease. Kidney Blood Press Res. 2011;34:235–44.
12. Bankir L, Bouby N, Ritz E. Vasopressin: a novel target for the prevention and retardation of kidney disease? Nat Rev Nephrol. 2013;9:223–39.
13. Abdel-Rahman EM, Mansour W, Holley JL. Thyroid hormone abnormalities and frailty in elderly patients with chronic kidney disease: a hypothesis. Semin Dial. 2010;23:317–23.
14. Lu Y, Ku E, Campese VM. Aldosterone in the pathogenesis of chronic kidney disease and proteinuria. Curr Hypertens Rep. 2010;12:303–6.
15. Liao MT, Sung CC, Hung KC, Wu CC, Lo L, Lu KC. Insulin resistance in patients with chronic kidney disease. J Biomed Biotechnol. 2012;2012:691369.
16. Siew ED, Ikizler TA. Insulin resistance and protein energy metabolism in patients with advanced chronic kidney disease. Semin Dial. 2010;23:378–82.
17. Wang AY. Clinical utility of natriuretic peptides in dialysis patients. Semin Dial. 2012;25:326–33.
18. Kolmakova EV, Haller ST, Kennedy DJ, Isachkina AN, Budny GV, Frolova EV, et al. Endogenous cardiotonic steroids in chronic renal failure. Nephrol Dial Transplant. 2011;26:2912–9.
19. El Ghonaimy E, Barsoum R, Soliman M, El Fikky A, Rashwan S, El Rouby O, et al. Serum gastrin in chronic renal failure: morphological and physiological correlations. Nephron. 1985;39:86–94.
20. Cheung WW, Mak RH. Ghrelin in chronic kidney disease. Int J Pept. 2010;2010.ID 567343.
21. Adamczak M, Wiecek A. The adipose tissue as an endocrine organ. Semin Nephrol. 2013;33:2–13.
22. Kidney Disease: Improving Global Outcomes (KDIGO) CKD-MBD Work Group. KDIGO clinical practice guideline for the diagnosis, evaluation, prevention, and treatment of chronic kidney disease-mineral and bone disorder. Kidney Int Suppl. 2009;76(113):S1–130.

Liver and Gastrointestinal Tract Problems in Chronic Kidney Disease

20

Michel Jadoul

Before You Start: Facts You Need to Know

- Nonspecific symptoms or signs, such as diarrhea or biochemical liver dysfunction, may in some patients be an important clue to the etiology of CKD.
- The level of some common biochemical tests such as ALT/AST is falsely low in the late CKD stages.
- Infection by the hepatitis B and C viruses is more common in CKD patients than in the general population.

Liver or gastrointestinal (GI) tract disease may sometimes be a cause or a consequence of CKD. In the first section, we discuss the etiologies of liver or GI tract disease that may be a clue to CKD etiology. In the second section, we discuss the liver and GI tract manifestations that are more prevalent or associated with CKD.

M. Jadoul, MD
Department of Nephrology, Cliniques Universitaires Saint-Luc, Université catholique de Louvain, Avenue Hippocrate 10, Brussels 1200, Belgium
e-mail: michel.jadoul@uclouvain.be

20.1 Liver and Gastrointestinal Tract Disease as Potential Clues to CKD Etiology

20.1.1 Liver Disease

20.1.1.1 Liver and Kidney Disease from the Same Cause

A number of diseases may cause both liver and kidney damage. The detection of biochemical or imaging evidence of both liver and kidney involvement may thus point to specific etiologies of CKD. These include among others amyloidosis (especially of the AL type), as well as autosomal dominant polycystic disease. The latter will easily be diagnosed by imaging, whereas the former should be investigated by the search for a paraprotein, a sign of clonal B cell lineage proliferation, followed by biopsy of an affected organ.

20.1.1.2 Liver Disease as Cause of CKD

Some liver diseases may not infrequently be complicated by significant glomerulonephritis (GN). These include hepatitis B and hepatitis C virus infection.

Hepatitis B virus (HBV) infection is an important cause of membranous nephropathy, especially in children and in emerging countries. A recent case series of biopsy-proven membranous nephropathy from China ascribed the disease to HBV in 12 % of cases [1]. The substantial reduction of the prevalence of HBV-associated membranous GN in several emerging countries since the advent of anti-HBV vaccination strongly supports

M. Arici (ed.), *Management of Chronic Kidney Disease*,
DOI 10.1007/978-3-642-54637-2_20, © Springer-Verlag Berlin Heidelberg 2014

the causal role of HBV. Thus, testing for HBV serological markers should be part of the etiologic investigation of any GN. Successful antiviral treatment is associated with improvement of the associated GN [2].

Similarly, the hepatitis C virus is one of the causal agents of type 1 membranoproliferative glomerulonephritis, with or without circulating cryoglobulins. Testing for HCV should thus be part of the etiologic investigation of a GN and successful antiviral treatment may improve the associated GN [3, 4]. Sometimes, immunosuppressive agents (corticosteroids, cyclophosphamide, rituximab) may be required to treat hyperactive lesions (such as crescents/capillary necrosis), prior to or associated with antiviral treatment or in case of failure of antiviral agents [3, 4].

20.1.2 Gastrointestinal Tract Disease

20.1.2.1 Kidney and GI Tract Disease from the Same Cause

Several diseases may concurrently affect both the GI tract and the kidney. This coexistence may thus be an important clue to the etiology of CKD. Such etiologies include among others Henoch-Schönlein purpura and atheroembolism.

The coexistence of signs of GN (hematuria and proteinuria) together with bouts of abdominal pain, with or without GI tract hemorrhage, not always accompanied by arthritis and/or skin purpura, should prompt consideration of Henoch-Schönlein purpura as a potential etiology of CKD. The diagnosis may ultimately be confirmed by the histological demonstration of IgA deposits in an affected organ. Management is supportive, with temporary steroids for symptomatic treatment of articular or digestive disease. The long-term prognosis is dependent on kidney involvement. A kidney biopsy should be performed if significant albuminuria persists.

Similarly, albeit much less frequently, atheroembolism is a more and more frequent cause or contributor to CKD in elderly patients with coexistent cardiovascular disease. Atheroembolism may affect various abdominal organs, including the bowel, in addition to the kidney. The coexistence of acute episodes of abdominal pain, sometimes with peritoneal irritation, in a patient with a recent potential trigger of atheroembolism (coronary or peripheral angiography, warfarin start, thrombolysis) should prompt, especially if peripheral eosinophilia is present, considering the diagnosis of atheroembolism. The management is supportive, together with withdrawal of warfarin and aggressive statin treatment.

20.1.2.2 Diseases of the GI Tract or Pancreas as a Cause of CKD

Diseases of the GI tract may cause acute, subacute, or sometimes chronic kidney disease (CKD). Indeed significant small bowel disease such as Crohn's disease but also in the postsurgical short bowel syndrome, chronic pancreatitis, as well as orlistat therapy (prescribed with the aim to favor weight loss) all can cause steatorrhea. The consequence of steatorrhea is that calcium binds to free fatty acids in the bowel lumen and there will thus be less calcium available to bind oxalate. Thus, more oxalate will be absorbed by the bowel, leading to hyperoxaluria and the so-called oxalate nephropathy. This is definitely an under-recognized cause of kidney disease. Kidney dysfunction may be partly reversible after etiologic treatment and oral calcium supplementation [5]. Thus, in the presence of unexplained CKD and concomitant diarrhea, oxaluria should be measured.

Preparations rich in sodium phosphate ("Fleet Phosphosoda") given orally are convenient to clean the large bowel prior to colonoscopy but have recently been recognized as a cause of acute kidney injury, sometimes with irreversible (chronic) kidney damage [6]. Their high phosphate content favors substantial phosphate absorption by the bowel, with the risk of renal deposition of calcium phosphate salts, especially in predisposed patients, such as CKD patients, the elderly, those under diuretics, and those with diabetes, hypertension, congestive heart failure, active colitis, etc. The recent KDIGO CKD Guidelines specifically recommend not to use oral phosphate-containing bowel cleaning preparations in patients with an eGFR <60 [7] (Box 20.1).

Box 20.1. What the Guidelines Say You Should Do

Oral phosphate-containing bowel preparations should not be used in people with a GFR <60 ml/min./1.73 m^2 or in those known to be at risk of phosphate nephropathy.

Source: Kidney Disease: Improving Global Outcomes (KDIGO) [7]

20.2 Liver and GI Tract Consequences/Implications of CKD

20.2.1 Liver

Patients with CKD can develop a variety of acute and chronic diseases of the liver. The most common and serious ones in CKD patients remain HBV and HCV infection.

20.2.1.1 HCV as a Cause of Liver Disease in CKD

Several studies, mostly small sized, have suggested that the prevalence of anti-HCV antibodies is high among patients with the late stages (mostly 4 and 5) of CKD non-D, ranging from 3.9 to 14 % [8–12]. These prevalence figures should be interpreted in the light of the known prevalence of HCV in the general population worldwide, known to be highest in Egypt; intermediate in Asia, the USA, and Southern/Eastern Europe; and lowest in Northern Europe [13].

The importance of HCV as cause of liver damage in patients with CKD stage 4–5 non-D has increased with the advent of preemptive kidney transplantation: understanding the characteristics of liver disease is important for the evaluation and management of potential renal transplant candidates. Lemos et al. [12] assessed the epidemiology and clinical significance of hepatitis C in a large cohort of uremic patients not yet receiving dialysis in Brazil. A total of 1,041 patients with a creatinine clearance of 36 ± 18 ml/min were enrolled (49 % had CKD stage 4–5). Forty-one (3.9 %) patients were anti-HCV positive (with viremia in 95 % of them). A population study conducted in the same region reported an anti-HCV prevalence of 1.4 % ($P<0.001$). Moreover, chronically HCV-infected patients presented significantly higher serum alanine aminotransferase (ALT) levels (1.3 vs. 0.4× ULN, $P<0.001$). By logistic regression analysis, a history of blood transfusion before 1992, intravenous drug abuse, and ALT level all had an independent and significant association with chronic HCV.

In a prospective, observational study in 860 US patients, the anti-HCV positivity rate was seven to eight times greater at dialysis start (14.4 %) than in the general population (1.8 %). In these US inner city units, much of the HCV burden (prevalence 16.8 %) was thus acquired prior to starting dialysis, particularly among those who are younger and black or have a history of drug use [10]. The authors concluded that risk factors for HCV infection in patients receiving dialysis now may differ substantially from those identified 20 years ago. Transmission of HCV in the HD setting has clearly decreased because of a now much safer blood supply, at least in developed countries, the availability of erythropoiesis-stimulating agents, and better hygienic precautions. Rather, most anti-HCV (+) dialysis patients may have become infected before the initiation of dialysis.

HCV infection results in an increase in serum aspartate (AST) and alanine (ALT) aminotransferase levels. Unfortunately, the diagnostic value of AST/ALT measurement to assess acute or chronic HCV is rather weak in CKD patients. Lower serum aminotransferase values in dialysis patients than in healthy controls have long been reported [14]. This phenomenon may extend to CKD non-D patients. In a large ($n=407$) cross-sectional survey of consecutive individuals with a serum creatinine >2 mg/dl, Fabrizi et al. [15] reported lower serum aminotransferase activity in comparison with healthy persons. The difference persisted in age-matched comparisons and after correction for viral markers (HBsAg and anti-HCV), AST 17.9±8 vs. 20.4±6 IU/l ($P=0.0001$) and ALT 17.5±10 vs. 21.7±11.3 IU/l ($P=0.0001$). Although this is a single cross-sectional study, it seems reasonable to state that in patients both with and without viral hepatitis, aminotransferase levels are higher in those with normal kidney function, probably intermediate in pre-dialysis, and lowest in patients on dialysis. Although the causes of this lower ALT/AST level in CKD are still disputed, the diagnostic implications are significant.

Regarding the management of HCV infection in CKD, the KDIGO Guidelines [16] recommend that all HCV-infected patients, regardless of treatment, be followed for HCV-associated comorbidities, including the onset of cirrhosis or hepatocellular carcinoma. Patients with clinical or histological evidence of cirrhosis should have follow-up every 6 months, whereas annual follow-up is suggested for patients without cirrhosis. Follow-up should include both alpha-fetoprotein measurement and liver imaging (Box 20.2).

The KDIGO Guidelines further suggest to base the decision to treat HCV infection on the potential benefits and risks of therapy, including life expectancy, candidacy for kidney transplantation, and comorbidities. The KDIGO Guidelines specifically suggest to treat HCV-infected patients accepted for kidney transplantation, but prior to kidney transplantation (Box 20.3).

Until recently, a liver biopsy was required before any antiviral treatment. Since the 2008 KDIGO Guidelines [16], both the APRI index (the ratio of AST level to platelets) and transient elastography (or "Fibroscan") have been shown to be good noninvasive markers of the extent of liver fibrosis [17, 18]. In particular, transient elastography has been validated both in the general population and in dialyzed patients so that despite the absence of large CKD non-D series, it probably works in CKD as well. It measures the velocity of a low-frequency elastic shear wave propagating through the liver. This velocity is directly related to tissue stiffness. The result of transient elastography and/or serum markers may in some cases make a liver biopsy unnecessary.

Finally it should be stressed that the main drugs (pegylated interferon and ribavirin) used hitherto in HCV antiviral treatment are eliminated by the kidney and their dosage should thus be adapted as a function of eGFR or CKD stage, along the general recommendations of Table 20.1.

Box 20.2. What the Guidelines Say You Should Do

All patients with HCV infection, regardless of treatment or treatment response, should be followed for HCV-associated comorbidities. Patients who have evidence of clinical or histological cirrhosis should have follow-up every 6 months. Annual follow-up for patients without cirrhosis is suggested.

Source: Kidney Disease: Improving Global Outcomes (KDIGO) [16]

Box 20.3. What the Guidelines Say You Should Do

It is suggested that the decision to treat CKD patients with HCV infection be based on the potential benefits and risks of therapy, including life expectancy, candidacy for kidney transplantation, and comorbidities. It is specifically suggested to treat HCV-infected patients accepted for kidney transplantation, but prior to kidney transplantation.

Source: Kidney Disease: Improving Global Outcomes (KDIGO) [16]

20.2.1.2 HBV in CKD

Like for HCV, the prevalence rates of HBV in CKD patients are related to the local general population prevalence, with a north-to-south and west-to-east gradient.

Thus, not surprisingly, small reports from India (7 %) or Turkey (10.5 %) showed high HBsAg-positive rates [11, 19], whereas the rate of chronic HBsAg seropositive individuals with pre-dialysis CKD from Spain and Italy was between 0 and 3.7 % [20].

Table 20.1 Recommended treatment of HCV infection in patients with CKD and associated adverse events

Stage of CKD	IFN	Ribavirin	Common adverse events
1 and 2	Pegylated IFN alfa-2a: 180 μg SQ q week	800–1,200 mg/day in two divided doses	IFN: headache, flu-like illness, depression
	Pegylated IFN alfa-2b: 1.5 μg/kg SQ q week		Ribavirin: worsened anemia due to hemolysis
3	Pegylated IFN alfa-2a: 180 μg SQ q week	eGFR 50–60: 400–800 mg/day	IFN: same as above
	Pegylated IFN alfa-2b: 1 μg/kg SQ q week	eGFR 30–50: 300 mg/day (200 mg and 400 mg alternating)	Ribavirin can cause hemolytic anemia, and its use must be supported with increased erythropoietin as needed
4	Pegylated IFN alfa-2a: 135 μg SQ q week	200 mg/day	Same as above
	Pegylated IFN alfa-2b: 1 μg/kg SQ q week		
5 non-D	Pegylated IFN alfa-2a: 90–135 μg SQ q week	200 mg/day	Same as above
	Pegylated IFN alfa-2b: 1 μg/kg SQ q week		

Source: Data from Fabrizi et al. [4]
Abbreviations: *SQ* subcutaneously, *q week* every week

Table 20.2 Dosage adjustment of nucleos(t)ide analogs and interferon according to creatinine clearance (CrCl)

CrCl (ml/min)	Lamivudine	Telbivudine	Adefovir	Entecavir	Tenofovir	Pegylated interferon α-2[a]
≥50	100 mg/day	600 mg/day	10 mg/day	0.5 mg/day	245 mg/day	180 μg SQ/week
30–49	100 mg first dose, then 50 mg/day	600 mg/day 2	10 mg/day 2	0.25 mg/day	245 mg/day 2	135 μg SQ/week
15–29	35 mg first dose, then 25 mg/day	600 mg/day 3	10 mg/day 3	0.15 mg/day	245 mg/day 2–3	
5–14	35 mg first dose, then 15 mg/day	600 mg/day 3	10 mg/day 3[b]	0.05 mg/day[b]	245 mg/week[b]	

Source: Adapted by permission from Macmillan Publishers Ltd: Pipili et al. [2], Copyright 2013
Abbreviation: *SQ* subcutaneous
[a]Recommendations only for nucleos(t)ide analog-naive patients
[b]Recommendation only for CrCl ≥10 ml/min

In a large cohort (n=405) of CKD non-D patients, the prevalence of HBsAg positivity was 3.7 % (15), thus lower than in dialysis (8.7 %) but greater than in healthy persons of the same region (0.5 %). Multivariate analysis showed an independent and significant association between AST level and HBsAg positivity.

Numerous risk factors may predispose predialysis patients to HBV and/or HCV infections: these include high-risk behaviors (recreational drug use or unsafe sex), prolonged hospitalizations or frequent health-care utilization potentially increasing nosocomial exposure to blood-borne agents, impaired immune response from chronic uremia, and decreased vaccine responsiveness.

The management of HBV infection in patients with CKD has recently been reviewed extensively [2]. It should be pointed out here again that the dosage of many of the anti-HBV drugs, eliminated by the kidney, should be adapted to eGFR/CKD stage, as detailed on Table 20.2.

20.2.1.3 Other Causes of Liver Disease in Chronic Kidney Disease

Any therapeutic drug has the potential of causing hepatic damage, although some drugs are far more likely than others to do so. In addition, susceptibility to developing such injury differs between patients. No firm evidence shows that patients with CKD stage 4 or 5 are more likely to develop drug-induced liver toxicity than other individuals. However, drug interactions have an important role in the pathogenesis of drug-induced liver disease in uremic patients, as these patients frequently receive multiple medications. Drug-induced hepatic injury can be either hepatocellular or cholestatic; a complete list of medications capable of producing hepatic damage is beyond the scope of this chapter. NSAIDs are widely used, although less so in CKD patients, and may, albeit infrequently, cause hepatic damage [21]. Allopurinol and anabolic steroids may be hepatotoxic in CKD patients; numerous antibiotics can also cause hepatic dysfunction, including tetracyclines, macrolides, trimethoprim-sulfamethoxazole, rifampicin, and isoniazid. Some cardiovascular medications are also hepatotoxic; for example, amiodarone and methyldopa cause cholestatic and hepatocellular injury, respectively. Monitoring of serum ALT and AST activity is recommended during treatment with HMG-CoA reductase inhibitors. Another potential cause of hepatic dysfunction is hepatic congestion due to heart failure. The diagnosis of drug-induced hepatotoxicity is made via a process of exclusion.

In the differential diagnosis of acute liver dysfunction in uremic patients, viral infections such as HBV and HCV, herpes simplex virus, Epstein-Barr virus, or cytomegalovirus should be considered, as should adverse effects of drugs. Patients with elevated levels of serum ALT, AST, and/or gamma-glutamyl transpeptidase should be rechecked after the patient has abstained from potentially toxic substances.

Ethanol-induced liver disease is an infrequent condition in uremic patients. Another form of liver disease receiving growing attention is non-alcoholic fatty liver disease. Risk factors include obesity, hyperlipidemia, and diabetes mellitus. All these factors have a growing prevalence and are associated with the prevalence of CKD, too. The diagnosis is a histological one, and disease management involves correcting the predisposing factors.

Another concern that is becoming prevalent is the frequent use of alternative medications, such as herbal and health food store products, by patients on complex medical regimens. The potential toxic effects of herbal products have been understudied, although at least some of these products may cause an elevation of serum levels of ALT, AST, or gamma-glutamyl transpeptidase. The recent KDIGO Guidelines for CKD specifically recommend not to use herbal remedies in CKD [7] (Box 20.4).

Box 20.4. What the Guidelines Say You Should Do

- Herbal remedies should not be used in people with CKD.

  Source: Kidney Disease: Improving Global Outcomes (KDIGO) [7]

20.2.2 GI Tract

20.2.2.1 Upper GI Tract

Upper GI Tract Symptoms

Nausea and vomiting are frequent symptoms in patients with CKD. These may derive from various categories of causes.

- Stage 5 ("terminal") CKD: Although some degree of anorexia and more rarely nausea, the latter typically in the morning before the breakfast, is common in CKD stage 4, such symptoms should not be ascribed to CKD per se until stage 5 CKD. And even in that late stage, alternative explanations should be searched for nausea/vomiting. Indeed, if symptoms are ascribed to terminal CKD, symptomatic treatment will usually be relatively unhelpful and renal replacement therapy will be required.

- Role of drugs: Many drugs commonly prescribed to CKD patients may cause nausea. In case of doubt, a short withdrawal (a week) may help clarify the impact of a specific drug. The most frequently incriminated drugs include phosphate binders (calcium based, sevelamer, and lanthanum), numerous antibiotics such as fluoroquinolones, digoxin, iron supplements, morphine derivatives, azathioprine, mycophenolate mofetil, sirolimus, etc. Obviously in patients under immunosuppressive drugs, the suspected causal drug should usually be temporarily replaced by an alternative immunosuppressive agent whenever feasible.

Upper GI Tract Disease More Prevalent in CKD Patients

Not surprisingly, in view of the high prevalence of diabetes in patients with CKD, diabetic gastroparesia is very common in CKD patients. Common symptoms are bloating, episodic vomiting, and early satiety. Delayed gastric emptying may adversely affect glycemic control as well as slow absorption of orally administered drugs. The ultimate diagnosis relies on nuclear medicine imaging of gastric emptying. Management is frequently difficult and includes use of prokinetic drugs such as domperidone, keeping in mind that many such drugs prolong the QT interval and should not be combined with other drugs having the same characteristic (such as sotalol, fluoroquinolones, amiodarone, etc.)

20.2.2.2 Lower GI Tract

Bowel Movement Disturbances

Many drugs may cause either constipation or diarrhea or not infrequently alternating constipation and diarrhea in CKD patients. These include the various phosphate binders, both calcium based as well as non-calcium based (sevelamer and lanthanum) and the more recent calcium and magnesium combination. Others are the calcium- and sodium-based potassium-binding resins and oral iron preparations. In a particular patient, a history of irregular bowel movements or constipation or diarrhea should trigger the question: is this drug-induced? A temporal relationship may often be disclosed by careful history taking. In case of doubt, temporary withdrawal of the suspected causal drug(s) may be very helpful.

Lower GI Tract Disease More Prevalent in CKD Patients

1. Ischemic colitis is definitely more prevalent in CKD as a result of the frequent association of CKD with multiple risk factors for atherosclerosis. Thus, this diagnosis should be considered rapidly in a CKD patient with abdominal pain, diarrhea, and bloody stools. Computerized tomography will usually establish the diagnosis.
2. Angiodysplasia is more prevalent too in CKD patients than in the general population. Although the reasons for this higher prevalence are disputed, angiodysplasia is not uncommon throughout the GI tract from the stomach to large bowel thus including the small bowel, much less accessible to investigation.

When managing a lower GI tract hemorrhage, unexplained despite colonoscopy, a small bowel enteroscopy or an angiography (after appropriate preparation to minimize the toxicity of the contrast agent) will be the next step, if bleeding persists.

When facing GI tract bleeding, drugs known to interfere with hemostasis (aspirin, warfarin, NSAIDs, clopidogrel) should be temporarily withdrawn if possible and the search for the causal lesion started. The efficacy of hormone (estrogen-based) therapy for GI tract bleeding due to angiodysplasia is debated. Endoscopic treatment may be possible for some lesions, especially as most patients with angiodysplasia are elderly and surgical resection is associated with a high risk [22].

Before You Finish: Practice Pearls for the Clinician

- The onset of GI tract symptoms/signs (nausea, diarrhea, constipation) in a CKD patient should trigger the suspicion of a drug-related side effect. Numerous drugs may be incriminated, including phosphate binders, K-binding resins, antibiotics, and various analgesics.
- CKD patients have an increased prevalence of GI tract angiodysplasia. This should be kept in mind when investigating GI tract hemorrhage in CKD.
- Testing for both HBV and HCV should be included in the serological assessment of unexplained glomerulonephritis.
- Significant steatorrhea (not always clinically overt) may cause oxalate nephropathy. Thus, when facing unexplained CKD in a patient with diarrhea, oxaluria should be measured.
- The dosage of many drugs used in the treatment of both HBV and HCV infection should be adapted to CKD stage.

References

1. Zeng CH, Chen HM, Wang RS, Chen Y, Zhang SH, Liu L, et al. Etiology and clinical characteristics of membranous nephropathy in Chinese patients. Am J Kidney Dis. 2008;52(4):691–8.
2. Pipili CL, Papatheodoridis GV, Cholongitas EC. Treatment of hepatitis B in patients with chronic kidney disease. Kidney Int. 2013;84(5):880–5.
3. Feng B, Eknoyan G, Guo ZS, Jadoul M, Rao HY, Zhang W, et al. Effect of interferon-alpha-based antiviral therapy on hepatitis C virus-associated glomerulonephritis: a meta-analysis. Nephrol Dial Transplant. 2012;27(2):640–6.
4. Fabrizi F, Aghemo A, Messa P. Hepatitis C treatment in patients with kidney disease. Kidney Int. 2013; 84(5):874–9.
5. Cartery C, Faguer S, Karras A, Cointault O, Buscail L, Modesto A, et al. Oxalate nephropathy associated with chronic pancreatitis. Clin J Am Soc Nephrol. 2011;6(8):1895–902.
6. Markowitz GS, Perazella MA. Acute phosphate nephropathy. Kidney Int. 2009;76(10):1027–34.
7. Kidney Disease: Improving Global Outcomes (KDIGO) CKD Work Group. KDIGO 2012 clinical practice guideline for the evaluation and management of chronic kidney disease. Kidney Int. Suppl. 2013;3:1–150.
8. Iwasa Y, Otsubo S, Sugi O, Sato K, Asamiya Y, Eguchi A, et al. Patterns in the prevalence of hepatitis C virus infection at the start of hemodialysis in Japan. Clin Exp Nephrol. 2008;12(1):53–7.
9. Fabrizi F, Marcelli D, Bacchini G, Guarnori I, Erba G, Locatelli F. Antibodies to hepatitis C virus (HCV) in chronic renal failure (CRF) patients on conservative therapy: prevalence, risk factors and relationship to liver disease. Nephrol Dial Transplant. 1994;9(7): 780–4.
10. Bergman S, Accortt N, Turner A, Glaze J. Hepatitis C infection is acquired pre-ESRD. Am J Kidney Dis. 2005;45(4):684–9.
11. Sit D, Kadiroglu AK, Kayabasi H, Yilmaz ME, Goral V. Seroprevalence of hepatitis B and C viruses in patients with chronic kidney disease in the predialysis stage at a university hospital in Turkey. Intervirology. 2007;50(2):133–7.
12. Lemos LB, Perez RM, Lemos MM, Draibe SA, Silva IS, Silva AE, et al. Hepatitis C among predialysis patients: prevalence and characteristics in a large cohort of patients. Nephron Clin Pract. 2008;108(2): c135–40.
13. Lavanchy D. The global burden of hepatitis C. Liver Int. 2009;29 Suppl 1:74–81.
14. Yasuda K, Okuda K, Endo N, Ishiwatari Y, Ikeda R, Hayashi H, et al. Hypoaminotransferasemia in patients undergoing long-term hemodialysis: clinical and biochemical appraisal. Gastroenterology. 1995; 109(4):1295–300.
15. Fabrizi F, Lunghi G, Finazzi S, Colucci P, Pagano A, Ponticelli C, et al. Decreased serum aminotransferase activity in patients with chronic renal failure: impact on the detection of viral hepatitis. Am J Kidney Dis. 2001;38(5):1009–15.
16. Kidney Disease: Improving Global Outcomes. KDIGO clinical practice guidelines for the prevention, diagnosis, evaluation, and treatment of Hepatitis C in chronic kidney disease. Kidney Int. 2008;73 (Suppl 109):S1–S99.
17. Liu CH, Liang CC, Huang KW, Liu CJ, Chen SI, Lin JW, et al. Transient elastography to assess hepatic fibrosis in hemodialysis chronic hepatitis C patients. Clin J Am Soc Nephrol. 2011;6:1057–65.
18. Castera L. Noninvasive methods to assess liver disease in patients with hepatitis B or C. Gastroenterology. 2012;142:1293–302.
19. Chandra M, Khaja MN, Hussain MM, Poduri CD, Farees N, Habeeb MA, et al. Prevalence of hepatitis B and hepatitis C viral infections in Indian patients with chronic renal failure. Intervirology. 2004;47(6):374–6.
20. Lopez-Alcorocho JM, Barril G, Ortiz-Movilla N, Traver JA, Bartolome J, Sanz P, et al. Prevalence of hepatitis B, hepatitis C, GB virus C/hepatitis G and TT viruses in predialysis and hemodialysis patients. J Med Virol. 2001;63(2):103–7.
21. Risser A, Donovan D, Heintzman J, Page T. NSAID prescribing precautions. Am Fam Physician. 2009;80(12):1371–8.
22. Chalasani N, Cotsonis G, Wilcox CM. Upper gastrointestinal bleeding in patients with chronic renal failure: role of vascular ectasia. Am J Gastroenterol. 1996;91(11):2329–32.

21 Pruritus and Other Dermatological Problems in Chronic Kidney Disease

Jenna Lester and Leslie Robinson-Bostom

Before You Start: Facts You Need to Know

- Pruritus is one of the most common cutaneous symptoms in patients with chronic kidney disease on dialysis. Treatments offer minimal relief.
- Xerosis cutis, another common finding in chronic kidney disease, can be treated with emollients.
- Disorders in calcium and phosphorus metabolism are common in patients with chronic kidney disease and include calciphylaxis and metastatic calcinosis cutis.

21.1 Pruritus

Pruritus is a commonly seen in patients with chronic kidney disease on dialysis. In the past, prevalence was reported to be as high as 90 % in patients with chronic kidney disease; however, more recently, rates of 20–50 % of patients have been described [1]. It seems to be independent of sex, ethnicity, type of dialysis, and underlying renal disease. Pruritus itself is not immediately threatening, but it is an independent predictor of mortality [1].

21.1.1 What Causes Pruritus in Chronic Kidney Disease?

The pathophysiologic mechanism of uremic pruritus is poorly understood, but hypotheses implicate immune system dysregulation that results in a proinflammatory state leading to itching [2]. The increase in levels of C-reactive protein and other inflammatory mediators contribute to itch. Additionally, the derangement in calcium and phosphate metabolism that occurs in CKD can cause accumulation of these substances in the skin, which can further exacerbate pruritus [1]. Some also postulate that changes in neurological perception that occur with chronic itching increase the perception and sensation of itch [1]. The middle molecule theory is based on the idea that nondialyzable substances accumulate and cause pruritus. This explains why the itching resolves after renal transplantation [3].

J. Lester, BA
Department of Dermatology, Warren Alpert Medical School of Brown University, 70 Ship Street, Box G-M 9075, Providence, RI 02903, USA
e-mail: jenna_lester@brown.edu

L. Robinson-Bostom, MD (✉)
Division of Dermatopathology, Warren Alpert Medical School of Brown University, Providence, RI, USA

Department of Dermatology, Rhode Island Hospital, APC 10, 593 Eddy Street, Providence, RI 02903, USA
e-mail: lrobinson-bostom@lifespan.org

M. Arici (ed.), *Management of Chronic Kidney Disease*,
DOI 10.1007/978-3-642-54637-2_21, © Springer-Verlag Berlin Heidelberg 2014

21.1.2 What Are the Important Clinical Characteristics?

Pruritus has a negative impact on quality of life. It is frequently disabling and can have a significant effect on mental well-being contributing to daytime fatigue, agitation, and depression [2]. Patients may have complaints ranging from intermittent itching to persistent pruritus, usually affecting the back [1, 2] and usually worse at night. The arms, head, and abdomen are also affected [2].

21.1.3 How Is Pruritus in CKD Treated?

Treatment for pruritus associated with CKD is limited. The evidence for the treatments described in the literature is mostly anecdotal or based on case series [4]. When approaching a patient with pruritus, a stepwise approach may be helpful. Treatment of xerosis with emollients is essential because pruritus can be worsened by dry skin. A trial of emollients containing menthol or pramoxine can be beneficial [1]. Topical capsaicin is also cited as being beneficial for localized pruritus but has not been effective in our clinical practice. Studies have demonstrated a dramatic reduction in pruritus with the use of topical tacrolimus [1], but this treatment may not be as effective and is not practical in patients with more diffuse pruritus.

Systemic treatments like gabapentin have been shown to be effective in some case studies [2, 4]. However, other studies have also failed to demonstrate any improvement with gabapentin [2]. In cases where it is effective, gabapentin was shown to decrease the mean pruritus score with a dosage of 300 mg three times a day. There is an increased risk of gabapentin toxicity in patients on dialysis; therefore, it is recommended to start with a low dose and gradually increase until the maximum dose is reached [2].

Broadband UVB phototherapy is another treatment option for pruritus in CKD and is regarded by many clinicians as the treatment of choice. UVB light decreases the levels of proinflammatory cytokines, which, as mentioned previously, may play a role in the pathogenesis of itch. Case series and pilot studies have shown UVB to be effective [2, 4]. It is important to consider the risk of skin cancer associated with UVB exposure because CKD patients are immunosuppressed and thus are predisposed to malignancy. This is especially important to consider if they have light skin types and are candidates for renal transplantation (Fig. 21.1).

Fig. 21.1 Lichenification in a CKD patient with pruritus

21.2 Xerosis

Xerosis is a common cutaneous manifestation of CKD and was shown in two different studies to be the most prevalent of skin changes observed [5, 6]. It is characterized by dryness of the skin, ichthyosis, roughness, and poor skin turgor [7]. The effects of this condition can lead to compromised functional integrity of the skin barrier resulting in increased susceptibility to contact irritants and infection. Some studies have reported a difference in prevalence of xerosis between patients receiving dialysis and those that are not receiving dialysis, but others have not observed any difference between these two groups [8].

21.2.1 What Causes Xerosis in CKD?

The cause of xerosis is unknown; however, many theories exist to explain its occurrence. The skin is a primary site of water homeostasis and with dialysis treatment and the associated high-dose diuretic therapies, water balance can be disturbed leading to skin dryness [7]. Other theories cite the reduction in size of sebaceous glands and eccrine sweat glands as the cause for xerosis [3].

21.2.2 What Are the Important Clinical Characteristics?

Xerosis can be generalized or localized and is most often located on the extremities. Patients complain of dry "cracked" skin that can be superimposed on uremic pruritus [3]. An important diagnosis to exclude is ichthyosis vulgaris as the clinical characteristics of this entity can closely resemble those of xerosis.

21.2.3 How Is Xerosis in CKD Treated?

It is important to ensure the skin is adequately lubricated. Gentle skin care and emollients can be helpful in treating xerosis and its associated symptoms [1]. In xerosis, there is a known decrease in glycerol content in the stratum corneum leading researchers to test the efficacy of emollients containing glycerol and paraffin [9]. One study showed a significant decrease in complaints of xerosis and xerotic lesions when using emollients with glycerol and paraffin. Glycerol has a hydrating effect, while paraffin protects the skin from irritants, thereby addressing two of the major components of xerosis [9] (Fig. 21.2).

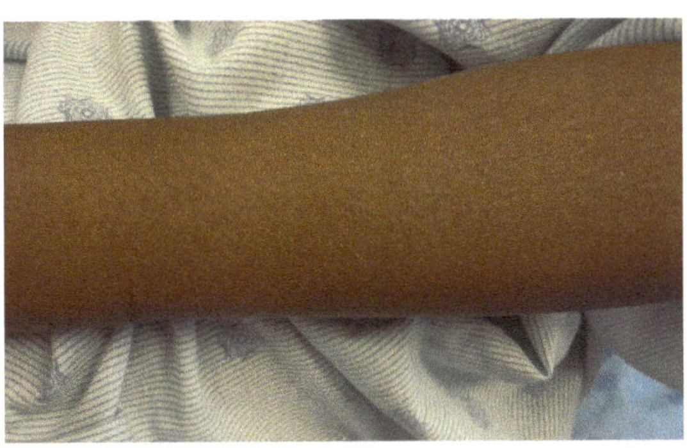

Fig. 21.2 Xerosis in a patient with CKD

21.3 Lindsay's (Half and Half) Nails

Lindsay's nails or half-and-half nails are a characteristic finding in patients with CKD. They are seen in patients with any degree of azotemia and present as a proximal white portion and distal reddish pink to brown portion of the nail. This specific nail finding is present in approximately 1/3 of patients with CKD [10]. Usually, this nail finding develops before patients need chronic dialysis, but it also is a frequent finding in patients on chronic dialysis [11].

21.3.1 What Causes Lindsay's Nails in CKD?

Although the condition is poorly understood, hypotheses include the increased tissue concentration of β-melanocyte-stimulating hormone due to its poor dialyzability [3].

21.3.2 What Are the Important Clinical Considerations in Lindsay's Nails?

There are nail changes that indicate other forms of disease that should be ruled out when a clinician suspects Lindsay's nails due to azotemia. Mees' lines, Beau's lines, and Terry's nails should all be ruled out in a patient with azotemia who presents with nail changes.

21.3.3 How Do You Treat Lindsay's Nails?

There are no treatments of Lindsay's nails, but the condition sometimes resolves with renal transplantation [3]. It has not been known to resolve with initiation of dialysis (Fig. 21.3).

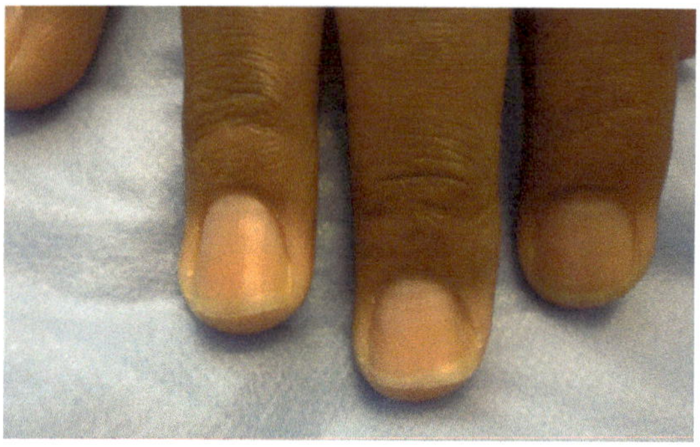

Fig. 21.3 Lindsay's (half and half) nails in a CKD patient. Note proximal white portion and distal reddish brown portion

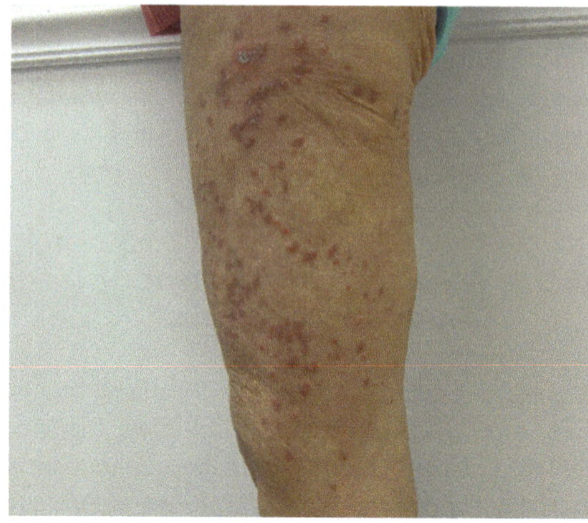

Fig. 21.4 Acquired perforating dermatosis with prominent Koebnerization in a patient with CKD (Image courtesy of Jessica Kirk, MD)

21.4 Acquired Perforating Dermatosis

This is an acquired pruritic disorder seen most commonly in patients with CKD with overlapping clinical and histologic features of the primary perforating disorders including perforating folliculitis, Kyrle's disease, elastosis perforans serpiginosa, and reactive perforating collagenosis [12]. This disorder is characterized by hyperkeratotic follicular papules.

21.4.1 What Causes Acquired Perforating Dermatosis?

The pathogenesis of this disorder is not well understood, but a common finding is the transepidermal elimination of altered dermal substances [12]. The theory suggests that acquired perforating dermatosis may be caused by the accumulation of dermal micro deposits containing substances like calcium salts that cause a foreign body reaction [13]. Another hypothesis cites local trauma induced by excoriation and microvasculopathy causing extrusion of substances through the dermis as another cause for acquired perforating dermatosis [3].

21.4.2 What Are Important Clinical Considerations of Acquired Perforating Dermatosis?

It is important to remember that acquired perforating dermatosis is a spectrum of clinical disorders, and thus the specific underlying disease may vary with a similar presentation. Furthermore, the patient may also have pruritus associated with acquired perforating dermatosis or due to uremic pruritus. Koebnerization, or the development of new lesions induced by trauma, can occur with acquired perforating dermatosis; thus, adequate treatment of pruritus as well as counseling to decrease scratching is appropriate.

21.4.3 How Do You Treat Acquired Perforating Dermatosis?

Topical and systemic retinoids, ultraviolet B phototherapy, psoralen and ultraviolet A, cryosurgery and photodynamic therapy, topical corticosteroids, and keratolytics should all be considered in the treatment of acquired perforating dermatosis [3]. Renal transplantation has also been known to clear acquired perforating dermatosis [13] (Fig. 21.4).

21.5 Calciphylaxis

Calciphylaxis is also known as calcific uremic arteriolopathy and is a cutaneous condition that typically presents in the setting of end-stage renal disease associated with secondary hyperparathyroidism. It results from arteriolar deposition of calcium leading to livedo reticularis and ultimately necrosis of the deep dermis and subcutaneous tissues. It is particularly seen in patients on hemodialysis, but even in this population, it is only present in 1–4 % [14]. Calciphylaxis is also seen in patients without uremia, specifically those with primary hyperparathyroidism, malignancy, connective tissue disease, previous corticosteroid use, alcoholic liver disease, and protein C or S deficiency [14].

21.5.1 What Causes Calciphylaxis?

The precise pathogenesis of calciphylaxis remains unknown, but small vessel endovascular fibrosis, fibrin thrombi, intimal proliferation, obliterative vasculopathy, tissue ischemia, calcification, panniculitis, and subcutaneous fat necrosis are all seen on histopathologic examination [14]. CKD also leads to decreased clearance of phosphorus resulting in extraosseous calcification [3]. This calcification decreases lumen diameter and can predispose to sudden vascular occlusion, which leads to the livedo reticularis and subsequent necrosis seen in calciphylaxis.

21.5.2 What Are the Important Clinical Considerations of Calciphylaxis?

Patients may report having exquisite tenderness over stellate-shaped lesions. The lesions are symmetric, and violaceous and progress to deep stellate ulcers. These ulcers may become gangrenous and are most commonly located on the proximal thighs and lower abdomen or distally on shins, digits, or penis [3]. There is a high morbidity and mortality associated with calciphylaxis. Death is usually secondary to sepsis.

21.5.3 What Are the Treatments of Calciphylaxis?

Treatment for calciphylaxis includes both medical and surgical modalities. Sodium thiosulfate, ordinarily used to treat cyanide toxicity, can be given intravenously. There are no standard dosages but case reports citing efficacy of sodium thiosulfate administered dosages ranging from 5 to 25 g IV three times a week, usually after hemodialysis [14]. This treatment is thought to work because it acts as an antioxidant, vasodilator, and calcium chelator.

It is also important to normalize serum phosphate and calcium. Studies using bisphosphonates to treat calcium and phosphate disturbances seen in calciphylaxis have found that they reduce pain and promote ulcer healing [14]. They are thought to have an anti-inflammatory effect by suppressing cytokine release and inhibiting macrophages.

The role for surgical debridement in calciphylaxis is an issue that is debated. Some advocate for aggressive surgical debridement. Studies do show an association between surgical debridement and significant improvement in survival rates [14]. Still, others advocate for the use of hydrocolloid dressing and atraumatic debridement methods as any skin trauma can lead to new lesions.

Parathyroidectomy is a potential surgical treatment for calciphylaxis in patients with hyperparathyroidism, but there are variable outcomes, and the evidence behind this treatment is not based on studies of large patient populations. Therefore, when considering this option, it is important to carefully consider the risk of the post-surgical effects of parathyroidectomy [14].

Hyperbaric oxygen therapy has also been studied as a treatment for calciphylaxis. Its purported benefits include stimulation of fibroblast proliferation, conversion to myofibroblasts, stimulation of neoangiogenesis, and toxicity to various organisms that have the potential to cause serious infection and impair wound healing [14] (Fig. 21.5).

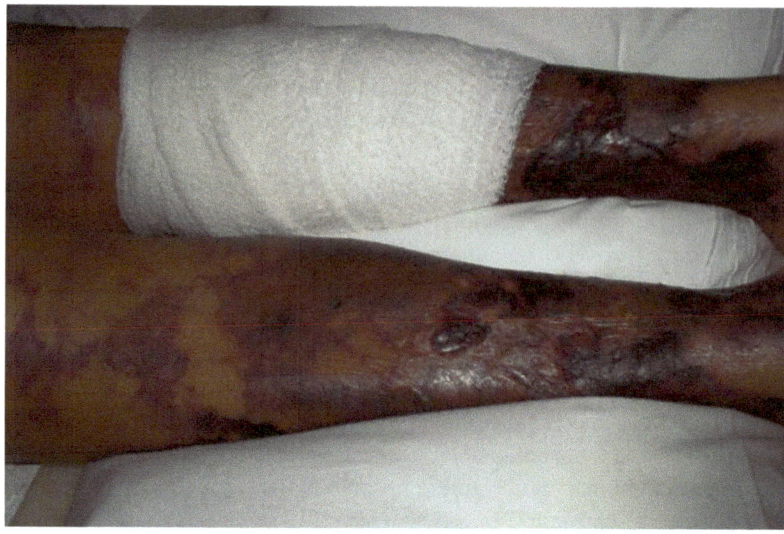

Fig. 21.5 Calciphylaxis in a patient with CKD (Image courtesy of Nathaniel Jellinek, MD)

21.6 Metastatic Calcinosis Cutis

Metastatic calcinosis cutis (MCC), also referred to as benign nodular calcification, is a condition presenting with firm nodules and plaques in the skin and subcutaneous tissue. They are usually painless but occasionally periarterial depositions or depositions near joints can be painful [15].

21.6.1 What Causes Metastatic Calcinosis Cutis?

Increased serum calcium or phosphate levels or both cause MCC. When the levels of these substances are increased in blood, they precipitate into the skin and subcutaneous tissues leading to palpable nodules and plaques [16]. Elevated calcium and phosphate is seen in renal failure due to poor renal excretion of phosphate and secondary hyperparathyroidism that develops as a result of poor intestinal reabsorption of calcium.

21.6.2 What Are the Important Clinical Considerations?

Patients may present with erythematous, firm, tender papules, nodules, or plaques with well-defined borders [16]. These lesions can undergo secondary change resulting in ulceration. They may also become fluctuant and extrude contents, which are chalky in nature. Calcium and phosphate deposition can extend beyond the skin and may occur in other organs.

21.6.3 What Are the Treatments for Calcinosis Cutis?

MCC lesions usually resolve after serum normalization of calcium and phosphate [3]. The surgical treatments of MCC lesions are similar to the treatments of calciphylaxis lesions including parathyroidectomy for hyperparathyroidism.

21.7 Nephrogenic Systemic Fibrosis (NSF)

This is a generalized fibrotic disorder that can occur in patients with CKD who have been exposed to gadolinium (see Chap. 3). Acute or chronic kidney dysfunction in combination with inflammation contributes to the development of NSF [3]. Liver disease, erythropoietin, and acidosis are suspected contributors.

21.7.1 What Causes NSF?

Gadolinium exposure in contrast MRA or MRI was recently identified as a potential trigger for NSF [3]. Precipitates of gadolinium are produced and serve as activating substances for macrophages and fibroblasts. These precipitates may be endocytosed by fibrocytes resulting in a fibrotic expression in fibroblasts subsequently leading to an activation of kappa B pathway and transforming growth factor beta, thus promoting fibrosis that is seen in this condition [3].

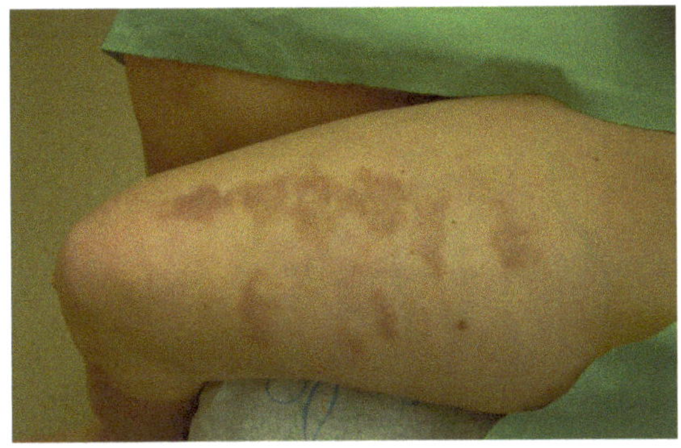

Fig. 21.6 Nephrogenic systemic fibrosis in a patient with CKD (Image courtesy of Seth Feder, MD)

21.7.2 What Are the Important Clinical Considerations in NSF?

Consider the diagnosis of NSF if the patient reports a recent history of undergoing a procedure requiring MRI or MRA with contrast. This condition can present with indurated plaques or diffuse areas of skin induration but can also involve joints causing contractures [3].

21.7.3 What Is the Treatment for NSF?

No treatments have proven effective in curing NSF, so it is important to counsel patients to avoid the known trigger of this disorder. There is anecdotal evidence that improvement of this condition can be observed with topical or systemic steroids, cyclophosphamide, thalidomide, plasmapheresis, immunoglobulin infusion, imatinib mesylate, and rapamycin [3] (Fig. 21.6).

21.8 Pseudoporphyria

Pseudoporphyria is a photodermatosis that is also known as bullous dermatosis of end-stage renal disease. It is seen in patients with CKD or in patients undergoing long-term dialysis [3].

21.8.1 What Causes Pseudoporphyria?

The exact pathophysiology of pseudoporphyria is unknown, but UV light is thought to play a role in this entity given its association with UVA light exposure and medications that sensitize the skin to damage in UV light. Furthermore, in patients with CKD, risk of injury due to free radicals is higher due to low levels of glutathione in the blood and red blood cells [3].

21.8.2 What Are the Important Clinical Considerations in Pseudoporphyria?

This condition usually affects sun-exposed areas, usually the dorsal aspect of the forearms and hands. The patient may describe having fragile skin and blisters.

21.8.3 What Is the Treatment for Pseudoporphyria?

Photoprotection and sun avoidance are important aspects of pseudoporphyria treatment. N-acetylcysteine can also be used as it is thought to increase the production of plasma glutathione, thus reducing the risk of damage due to free-radical injury. These symptoms are slow to resolve and may recur with discontinuation of treatment [3].

21.9 Porphyria Cutanea Tarda

Porphyria cutanea tarda (PCT) is a disorder caused by a deficiency in uroporphyrinogen decarboxylase. This results in accumulation of heme substances in the blood causing skin changes on exposure to UV light. Scarring, fragility, hyperpigmentation, hypertrichosis, and milia are common changes seen in PCT [17]. PCT can occur in many disease states and has an estimated prevalence of 1.2–18 % in CKD [17].

21.9.1 What Causes PCT?

As mentioned above, an accumulation of heme products in the blood leads to skin changes upon sun exposure. The cause of PCT in patients with CKD is not well understood but is likely multifactorial. Hypotheses implicate the disturbance of iron balance that can be seen in patients on dialysis.

21.9.2 What Are Some Important Clinical Considerations?

There are two types of PCT: type I (sporadic) and type II (familial). Patients presenting in their twenties likely have familial PCT, while those presenting in middle age are more likely to have sporadic PCT [3]. In addition to the skin changes mentioned above, patients may also have complaints of dark urine and pruritus [3].

21.9.3 How Do You Treat PCT?

Photoprotection and avoidance of sun exposure are key components to the management of PCT. Phlebotomy is an effective treatment of PCT and can be a treatment consideration in patients with CKD. However, some patients with CKD cannot tolerate the removal of 250–500 mL of blood twice weekly. For these patients, small-volume phlebotomy is an option [18]. Research has also shown efficacy of deferoxamine treatment administered concurrently with dialysis. There is also a reported synergistic effect when deferoxamine is given with erythropoietin treatment [17] (Fig. 21.7).

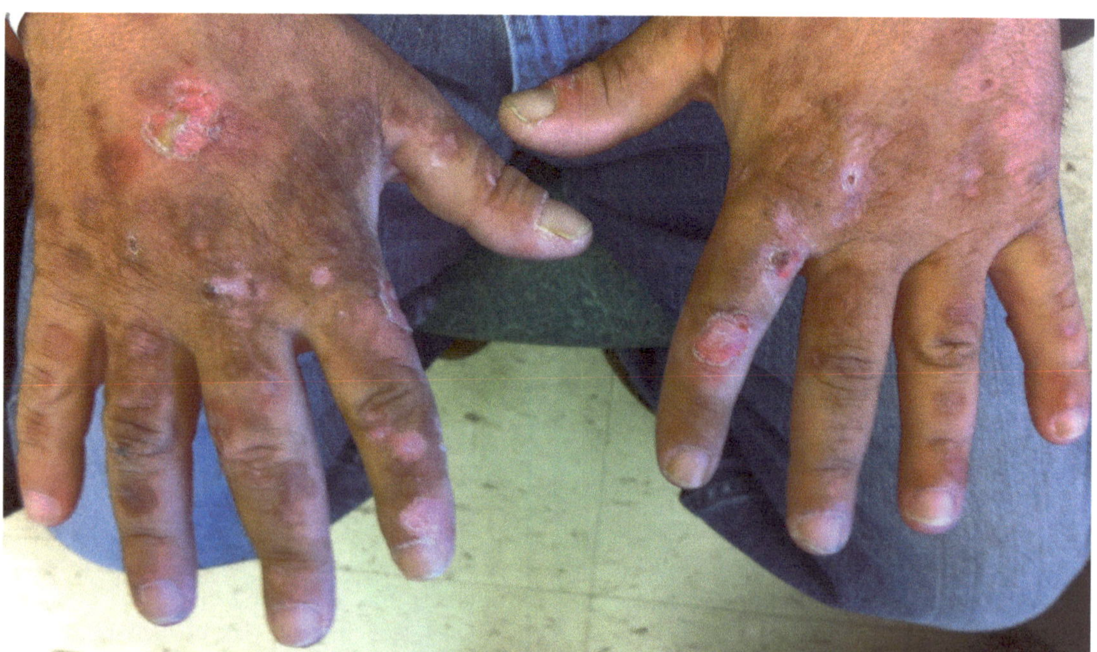

Fig. 21.7 Porphyria cutanea tarda in a patient with CKD (Image courtesy of Sandy Chai, MD)

Before You Finish: Practice Pearls for the Clinician

- There is no treatment for Lindsay's nails but sometimes it resolves with renal transplantation.
- Normalization of serum calcium and phosphate levels is the cornerstone of treatment in calciphylaxis and MCC.
- There are no effective treatments for NSF and therefore it is best to avoid gadolinium, a known trigger of the condition.
- Photoprotection is an important component of PCT and pseudoporphyria treatment. Deferoxamine and small-volume phlebotomy have also been effective in past studies.

References

1. Berger TG, Steinhoff M. Pruritus and renal failure. Semin Cutan Med Surg. 2011;30(2):99–100.
2. Patel TS, Freedman BI, Yosipovitch G. An update on pruritus associated with CKD. Am J Kidney Dis. 2007;50(1):11–20.
3. Markova A, Lester J, Wang J, Robinson-Bostom L. Diagnosis of common dermopathies in dialysis patients: a review and update. Semin Dial. 2012; 25(4):408–18.
4. Mettang M, Weisshaar E. Pruritus: control of itch in patients undergoing dialysis. Skin Therapy Lett. 2010;15(2):1–5.
5. Khanna D, Singal A, Kalra OP. Comparison of cutaneous manifestations in chronic kidney disease with or without dialysis. Postgrad Med J. 2010; 86(1021):641–7.
6. Falodun O, Ogunbiyi A, Salako B, George AK. Skin changes in patients with chronic renal failure. Saudi J Kidney Dis Transpl. 2011;22(2):268–72.
7. Szepietowski JC, Balaskas E, Taube KM, Taberly A, Dupuy P. Quality of life in patients with uraemic xerosis and pruritus. Acta Derm Venereol. 2011;91(3):313–7.
8. Amatya B, Agrawal S, Dhali T, Sharma S, Pandey SS. Pattern of skin and nail changes in chronic renal failure in Nepal: a hospital based study. J Dermatol. 2008;35(3):140–5.
9. Balaskas E, Szepietowski JC, Bessis D, Ioannides D, Ponticelli C, Ghienne C, Taberly A, Dupuy P. Randomized, double-blind study with glycerol and paraffin in uremic xerosis. Clin J Am Soc Nephrol. 2011;6(4):748–52.
10. Sharma V, Kumar V, Sharma A. Half-and-half nails. Iran J Kidney Dis. 2011;5(4):228.
11. Jamal A, Subramanian PT, Hussain KS. Nail changes in end-stage renal failure on hemodialysis. Saudi J Kidney Dis Transpl. 2000;11(1):44–7.
12. Udayakumar P, Balasubramanian S, Ramalingam KS, Lakshmi C, Srinivas CR, Mathew AC. Cutaneous manifestations in patients with chronic renal failure on hemodialysis. Indian J Dermatol Venereol Leprol. 2006;72(2):119–25.
13. Saray Y, Seckin D, Bilezikci B. Acquired perforating dermatosis: clinicopathological features in twenty-two cases. J Eur Acad Dermatol Venereol. 2006;20(6): 679–88.
14. Vedvyas C, Winterfield LS, Vleugels RA. Calciphylaxis: a systematic review of existing and emerging therapies. J Am Acad Dermatol. 2012; 67(6):e253–60.
15. Cordova KB, Oberg TJ, Malik M, Robinson-Bostom L. Dermatologic conditions seen in end-stage renal disease. Semin Dial. 2009;22(1):45–55.
16. Tan O, Atik B, Kizilkaya A, Ozer E, Kavukcu S. Extensive skin calcifications in an infant with chronic renal failure: metastatic calcinosis cutis. Pediatr Dermatol. 2006;23(3):235–8.
17. Labidi J. Porphyria cutanea tarda in a chronic hemodialysis patient. Pediatr Dermatol. 2010;21(5):919–22.
18. Shieh S, Cohen JL, Lim HW. Management of porphyria cutanea tarda in the setting of chronic renal failure: a case report and review. J Am Acad Dermatol. 2000;42(4):645–52.

Pain Management in Chronic Kidney Disease

22

Edwina A. Brown and Sara N. Davison

Before You Start: Facts You Need to Know

- Pain is common in patients with chronic kidney disease (50–70 % patients depending on study) and is often not recognized.
- Pain is related to comorbidities and causes and complications of chronic kidney disease.
- Pain can be controlled safely in patients with kidney disease, including those on dialysis.
- Pain medication should be prescribed in a logical manner using a pain-control ladder.
- Pain adversely affects quality of life so must not be ignored.

22.1 Pain in CKD

Pain is common – we have all experienced it. Unlike most things treated in medicine, the experience of pain is entirely subjective. We can recognize situations where we expect pain, such as fractures, tissue damage due to surgery, ischaemia, etc., but the pain itself is perceived differently by each individual. Pain can therefore only be diagnosed if we ask patients whether they have pain and how this is affecting them. How pain is experienced depends on many factors including culture, social support, mood as well as the pathology causing the pain. Often patients will not complain about chronic pain as they feel that this is part of their illness, that the healthcare team is not interested, or that any medication they have tried has been ineffective or has had side effects. Ideally, this should not happen as pain is known to be associated with depression and adversely affects quality of life.

22.1.1 Causes of Pain

It is not surprising that patients with CKD have such a high pain burden. As shown in Table 22.1, pain can be due to the underlying kidney disease, complications of poor kidney function, dialysis itself and comorbidities [1–3]. Determining the cause of pain therefore requires careful history taking. Indeed, patients may have often more than one cause of pain [1–3].

E.A. Brown, DM (Oxon), FRCP
Imperial College Kidney and Transplant Centre, Hammersmith Hospital, Du Cane Road, London W12 0HS, UK
e-mail: e.a.brown@imperial.ac.uk

S.N. Davison, MD, MSc (✉)
Department of Medicine and Dentistry, University of Alberta Hospital, 11-107 Clinical Sciences Building, Edmonton, AB T6G2G3, Canada
e-mail: sara.davison@ualberta.ca

M. Arici (ed.), *Management of Chronic Kidney Disease*,
DOI 10.1007/978-3-642-54637-2_22, © Springer-Verlag Berlin Heidelberg 2014

Table 22.1 Causes of pain related to CKD

Primary kidney disease	Some specific causes of kidney disease can be associated with significant and often severe pain, even at stages when kidney function itself is not impaired. Examples include: Polycystic kidneys Pain from bleeding into or rupture of cysts in kidney or liver Infection of cysts in kidney or liver Back pain from lumbar lordosis caused by abdominal distension from size of kidneys and/or liver Renal calculi – infection and obstruction
Comorbidity	Ischaemic heart disease – angina Peripheral vascular disease – claudication, ischaemic ulcers Diabetes – peripheral neuropathy Malignancy
Complications of CKD	Renal bone disease Peripheral neuropathy Gout Calciphylaxis
Haemodialysis	Steal syndrome related to arteriovenous fistula access Cramps during dialysis Dialysis amyloid arthropathy Discitis secondary to access infection Femoral vein thrombosis following femoral vein access
Peritoneal dialysis	Abdominal pain related to dialysate inflow or outflow or distension Lower back pain related to increased intra-abdominal pressure Peritonitis Bowel obstruction secondary to encapsulating peritoneal sclerosis
Transplant	Surgery related Acute rejection Lymphocele

Table 22.2 Causes of pain related to ageing

Musculoskeletal	Osteoarthritis Spinal stenosis Disc protrusion – sciatica Cervical spondylosis Vertebral fractures and collapse
Immobility	Decubitus ulcers

Increasingly, CKD is a disease of the elderly. Over 30 % of people over 80 years old have impaired kidney function. The majority of patients attending a general CKD clinic are therefore elderly and will have the general features and complications of ageing. Many of these are associated with pain as shown in Table 22.2.

22.1.2 Types of Pain

It is important to differentiate between acute and chronic pain. *Acute pain* is often associated with tissue damage, e.g. after injury or surgery. Dialysis patients may also experience episodes of acute pain during dialysis, such as headaches and cramps. Acute pain can be episodic but with periods without pain. In contrast, *chronic pain* is present for long periods of time and is often out of proportion with the extent of the originating injury. Experience of chronic pain by the patient will be affected by psychosocial factors as well as the underlying pathology causing the pain.

For the purpose of management, it is helpful to categorize pain into:

- *Nociceptive* – pain due to tissue damage
- *Neuropathic* – pain due to nerve damage
- *Mixed nociceptive and neuropathic* – e.g. pain of peripheral ischaemia
- *Incident or movement related* – caused by bone or joint damage; pain often absent at rest but more severe on movement
- *Other specific causes* – such as renal colic, bowel obstruction

22.2 Screening and Assessment of Pain (Box 22.1)

Pain is not assessed routinely by renal clinicians and is therefore frequently not recognized. Routine and proactive assessment of pain is important [2, 3]. There are three global symptom assessment tools in regular use, which have been adapted and validated specifically for use in those with CKD. These are the renal version of the Palliative Outcome Scale – symptom module (POSs renal), the renal modified Edmonton Symptom Assessment Scale (ESAS) and the Dialysis Symptom Index (DSI). All three tools ask the patient about the presence and severity of common physical and psychosocial symptoms in CKD [4–7].

Understanding the nature, severity and need for treatment of pain is a challenge and takes time. Many patients do not discuss their pain if they feel that the healthcare team is not interested, is rushed, or that treatment is ineffective or carries too many side effects. A proper assessment of pain can greatly improve the relationship between patient and their doctor or nurse. It is also important that this is ongoing with repeat assessments to assess efficacy and the need for potential changes of management.

Box 22.1. Screening and Assessment of Pain in CKD

- Key Facts
- Pain is perceived only by the patient, so can only be described by the patient.
- Perception of pain is affected by mood and the meaning of pain for the patient.

22.2.1 Obtaining a Pain History

A pain history should determine the site of pain, duration, whether constant or intermittent, what makes it worse or better, radiation, intensity and nature of the pain. It is also important to determine the mood of the patient, particularly whether depressed or not, and the meaning of the pain to the person [8]. A full pain assessment is shown in Table 22.3.

22.3 Management of Pain

22.3.1 Barriers to Pain Management

A combination of clinician and patient factors contribute to poor pain recognition and management in patients. This is true for all patients, but probably happens more frequently for patients with CKD owing to the complexity of the causes of pain, the fact that many nephrologists are not trained in pain management and the difficulty of prescribing analgesia with impaired *kidney* function. Table 22.4 lists potential clinician and patient factors and how these could be overcome.

22.3.2 Non-pharmacological Management

Pain perception and analgesic requirement vary between patients and with time in individual patients. Many factors can exacerbate pain including depression, loneliness, inactivity, fear and anxiety about meaning of pain. Pain management therefore includes exploring psychosocial issues with patients and eliciting potential depression and anxiety which should then be appropriately managed with psychological support and/or

Table 22.3 Scheme for pain assessment

	Useful questions
Site of pain	Where is pain?
Radiation	Does the pain go anywhere else?
History of pain	When did pain start? Was there anything that caused pain to start such as an injury, surgical procedure and infection? Has the pain got better or worse over time or does it fluctuate? Is the pain worse during the day or at night? Does the pain keep you awake?
Nature of pain	What is the pain like? Is it burning, stabbing, sharp, colicky, dull, etc.? Note: *nociceptive pain* is usually described as sharp; *neuropathic pain* is commonly described as burning, shooting and stabbing
Aggravating factors	What makes the pain worse – movement, position, eating, etc.?
Relieving factors	What makes the pain better – position, eating, temperature, etc.?
Severity	How severe would you say the pain is – mild, moderate, severe? Can you grade the pain on a scale of 1–10, with 10 being worst? Does the severity vary and if so how?
Impact of pain	How does the pain impact on daily activities, exercise, etc.? Does the pain stop you from sleeping? Do you ever feel down because of the pain?
Effect of treatment	What have you done to try and make the pain less? Do you take any painkillers, and if so what? Do you find the painkillers helpful?

Table 22.4 Potential barriers to pain management

Potential barriers	Overcoming barrier
Clinician factors	
Focus of care on management of medical problems – kidney disease, dialysis, transplant and comorbidity, so limited time for focus on other issues such as pain	Ensure that pain and its management in CKD is included in curriculum for all trainee renal healthcare professionals
Lack of awareness of potential pain, so not asked about	Arrange local CPD and conferences about pain management
Not sure how to manage pain if any is reported	Make "renal" pain-control ladder readily available on wards and in clinics
Failure to monitor response to any treatment Fear of drug toxicity because of impaired kidney function Fear of using opiates in noncancer pain More than one cause of pain so management complex	Audit pain assessment and management as quality improvement project
Patient factors	
Underreporting of pain – particularly if pain is chronic and thought by patient not to be related to kidney disease	Clinician should remember to ask patient about pain
Analgesia not taken because of fear of side effects	Routine symptom survey questionnaires that include pain – though these must then be reviewed by clinical team and acted upon
Analgesia stopped because of side effects – and not reported to clinician	Availability of pamphlets about pain control in kidney disease
Anxiety about taking opiates because of fear of addiction Delaying procedures that may relieve pain, e.g. amputation for ischaemic limbs	Availability of healthcare professional from renal and/or palliative care team who can talk to patient about pain control and alleviate concerns

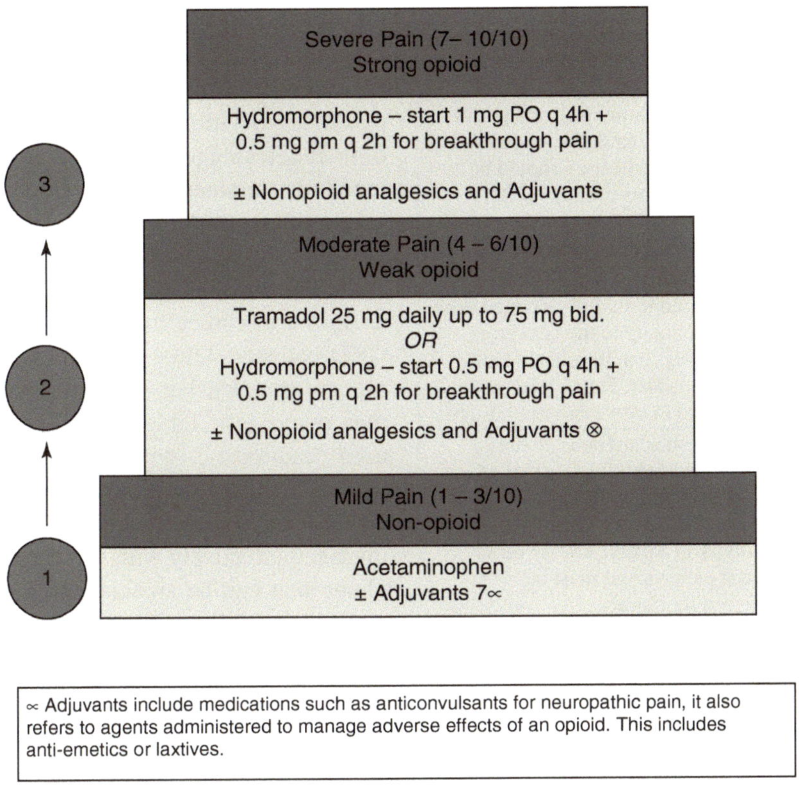

Fig. 22.1 Adapted World Health Organization 3-step analgesic ladder for patients with advanced chronic kidney disease

medications such as antidepressants [1]. Other nondrug measures for pain relief include:

Transcutaneous nerve stimulation (*TENS*): The rationale for TENS is based on the gate theory for pain. TENS should only be used for chronic pain, including neuropathic pain – there is no evidence of benefit for acute pain. It should only be administered by specialist pain clinics as how electrodes are placed makes considerable difference to efficacy.

Acupuncture: Although evidence of benefit is equivocal, some patients find acupuncture beneficial for management of chronic pain. Theories for its mode of action include the production of endorphins.

Physiotherapy and manipulation: Many people will try these methods, particularly for back pain, despite lack of evidence of benefit. Physiotherapy for patients with reduced mobility can also improve general well-being and mood, both of which may alleviate perception of pain.

22.3.3 Drug Management

The World Health Organization (WHO) analgesic ladder uses a stepwise approach to prescribing analgesics that selects initial analgesia according to the severity of the pain, starting at the lowest appropriate level and titrating as required to alleviate pain. An example of such an approach adapted for patients with advanced CKD is shown in Fig. 22.1 [9]. This approach has been found to be useful and efficacious for cancer pain as is now advocated for use in patients with non-malignant chronic pain, including patients with advanced CKD and those on dialysis [10, 11]. Table 22.5 outlines the five key principles to keep in mind when prescribing analgesics. Sustained-release preparations are generally not recommended in advanced CKD patients.

Most analgesics, including opioids and their active metabolites, are cleared renally. The selection of analgesics for patients with

Table 22.5 Principles of pain management

By mouth	Use the oral or transdermal route whenever possible
By the clock	Where pain is continuous, analgesics should be given regularly. Additional breakthrough medication should be available on an "as needed" (PRN) basis
By the ladder	Use the WHO analgesic ladder level based on severity of pain. The analgesic should be used to its full-tolerated dose before stepping up to the next level. Adjuvant drugs can be added to all 3 steps of the ladder. Step 1 analgesics can be added to step 2 or step 3 drugs
For the individual	There is no standard dose of strong opiates. The "right dose" is that which relieves pain without causing unacceptable adverse effects. Sensitivity to adverse effects varies between patients and must be monitored for closely
Attention to detail	Pain changes over time; thus, there is a need for ongoing reassessment

advanced CKD is therefore challenging and must take into account the altered pharmacokinetics and pharmacodynamics, especially when eGFR is <30 ml/min. Table 22.6 outlines recommended analgesics in CKD. Even for recommended analgesics, adverse effects are common; so ongoing monitoring is important [12–15].

Acetaminophen is considered the non-narcotic analgesic of choice for mild to moderate pain in CKD patients. All of the opioids can cause significant toxicity, but some are less problematic than others (see Table 22.6). They should all be used cautiously, with both dose reduction, increase in the dosing interval and regular monitoring. Patients requiring step 3 analgesics can be managed effectively with short-acting hydromorphone that can be switched to transdermal fentanyl if the daily hydromorphone dose exceeds 8 mg.

Table 22.6 Analgesic use in advanced chronic kidney disease based on the WHO analgesic ladder

Recommended but use with caution	
Step 1	
Acetaminophen	Metabolized by the liver with only 2–5 % excreted in the urine and does not require dose adjustment in CKD. Recommended maximum daily dose of 3.2 g/day. In high-risk patients (chronic stable liver disease, alcoholics and malnourished patients), limit the maximal dose to 2.6 g/day
Step 2	
Tramadol	May induce fewer adverse effects for a given level of analgesia compared with traditional opioids. Parent drug and metabolites are excreted renally with increased risk of seizure in advanced CKD, so dose adjustments are required. Maximum dose of 200 mg/day with an eGFR <30 ml/min and 100 mg/day with an eGFR <15 ml/min
Oxycodone	Limited pharmacokinetic evidence for safety in advanced CKD with conflicting case reports. While not contraindicated, use with extreme caution and never use slow-release formulations. Consider a starting dose of 2.5 mg by mouth every 8–12 h
Step 3	
Hydromorphone	Metabolites removed by dialysis, and if followed carefully, patients can tolerate well if doses started low and titrated slowly. Consider a starting dose of 0.5 mg by mouth every 6 h. Active metabolites accumulate without dialysis therefore may not be an appropriate analgesic for patients with stage 5 CKD not on dialysis
Fentanyl patch	Rapidly metabolized in the liver, with only 5–10 % excreted unchanged in the urine. Its metabolites are considered to be inactive. There does not appear to be clinically significant accumulation in advanced CKD and transdermal preparations have been used successfully. Not appropriate for opioid-naïve patients
Methadone	Extensively distributed in the tissues where it accumulates. Slow release from the tissues can result in prolonged pharmacological action of up to 60 h. In advanced CKD it is excreted mainly in the faeces and does not appear to accumulate appreciably in plasma. It may be more effective for neuropathic pain than other strong opioids because of its NMDA receptor antagonism

(continued)

Table 22.6 (continued)

Buprenorphine patch	Limited experience in advanced CKD, but the liver metabolizes it with little parent drug found in the urine. Pharmacokinetics appears minimally altered in CKD. Metabolites, however, accumulate in CKD but appear relatively inactive. It can be administered via a transdermal patch, but might be difficult to antagonize with opioid antagonists. Additional care should be taken when used with benzodiazepines
Adjuvants	
Gabapentin and pregabalin	First-line therapy for neuropathic pain in advanced CKD. Titrate slowly. Doses up to 300 mg/day are generally safe but monitor for side effects (nystagmus, ataxia, tremor, somnolence and reduced level of consciousness)
TCA antidepressants (e.g. nortriptyline, desipramine)	Use may be limited due to anticholinergic, histaminergic and adrenergic side effects resulting in symptoms such as dry mouth, orthostatic hypotension and somnolence. Tachyarrhythmias are also a concern. Considered second-line therapy for neuropathic pain in CKD. Initiate at low dose, give in divided daily doses and titrate slowly
Do not use	
Step 1	
NSAIDs	Risks include irreversible reduction in GFR for those with residual renal function, an increased risk of gastrointestinal bleeding and possible increased risk of myocardial infarction. Use is best reserved for specific indications of acute pain such as gout or renal colic
Step 2	
Codeine	Metabolites accumulate and can cause prolonged narcosis and respiratory depression, even at trivial doses. This appears to be an idiosyncratic and unpredictable phenomenon with some patients able to tolerate regular doses for prolonged periods without experiencing toxicity
Step 3	
Morphine, propoxyphene, meperidine (pethidine)	Neurotoxic metabolites are excreted renally and accumulate in CKD. Patients are at high risk of neurotoxicity, including seizures

22.3.4 Neuropathic (Nerve) Pain

Neuropathic (nerve) pain is unlikely to respond to opioids alone. Adjuvants such as anticonvulsants and antidepressants have proven successful in this regard, though studies specific to patients with advanced CKD are lacking. Opioids may be required in addition to adjuvant therapy. Methadone may be more useful than other step 3 opioids for treating neuropathic pain. There are insufficient data or clinical experience with selective serotonin reuptake inhibitors (SSRI) and selective serotonin-norepinephrine reuptake inhibitors (SSNRI) for neuropathic pain in CKD to make a recommendation.

22.3.5 Other

Opioids can be abused so safe prescribing requires consideration of the risks associated with drug abuse and addiction. These issues need to be separated from physiological physical dependence, which is defined as the occurrence of withdrawal symptoms if the dose is abruptly reduced or after administration of an opiate antagonist. Experience suggests that less than 10 % of patients have the biological characteristics that put them at risk of becoming addicted. Risk is highest in patients who have a personal or family history of alcohol or drug abuse. Such patients will benefit from careful monitoring by a specialist pain team.

Conclusion

Pain is common in patients with chronic kidney disease and can be caused by the kidney disease itself, complications related to kidney disease and comorbidities. It is therefore important that all patients should be asked about the existence and nature of any pain, that the cause of the pain is identified and that patients are given adequate and appropriate pain control. Management of pain also includes addressing psychosocial issues as pain can adversely affect quality of life, and this in turn can impact negatively on the perception of pain severity by the patient. Renal clinicians should be aware of the complex manner in which analgesic dosing is affected by kidney function and therefore become familiar with a few analgesics for each stage of the WHO pain-control ladder. Referral to palliative care or specialist pain services should be considered for management of complex pain or when drug abuse or addiction is suspected.

Before You Finish: Practice Pearls for the Clinician

- Regularly ask all patients with kidney disease about the existence of pain.
- Take a full pain history to determine nature, cause and severity of pain and its psychosocial impact.
- Ask patients about existing analgesia to determine whether this is sufficient and/or appropriate for level of kidney function.
- Become familiar with one or two drugs in each analgesic class regarding dosage related to kidney function and likely side effects.
- Collaborate with your local specialist pain service and refer patients.

References

1. Davison SN, Chambers EJ, Ferro CJ. Chapter 8. Management of pain in renal failure. In: Chambers EJ, Brown EA, Germain MJ, editors. Supportive care for the renal patient. 2nd ed. Oxford: Publ Oxford University Press; 2010.
2. Davison SN. Pain in hemodialysis patients: prevalence, cause, severity, and management. Am J Kidney Dis. 2003;42:1239–47.
3. Murtagh FE, Addington-Hall J, Higginson IJ. The prevalence of symptoms in end-stage renal disease: a systematic review. Adv Chronic Kidney Dis. 2007;14(1):82–99.
4. Saini T, Murtagh FE, Dupont PJ, McKinnon PM, Hatfield P, Saunders Y. Comparative pilot study of symptoms and quality of life in cancer patients and patients with end stage renal disease. Palliat Med. 2006;20(6):631–6.
5. Weisbord SD, Fried L, Mor MK, Resnick AL, Unruh ML, Palevsky PM, et al. Renal provider recognition of symptoms in patients on maintenance hemodialysis. Clin J Am Soc Nephrol. 2007;2:960–7.
6. Davison SN, Jhangri GS, Johnson JA. Longitudinal validation of a modified Edmonton symptom assessment system (ESAS) in haemodialysis patients. Nephrol Dial Transplant. 2006;21(11):3189–95.
7. Murphy EL, Murtagh FE, Carey I, Sheerin NS. Understanding symptoms in patients with advanced chronic kidney disease managed without dialysis: use of a short patient-completed assessment tool. Nephron Clin Pract. 2009;111(1):c74–80.
8. Weisbord SD, Fried LF, Arnold RM, Rotondi AJ, Fine MJ, Levenson DJ, et al. Development of a symptom assessment instrument for chronic hemodialysis patients: the Dialysis Symptom Index. J Pain Symptom Manage. 2004;27(3):226–40.
9. Davison SN, Jhangri GS. The impact of pain and symptom burden on the health-related quality of life of hemodialysis patients. J Pain Symptom Manage. 2010;39(3):477–85.
10. World Health Organisation. Cancer pain relief and palliative care. Geneva: World Health Organisation; 1990.
11. Barakzoy AS, Moss AH. Efficacy of the world health organization analgesic ladder to treat pain in end-stage renal disease. J Am Soc Nephrol. 2006;17:2198–203.
12. Launay-Vacher V, Karie S, Fau JB, Izzedine H, Deray G. Treatment of pain in patients with renal insufficiency: the World Health Organization three-step ladder adapted. J Pain. 2005;6(3):137–48.
13. Murtagh FE, Chai MO, Donohoe P, Edmonds PM, Higginson IJ. The use of opioid analgesia in end-stage renal disease patients managed without dialysis; recommendations for practice. J Pain Palliat Care Pharmacother. 2007;21:5–16.
14. King S, Forbes K, Hanks GW, Ferro CJ, Chambers EJ. A systematic review of the use of opioid medication for those with moderate to severe cancer pain and renal impairment: a European Palliative Care Research Collaborative opioid guidelines project. Palliat Med. 2011;25:525–52.
15. Dean M. Opioids in renal failure and dialysis patients. J Pain Symptom Manage. 2004;28(5):497–504.

Depression and Other Psychological Issues in Chronic Kidney Disease

23

Nishank Jain and S. Susan Hedayati

Before You Start: Facts You Need to Know

- Depression, anxiety, and other psychological disorders are prevalent in patients with CKD.
- Patients with CKD commonly present with somatic symptoms, such as sleep disturbances, sexual dysfunction, low energy level, easy fatigability, and weight and appetite changes, which may be related to uremia and difficult to differentiate from depressive symptoms.
- The presence of depressive symptoms and major depressive disorder predicts adverse clinical outcomes in patients with CKD.
- Depression is a less commonly recognized problem in patients with CKD and ESRD.
- Depression is often treated inadequately.
- Clinicians need to know the nuances in recognizing, diagnosing, and treating depression in patients with CKD in order to improve adverse clinical outcomes and quality of life.

Major depressive disorder (MDD) is a constellation of symptoms that a patient experiences for 2 weeks or more, comprised of either depressed mood or *anhedonia* plus at least five of the nine *Diagnostic and Statistical Manual of Mental Disorders (DSM) criteria* symptom domains [1] (Box 23.1). Patients with chronic kidney disease (CKD) and end-stage kidney disease (ESKD) experience decreased energy, poor appetite, and sleep disturbance commonly that may not necessarily reflect an episode of MDD but represent symptoms of uremia or burden of other comorbid illnesses, such as congestive heart failure. In addition, other symptom burdens, psychiatric conditions, or cognitive impairment experienced commonly by patients with advanced CKD or ESKD may be present such as anxiety, chronic pain, erectile dysfunction, dementia, and delirium that need to be differentiated from a depressive disorder [2]. It is even more challenging for clinicians to manage MDD in CKD and ESRD patients once it is identified due to limited data on safety and efficacy of antidepressant medications in this high-risk population, which leads to only a minority of such patients getting treated appropriately

N. Jain, MD, MPH
Division of Nephrology,
Department of Internal Medicine,
University of Texas Southwestern Medical Center,
4500 S. Lancaster Rd., MC 111G1,
Dallas, TX 75126, USA
e-mail: nishank.jain@utsouthwestern.edu

S.S. Hedayati, MD, MHSc (✉)
Division of Nephrology,
Department of Internal Medicine,
University of Texas Southwestern Medical Center
and Veterans Affairs North Texas Health Care System,
4500 S. Lancaster Rd., MC 111G1,
Dallas, TX 75126, USA
e-mail: susan.hedayati@utsouthwestern.edu

M. Arici (ed.), *Management of Chronic Kidney Disease*,
DOI 10.1007/978-3-642-54637-2_23, © Springer-Verlag Berlin Heidelberg 2014

Box 23.1. Clinicians Must Know the Nine Criterion Symptom Domains for Major Depressive Disorder Based on the Diagnostic and Statistical Manual of Mental Disorders (DSM) [1]

1. Depressed mood
2. Loss of interest or pleasure (anhedonia)
3. Appetite disturbance
4. Sleep disturbance
5. Psychomotor agitation or retardation
6. Fatigue and tiredness
7. Worthlessness, feeling like a burden, or guilty
8. Difficulty concentrating
9. Recurring thoughts of death or suicide

and adequately [2]. Pain, sexual dysfunction, and quality of life issues in patients with CKD are discussed in other chapters and will not be further discussed here.

23.1 Prevalence of Depression in Patients with CKD

There is a high prevalence of depression in patients with chronic illnesses such as cardiovascular diseases (CVD) and ESKD. The point prevalences of depression in the general population and the primary care setting are estimated to be 2–4 % and 5–10 %, respectively [2]. On the other hand, the point prevalences of depression in patients with chronic diseases such as post-myocardial infarction (MI), congestive heart failure (CHF), and ESKD on chronic dialysis are much higher at 16, 14, and 26 %, respectively [2].

A distinction must be made between the presence of depressive affect or depressive symptoms ascertained from patients by the use of self-report scales and a depressive disorder diagnosis (such as MDD) made by a physician using an interview. The majority of studies reporting the prevalence of depression in patients with CKD and ESKD used self-report questionnaires to assess depressive symptoms instead of reports by a physician or interview-based diagnosis. Unfortunately, the estimates by self-reported rating scales may overestimate the presence of MDD, particularly in patients with advanced CKD or ESKD treated with maintenance dialysis, given the overemphasis of the somatic symptoms of depression, such as appetite changes, sleep disturbance, and fatigue that are commonly present in such patients. This was illustrated in a recent meta-analysis [3], where the prevalence of depression in ESKD patients on maintenance dialysis when ascertained by self-report scales was much higher at 39.3 %; 95 % CI 36.8–42.0 vs. by interview at 22.8 %; 95 % CI 18.6–27.6. In addition, point prevalence estimates of interview-based depression were also high in CKD stages 1–5 patients not treated with maintenance dialysis (21.4 %; 95 % CI 11.1–37.2), as well as in kidney transplant recipients (25.7 %; 95 % CI 12.8–44.9), but not as precise as those for patients with ESKD, as reflected in the wide confidence intervals. This could be due to a lesser number of studies evaluating the point prevalence of depression in early-stage CKD patients and transplant recipients.

23.2 Association of Depression with Adverse Clinical Outcomes

CKD or ESKD patients experiencing either depressive symptoms based on self-report scales or a clinical diagnosis of MDD are at a much higher risk of adverse clinical events as compared to similar patients without such symptoms or diagnosis (Box 23.2) [4–7]. These findings were not only reported in the kidney but also in the cardiovascular literature. The risk of death and hospitalization within a year doubles in ESKD patients on chronic dialysis with an interview-based clinical diagnosis of depression compared to those without it [4]. In addition, a clinical diagnosis of depression may increase cumulative hospital days and number of admissions to the hospital by 30 % independent of other comorbidities (Box 23.2) [2].

Box 23.2. Clinicians Must Know That Depressive Symptoms and a Clinical Diagnosis of Major Depressive Disorder in CKD and ESKD Patients Are Independently Associated with Adverse Clinical Outcomes

1. Death
2. Hospitalization (increased cumulative hospital days and number of admissions)
3. Progression of kidney disease
4. Initiation of dialysis
5. Poor quality of life
6. Physical and sexual dysfunction

Furthermore, depression is an independent risk factor for recurrent cardiac events, rehospitalization, and death in many chronic diseases including CVD and CHF, similar to its independent association with the risk of hospitalization, progression of kidney disease, initiation of dialysis, and death in patients with CKD and ESKD (Box 23.2) [4–7]. Noticeably, the strength of association of depression with adverse outcomes is as high as some of the other comorbidities including diabetes mellitus, peripheral vascular disease, and congestive heart failure. Depression not only predicts adverse clinical outcomes, it decreases quality of life (QOL) and aggravates physical and sexual dysfunction in patients with CKD and ESKD substantially (Box 23.2) [8, 9]. It is, therefore, important to identify and manage levels of depression and functional impairment without which such problems fail to remit spontaneously in untreated CKD and ESKD patients.

23.3 Risk Factors for Depression in Patients with CKD

As depressive symptoms and MDD prognosticate poor clinical outcomes and decreased QOL in patients with CKD and ESKD, clinicians must be able to recognize the risk factors for depression (Box 23.3). Several risk factors for depression in this high-risk population are similar to those in the general population and include younger age, female gender, low household income, lower education level, and unemployment (Box 23.3) [2, 8–10]. Although white race has been reported as a risk factor, a high level of depressive affect has also been reported among urban African American ESKD patients treated with maintenance hemodialysis [6]. Dialysis-related factors such as nonadherence to diet and interdialytic weight gain are associated with depression, but it is not clear whether they are risk factors for or result from the presence of depression [2, 6, 8–10]. Other clinical conditions such as diabetes mellitus, hypoalbuminemia, cerebrovascular and cardiovascular diseases, and comorbid psychiatric disorders, commonly associated with CKD and ESKD, add medical complexities and increase the risk for depression [2, 6, 8–10]. The association between medical comorbidities and depression is similar to the general population. Depression makes

Box 23.3. Clinicians Must Be Able to Recognize the Risk Factors Associated with Depression in CKD and ESKD Patients

1. *General factors*:
   (a) Younger age
   (b) White race
   (c) Female gender
   (d) Low household income
   (e) Lower education level
   (f) Unemployment
2. *Dialysis-related factors*:
   (a) Nonadherence to recommended diet
   (b) Nonadherence to interdialytic weight gain
3. *Other comorbid illnesses/conditions*:
   (a) Diabetes mellitus
   (b) Hypoalbuminemia
   (c) Cerebrovascular disease
   (d) Cardiovascular disease
   (e) Other psychiatric disorders
4. *Psychosocial factors*:
   (a) Impaired social interactions
   (b) Estranged spouse
   (c) Estranged family members

social interactions and relationships more difficult for patients, leading to estrangement from spouse, family, work, community, and religious organizations (Box 23.3) [8]. Post-dialysis fatigue, time spent on dialysis, cognitive impairment, and comorbid illnesses may be further impediments to social interactions and impair ability to build relationships. An attempt should be made by clinicians to identify interrelated risk factors for depression in order to best manage their patients with CKD or ESKD diagnosed with depression.

23.4 Potential Mechanisms for the Association of Depression with Adverse Outcomes

It is unclear whether depression itself has a direct mechanistic role in the development of cardiac events and other adverse clinical outcomes or whether it is merely a surrogate marker of comorbid illness (Fig. 23.1). However, specific biological factors were proposed and investigated as potential mechanisms by which depression may lead to cardiac events that are compelling. First, both depression and CVD appear heritable in twin studies. In a study that included 2,700 male twin pairs from the Vietnam era, there was a correlation between genetic influences on depression and CVD, suggesting a common genetic link [2]. Second, depression leads to nonadherence with medications, unhealthy lifestyle, malnutrition, and loss of social network that can precipitate adverse events such as increase in peritonitis events noted in depressed chronic peritoneal dialysis patients compared to those who are not depressed [2]. Third, there are reports of altered autonomic tone, such as lower heart rate variability, in patients with recent MI with depression leading to coronary vasoconstriction and tachyarrhythmias. Therefore, autonomic dysfunction may be a potential pathophysiologic mechanism that can explain how depression leads to adverse clinical outcomes [2]. Fourth, several studies observed enhanced activity of the hypothalamic–pituitary axis, specifically increase in cortisol and norepinephrine secretion, in patients with CVD and depression. It is hypothesized that increase in the levels of inflammatory cytokines due to depression may result in hyperactive hypothalamic–pituitary–adrenal axis and increase in cortisol and norepinephrine secretions. It is further postulated that increase in cortisol and norepinephrine levels may be important in decreasing the availability of tryptophan, an important precursor for neurocellular function, and thus precipitate depressive symptoms by decreasing the availability of neurotransmitters such as dopamine and serotonin [2]. Fifth, inflammation has

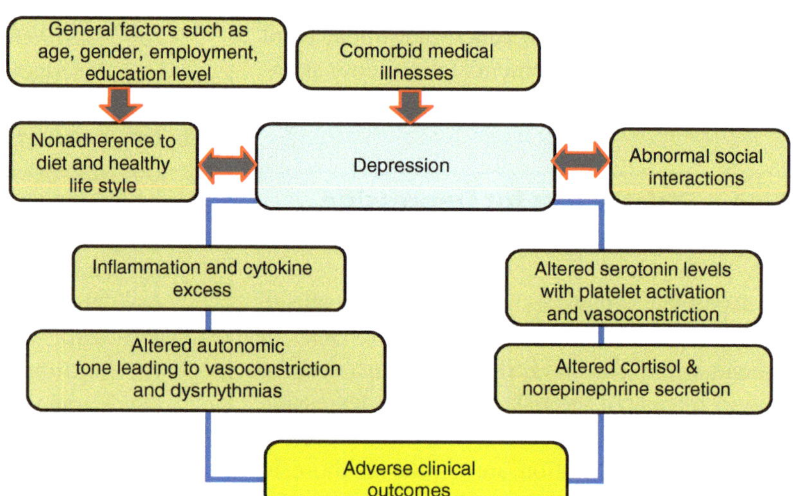

Fig. 23.1 Risk factors for depression and potential mechanisms by which depression may lead to adverse clinical outcomes

been implicated, such as an increase in serum C-reactive protein (CRP) and decrease in omega-3-fatty acid serum concentrations. There is an association between inflammation and depression as shown in some patients treated with interferon alpha who show a decrease in brain dopamine and serotonin levels that is treatable with paroxetine. To further support the role of inflammation, it was reported that depressed patients with psoriatic arthritis show improvement in their disease activity and depression when treated with etanercept [2]. Finally, the most compelling proposed mechanism of depression predicting adverse clinical outcomes is the association of altered serotonin levels seen in depression, with resultant increased platelet activation and vasoconstriction that can then lead to coronary events [2]. However, all of the above are potential mechanisms to explain how depression predicts poor outcomes. Future studies are needed to confirm the mechanistic pathways involved in adverse clinical outcomes in depressed patients with kidney disease, such as higher rates of cardiovascular events, progression to ESKD, death, and hospitalizations.

23.5 How to Identify Depression in Patients with CKD

Given one out of four or five patients with CKD or ESKD may be depressed, which puts them at increased risk for adverse clinical outcomes, poor QOL, and functional impairment, it is important for clinicians to screen such patients for depression. It is suggested that screening should be performed at the first outpatient evaluation in the CKD or dialysis clinic and then repeated annually or semiannually. Self-report questionnaires that assess depressive symptom severity perform well as screening tools with high sensitivity and average specificity (Table 23.1) [12, 13]. These can be administered easily and consume no significant extra time during a patient visit. The 20-item Center for Epidemiological Studies Depression Scale (CES-D), the 21-item Beck Depression Inventory (BDI-II), and the 9-item Patient Health Questionnaire (PHQ-9) are screening tools that were specifically validated against DSM-IV-based structured interviews to diagnose MDD in patients with ESKD (Table 23.1). Similarly, the BDI-II and 16-item Quick Inventory for Depressive Symptomatology Self-Report (QIDS-SR_{16}) are validated screening tools in CKD patients not yet initiated on maintenance dialysis (Table 23.1).

Compared to patients without kidney disease, those with ESKD requiring maintenance dialysis have higher cutoffs on the self-report rating scales to diagnose MDD, perhaps due to the presence of somatic symptoms associated with uremia or chronic disease. For example, the cutoffs on the 21-item BDI-II validated for the diagnosis of MDD in the general population, CKD and ESKD are ≥10, ≥11 and ≥14–16, respectively [12, 13]. The 20-item CES-D cutoffs in the general population and ESKD are ≥16 and ≥18, respectively. There is no difference in the PHQ-9 and QIDS-SR_{16} cutoffs between the general population and patients with kidney disease (Table 23.1).

Given the coexistence of somatic symptoms of depression in CKD patients with uremic symptoms and other comorbid medical conditions, those who screen positive on self-report scales need to be further assessed with a structured interview to confirm a clinical diagnosis of

Table 23.1 Clinicians should be familiar with the available validated screening tools to screen for and rate depressive symptoms in patients with CKD and ESKD [11]

Rating scale	Cutoff score in non-CKD patients	Cutoff in CKD patients	Remarks
21-item BDI-II	≥10	≥11 in CKD	Higher cutoff of ≥14–16 is used in ESKD
16-item QIDS-SR	≥10	≥10 in CKD	Not validated in ESKD
20-item CES-D	≥16	≥18 in ESKD	Not validated in CKD
9-item PHQ	≥10	≥10 in ESKD	Not validated in CKD

BDI-II Beck Depression Inventory, *QIDS-SR* Quick Inventory for Depressive Symptomatology Self-Report, *CES-D* Center for Epidemiological Studies Depression Scale, *PHQ* Patient Health Questionnaire, *CKD* chronic kidney disease, *ESKD* end-stage kidney disease depressive disorder, such as MDD. In research, clinician-administered structured interviews such as the *Structured Clinical Interview for Depression* (SCID) or the *Mini-international Neuropsychiatric Interview* (MINI) have been used to establish diagnosis [12, 13]. These interviews take a significant amount of time (30–60 min) and require a certain level of training to administer. Therefore, in the clinical setting, eliciting the presence of 5 or greater of the depression symptom domains, including the presence of sadness or anhedonia, for a period of at least 2 weeks would confirm the presence of a clinical depressive disorder (Box 23.1).

23.6 Differential Diagnosis of Depression in Patients with CKD

Of the psychiatric illnesses identified among the US Medicare ESKD patients admitted to hospitals, the prevalences of depression, dementia, and substance or alcohol abuse could be found in as high as 26, 26, and 15 % of such patients, respectively [10, 14]. Therefore, it is important for providers to recognize the differential diagnosis of depression in an attempt to manage patients appropriately (Fig. 23.2) [11].

Importantly, there is a need to simultaneously identify cognitive impairment commonly seen in CKD and ESKD patients. Persistent and/or progressive impairment in memory and other cognitive functions such as attention, language, orientation, reasoning, or executive functioning, the cognitive skill necessary for planning and sequencing tasks, is defined as dementia [14]. A score of <24 on the Mini-Mental State Examination (MMSE) is commonly used to suggest dementia, which has limited sensitivity and specificity in patients with CKD and ESKD. The prevalence of dementia may be as high as 16–38 % in such patients. This too should be appropriately recognized by clinicians, as it also predicts poor outcomes. In addition, cognitive dysfunction acts as an impediment to decision-making, adhering to complex medicine dosing schedules, and self-care. Dementia is more insidious in onset, progressive in course over months to years, usually not reversible, and impairs consciousness in advanced stages. Interestingly, many of the risk factors associated with MDD are similar to those for dementia [14].

Delirium can masquerade dementia and depression and should be part of the differential [14]. Clinicians should recognize the fluctuating course of delirium that develops over a short period of time associated with lack of attention and consciousness. Usually, there is no complaint pertaining to loss of memory, and it occurs as a result of medical conditions (e.g., cardiac disease, liver disease, hypertensive encephalopathy, infections, hypoglycemia, hyponatremia, and hypercalcemia), side effects of certain medications (e.g., opioids, benzodiazepines, antihistamines, antipsychotics, and anticholinergics), or intoxications. Unlike dementia, delirium and depression are usually reversible. In addition, depression can be acute or insidious in onset and is associated with intact consciousness unlike delirium. Therefore, it is very important to differentiate dementia, delirium, and depression so that management can be tailored accordingly. Box 23.4 shows important differences in dementia, delirium, and depression. Proper workup to rule out other disorders includes (a) medication review; (b) obtaining laboratory data to rule out vitamin B12 and folate deficiency, thyroid dysfunction, acquired immunodeficiency syndrome, and substance abuse; (c) obtaining brain imaging for presence of significant atherosclerotic cerebrovascular disease; (d) assessing sleep disorders (such as restless legs and obstructive sleep apnea) by history and physical examination; and (e) assessing dialysis adequacy, anemia, and aluminum toxicity in ESKD patients.

Apart from delirium and dementia, generalized anxiety is quiet common in patients with kidney disease and should be distinguished from depression by identifying patients who worry excessively on more days than not about a number of topics that has persisted for more than 6 months and with the self-perception that they are worried and lack control to modify its intensity and

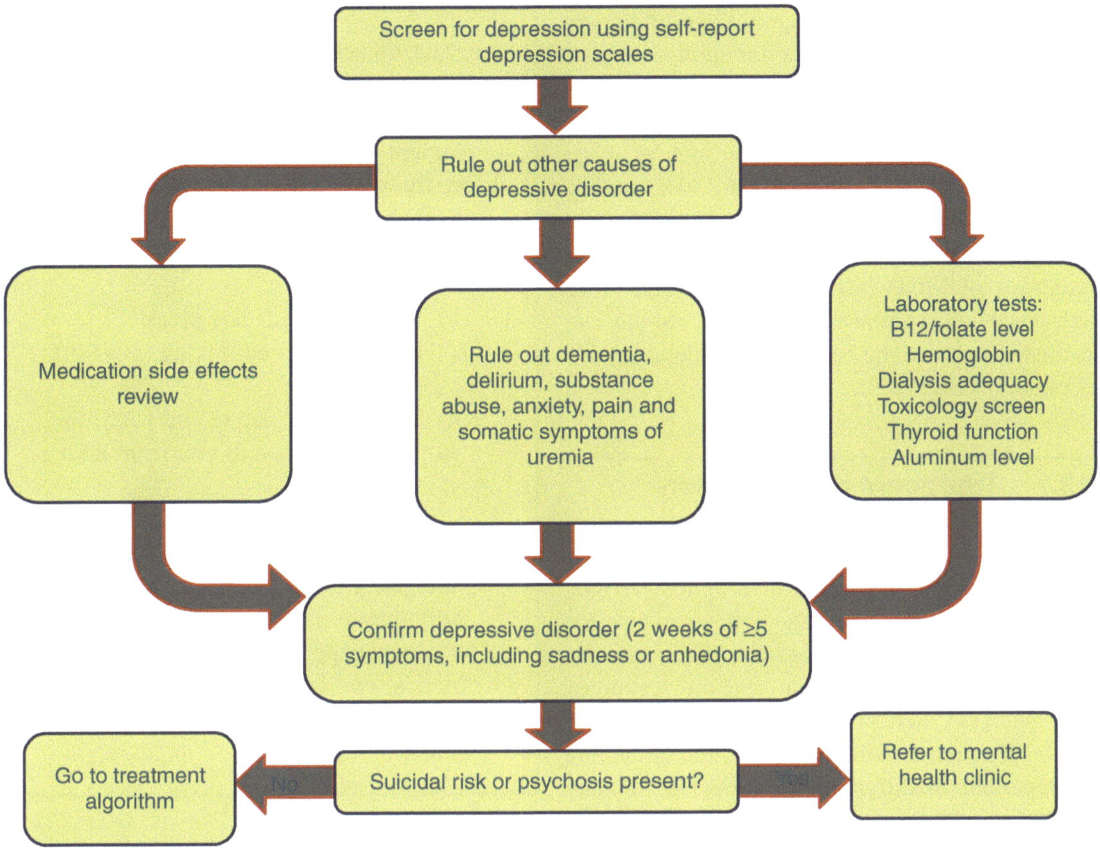

Fig. 23.2 Diagnostic algorithm

Box 23.4. Clinicians Must Be Able to Differentiate Delirium and Dementia from Depression [14]

1. *Delirium*:
   (a) Develops over a short period of time
   (b) Lack of attention and consciousness
   (c) No complaints pertaining to loss of memory
   (d) Occurs as a result of:
      (i) Medical conditions
      (ii) Side effects of certain medications
      (iii) Intoxications
   (e) Reversible
2. *Dementia*:
   (a) Develops over months to years, insidiously and progressively
   (b) Altered consciousness in advanced disease
   (c) Loss of memory common, along with loss of at least one other cognitive function such as:
      (i) Attention
      (ii) Language
      (iii) Orientation
      (iv) Reasoning
      (v) Executive functioning
   (d) Rarely reversible
3. *Depression*:
   (a) Can develop acutely or insidiously
   (b) Not associated with altered consciousness
   (c) Complaints of memory loss can be present
   (d) Reversible

frequency [1]. This accompanies three of the six criterion symptom domains including fatigue, irritability, muscle tension, sleep disturbance, psychomotor agitation, and disturbed concentration [1]. Similarly, somatic symptoms such as sleep disturbances, sexual dysfunction, low energy level, easy fatigability, and weight and appetite changes can be present with uremia and make the diagnosis of MDD difficult. Alcohol and other substance abuse-related disorders should be excluded, as these are commonly associated with depression (Fig. 23.2).

23.7 Treatment of Depression in Patients with CKD

A diligent clinician should recognize MDD, identify its risk factors, triage patients at risk for suicide, and tailor management based on the needs of the specific patient and the resources available [11]. Screening tools enable clinicians to identify patients who are at risk for suicide. It is important to differentiate "thoughts for suicide" from "thinking about death" in patients with end-stage and terminal diseases such as ESKD and cancer in order to triage patients appropriately. Given that a majority of patients with kidney disease are elderly, "thoughts of death" may be common without depressive symptoms or thoughts of suicide. Furthermore, those who screen positive for suicidal thoughts should be queried for presence of suicidal intent or plan (Box 23.5). Those with suicidal intent or plan should be referred to an emergency room or urgent care facility that can provide further urgent psychiatric clinical assessment and triage and appropriate support groups.

Pharmacological and non-pharmacological interventions can be implemented to treat MDD in CKD and ESKD patients [11]. Unfortunately, proposed interventions are not completely evidence-based due to a paucity of large enough studies and placebo-controlled randomized trials to establish the safety and efficacy of antidepressant medications and other interventions for the treatment of depression in CKD and ESKD patients [11]. Second, a high medication discontinuation rate is commonly observed in depressed patients with kidney disease [11]. Third, safety concerns of adverse events drive clinicians to either undertreat MDD or underdose antidepressants in CKD and ESKD patients (Box 23.6) [11]. Encouraging results of efficacy for the use of antidepressants in treating MDD associated with chronic diseases such as CVD come from a double-blind, placebo-controlled, randomized trial, the *Sertraline Antidepressant Heart Attack Trial* (*SADHART*), which showed sertraline to be safe and efficacious in patients with acute coronary syndrome. Based on these results, sertraline may be considered for treating MDD in CKD and ESKD individuals [11]. Sertraline is being currently evaluated by the double-blind, placebo-controlled, randomized, flexible-dose *Chronic Kidney Disease Antidepressant Sertraline Trial* (*CAST*) (clinical trials identifier number, NCT00946998). Despite the paucity of

Box 23.5. Clinicians Must Be Able to Recognize Those at Risk for Suicide So That Time-Dependent Interventions Can Be Implemented

1. In those with thoughts of suicide or death, ask about suicidal intent or plans:
   (a) How often do you think about suicide?
   (b) Have you made any plans?
   (c) Have you tried taking your life before?
   (d) How do you plan to end your life?
   (e) What will prevent you from taking your life?
2. Those patients who have suicidal intent should be immediately referred to an emergency room for further evaluation. Appropriate steps should be taken to organize support groups from family, friends, community, and religious and social organizations based on the availability of resources.

data in patients with advanced CKD and ESKD, guidelines were developed by the European Renal Best Practice recommending the use of antidepressants in patients with CKD stages 3–5, which are summarized in Box 23.7 [15].

Table 23.2 describes the potential side effect profiles of several classes of common antidepressants that can occur at increased frequency in CKD and ESKD patients compared to those with no kidney disease [11]. Although there is lack of significant data on the safety and efficacy for the use of antidepressant medicines in advanced CKD stages 3b-5 and ESKD patients, this should not discourage clinicians from treating depression appropriately until more data becomes available. Management strategies require discussion of risks vs. benefits of antidepressant medications with patients, the use of a class of antidepressant with the least possible drug–drug interactions, starting antidepressants at a lower dose than that recommended for patients without kidney disease, and close follow-up to monitor treatment response, side effects, and need for dose adjustment. Providers should pay special attention to drug–drug interactions that are highly likely in chronic hemodialysis patients due to polypharmacy. Typically, antidepressants should be started at low doses and dose escalation should be based on response and tolerability after at least 1–2 weeks of treatment on a particular dose.

Non-pharmacological interventions hold promise for the management of MDD in CKD and ESKD patients without increasing pill burden or raising concerns regarding adverse events and drug–drug interactions [11]. Such interventions include changes in dialysis prescription, exercise, and cognitive behavioral therapies that were

Box 23.6. Clinicians Face Day-to-Day Challenges in Treating Depression Because of Lack of Data Regarding Safety and Efficacy of Antidepressant Medication Use in Patients with CKD and ESKD

1. Lack of large studies and placebo-controlled randomized antidepressant trials in CKD stage 3b-5 and ESKD
2. High rate of medication discontinuation seen in small studies
3. Safety concerns related to adverse events from antidepressant medications thought to be due to:
   (a) Renally excreted active metabolites and risk of accumulation to toxic levels
   (b) Risk of drug–drug interactions given the presence of other comorbid conditions and high pill burden
   (c) Cardiac side effects of several classes of antidepressants that may worsen the disproportionate burden of cardiovascular disease seen in CKD and ESKD patients
   (d) Increased risk of bleeding in the setting of uremic platelet dysfunction
   (e) Side effects of nausea and vomiting that may exacerbate uremic symptoms
   (f) CNS depression that may increase risks of cognitive dysfunction or delirium

Box 23.7. What the Guidelines Say You Should Do: Use of Antidepressants in CKD Stages 3–5 Patients [15]

1. Active treatment should be started for patients with CKD stages 3–5 who meet the DSM-IV criteria for major depressive disorder—level of evidence and recommendation: 2D.
2. Treatment effect should be reevaluated after 8–12 weeks of treatment with antidepressant drug therapy—level of evidence and recommendation: 2D.
3. Selective serotonin reuptake inhibitors should be the first line of therapy if pharmacological intervention is considered for patients with CKD stages 3–5—level of evidence and recommendation: 2C.

Table 23.2 Clinicians should be aware of the safety profiles and dose adjustments recommended for different classes of antidepressants to be used in patients with CKD and ESKD

Medication	Dose (mg/day)	Metabolism	Potential side effects	Dose adjustment
Selective serotonin reuptake inhibitors				
Sertraline	50–200	Active metabolite is excreted by the kidney	Increased risk of bleeding; GI side effects (nausea and diarrhea); hyponatremia; sexual dysfunction	Start at lower doses and escalate slowly
Paroxetine	10–40	Prolonged half-life	Same as the class side effects	Lower maximum dose recommended
Fluoxetine	20–80	Prolonged half-life	Same as the class side effects	Use with caution
Citalopram	10–40	Active metabolite accumulates	Higher doses prolong QT_c and increase risk of torsades de pointes	Not recommended for eGFR <20 mL/min
Escitalopram	10–20	Active metabolite accumulates	Same as the class side effects	Use with caution in severe kidney disease
Dopamine/norepinephrine reuptake inhibitors				
Bupropion	200–450	Active metabolite can accumulate to toxic levels	Cardiac dysrhythmias, wide QRS complex, nausea, insomnia, and dizziness	Reduce frequency or maximum dose
Noradrenergic and serotonergic agonists				
Mirtazapine	15–45		CNS side effects include somnolence and weight gain	Reduce by 30 % if CrCl 11–39; by 50 % if CrCl <10
Tricyclics (TCAs)				
Amitriptyline	75–150		QTc prolongation, arrhythmias, orthostatic hypotension, and CNS and anticholinergic side effects	None; avoid in CKD and ESKD
Serotonin/norepinephrine reuptake inhibitors				
Venlafaxine	75–225	Accumulation of toxic metabolite	Hypertension, neuroleptic malignant syndrome, serotonin syndrome, sexual dysfunction	Reduce dose by 25–50 % in mild–moderate CKD
Serotonin modulators				
Trazodone	150–400		Cardiac dysrhythmias, priapism, liver failure, Stevens–Johnson syndrome	Reduce dose and use with caution in advanced CKD and ESKD

CrCl creatinine clearance, *GI* gastrointestinal, *CNS* central nervous system, *eGFR* estimated glomerular filtration rate, *CKD* chronic kidney disease, *ESKD* end-stage kidney disease

shown to be efficacious in the general population (Box 23.8). The *Following Rehabilitation, Economics and Everyday-Dialysis Outcome Measurements* (*FREEDOM*) cohort observational study reported improvements in the depressive symptom severity scores measured by the BDI-II scale and health-related QOL measured by the Short Form-36 (SF-36) with six times weekly hemodialysis [11]. However, although in the *Frequent Hemodialysis Network* (*FHN*) trial, frequent hemodialysis (six times a week as compared with three times a week) was associated with significant benefits with respect to both co-primary composite outcomes of death or increase in left ventricular mass and death or a decrease in the physical-health composite score, there were no significant effects of frequent hemodialysis on cognitive performance or self-reported depression [16].

Weekly cognitive behavioral therapy (CBT) by a trained professional for 12 weeks or more was reported to improve depressive symptom severity on the BDI-II scale and overall QOL on the Kidney Disease QOL Questionnaire-Short Form (KDQOL-SF). A trained psychologist attempts to restructure negative thoughts and encourage logical thinking so as to modify behavior and mood. Those who ineffectively handle problems and/or make poor decisions are able to better cope with adversities and improve their

Box 23.8. Clinicians Should Be Aware of the Non-pharmacological Interventions That Can Be Used to Treat Major Depressive Disorders in Patients with CKD and ESKD

1. *Alterations in dialysis prescription*
   (a) Frequent dialysis, six times vs. three times per week
2. *Cognitive behavioral therapy* (*CBT*)
   (a) Trained psychologist to administer therapy
   (b) Trained social worker to administer support and therapy
3. *Exercise training therapy*
   (a) Resistance training exercises (e.g., ankle weights)
   (b) Aerobic exercises
4. *Treatment for anxiety, pain, sleep disorders, and sexual dysfunction*
5. *Alternative approaches*:
   (a) Music and art therapy
   (b) Involving community and religious organizations
   (c) Social interventions to gain support from family and friends

depressive symptom severity [11]. This technique administered by trained social workers to the ESKD patients after Hurricane Katrina showed encouraging results in assuaging depressive symptoms. Combined pharmacological intervention and CBT may be also considered, as used in the general population, based on the availability of resources [11]. Decreased functional capacity is common in patients with ESKD and is associated with poor QOL measures. Resistance exercise training by ankle weights was reported to improve QOL in patients on chronic maintenance hemodialysis. Similarly, aerobic exercise over 10 months was effective in improving heart rate variability, depressive symptom severity and QOL measures in a small group of chronic hemodialysis patients. Therefore, exercise training can potentially function as a non-pharmacological intervention that clinicians can prescribe to treat MDD in CKD and ESKD patients.

Other potential approaches to treat MDD in CKD and ESKD patients focus on pain management, improving sexual function, and management of anxiety (Box 23.8) [11]. Future research is required to evaluate if community and religious organizations may intervene and ameliorate depressive symptoms of CKD and ESKD patients by improving their social interaction skills. This may also help in addressing and overcoming marital and family discord that is commonly found in this patient population. Music and art therapy is an exciting field that remains to be more fully explored in patients on chronic hemodialysis while they remain idle on the dialysis machine for a long period of time. It remains to be investigated whether treatment of depression in patients with CKD can result in improvements in QOL and survival (Fig. 23.3) [11].

23.8 Recommendations and Conclusions

Depression is common in patients with kidney disease but less frequently recognized and inadequately treated. It is well established that a diagnosis of current MDD or depressive symptoms independently predicts adverse clinical outcomes in patients with kidney disease. Therefore, it becomes imperative for clinicians who are involved in the care of such patients to screen for and diagnose depression accurately. Several quick and easily administered self-report scales are validated to screen for depression in these patients. However, those who screen positive for depression on screening need to be further evaluated so that dementia, delirium, anxiety disorders, medication side effects, and other medical conditions that may lead to the presence of somatic symptoms, such as underlying sleep disorders, thyroid dysfunction, or dialysis inadequacy, can be excluded. Finally, appropriate management strategies should be implemented to maximize efficacy and safety of depression treatment using available pharmacological and non-pharmacological interventions that are acceptable to specific patients. The ultimate goal of a clinician should be to assuage depressive symptoms and potentially achieve complete remission of depression.

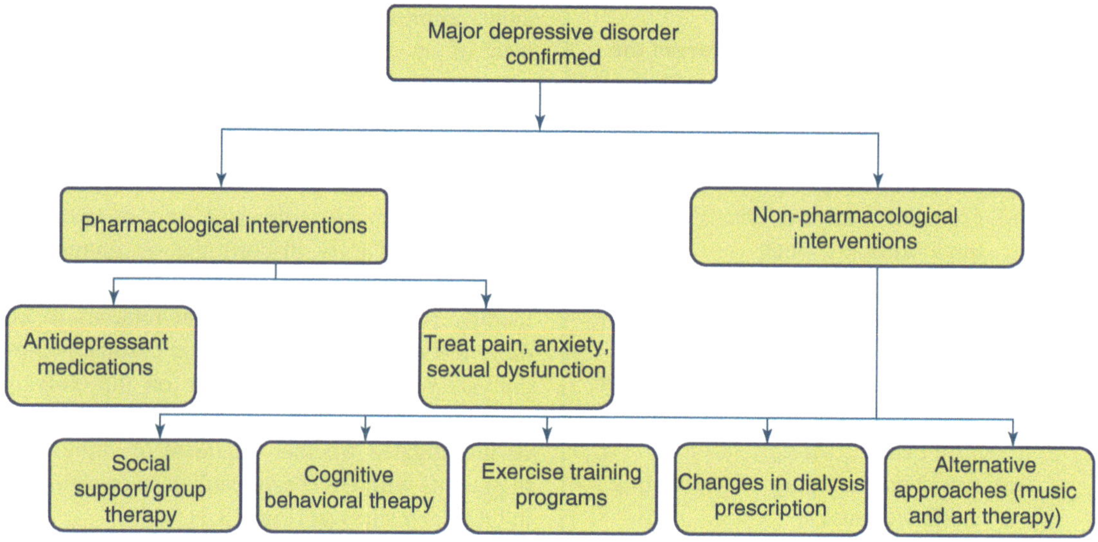

Fig. 23.3 Treatment algorithm

Before You Finish: Practice Pearls for the Clinician

- Clinicians should be able to recognize the risk factors for depression.
- Clinicians should understand the differences between depressive symptoms and a clinical diagnosis of major depressive disorder.
- Screening for depression should be performed at the first outpatient evaluation in the chronic kidney disease or dialysis clinic and then repeated annually.
- Validated self-report tools exist that can be easily administered to screen for depression. Subsequently, a current major depressive disorder should be confirmed by a clinician interview in those who screen positive.
- Those at risk for suicide should be identified for urgent triage and further management.
- A broad differential diagnosis should be considered, based on appropriate physical examination, Mini-Mental State Examination and laboratory data.
- Once a diagnosis of major depressive disorder is confirmed, a thorough review of risks vs. benefits of pharmacological and non-pharmacological interventions should be discussed with patients to tailor individualized management strategies.
- To start an antidepressant medication, the lowest possible dose should be initially prescribed, followed by frequent monitoring and gradual dose escalation every 1–2 weeks based on patient's response to and tolerability of the medication.

Acknowledgments Work from Dr. Hedayati's laboratory was supported by grant number R01DK085512 from the National Institute of Diabetes and Digestive and Kidney Diseases (NIDDK) and VA MERIT grant (CX000217-01). The content is solely the responsibility of the authors and does not necessarily represent the official views of the NIDDK, the National Institutes of Health, or the Department of Veterans Affairs.

References

1. American Psychiatric Association. Diagnostic and statistical manual of mental disorders. 4th ed. Washington, DC: American Psychiatric Association; 1994.
2. Hedayati SS, Finkelstein FO. Epidemiology, diagnosis, and management of depression in patients with CKD. Am J Kidney Dis. 2009;54:741–52.

3. Palmer S, Vecchio M, Craig JC, Tonelli M, Johnson DW, Nicolucci A, et al. Prevalence of depression in chronic kidney disease: systematic review and meta-analysis of observational studies. Kidney Int. 2013;84:179–91.
4. Hedayati SS, Bosworth H, Briley L, et al. Death or hospitalization of patients on chronic hemodialysis is associated with a physician-based diagnosis of depression. Kidney Int. 2008;74:930–6.
5. Lopes AA, Bragg J, Young E, Goodkin D, Mapes D, Combe C, et al. Depression as a predictor of mortality and hospitalization among hemodialysis patients in the United States and Europe. Kidney Int. 2002;62:199–207.
6. Kimmel PL, Peterson RA, Weihs KL, Simmens SJ, Alleyne S, Cruz I, et al. Multiple measurements of depression predict mortality in a longitudinal study of chronic hemodialysis outpatients. Kidney Int. 2000;57:2093–8.
7. Hedayati SS, Minhajuddin AT, Afshar M, Toto RD, Trivedi MH, Rush AJ. Association between major depressive episodes in patients with chronic kidney disease and initiation of dialysis, hospitalization, or death. JAMA. 2010;303:1946–53.
8. Cohen SD, Norris L, Acquaviva K, Peterson RA, Kimmel PL. Screening, diagnosis, and treatment of depression in patients with end-stage renal disease. Clin J Am Soc Nephrol. 2007;2:1332–42.
9. Cohen SD, Patel SS, Khetpal P, Peterson RA, Kimmel PL. Pain, sleep disturbance, and quality of life in patients with chronic kidney disease. Clin J Am Soc Nephrol. 2007;2:919–25.
10. Kimmel PL, Peterson RA, Weihs KL, Simmens SJ, Boyle DH, Umana WO, et al. Psychologic functioning, quality of life, and behavioral compliance in patients beginning hemodialysis. J Am Soc Nephrol. 1996;7:2152–9.
11. Hedayati SS, Yalamanchili V, Finkelstein FO. A practical approach to the treatment of depression in patients with chronic kidney disease and end-stage renal disease. Kidney Int. 2012;81(3):247–55.
12. Hedayati SS, Minhajuddin AT, Toto RD, Morris DW, Rush AJ. Validation of depression screening scales in patients with CKD. Am J Kidney Dis. 2009;54:433–9.
13. Watnick S, Wang PL, Demadura T, Ganzini L. Validation of 2 depression screening tools in dialysis patients. Am J Kidney Dis. 2005;46:919–24.
14. Kurella Tamura M, Yaffe K. Dementia and cognitive impairment in ESRD: diagnostic and therapeutic strategies. Kidney Int. 2011;79:14–22.
15. Nagler EV, Webster AC, Vanholder R, Zoccali C. Antidepressants for depression in stage 3-5 chronic kidney disease: a systematic review of pharmacokinetics, efficacy and safety with recommendations by European Renal Best Practice (ERBP). Nephrol Dial Transplant. 2012;27(10):3736–45.
16. The FHN Trial Group. In-Center hemodialysis six times per week versus three times per week. N Engl J Med. 2010;363:2287–300.

Sexual Dysfunction in Chronic Kidney Disease

24

Domenico Santoro, Ersilia Satta, and Guido Bellinghieri

Before You Start: Facts You Need to Know

- Physiology of erectile function is dependent on a balanced vascular, neurologic, hormonal, and psychological system.
- Prevalence of erectile dysfunction (ED) in the Western industrialized countries amounts to 20–30 % in the general male population and probably higher, about 75 % in patients at high risk for cardiovascular disease.
- Sexual dysfunction (SD) in patients with CKD should be thought as a multifactorial problem that is caused by a variety of physiological and psychological factors, as well as by comorbid conditions. For example, diabetes and vascular disease (commonly encountered in patients with CKD) can impair the ability of male patients to achieve an erection and of female patients to become sexually aroused.
- Drugs that sustain cyclic-GMP-mediated smooth muscle relaxation in the corpus cavernosum, such as sildenafil, vardenafil, and tadalafil, can improve erectile function in male patients.

Sexual dysfunction (SD) is a common problem in people with chronic kidney disease (CKD). SD in these patients should be considered as a multifactorial problem, caused by a variety of physiological and psychological factors, as well as by comorbid conditions [1]. Male patients with CKD suffer from reduced libido, erectile dysfunction (ED), and difficulty reaching the orgasm. In females with CKD, dyspareunia, amenorrhea, reduction of libido, and a delay in sexual development are frequently observed (Table 24.1) [1]. Approximately 50 % of male predialysis CKD patients and 80 % of male dialysis patients have ED [2]. These patients have diffuse atherosclerotic disease of the penile arteries and hypoxic changes of the contractile and structural components of the erectile tissue. In 1972, the first epidemiological survey of sexual function in patients with CKD was conducted. Since then, multiple studies confirmed that SD in CKD patients is highly prevalent. Although it is a major factor that impacts quality of life in end-stage renal disease (ESRD), SD in dialysis patients receives very limited attention from the patients' attending medical team. Despite its importance, only 25 % of patients discuss about SD with their physicians [2–4].

24.1 Male Sexual Dysfunction

Erection is a neurovascular event. Under sexual stimulation, vasodilation and relaxation of trabecular smooth muscle allows blood flow into the cavernosal sinusoids and increase the intracavernosal

D. Santoro, MD (✉) • E. Satta, MD • G. Bellinghieri, MD
Department of Clinical and Experimental Medicine, University of Messina, Messina, Italy
e-mail: dsantoro@unime.it; ersiliasat@libero.it; gbellinghieri@hotmail.com

M. Arici (ed.), *Management of Chronic Kidney Disease*,
DOI 10.1007/978-3-642-54637-2_24, © Springer-Verlag Berlin Heidelberg 2014

Table 24.1 Clinical manifestations of SD in CKD patients

Women	Men
Premature menopause	Erectile dysfunction
Decreased libido	Decreased libido
Sexual aversion disorder	Oligospermia
Hypoactive sexual desire	Decrease in muscle mass
Endocrine abnormality: decrease in estrogen production, vaginal dryness, dyspareunia	Azoospermia, infertility
Irregular menstrual cycles, anovulatory cycles, infertility	Depression, anxiety
Depression, anxiety	

pressure (ICP) [1, 5]. Erection is maintained by the compression of subtunical venules against tunica albuginea. Relaxation of the smooth muscle of the corpus cavernosum is the crucial physiological event in penile erections. Nitric oxide/cyclic guanosine monophosphate (NO/cGMP) pathway had been acknowledged as a classic pathway in mediating relaxation of corpus cavernosum smooth muscle. Cavernous nerve activation induces the release of NO from the nerve terminals in the corpus cavernosum. Additionally, NO is released from the endothelium in response to shear stress. NO is synthesized by neuronal nitric oxide synthase (nNOS) in the corpus cavernosum nerve terminals and by endothelial oxide synthase (eNOS) in endothelium, which utilizes L-arginine and oxygen as substrate to produce NO. Subsequently, NO activates soluble guanylate cyclase (GC) and increases cGMP levels in smooth muscle cells. The increase in blood flow required for erection is comparable to that required by the heart for vigorous exercise [5, 6].

ED is the persistent inability to achieve and/or maintain an erection sufficient for satisfactory sexual intercourse [6, 7]. ED can mask as yet undiagnosed comorbid conditions such as cardiovascular disease and diabetes. Irrespective of the etiology, ED will almost be accompanied by psychological symptoms if the man is "bothered" by his condition (performance anxiety). Risk factors for ED can be grouped into those that have an effect upon the vasculature, those in which the mode of action is nonvascular in nature, and age. Causes of vasculogenic ED include diabetes, dyslipidemia, and hypertension, while causes of nonvascular ED include surgery for prostate cancer and diseases of the central nervous system (CNS).

Aging is one of the most important and well-defined risk factors for ED and mediates its effect through both vascular and nonvascular modes. The increasing incidence of atherosclerosis with age is matched by the negative impact of age on sexual desire and libido. These categories are, therefore, not mutually exclusive; indeed, there is a high degree of overlap.

It is well documented that hormonal alterations characterized by prolactin, gonadotropins, and gonadal hormone change are present in men and women [5].

In male CKD patients, there are abnormalities in testicular structure and function. Common histological findings show damage to the testes in the seminiferous tubules, interstitial fibrosis, calcifications, thickening of the basement membrane, and stopped germinal maturation but also decreased volume of ejaculate, low or complete azoospermia, and low percentages of motility and infertility [1]. High levels of prolactin hormone in CKD are responsible for reduced libido. Modification of androgen synthesis and metabolism begin to appear early in the course of CKD. Reduction of testosterone level is correlated to Leydig cell dysfunction. Today there is a new field of interest, represented by molecular mechanism of testosterone and its role in the pathogenesis of cardiovascular diseases. Recent studies have been carried out in order to correlate the blood levels of testosterone in patients with ED with different degrees of CKD (stages I–IV) [5]. Autonomic nervous system alterations are a frequent cause of SD in CKD; the integrity of this system can decrease sensation and arousal stimuli during sexual activity. Anemia, a common complication of CKD, has been linked with a reduction of libido and ED [6, 7]. The decrease of oxygen that accompanies reduction of hemoglobin levels has been associated with a decrease of NO synthesis and an increase in endothelium-derived contracting factor, which results in inhibition of erectile capacity. Recombinant human EPO therapy has been shown to improve erectile function and sexual performance in some, but not all, patients with CKD [8].

24.2 Female Sexual Dysfunction

In women, with CKD, decrease of libido, amenorrhea, and irregular menstrual and anovulatory cycles are caused by elevated levels of follicle-stimulating hormone (FSH) and luteinizing hormone (LH). Midcycle LH surge cannot be mitigated with endogenous administration of estrogen, confirming a central hypothalamic derangement. Clinical manifestations of SD in women include premature menopause, skin wrinkling, urinary incontinence, hot flushes, sleep and cognitive disorders, and cardiovascular disease. The reduction of libido is frequently observed, while pregnancy is rare (spontaneous abortion is a common eventuality). Few studies carefully examined ovarian function in women with CKD; this lack of data reflects probably the complexity of studying the reproductive system in women [5].

The high prevalence of SD in patients with ESRD emphasizes the need to investigate the impact of SD at all stages of CKD [9, 10].

Psychosocial factors can have a substantial effect on the sexual function in patients with CKD. It has been noted in several studies that 20–30 % of patients with CKD suffer from clinical depression. Studies have also shown an association between SD and a variety of other quality-of-life parameters, such as mental and physical components of the 36-item short-form (SF-36) health survey, and depression scores [5].

24.3 Diagnosis and Evaluation of Sexual Dysfunction

The first step in the evaluation of SD in patients with CKD is to obtain a detailed sexual history about the sexual desire, arousal and orgasmic capabilities, fertility, and ED in men. Changes in the frequency of intercourse need to be determined. Often the patients are very reluctant to tell such concerns. The physicians should determine the time of the onset of these problems in relation to the stage of CKD. In addition, the medical history should focus on the patient's past and present medical illness, i.e., chronic/medical illness, such as diabetes; anemia; neurological illness or lumbosacral disk disease; endocrinological disease, like hypogonadism, hyperprolactinemia, and thyroid disorders; and atherosclerotic vascular risk, such as diabetes, hypercholesterolemia, hypertension, hyperhomocysteinemia, smoking habits, or family history. Current drug therapy should also be reviewed in detail. Drugs such as cimetidine, tricyclic antidepressant, phenothiazines, and metoclopramide are often implicated in ED.

Finally, it is important to investigate patients for presence of psychosocial problems (depression, psychiatric illness) and current stress factor (loss of job or home and so on).

24.3.1 In Men

The physical examination is important for assessment of the male patient's sexual function. These assessments should include vascular disease, autonomic disease, autonomic dysfunction, and hypogonadism [1, 5]. The lack of secondary sexual characteristics and the presence of small and soft testicles suggest hypogonadism. The test of nocturnal penile tumescence (NPT) may be used to discriminate organic and psychological causes of impotence. A patient with normal nocturnal erections during rapid eye movement (REM) sleep may benefit from psychological testing and evaluation [11]. Consideration should be given to laboratory assessment of hormone levels (testosterone, estrogen, FSH, LH, TSH, PTH, prolactin levels) and zinc levels, on the basis of the specific complaints of each patient. The test that discriminates between a neurogenic and a vascular cause of impotence includes Doppler studies to measure penile blood flow, measurement of penile blood pressure, and penile pulse palpation. The NIH Consensus Panel on ED outlined several goals for basic and clinical research on ED. One of these goals was to create a staging system for the quantitative and qualitative classification of ED. Such a system would assist research and patient management by (1) quantifying the specific type of patient population to include in a clinical trial, (2) determining and comparing responder rates associated with different treatments, (3) improving clinical decision-making and patient care, (4) fostering educational initiatives, and (5) supporting claims for reimbursement. The EF domain of the International Index of Erectile Function (IIEF) was considered for such purpose. This subscale in particular showed a high degree of reliability, as well as excellent sensitivity and specificity to treatment effects in validation studies [8]. The IIEF was developed in conjunction with the clinical trial program for sildenafil, and since that period, it has been adopted as the "gold standard" measure for efficacy assessment in clinical trials of ED. Total scores of 22–25 suggest a normal EF, while lower scores indicate ED (mild ED, 17–21; mild to moderate ED, 12–16; moderate ED, 8–11; and severe ED, less than 8 points). The Arizona Sexual Experiences Scale (ASEX) is a five-item rating scale, which quantifies sexual drive, arousal, vaginal lubrication or penile erection, ability to reach orgasm, and satisfaction from orgasm. Possible total scores range from 5 to 30, with the higher scores indicating more SD. Its reliability has been positively assessed for use in dialyzed patients [8]. The Mell–Krat scale is commonly used in Poland and Czech Republic as a validated tool helpful in a complex assessment of sexual function and quality of sexual life. The version for males includes 13 and that for females includes 20 questions with answers scoring from 0 to 4. The higher the score, the better the sexual function. Optimal results for men are 38 points or higher, for women 55 points or higher. Beck Depression Inventory (BDI) is one of the most widely used instruments for measuring the severity of depression. It is composed of 21 questions scored from 0 to 3, each evaluating a specific symptom commonly existing in people with depression. Total scores of 10 or higher indicate depression (10–18 for mild, 19–29 for moderate, and more than 30 points for severe depression).

24.3.2 In Women

Assessing sexual function in women perhaps is more difficult than in men, which may be one explanation for the lack of studies of SD in women with CKD [1–5]. The domains of sexual function in women include desire, arousal, pain, and satisfaction. These can be assessed using the 9-item FSFI. There are several validated screening tools that focus on hypoactive sexual desire disorder (HSDD), which is the most common sexual concern of women of all ages. These screening tools will vary in their usefulness depending upon your clinical specialty and the patient population you serve (Box 24.1). Menstrual abnormalities are common in CKD and many women are anovulatory. The hormonal alterations that lead to premature menopause in women with CKD likely contribute to SD and are, at least, partially responsible for higher reported prevalence of sexual dysfunction in women with CKD compared with general population. The ovarian failure in women with CKD can be associated with abnormalities in the hypothalamic–pituitary–ovarian axis [9, 11].

Box 24.1. Screening Tools for Female SD

- Decreased Sexual Desire Screener (DSDS): 5 questions, self-administered; assesses for generalized acquired HSDD [12].
- Female Sexual Function Index (FSFI): 19 questions, self-administered; assesses all of the dimensions of female sexual function including sexual satisfaction [13].
- Sexual Interest and Desire Inventory – Female (SIDI-F): 13 items, clinician administered; assesses severity of female HSDD [14].
- Brief Hypoactive Sexual Desire Disorder Screener: 4 questions, self-administered HSDD in postmenopausal women [15].
- Brief Profile of Female Sexual Function (B-PFSF): 7 questions, self-administered HSDD in postmenopausal women [16].
- Female Sexual Distress Scale – Revised (FSDS-R): 13 questions, self-administered; assesses distress associated with female SD [17].

24.4 Management of Sexual Dysfunction in Men and Women

24.4.1 In Men

In the general population, drugs that sustain cyclic-GMP-mediated smooth muscle relaxation in the corpus cavernosum, such as sildenafil, vardenafil, and tadalafil, can improve ED in male patients.

The introduction of sildenafil has completely changed the approach to evaluating the subjects with SD, because this drug is considered an effective well-tolerated treatment for men with ED (Table 24.2). It is important to avoid the use of sildenafil in selected conditions (Box 24.2). In the past, we proposed an algorithm in CKD patients that gave the opportunity to explore the previously mentioned factors using some instrumental interventions, such as the NPT test, penile echo color Doppler, nervous conduction velocity, or cavernous body biopsy, addressed to prescribe needed surgical or medical interventions [6, 7]. The complexity of the proposed algorithm requires many diagnostic procedures and much time and economic resources to localize the pathological lesions responsible for the ED. Because of the new oral drug sildenafil, we proposed in the past an algorithm to test the possibility of obtaining an erection and classify patients as responders or nonresponders to the sildenafil test (Fig. 24.1). In nonresponders, it is necessary to explore other factors (hormonal, psychological, neurological, vascular, cavernous body alteration, or particular drugs) involved in inducing or maintaining the ED [7] (Box 24.3).

Table 24.2 Common adverse effects of medical treatment of SD

Sildenafil	Testosterone
Headache	Decrease in high-density lipoprotein, fibrinogen, lipoprotein (a)
Nasal congestion	Increase prostate volume, prostate cancer, exacerbating symptoms of benign prostate hypertrophy
Gastric reflux	Alterations in liver function
Muscle/back pain	Polycythemia
Flushed face	Exacerbation of sleep apnea

Box 24.2. Precautions to the Use of PDE5 Inhibitors

- Nitrates and PDE5 inhibitors must not be used together.
- Amyl nitrate should not be used together with sildenafil.
- Any treatment for ED is contraindicated in men for whom sexual intercourse is inadvisable due to cardiovascular risk factors.

Testosterone therapy is indicated in adult men with diagnosis of hypogonadism. Clomiphene citrate has also been used to increase testosterone levels, with improvement in sexual function. Oral testosterone and testosterone derivatives are not used because of their lack of efficacy and adverse

Box 24.3. What the Guidelines Say You Should Do: Workup on ED [18]

- Sexual history and physical examination are needed in the initial assessment of ED to identify underlying medical conditions associated with ED.
- Clinical use of a validated questionnaire related to ED may help assess all sexual function domains.
- Routine laboratory tests, including glucose–lipid profile and total testosterone, are required to identify and treat any reversible risk factors and modifiable lifestyle factors.
- Specific diagnostic tests are indicated by only a few conditions: nocturnal penile tumescence and rigidity testing using RigiScan, intracavernous vasoactive drug injection, duplex ultrasound of the cavernous arteries, dynamic infusion cavernosus arteries, dynamic infusion cavernosometry, and cavernosography.

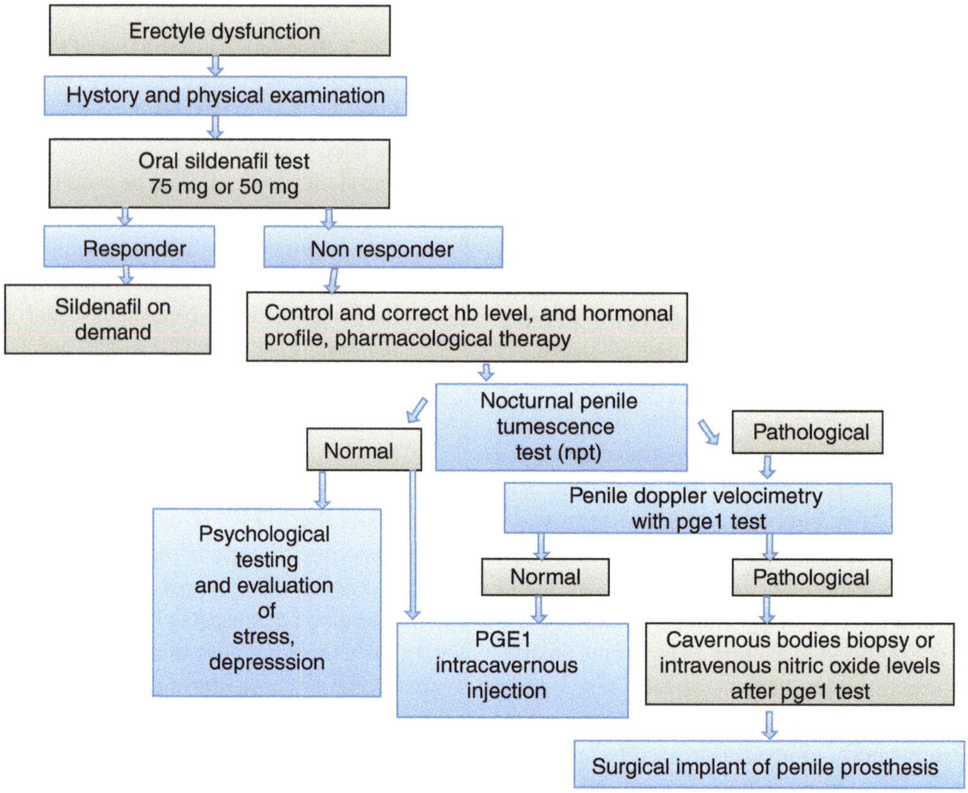

Fig. 24.1 Diagnostic and therapeutic algorithm for the evaluation of ED in CKD patient

Box 24.4. What the Guidelines Say You Should Do: Treatment of ED [18]

- Lifestyle changes and risk factor modification must precede or accompany ED treatment.
- The American College of Physicians recommends that clinicians initiate therapy with a PDE-5 inhibitor in men who seek treatment for ED and who do not have a contraindication to PDE-5 inhibitor use.
- Clinicians must base the choice of a specific PDE-5 inhibitor on the individual preferences of men with ED, including ease of use, cost of medication, and adverse effects profile.
- The evidence is insufficient to compare the efficacy and adverse effects of different PDE-5 inhibitors for the treatment of ED because only few head-to-head trials are available.
- Pro-erectile treatments must be given at the earliest opportunity after radical prostatectomy.
- Testosterone replacement restores efficacy in hypogonadic nonresponders to PDE5-Is.
- Apomorphine can be used in mild to moderate ED, psychogenic ED, or in patients with contraindications to PDE5-Is.
- A vacuum constriction device can be used in patients with stable relationship.
- Intracavernous injection is second-line therapy.
- Penile implant is third-line therapy.

effects on liver function and lipid profile and thus are used as parenteral and transdermal preparation (Boxes 24.4 and 24.5). Studies on the use of testosterone in patients with CKD are few, and several studies suggest that ED in the CKD does not improve with testosterone (Table 24.2 Boxes 24.4 and 24.5) [11, 19–22].

24.4.2 In Women

Few studies address decreased libido and sexual function in women with CKD. Quality-of-life surveys suggest that discussion of sexual function and other reproductive issues are a key component of psychosocial assessment and that education on sexual function in the setting of CKD is widely needed (Box 24.5). Pharmacologic therapy with estrogen/progesterone and androgens along with correction of anemia, ensuring adequate dialysis delivery, and treatment of underlying depression is important [1, 4]. Changes in lifestyle such as smoking cessation, strength training, and aerobic exercises may decrease depression, enhance body image, and have positive impacts on sexuality. Women with CKD who suffer from chronic anovulation and lack of progesterone secretion may be treated with oral progesterone at the end of each menstrual cycle to restore menstrual cycles. It is not clear whether unopposed estrogen stimulation of the endometrium (due to anovulatory cycles) predisposes women with CKD to endometrial hyperplasia or endometrial cancer. Routine gynecologic follow-up is recommended in these cases, and some women may also benefit from the use of a progestational agent several times a year to mitigate the effects of estrogen on the endometrium (Boxes 24.5 and 24.6) [24, 25].

Box 24.5. Relevant Guidelines on Sexual Dysfunction

1. European Association of Urology for diagnostic workup and treatment of ED in general population [18]
2. Hormonal testing and pharmacologic treatment of erectile dysfunction: a clinical practice guideline from the American College of Physicians [23]
3. Practice guidelines on sexual dysfunction in women from American College of Obstetricians and Gynecologists (ACOG) [24]
4. British Society for Sexual Medicine (BSSM). Guidelines on the management of sexual problem in women: the role of androgens [25]

Box 24.6. What the Guidelines Say You Should Do: Treatment of SD in Women and the Opportunity for Psychosexual and/or Couples Counseling [24, 25]

- The generalized use of testosterone by women has been advised against, because of inadequate indications and lack of long-term data. However, postmenopausal women who are distressed by their decreased sexual desire and who have other identifiable cause may be candidates for testosterone therapy. Androgens may also be used by those women who are hypogonadal as a result of pituitary problems in premenopause.
- Although there is no consistent correlation between sexual functioning and levels of androgens (free and total testosterone, androstenedione, dehydroepiandrosterone, and SHBG) across wide age range, in some women androgen therapy can improve sexual desire.
- Transdermal patches and topical gel or creams are preferred over oral products because of first-pass hepatic effects documented with oral formulation.
- The major side effects of androgens are hirsutism and acne. No safety with regard to testosterone implants. There is no indication for increased frequency of breast cancer.

Low estradiol levels in amenorrhoeic women on dialysis leads to vaginal atrophy and dyspareunia. Topical estrogen cream and vaginal lubricants may be helpful in this situation. Women with CKD who do have menstrual cycles should be encouraged to use contraception; because of poor pregnancy outcomes, restoring fertility is not an advisable therapeutic goal. HSDD is the most common sexual problem reported by women with CKD. Testosterone replacement therapy to treat HSDD has been effective in some women without CKD. However, long-term safety data on the use of androgens in women with CKD and ESRD are very limited [21, 22, 26].

Before You Finish: Practice Pearls for the Clinician

- A detailed history of menstrual patterns should be obtained for women and history of ED obtained for men.
- Consideration should be given to laboratory dosage of hormone levels (testosterone, estrogen, FSH, LH, thyroid-stimulating hormone, PTH, and prolactin level).
- For male and female patients, it is important to address the psychosocial factors that might contribute to SD.
- As first-line therapy, phosphodiesterase inhibitors are recommended for their effectiveness, ease of use, and good side-effect profile.
- Sildenafil, vardenafil, and tadalafil equally seem to be effective; tadalafil is preferable for a longer duration of action.
- As a second-line therapy, recommended drugs are injectable intrauretral/intracavernous, such as alprostadil, according to the preferences of the patient.
- As third-line therapy, surgical implantation of penile prosthesis is reserved for patients who cannot use or which have not responded to the first- and second-line therapies.
- Androgen replacement therapy may be indicated only in cases of documented hypogonadism.

References

1. Palmer BF. Sexual dysfunction in uremia. J Am Soc Nephrol. 1999;10(6):1381–8.
2. Finkelstein SH, Finkelstein FO. Evaluation of sexual dysfunction in dialysis patients. In: Dialysis therapy. 3rd ed. Philadelphia: Hanley & Belfus; 2002. p. 368–73.
3. Levy NB. Sexual adjustment to maintenance hemodialysis and renal transplantation: national survey by questionnaire: preliminary report. Trans Am Soc Artif Intern Organs. 1973;19:138–43.
4. Anantharaman P, Schmidt RJ. Sexual function in chronic kidney disease. Adv Chronic Kidney Dis. 2007;14(2):119–25.
5. Finkelstein FO, Shirani S, Wuerth D, Finkelstein SH. Therapy insight: sexual dysfunction in patients with chronic kidney disease. Nat Clin Pract Nephrol. 2007;3(4):200–7.
6. Bellinghieri G, Santoro D, Mallamace A, Savica V. Sexual dysfunction in chronic renal failure. J Nephrol. 2008;21 Suppl 13:S113–7.
7. Bellinghieri G, Santoro D, Lo Forti B, Mallamace A, De Santo RM, Savica V. Erectile dysfunction in uremic dialysis patient: diagnostic evaluation in the sildenafil era. Am J Kidney Dis. 2001;38(4 Suppl 1): S115–7.
8. Rosen RC, Riley A, Wagner G, Osterloh IH, Kirkpatrick J, Mishra A. The international index of erectile function (IIEF): a multidimensional scale for assessment of erectile dysfunction. J Urol. 1997;49(6): 822–30.
9. Holley JL, Schmidt RJ. Sexual dysfunction in CKD. Am J Kidney Dis. 2010;56(4):612–4.
10. Holley JL, Schmidt RJ, Bender F, Dumler F, Schiff M. Gynecologic and reproductive issues in women on dialysis. Am J Kidney Dis. 1997;29(5):685–90.
11. Palmer BF. Sexual dysfunction in men and women with chronic kidney disease and end stage renal disease. Adv Ren Replace Ther. 2003;10(1):48–60.
12. Clayton AH, Goldfischer ER, Goldstein I, Derogatis L, Lewis-D'Agostino DJ, Pyke R. Validation of the decreased sexual desire screener (DSDS): a brief diagnostic instrument for generalized acquired female hypoactive sexual disorder (HSDD). J Sex Med. 2009;6(3):730–8.
13. Rosen R, Brown C, Heiman J, Leiblum S, Meston C, Shabsigh R. The Female Sexual Function Index (FSFI): a multidimensional self-report instrument for the assessment of female sexual function. J Sex Marital Ther. 2000;26(2):191–208.
14. Clayton AH, Segraves RT, Leiblum S, Basson R, Pyke R, Cotton D, et al. Reliability and validity of the Sexual Interest and Desire Inventory Female (SIDI-F), a scale designed to measure severity of female hypoactive sexual desire disorder. J Sex Marital Ther. 2006;32(2):115–35.
15. Leiblum S, Symonds T, Moore J, Soni P, Steinberg S, Sisson M. A methodology study to develop and validate a screener for hypoactive sexual desire disorder in postmenopausal women. J Sex Med. 2006;3(3): 455–64.

16. Rust J, Derogatis L, Rodenberg C, Koochaki P, Schmitt S, Golombok S. Development and validation of a new screening tool for hypoactive sexual desire disorder: the brief profile of the Female Sexual Function (B-PFSF). Gynecol Endocrinol. 2007; 23(11):638–44.
17. De Rogatis LR, Allgood A, Rosen RC, Leiblum S, Zipfel L, Guo CY. Development and evaluation of the women's sexual interest diagnostic interview (WSID):a structured interview to diagnose hypoactive sexual desire disorder (HSDD) in standardized patients. J Sex Med. 2008;5(12):2827–41.
18. Hatzimouratidis K, Amar E, Eardley I, Giuliano F, Hatzichriston D, Montorsi F, et al. Guidelines on male sexual dysfunction and premature ejaculation. Eur Urol. 2010;57(5):804–14.
19. Schmidt RJ, Holley JL. Fertility and contraception in end stage renal disease. Adv Ren Replace Ther. 1998;5(1):38–44.
20. Leavey SF, Weitzel WF. Endocrine abnormalities in chronic renal failure. Endocrinol Metab Clin North Am. 2002;31(1):107–19.
21. Holley JL, Schmidt RJ. Hormone replacement therapy in postmenopausal women with end stage renal disease: a review of the issues. Semin Dial. 2001; 14(3):146–9.
22. Berman JR, Berman LA, Toler SM, Gill J, Haughie S, Sildenafil Study Group. Safety and efficacy of sidenafil citrate for the treatment of female sexual arousal disorder: a double-blind, placebo controlled study. J Urol. 2003;170(6 Pt 1):2333–8.
23. Qaseem A, Snow V, Denberg TD, Casey DE, Fornea MA, Owens DK, Clinical Guidelines Committee of the American College of Physicians. Hormonal testing and pharmacologic treatment of erectile dysfunction. Ann Intern Med. 2009;151(9):639–49.
24. Armostrong C. ACOG Guideline on sexual dysfunction in women. Am Fam Physician. 2011;84(6): 705–9.
25. Wylie K, Rees M, Hackett G, Anderson R, Boulaux PM, Cust M, et al. Androgens, health and sexuality in women and men. Hum Fertil. 2010;13(4): 277–97.
26. Vecchio M, Navaneethan SD, Johnson DW, Lucisano G, Graziano G, Querques M, et al. Treatment options for sexual dysfunction in patients with chronic kidney disease: a systematic review of randomized controlled trials. Clin J Am Soc Nephrol. 2010;5(6):985–95.

25 Sleep Disorders in Chronic Kidney Disease

Rosa Maria De Santo

Before You Start: Facts You Need to Know

- More than 80 % of patients with ESRD on dialysis lack the benefits of a refreshing sleep. Sleep complaints include insomnia, daytime somnolence, delayed sleep onset, frequent awakenings, restless legs syndrome (RLS), periodic limb movements in sleep (PLMS), obstructive sleep apnea syndrome (OSAS), central sleep apnea (CSA), frequent nightmares, sleepwalking, and narcolepsy.
- The dialysis schedule has a significant influence on sleep quality. Patients dialyzed in the morning shift reported a shortest nocturnal sleep and worst sleep efficiency than those treated in the afternoon (like a disease of shift workers). The best and longest sleep is achieved in the night immediately after dialysis. Total sleep time (TTS) tends to decrease with the time distance from hemodialytic treatment being minimal in the night with the longest interdialytic interval. The worst sleepers are the patients on hemodialysis with medically intractable hyperparathyroidism and in need of surgery.
- Disordered sleep occurs in association with depression, pain, hypertension, cardiovascular events, low quality of life (QOL), and mortality.
- Even successful renal transplantation does not restore poor sleep to normalcy.
- Hypertension and the use of antihypertensive drugs have an independent role in the genesis of poor sleep.
- Awareness of sleeping disorders in patients with ESRD is preliminary to any intervention to improve their QOL. Patients with the worst sleep score have a 16 % higher mortality risk than that in good sleepers.
- Patients with a disordered sleep use more health resources.

25.1 Introduction

Sleep quality has been extensively studied in patients with end-stage renal disease (ESRD). A vast literature exists; however, the exact knowledge of the pathophysiological mechanisms is still lacking, and therapy is limited to the worst cases. Sleeping pills are rarely prescribed but are used by patients who also make use of various herbals.

R.M. De Santo
Italian Institute for Philosophical Studies,
20 Salita Scudillo, Parco La Collinetta,
Naples 80131, Italy
e-mail: bluetoblue@libero.it

M. Arici (ed.), *Management of Chronic Kidney Disease*,
DOI 10.1007/978-3-642-54637-2_25, © Springer-Verlag Berlin Heidelberg 2014

In contrast to the huge amount of data on sleep disorders in ESRD, data on sleep disorders in chronic kidney disease (CKD) are limited due to the recent onset of interest in the topic. The data available, however, provide stringent evidence for the existence of a disordered sleep with CKD, which will be discussed in this chapter.

25.2 Sleep Disorders in CKD: Definitions

Short definitions of the principal and most frequent sleep disorders encountered in CKD are given as a guide to identifying the vastness of this under-recognized burden affecting patients with many losses and dependences.

Insomnia is defined by experts as repeated complaints of unsatisfactory sleep, despite having adequate opportunity for sleep. The complaints can consist of difficulty initiating or maintaining sleep, waking up too early, and/or having unrefreshing sleep. Additionally, daytime consequences such as fatigue and lack of energy, impairment of concentration or memory, social or vocational dysfunction, or disturbances in mood or motivation must follow disturbed sleep. Chronic insomnia is generally defined as lasting at least 30 days [1].

Restless legs syndrome (*RLS*) is a sensorimotor disorder characterized by an almost irresistible urge to move one's legs or, more rarely, one's arms. RLS is usually associated with disagreeable leg sensations that are exacerbated during inactivity and have a profound impact on sleep. It is diagnosed by interview and based on the presence of the following criteria: (1) an urge to move the limbs, usually accompanied or caused by uncomfortable and unpleasant feelings in the limbs; (2) rest or inactivity precipitates or worsens symptoms; (3) getting up or moving improves the sensation; and (4) the urge to move or unpleasant sensations are only present or are worse in the evening or night. RLS is a common cause of sleep disorder in CKD [1].

Periodic limb movements in sleep (*PLMS*) are stereotyped, repetitive movements that primarily involve the legs. Each movement lasts from 0.5 to 5.0 s and occurs in regular intervals of 20–40 s during episodes that may last from minutes to almost all night. Many normal sleepers have such movements without ill effects. Periodic limb movement disorder (PLMD) is only diagnosed as a clinical condition when the PLMS (or their associated short arousals) exceed the norms for age and cause an otherwise unexplainable insomnia and/or excessive daytime fatigue [1].

Sleep apnea (*SA*) is an intermittent interruption of air flow during sleep, at the level of nose and mouth. It may be obstructive (OSA), central (CSA), or mixed (MSA).

Obstructive sleep apnea syndrome (*OSAS*) is characterized by repetitive partial or complete upper airway obstructions during sleep that cause apneas and hypopneas. A diagnosis of OSAS requires at least 15 obstructive events (apneas, hypopneas, and respiratory event-related arousals) per hour of sleep or greater than 5 such episodes per hour in a patient who reports excessive sleepiness, insomnia, and gasping during sleep or has a bed partner who reports loud snoring, breathing interruptions, or both during the patient's sleep [1].

Central sleep apnea syndrome (*CSAS*) consists of repetitive diminished or absent (10 s or less) respiratory efforts due to the failure of central respiratory centers to signal to breathe. This can result from the inability of the medulla and carotid chemoreceptors to correctly sense O_2 and CO_2 blood concentrations or in the inability of newly oxygenated blood to get from the lungs to these sensory centers (e.g., by impaired cardiac output). In contrast to OSAS, where arousals are typically required to terminate the apnea, CSAs often end gradually, when the signal to breathe returns. CSAs often cause arousals from sleep [1].

Excessive daytime sleepiness (*EDS*) interferes with daytime functioning. EDS can manifest itself as a tendency to fall asleep during normal waking hours when unstimulated (e.g., when driving long distances or when reading). EDS is objectively diagnosed when the average sleep latency on the multiple sleep latency test drops to $\leq$8 min. EDS and hypersomnia are currently used interchangeably [1].

Sleep quality is defined as one's satisfaction of the sleep experience, integrating aspects of sleep initiation, sleep maintenance, sleep quantity, and refreshment upon awakening [2].

Cognitive behavioral therapy focuses on addressing factors that contribute to the persistence of insomnia: (1) conditioned arousal, (2) identifying and eliminating habits that were developed in an effort to improve sleep but have become ineffective, and (3) reducing sleep-related worry and other sources of heightened arousal [3].

25.3 Prevalence and Predictors of Sleep Disorders in CKD

Evidence obtained in cross-sectional studies indicates that disordered sleep occurs very early in the natural course of chronic kidney disease and may affect the lives of 89.5 % of patients with a mean eGFR of 58.6 ml/min within 4 weeks following the first diagnosis of CKD [4]. One of three patients received hypnotic drugs. Longitudinal studies [5, 6] in turn suggest that blood pressure control may be a key element in the prevention and cure of sleep disorders.

Sabbatini et al. [5] performed a 3-year longitudinal study. Patients who completed the study had baseline mean creatinine clearance of 45 ml/min and a mean diastolic blood pressure of 95.2 mmHg and were using 1.36 antihypertensive drugs a day. Sixty-two percent of patients suffered from poor sleep. At completion of the study (3 years), there was an additional loss of creatinine clearance (13.25 ml over baseline), and the mean arterial blood pressure averaged 103.7 mmHg. The use of hypotensive drugs significantly increased to 1.78 ± 1.10, and 97.5 % were poor sleepers (Fig. 25.1). Since progression of kidney disease was accompanied by worsening sleep quality, pharmacological intervention to treat sleep disorders seemed appropriate.

A 4-year longitudinal study in early-CKD patients, eGFR 84 ± 21.1 ml/min/1.73 m^2, disclosed that 1 month after receiving CKD diagnosis, 85.5 % of patients were poor sleepers [6]. Sleep habits improved with time by accurate control of blood pressure with various hypotensive drugs. Also, the score of Beck Depression Inventory (BDI) improved with time. The use of hypnotic drugs also reduced over time (Table 25.1).

Thus, the high prevalence of poor sleepers in early-stage CKD is viewed as a marker of the process of coping with the idea of a chronic disease associated with lifelong dependencies and

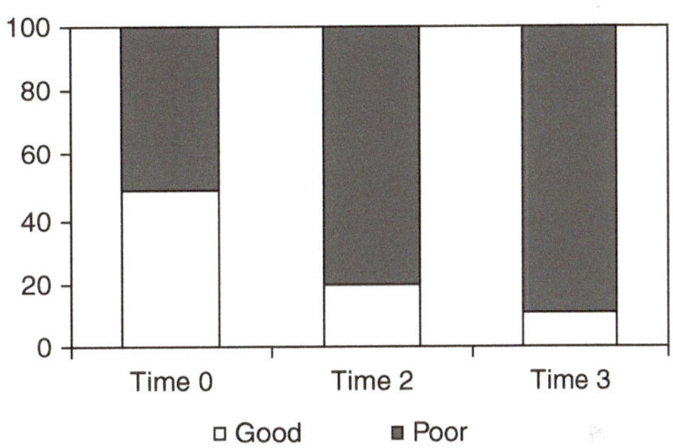

Fig. 25.1 Percent distribution of good (*white columns*) and poor (*dark columns*) sleepers during the time course of the study. *$p < 0.001$ vs Time 2 and Time 0 (minimum value) (Reprinted with permission from Sabbatini et al. [5])

Table 25.1 Longitudinal follow-up (4 years) of patients with early-stage CKD

	Baseline	2 years	4 years
Pts, no	220	210	200
eGFR, ml/min	84.1 ± 21.1	86.3 ± 22.10	83.7 ± 9.6
SBP, mmHg	139.6 ± 12.1	132.2 ± 10.7*	131.9 ± 10.7*
DBP, mmHg	83.9 ± 111	78.1 ± 8.7	77.9 ± 8.8*
On hypotensive drugs (%)	80	81.9	80.5
PSQI <5 (%)	15.5	19.0	50*+
BDI <11 (%)	36.4	50*	70*+
On hypnotics (%)	30 %	26.3	15.0*+

Source: Data from De Santo et al. [6]
*$p < 0.001$ vs basal +$p < 0.001$ vs. 2 years
eGFR estimated glomerular filtration rate, *SBP* systolic blood pressure, *DBP* diastolic blood pressure, *PSQI* Pittsburgh Sleep Quality Index, *BDI* Beck Depression Inventory

losses. This explains the high percentage of patients needing sleeping pills, a number that exceeds the percentage observed in patients on hemodialysis. A chronic disease potentially amenable to dialysis, or at best, to renal transplantation, is the disrupting event to which patients must adapt. So the time of diagnosis is crucial for the kidney patient, since they must generate and develop a coping mechanism.

25.3.1 Is Pain a Determinant of Poor Sleep in CKD?

Cohen et al. [7] studied pain, sleep disorders, and quality of life in predialysis patients (eGFR 33.4±23.7 ml/min) along with 61 general medical outpatients (eGFR 71.9±26.7 ml/min ($p<0.0001$). A total of 55.2 % of CKD patients had disordered sleep, which correlated with poorer quality of life, perception of pain, illness burden, and social support but was not associated with eGFR. In CKD patients, both the prevalence of sleep disturbances and pain were similar to those observed in general medical outpatients. Unfortunately, blood pressure was not measured—a rare occurrence in studies on CKD patients—and no reference was made available about the use of antihypertensive drugs.

25.3.2 Restless Leg Syndrome (RLS)

A 10.9 % prevalence of RLS was reported [8] in CKD patients (eGFR 41.6±19 ml/min, range 10–86) and was compared to healthy control subjects (3.3 % ($p<0.01$)). In CKD, the prevalence of hypertension was 91.8 % and that of anemia was 38.8 %. Patients with RLS used more benzodiazepines. A total of 86.9 % of the patients in this study were on drugs active on the cardiovascular system; however, it is not known whether hypertension was under control and, if so, by which drug. Independent predictors of RLS were sex (female) and percent transferrin saturation. Statistically significant findings show that patients with RLS had longer sleep latency, lower total sleep time, took more and longer naps, were more likely to be insomniacs, and had more daytime sleepiness. In multivariate analysis, RLS was independently associated with CKD. The study suggests that physicians caring for CKD patients with RLS should recognize female gender and iron deficiency as important indications.

25.3.3 Sleep Disordered Breathing (SDB)

Home polysomnographic studies [9] in CKD patients with eGFR <40 ml/min/1.73 m^2 (CKD 4 and 5), healthy controls, and HD (conventional three times a week) disclosed that severe sleep disordered breathing was highly prevalent not only in HD but also in CKD. Males were at higher risk of SDB. Potential pathophysiological mechanisms and mediators were increased pharyngeal cross-sectional area and abdominal circumference, overhydration, metabolic acidosis, and high levels of proinflammatory cytokines, C-reactive protein, and triglycerides. The study suggests that nephrologists should have a high index of suspicion of the diagnosis and treatment of SDB in CKD. In CKD patients in stages 3–5 and who have a mean eGFR of 24.9±10.6 ml/min who completed the self-reported Kidney Disease Quality of Life Instrument (KDQOL), the prevalence of poor sleepers was 57 % in the study of Kumar et al. [10]. Self-reported daytime sleepiness was associated with a higher risk of mortality prior to ESRD and with a lower quality of life and several modifiable symptoms. The prevalence of poor sleep was comparable to that in HD patients in the Dialysis Outcomes and Practice Patterns Study Program (DOPPS). Poor sleep was associated with lower age, pain, dyspnea, depressive symptoms, nausea, cramps, and itching. A group of 382 patients was restudied after 1 year, but no correlation was seen between delta changes in sleep quality (SQ) and delta changes in eGFR. The data indicate the necessity to give great attention to pain, dyspnea, depression, nausea, cramps, itching, and daily sleepiness in patients with CKD grades 3–5. The study also points to a wider utilization of the KDQOL to screen unsuspected sleep disturbances by just asking the patients to complete the questionnaire.

In a study of the Kaiser Permanente cohort [11], SA was investigated for over 1,102,089 persons (61.37 % F) aged >18 years, 37.11 % hypertensive, 15.67 % with diabetes, and 3.45 % with congestive heart failure (CHF). The prevalence of SA was 2.54 %, a figure closer to the 2 % in females in the normal population than to the 4 % of males. A high risk for SA was found for eGFR <60 ml/min/1.73 m^2 when compared to persons with normal kidney function. The risk was not eliminated by controlling for hypertension, diabetes, and CHF.

In Japan, the prevalence of obstructive sleep apnea (OSA) was studied on 100 consecutive in-hospital CKD patients (mean eGFR of 28.5 ml/min/1.73 m^2), 80 % of whom were hypertensive [12]. The prevalence of OSA was 65 %. In univariate analysis, an association was found between AHI and eGFR, which persisted in multivariate analysis. The finding was explained by narrowing airway dimensions, enhanced chemoresponsiveness, and an effect on BP through heightened sympathetic nerve tone, which in turn activates the renin-angiotensin-aldosterone systems and leads to hyperfiltration. In addition, it was speculated that OSA promotes oxidative stress, micro-inflammation, and endothelial dysfunction leading to renal ischemia, CKD progression, and cardiovascular disease. Every 10 ml/min/1.73 m^2 decrease in eGFR is associated with a 42 % increased risk for OSA.

25.3.4 The Poor Sleep of Old Persons with CKD5

Data in patients aged 82 ± 6.6 years with the lowest GFR not treated with dialysis (11.2 ± 2.8 ml/min) disclosed a prevalence of disordered sleep in 41 %, of restless leg syndrome in 48 %, and of pain in 58 % [13].

25.3.5 Is Sleep Disordered Breathing a Risk for CKD?

The prevalence of CKD defined as eGFR <60 ml/min/1.73 m^2 was evaluated in 1,624 persons undergoing in-hospital polysomnography (PSG) and compared with that in 7,454 age- and sex-matched persons from the general population [14]. The prevalence of CKD was 30.9 % in the group with OSA and 9.1 % in the general population ($p < 0.0001$). In contrast with the screened population, the prevalence of CKD was inversely related to Beck Depression Inventory (BDI). The prevalence of CKD in the population in nondiabetic, non-hypertensive people was 5 %, whereas in diabetic and hypertensive persons, it was 13.8 %. Unfortunately, blood pressure and blood glucose were not studied in the OSA group. The study suggests the value of investigating renal function in non-obese patients with OSA on and off CPAP in order to prevent progression to ESRD.

A group of 158 consecutive patients, aged 61.2 ± 12.7 years, referred for full-night-observed-in-hospital PSG, was stratified according to the presence of sleep apnea [15]. After examination, a total of 25 persons were apnea-free and their eGFR averaged 94.67 ml/min/1.73 m^2, whereas in those with apnea, eGFR averaged 84.57 ml/min/1.73 m^2 ($p < 0.037$). All patients were stratified according to eGFR in CKD groups. Sleep apnea was present in 86 % of persons in CKD1, 80 % in CKD2, and 94 % in CKD3 (differences not statistically significant). Statistically significant results show, however, that the number of central sleep apneas (CSA) in CKD3 averaged 5.9 ± 12.2, six times greater than in patients with GFR >60 ml/min (averaging only 1.0 ± 2.1) (Fig. 25.2). In patients with central sleep apnea, then, eGFR must be calculated for appropriate treatment and improved outcomes.

Non-hypertensive nondiabetic OSA patients studied by in-hospital overnight PSG showed a prevalence of 18 % for CKD1-2 and 14 % prevalence of urine albumin-to-creatinine ratio (UACR) >30 mg/g. AHI was an independent risk factor for both CKD1-2 and UACR [16].

These studies indicate that patients with SDB are at risk of CKD. This, obviously, renders the measurement of plasma creatinine concentration mandatory in all patients with SDB.

25.3.6 Lessons from Population-Based Studies

Inadequate sleeping (<6 h per night) differed by CKD severity in a population-based study [17].

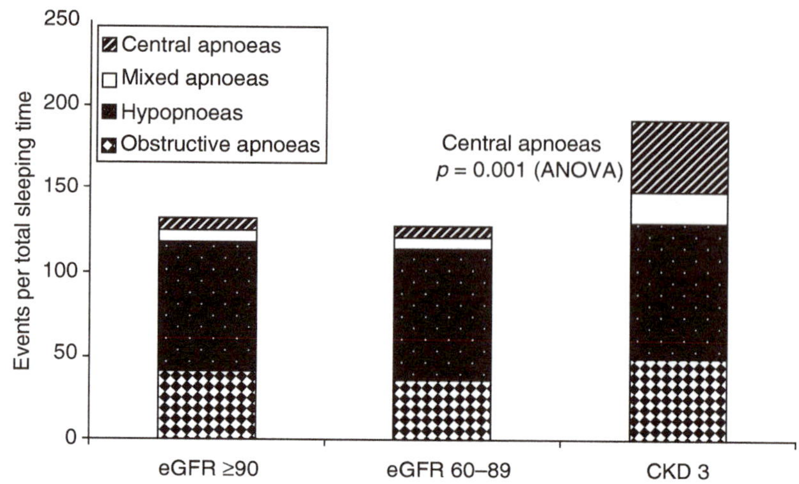

Fig. 25.2 Respiratory event per total sleep time (Reprinted with permission from Fleischmann et al. [15])

Sleeping pills use, legs symptoms, and nocturia also differed according to CKD severity. After adjustment for age, sex, race/ethnicity, obesity, diabetes, and cardiovascular disease, the prevalence of sleep-related problems remained higher in people with CKD 1 and 2 relative to no CKD. Primary care providers should know that nearly 9 % of the US adult population reported using sleep pills 5 or more times a month, although few of these reported having a prescription for sleep aid, indicating that the most sleeping aids used are available over-the-counter. Patients with moderate to severe CKD reported more frequent use of sleeping pills. Thus, providers of primary care should not forget to ask about the use of herbal, off-label, and over-the-counter drugs for sleep to ensure their patients' safety and prevent kidney-related complications. In patients with moderate CKD who used a prescription sleep aid, nearly 25 % were using medications contraindicated for kidney disease, likely because their physicians were unaware of their disease.

25.3.7 Reviewing the Topic of Poor Sleep in CKD

Sleep disorders in non-dialyzed CKD patients have been thoroughly followed up [18, 19]. Sim et al. [18] mainly focused on the relation of SA to CKD and point to a complex interaction of two disease processes where hypertension may represent an intermediary variable as depicted in Fig. 25.3, showing the overlapping of SA, CKD, and hypertension. Apnea per se may induce hypertension which in turn may cause CKD. Strong emphasis must be given to focal segmental glomerular sclerosis (FSGS) in sleep apnea (a disease characterized by renal hypoperfusion and ischemia), increased vascular endothelial growth factor (VEGF) levels, and reduced concentrations of nitric oxide. Patients with FSGS should be studied and treated according to the rules valid for the general population, namely, treatment of obesity, changes of lifestyles, adoption of an appropriate sleep position, and the use of medication. Control of blood pressure is also recommended to achieve target levels. Proteinuria and increased blood glucose must be also treated. Finally, one should not neglect that poor sleep exacerbates three risk factors for CKD (Fig. 25.4): hypertension, type 2 diabetes mellitus, and obesity [19].

25.3.8 Is Melatonin Circadian Rhythm Important?

In hemodialysis patients, the nocturnal melatonin rise associated with sleep propensity is absent. In CKD patients (mean GFR 50 ± 30 ml/min), the time course of melatonin concentration [20] varied according to renal function; those with highest GFR had the highest melatonin concentration

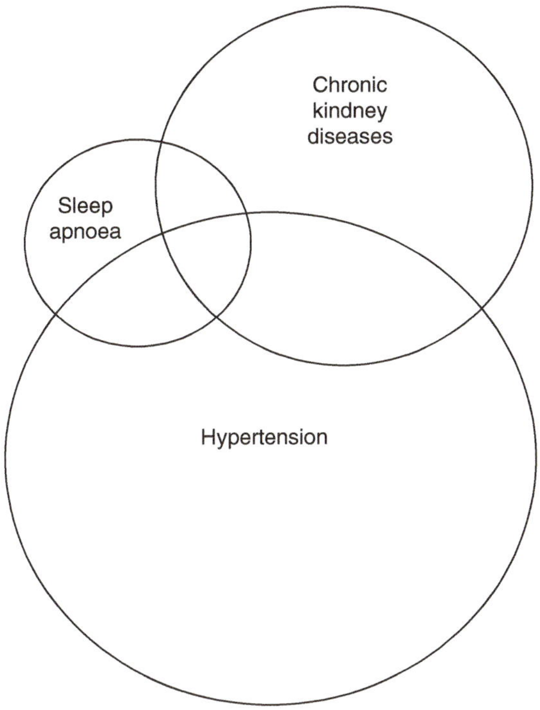

Fig. 25.3 Overlapping of CKD, hypertension, and sleep apnea (Reprinted with permission from Sim et al. [18])

and those with the lowest GFR had also the lowest melatonin (Fig. 25.5). In addition, the amplitude of the melatonin rhythm correlated with GFR (Fig. 25.6), as was the case for total melatonin production. The relation is not age and gender dependent. Melatonin is, however, under the influence of anemia, acidosis, and suppressed N-acetyltransferase (NAT)—which are markers of CKD—as well as beta-blockers and benzodiazepines, drugs frequently used by kidney patients. Acidosis and anemia are among the features of CKD, a condition which occurs with NAT suppression. In addition, beta-blockers are fundamental drugs to treat blood pressure, and benzodiazepines are used to treat insomnia. The same authors have reported that exogenous melatonin administration, in daytime hemodialysis patients characterized by absent nocturnal melatonin rise, caused a recovery of the melatonin rise and an improvement of subjective and objective sleep measurements in a placebo-controlled crossover study. The melatonin studies suggest that more research is needed in experiments with CKD persons following exogenous melatonin

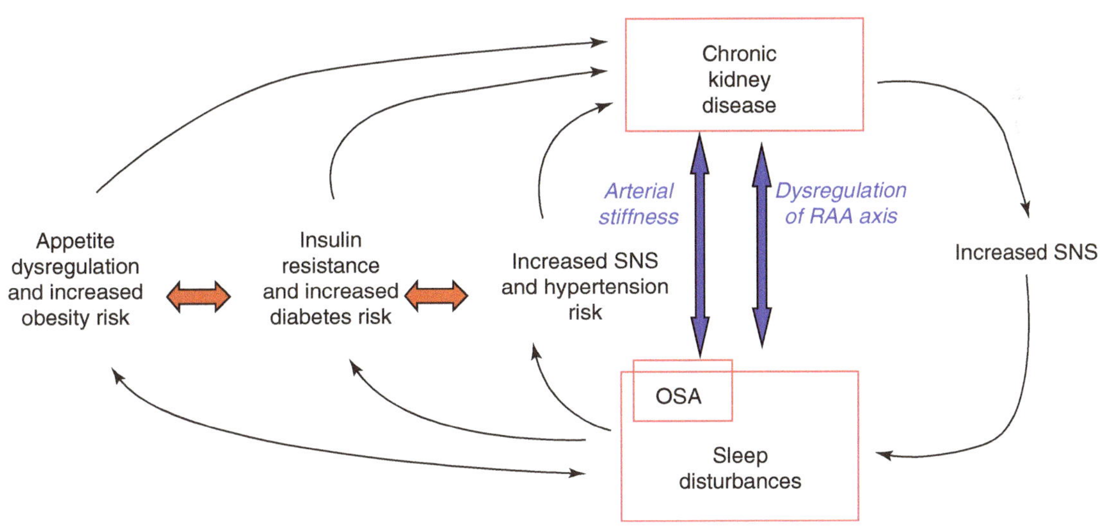

Fig. 25.4 Putative mechanisms linking sleep disturbances with CKD progression. *RAA* renin-angiotensin-aldosterone, *OSA* obstructive sleep apnea, *SNS* sympathetic nervous system activity (Reprinted with permission from Turek et al. [19])

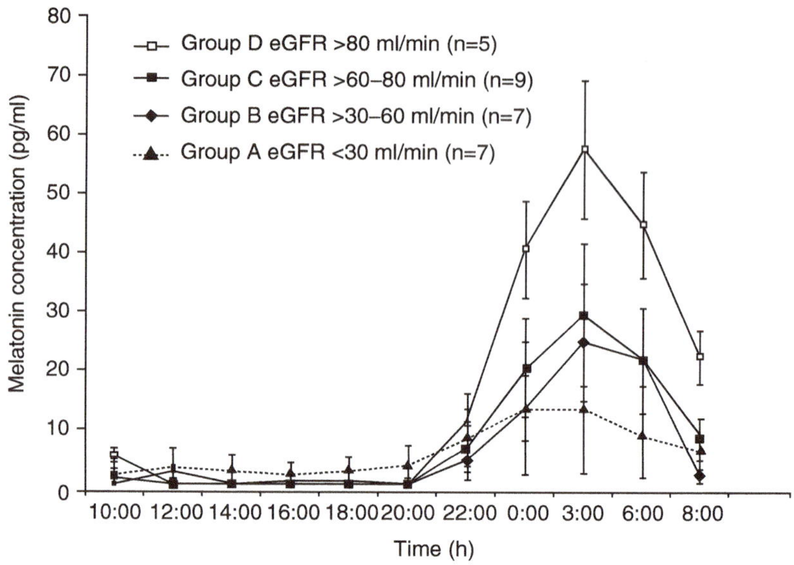

Fig. 25.5 Time course of melatonin concentration according to eGFR (Reprinted from Koch et al. [20] by permission of Oxford University Press)

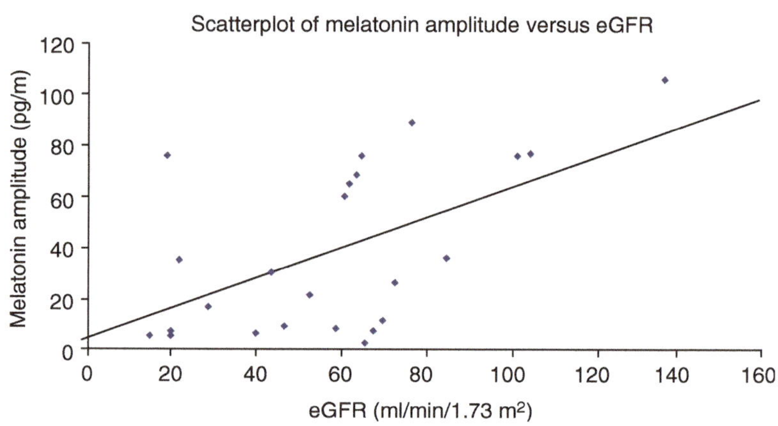

Fig. 25.6 Melatonin amplitude vs. eGFR in patients with melatonin rhythm (Reprinted from Koch et al. [20] by permission of Oxford University Press)

administration to mimic the endogenous melatonin rhythm.

25.4 Diagnosis and Therapy of Sleep Apnea

25.4.1 In the General Population

In a statement paper of the American Heart Association and of the American College of Cardiology [21], the whole topic has been reviewed in order to scrutinize (1) the pathophysiological components of OSA, (2) the activation of cardiovascular disease components, and (3) cardiovascular diseases. Table 25.2 differentiates central and obstructive sleep apnea.

25.4.2 In CKD Patients

OSA has negative influence on disease outcomes in various branches of clinical medicine including ESRD and CKD. It increases the utilization of health services, lowers the quality of life, and increases mortality. In CKD patients, sleep apnea deteriorates with nephron loss since it activates (Fig. 25.7) the sympathetic nervous system, the angiotensin-aldosterone system, cardiovascular hemodynamics, and the generation

Table 25.2 Sleep, signs, diagnosis, and therapy of obstructive sleep apnea (OSA) and central sleep apnea (CSA)

	Obstructive sleep apnea	Central sleep apnea
Sleep	Apnea Hypersomnolence Nocturia Snoring	Apnea Cheyne-Stokes respiration
Signs	Behavioral changes Enlarged neck size Headache in the morning Hypertension Male gender Obesity Reduced section of pharyngeal airway Sexual dysfunction Weakness	Cheyne-Stokes respiration during awakening Male gender Older age Heart failure Mitral regurgitation, atrial fibrillation Hyperventilation with hypocapnia
Diagnosis	Berlin questionnaire Epworth Sleepiness Scale 24-h Blood pressure recording Overnight oximetry In-hospital PSG +ECG monitoring Unattended PSG (?)	24-h Blood pressure recording Overnight oximetry In-hospital PSG Unattended PSG (?)
Therapy	Body weight loss, No alcohol No sedatives Positional therapy CPAP Surgery on uvula, tonsils, trachea	Strict control of heart failure CPAP Supplemental oxygen

Source: Data from Somers et al. [21]

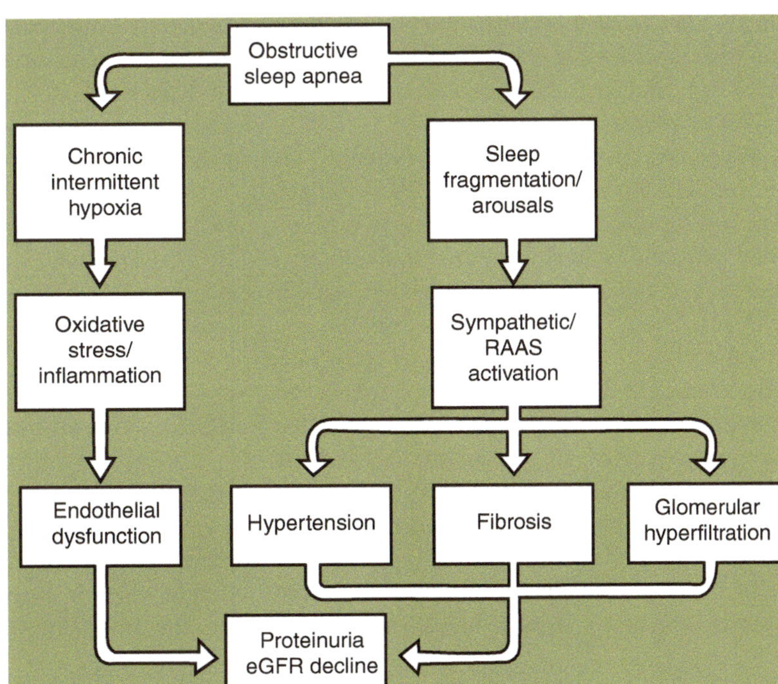

Fig. 25.7 Impact of obstructive sleep apnea on CKD (Reprinted with permission from Adeseun and Rosas [22])

of free radicals. The latter, in turn, triggers endothelial dysfunction, inflammation, platelet aggregation with thrombosis, increased negative intrathoracic pressure, atherosclerosis and fibrosis, insulin resistance, age and body mass index (BMI) independent hypertension, renal damage, proteinuria, CKD progression, nocturia, and increased blood atrial natriuretic peptide (ANP) concentrations [22].

Although there are no guidelines for sleep disorders in CKD, indications for treatment exist at least for SA [23]. It is known that SA and hypertension are associated. In addition, SA is a risk for CKD patients. SA and CKD are associated with a higher risk of hypertension. SA is a risk for mortality and progression of CKD because of the detrimental effects of anoxia, which also promotes tubulointerstitial lesions. Finally, the respiratory adaptation to metabolic acidosis may produce hypocapnia. Much can also be learned from available data in CKD patients following renal transplantation in whom SA may develop de novo (i.e., transplantation may represent a risk for SA). Steroids are, in fact, associated with increased body weight, total body water, total body sodium, and obesity. All of these may have a causal role for SA in these patients. Therefore, newer sleep complaints after renal transplantation should stimulate awareness for SA. Physicians should also be aided by the fact that proteinuria with SA improves after treatment of SA.

Psychiatric/psychological assessment and intervention are recommended; PSG is the gold standard for diagnosis and may help to differentiate between central and obstructive SA. It becomes mandatory in hypertensive patients with suspected SA. PSG also has a role to control the effects of therapy. PSG is associated with overnight assessment of electroencephalography (EEG), electrooculography (EOG), electromyography (EMG), respiratory parameters and electrocardiogram (ECG), pulse oximetry, and noninvasive measurements of CO_2 blood levels.

In patients with SA and early CKD, with/without proteinuria, a renal biopsy may help in disclosing glomerulomegaly and the lesions of focal segmental glomerular sclerosis leading to hyperfiltration. Nasal continuous airway positive pressure (nCPAP) is the therapy of choice in moderate sleep apnea. It reduces daytime sleepiness, improves quality of life (QOL), and reduces the rate of cardiovascular accidents. Surgery, including tracheostomy, may be needed. Additional rules may be found in a recent paper of Kuhlmann et al. [23], where indications on signs, diagnosis, and therapy are available (Table 25.3).

Table 25.3 Therapy for obstructive sleep apnea

No evidence for effectiveness
Reduce body weight
Abstain from alcohol and drinks containing caffeine
Caveats
Tranquilizers induce and intensify obstruction
Beta-blockers are usable in the absence of bradycardia
Oxygen may prolong apnea periods
Evidence for effectiveness
Avoid supine sleeping
Lateral and abdominal sleeping reduces sleep apneas (aids may be needed)
Diuretics
Nasal CPAP reduces hypertension and daytime sleepiness
Side effects of CPAP
Hypoventilation, acute cardiac insufficiency, and a 25 % prevalence of rhinitis may make CPAP intolerable
Noncompliance is associated with increased mortality risk

Source: Data from Somers et al. [21]

For patients who cannot adapt/or refuse nCPAP, pharmacological treatment of the sympathetic overactivity may represent the last resort in managing the high risk carried by SDB, and clinical trials are warranted [24].

25.5 The Management of RLS/PLMS

RLS/PMLS occur with sympathetic hyperactivity, increased blood pressure and pulse rate, heart disease, and stroke, due to a dopaminergic deficit which is the primary target of dopaminergic therapy [25]. We know that RLS may not increase through CKD 1–5, with the exception of diabetic patients, and is always associated with daytime sleepiness. Its pathophysiology is unknown but at a certain extent is related to iron deficiency. We also know that it improves after renal transplantation. In CKD, the prevalence of PLMS, in comparison with normal population (prevalence of 3–4 %), is increased by a factor of ten. Dopaminergic mechanisms have been identified.

Patients are recommended to abstain from alcohol and nicotine and to adopt specific physical exercises. In cases associated with depletion of body iron stores, a repletion is mandatory. Dopamine, dopamine receptor agonists, anticonvulsants, and opioids may be used. Benzodiazepines and various central depressants of the nervous system may however depress the respiratory drive and negatively affect the patency of the airways. Drugs must be dosed—when necessary—according to kidney function. For benzodiazepines and various central depressants of the nervous system, patients may have reduced capability in decreasing respiratory drive and also see effects to the patency of the airways. Drugs must be dosed—when necessary—according to kidney function.

25.6 Nephrologist's Role in the Work-up and Therapy of Sleep Disorders in CKD

For the American Academy of Sleep Medicine, sleep is a vital and necessary function, and sleep needs (like hunger and thirst) must be met. Sleep disorders are associated with low quality of life and impaired social and occupational functioning, are a risk for depression, and increase health care utilization. There are no specific guidelines for diagnosis management of sleep disorders in CKD (Box 25.1). However, the status of the art has reached a niveau that allows to appropriately assist the insomniac CKD patients (Box 25.2).

Nephrologists have a driving role for diagnosis (Box 25.3) which can be made either by means of clinical interviews or using sleep logs and/or questionnaires. The Pittsburgh Sleep Quality Index [26] has provided convincing results and is easy to handle. There are 19 questions with seven "component" scores. A global PSQI >5 has an 89.6 % sensitivity and 86.5 % specificity. Polysomnography (the gold standard) is usually performed on a single night and

Box 25.1. Relevant Guidelines

No guidelines are available for sleep disorders in CKD; however, relevant information is available in various papers which deal with insomnia, restless legs syndrome, and sleep apnea:

Insomnia

1. Schutte-Rodin S, Broch L, Buysse D, Dorsey C, Sateia M. Clinical guideline for the evaluation and management of chronic insomnia in adults. J Clin Sleep Med. 2008;4:487–504.

Restless Legs Syndrome and Periodic Limb Movement Disorder

2. Aurora RN, Kristo DA, Bista SR, Rowley JA, Zak RS, Casey KR, et al. The treatment of restless legs syndrome and periodic limb movement disorder in adults – an update for 2012: practice parameters with an evidence-based systematic review and meta-analyses. Sleep. 2012;35:1039–62.

Sleep Apnea

3. Sim JJ, Rasgon SA, Derose SF. Managing sleep apnoea in kidney diseases. Nephrology. 2010;15:146–52.

Antidepressants

4. Nagler EV, Webster AC, Vanholder R, Zoccali C. Antidepressant for depression in stage 3–5 chronic kidney disease: a systematic review of pharmacokinetics, efficacy and safety with recommendations by European Renal Best Practice (ERBP). Nephrol Dial Transplant. 2012;27:3736–45.

in a sleep laboratory, which may not be indicative of normal sleep patterns. Actigraphy is a valid noninvasive method measuring sleep parameters at home and over multiple days. It is complementary to PSG. Hypnotics in CKD are used sparingly; however, the highest usage was reported in early-CKD patients immediately after receiving a diagnosis of chronic kidney disease. Recently, electrostimulation of leg extensors in ESRD reduced pain and improved QOL and quality of sleep [27].

Nephrologists, before asking for the help of the sleep specialist, should be aware that hemoglobin concentration and systolic and diastolic blood pressure must be kept within targets and pain cured according to WHO ladders. This is a prerequisite to the cure of the disordered sleep which is detailed in Box 25.4.

Box 25.2. What the Guidelines Say You Should Do

- Clinical assessment must be achieved through self-administered questionnaires, at-home sleep logs, symptoms checklists, psychological screening tests, and bed partner interviews. The Pittsburgh Sleep Quality Index has been translated into 56 languages. Actigraphy is becoming of age. Polysomnography is the gold standard.
- Sleep hygiene (caffeine, alcohol, nicotine) must be checked and followed up.
- If pain coexists, specific drugs must be given.
- Cognitive behavioral therapy is the first approach.
- Hypnotics have a role.
- nCPAP is an effective therapy for apnea.
- For RLS, start with iron replacement therapy. Medications include low-potency opioids, dopamine agonists, and gabapentin.

Box 25.3. The Role of the Nephrologists in the Work-up of Sleep Disorders in CKD

- CKD patients usually complain of their sleep problems and ask for help. Usually they complain of difficulties in initiating and maintaining sleep, early waking up, and unrefreshing sleep, which causes stress. The nursing staff is the most frequent target of these complaints. Sometimes, either the bed partner, family members, accompanying persons, or the patients hosted in the same hospital bedroom disclose RLS, PLMS, snoring, and OSAS.
- Nephrologists may get a direct insight in the sleeping problems by listening to the patient's narrative.
- The use of the PSQI may help.
- Daytime sleepiness with inability to maintain wakefulness may cause accidents.
- OSA may cause reduction of renal function.
- In the case that a sleep problem emerges, it might be appropriate to look for the coexistence of depression by using the Beck Depression Index (BDI). BDI is structured on 21 items. Each question is scored from 0 to 3. In the general population, a BDI score of 11 or greater indicates depression. In CKD, the cutoff for depression is score >14.
- In case of snoring, an overnight pulse oximetry—now easily available in any hospital—will monitor SaO_2. Further decision to proceed to PSG should be made in association with the sleep expert in the hospital.

Box 25.4. Therapy of Sleep Disorders in CKD

- Hemoglobin should be kept within the targets.
- Strict blood pressure control by low salt intake and drugs may have a beneficial effect.
- Be aware that beta-blockers have negative effects on sleep.
- Pain requires treatment according to WHO suggestions.
- Cognitive behavioral therapy is an effective nonpharmacological therapy which can improve the quality of sleep and decrease fatigue.
- The use of bright light (1,000 lux) may be appropriate in the old patients.
- Melatonin administration carries no risk and potentially may help circadian resynchronization.
- For insomnia, hypnotics must be used. The general practitioners and nephrologists, for unknown reasons, make a spare use of them which causes underdosage. The sleep specialist should advise for appropriate dosage and length of treatment. Benzodiazepines induce sleep, reduce sleep latency, and suppress REM and slow-wave sleep, but their effect is unwarranted. Non-benzodiazepine hypnotics should be preferred. Zolpidem is effective and does not cause apnea. The antidepressant mianserin may be advantageous as sleep inducer; however, a guide to use antidepressant is provided by European Renal Best Practice (See Box 25.1) [4].
- In presence of RLS and PMLS correct iron deficiency, forbid alcohol and smoking. L-dopa, and dopamine receptor agonists, anticonvulsants, and opioids may be used. Benzodiazepines may decrease the respiratory drive and also reduce airway patency. Drugs must be dosed—when necessary—according to renal function.
- OSAS may require nasal CPAP (i.e., delivering compressed air), which is not always tolerated.
- Daytime sleepiness renders patients unable to maintain wakefulness and is a reason for indoor and outdoor accidents.

Before You Finish: Practice Pearls for the Clinician

- SA in CKD is now considered a warning and deteriorates with the severity of nephron loss. The concept may be extended to all causes of disordered sleep in CKD.
- RLS is an important source of sleep disruption in CKD patients.
- Wake and sleep functions should be viewed as a vital sign: every patient should be asked about sleep and daytime alertness. Any complaint should be taken seriously and not simply attributed to the underlying renal disease and/or medications.
- Impaired quality of sleep impairs quality of life in CKD patients.
- A clinical suspicion of non-refreshing sleep should be followed by further assessment.
- Questionnaires are the cheapest and most easily available at every bedside. The PSQI is a good instrument. Actigraphy is simple and coming of age. PSG is the gold standard.
- The kidney specialist and the sleep specialist must interact to solve sleep problems in CKD.
- Awareness of sleep problems in CKD patients is the starting point to improve their QOL.
- Sleeping medications (usually benzodiazepines) are used with a warning for patients with SA..Nasal CPAP is the therapy of choice for severe SA.
- Poor sleep quality is associated with lower QOL and risk of pre-ESRD mortality.

References

1. The sleep disorders. A publication of the National Sleep Foundation. Accessed on line 29 April 2014 at http://sleepdisorders.sleepfoundation.org/chapter-2-insomnia/definitions/what-is-insomnia/.
2. Kline C. Sleep quality. In: Gellman MD, Turner JR, editors. Encyclopedia of behavioral medicine. New York: Springer; 2013. p. 1811–3 (accessed on line, July 12, 2013).
3. Stanford Center for Sleep Sciences and Medicine [internet]. Redwood City: Stanford Hospitals and Clinics; 2013. Cognitive and Behavioral therapy for Insomnia. Available from: http://stanfordhospital.org/clinicsmedServices/clinics/sleep/treatment_options/cbt.html. Cited 12 Aug 2013.
4. De Santo RM, Bartiromo M, Cesare CM, Cirillo M. Sleep disorders occur very early in chronic kidney disease. J Nephrol. 2008;21 Suppl 13:S59–65.
5. Sabbatini M, Pisani A, Crispo A, Ragosta A, Gallo R, Pota A, Serio V, Tripepi G, Cianciaruso B. Sleep quality in patients with chronic renal failure: a 3-year longitudinal study. Sleep Med. 2008;9:240–6.
6. De Santo RM, Bilancio G, Santoro D, Li Vecchi M, Perna A, De Santo NG, Cirillo M. A longitudinal study of sleep disorders in early-stage chronic kidney disease. J Ren Nutr. 2010;20:S59–63.
7. Cohen SD, Patel SS, Khetpal P, Peterson RA, Kimmel PL. Pain, sleep disturbance and quality of life in patients with chronic kidney disease. Clin J Am Soc Nephrol. 2007;2:919–25.
8. Merlino G, Lorenzut S, Gigli GL, Romano G, Montanaro D, Moro A, Valente M. A case–control study on restless legs syndrome in nondialyzed patients with chronic renal failure. Mov Disord. 2010;25:1019–25.
9. Roumelioti ME, Buysse DJ, Sanders MH, Strollo P, Newman AB, Unruh ML. Sleep disordered – breathing and excessive daytime sleepiness in chronic kidney disease and hemodialysis. Clin J Am Soc Nephrol. 2011;6:986–94.
10. Kumar B, Tilea A, Gillespie BW, Zhang X, Kiser M, Eisele G, Finkelstein F, Kotanko P, Levin N, Rajagopalan S, Saran R. Significance of self-reported sleep quality (SQ) in chronic kidney disease (CKD): the Renal Research Institute (RRI)-CKD study. Clin Nephrol. 2010;73:104–14.
11. Sim JJ, Rasgon SA, Kujubu DA, Kumar VA, Liu IL, Shi JM, Pham TT, Derose SF. Sleep apnea in early and advanced chronic kidney disease: Kaiser Permanente Southern California cohort. Chest. 2009;135:710–6.
12. Sakaguchi Y, Shoji Y, Kawabata H, Niihata K, Suzuki A, Kaneko T, Okada N, Isaka Y, Rakugi H, Tsubakihara Y. High prevalence of obstructive sleep apnea and its association with renal function among nondialysis chronic kidney disease patients in Japan: a cross-sectional study. Clin J Am Soc Nephrol. 2011;6:995–1000.
13. Murtagh FE, Addington-Hall JM, Edmonds PM, Donohoe P, Carey I, Jenkins K, Higginson IJ. Symptoms in advanced renal disease: a cross-sectional survey of symptom prevalence in stage 5 chronic kidney disease managed without dialysis. J Palliat Med. 2007;10:1266–76.
14. Iseki K, Tohyama K, Matsumoto T, Nakamura H. High prevalence of chronic kidney disease among patients with sleep related breathing disorder (SRBD). Hypertens Res. 2008;31:249–55.
15. Fleischmann G, Fillafer G, Matterer H, Skrabal F, Kotanko P. Prevalence of chronic kidney disease in patients with suspected sleep apnoea. Nephrol Dial Transplant. 2010;25:181–6.
16. Chou YT, Lee PH, Yang CT, Lin CL, Veasey S, Chuang LP, Lin SW, Lin YS, Chen NH. Obstructive sleep apnea: a stand-alone risk factor for chronic kidney disease. Nephrol Dial Transplant. 2011;26:2244–50.
17. Plantinga L, Lee K, Inker LA, Saran R, Yee J, Gillespie B, Rolka D, Saydah S, Powe NR, CDC CKD Surveillance Team. Association of sleep-related problems with CKD in the United States, 2005–2008. Am J Kidney Dis. 2011;58(4):554–64.
18. Sim JJ, Rasgon SA, Derose SF. Review article: managing of sleep apnoea in kidney diseases. Nephrology (Carlton). 2010;15:146–52.
19. Turek NF, Ricardo AC, Lash JP. Sleep disturbances as nontraditional risk factors for development and progression of CKD: review of the evidence. Am J Kidney Dis. 2012;60:823–33.
20. Koch BC, van der Putten K, Van Someren EJ, Wielders JP, Ter Wee PM, Nagtegaal JE, Gaillard CA. Impairment of endogenous melatonin rhythm is related to the degree of chronic kidney disease (CREAM study). Nephrol Dial Transplant. 2010;25:513–9.
21. Somers VK, White DP, Amin R, Abraham WT, Costa F, Culebras A, Daniels S, Floras JS, Hunt CE, Olson LJ, Pickering TG, Russel R, Woo M, Young T. Sleep apnea and cardiovascular disease. J Am Coll Cardiol. 2008;52:686–717.
22. Adeseun GA, Rosas SE. The impact of obstructive sleep apnea on chronic kidney disease. Curr Hypertens Rep. 2010;12:378–83.
23. Kuhlmann U, Bormann FG, Becker HF. Obstructive sleep apnoea: clinical signs, diagnosis and treatment. Nephrol Dial Transplant. 2009;24:8–14.
24. Mallamaci F, Tripepi G. Comment accompanying: obstructive sleep apnea: a stand-alone risk factor for chronic kidney disease by Chou Yu-Ting. Nephrol Dial Transplant. 2011;26:2072–4.
25. Walters AS, Rye DB. Review of the relationship of restless legs syndrome and periodic limb movements in sleep to hypertension, heart disease and stroke. Sleep. 2009;32:589–97.
26. Iliescu EA, Yeates KE, Holland DC. Quality of sleep in patients with chronic kidney disease. Nephrol Dial Transplant. 2004;19:95–9.
27. Klassen A, Di Iorio BR, Guastaferro P, Bahner U, Heidland A, De Santo NG. High-tone external muscle stimulation in end-stage renal disease: effects on symptomatic diabetic and uremic peripheral neuropathy. J Ren Nutr. 2008;18:46–51.

26 Neuropathy and Other Neurological Problems in Chronic Kidney Disease

Ria Arnold and Arun V. Krishnan

Before You Start: Facts You Need to Know

- Neurological complications are highly prevalent in CKD and contribute substantially to patient morbidity and mortality risk.
- The uremic state can potentially affect all levels of the nervous system, from central nervous system disorders, such as encephalopathy and cognitive dysfunction, to peripheral disorders such as myopathy and autonomic and peripheral neuropathies.
- Neurological complications often become clinically apparent with severe kidney disease; however, detection and management of these conditions in earlier stages of CKD may reduce their impact at later stages.

26.1 Neuropathy in CKD

Neurological complications are highly prevalent in patients with CKD. The systemic nature of uraemia causes a variety of neurological disorders potentially affecting all levels of the nervous system [1] (Fig. 26.1). These may manifest as central nervous system disorders, such as encephalopathy and cognitive dysfunction, to peripheral disorders such as myopathy and autonomic and peripheral neuropathies (Table 26.1). It is evident that these conditions have significant impacts on patient morbidity and mortality [2, 3]. While quality of life is profoundly affected by these conditions, increased mortality is also a significant concern, particularly where there is severe encephalopathy causing coma or advanced neuropathy, which may lead to skin ulceration and even gangrene [4]. Furthermore, less common causes of CKD may also affect the central and/or peripheral nervous system independent of uraemia such as amyloidosis, systemic lupus erythematosus, hepatic failure, Wilson's disease and Fabry's disease [5]. Despite this, there are currently no clinical guidelines for the management of neurological complications in CKD and only brief mentions of this topic in K/DOQI Clinical Practice Guidelines (Box 26.1). Given that most neurological complications manifest with an eGFR of less than 20 mL/min, their prevalence is only clearly documented in stage 5 CKD and dialysis populations. However, the association between declining kidney function and severity of neurological complications [4] suggests that

R. Arnold, BS
Department of Neurological Sciences, Prince of Wales Hospital, High Street, Randwick, Sydney, NSW 2031, Australia
e-mail: r.arnold@neura.edu.au, ria.arnold@unsw.edu.au

A.V. Krishnan, MBBS, PhD, FRACP (✉)
Department of Neurology, Prince of Wales Hospital, High Street, Randwick, Sydney, NSW 2031, Australia
e-mail: arun.krishnan@unsw.edu.au

M. Arici (ed.), *Management of Chronic Kidney Disease*,
DOI 10.1007/978-3-642-54637-2_26, © Springer-Verlag Berlin Heidelberg 2014

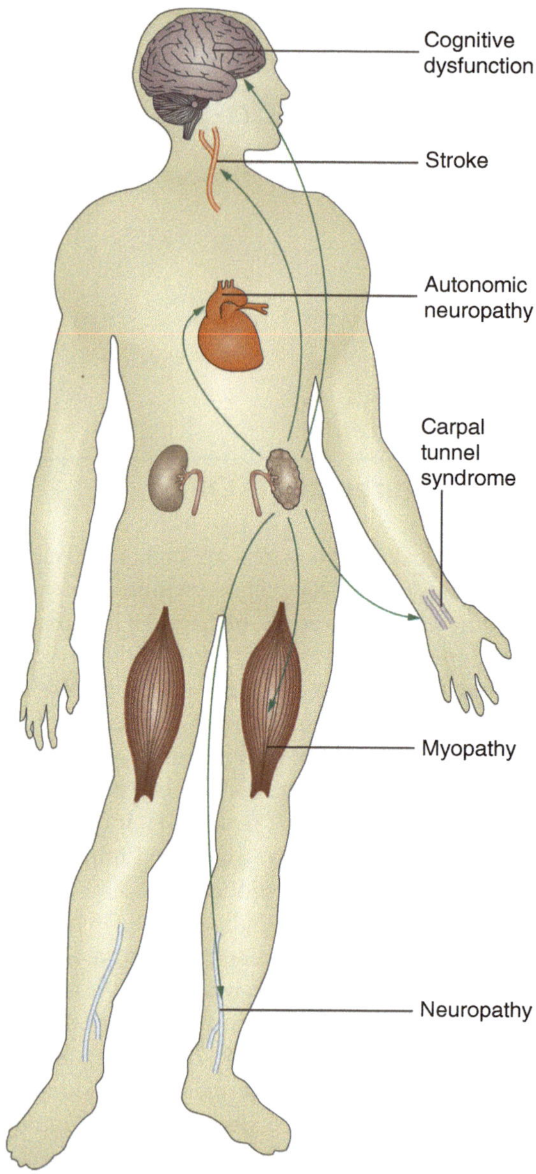

Fig. 26.1 The spectrum of neurological complications in chronic kidney disease (Reprinted from Krishnan and Kiernan [1])

pathological changes occur in earlier stages of CKD. As such, detection and management of these conditions in earlier stages of CKD may provide a window of opportunity to reduce their impact at later stages.

26.1.1 Peripheral Neuropathy

26.1.1.1 Definition

The most common neurological complication of CKD is peripheral neuropathy, also known as uremic neuropathy, which affects 60–90 % of dialysis patients [1]. The onset and severity of uremic neuropathy closely relates to the severity of kidney dysfunction with most cases becoming clinically evident at glomerular filtration rates of <12 mL/min [7]. The prevalence of uremic neuropathy in earlier stages of CKD has not been systemically investigated. However, the increasing incidence of diabetic nephropathy introduces a highly susceptible patient cohort that may have pre-existing neuropathy and are thus likely to have neuropathy of greater severity [2, 8]. Patients typically experience symptoms such as pain, paraesthesia and numbness, which may become functionally disabling [9]. Furthermore, this disorder negatively impacts on quality of life, increases risk of lower extremity amputation and thereby increases morbidity and mortality risk, especially for those with diabetic nephropathy [2, 8].

26.1.1.2 Clinical Presentation

Peripheral neuropathy typically manifests as a slowly progressive, symmetrical, length-dependent neuropathy of insidious onset. Given the length-dependent nature of peripheral neuropathy, there is preferential involvement of distal nerves and more severe involvement of the lower limbs than upper limbs [9]. As such, clinical examination in early stages reveals symptoms and signs confined to the lower limbs, including distal sensory loss to pinprick and vibration and reduced or absent ankle deep tendon reflexes [2, 9]. With more severe disease, sensory involvement progresses proximally and upper limb involvement may occur in a 'stocking-and-glove' distribution. In advanced cases, motor nerve involvement can develop resulting in muscle atrophy and weakness, which is again most prominent distally [9] (Fig. 26.2). Assessment of power in intrinsic foot muscles, such as extension

Table 26.1 Neurological disorders in patients with CKD

Neurological disorder	Prevalence	Clinical features	Management
Uremic neuropathy	90 % of patients with CKD	Sensory loss, weakness and wasting, maximal distally; absence of ankle jerks; lower limbs more severely affected than upper limbs	Most effective: transplantation, adequate dialysis (increase frequency or use high flux dialysis); neuropathic pain therapy Other options: vitamin supplementation; potassium restriction; erythropoietin; exercise programmes
Autonomic neuropathy	50–60 % of patients with CKD	Impotence; postural hypotension; cardiac arrhythmia; symptomatic intradialytic hypotension	Most effective: transplantation; adequate dialysis; sildenafil to treat impotence Other option: midodrine to treat intradialytic hypotension
Cognitive dysfunction	30–40 % of patients on dialysis	Impairments in memory and executive function	Most effective: renal transplantation Other option: erythropoietin
Encephalopathy	–	Sensorial clouding, apathy, irritability; confusion, disorientation, coma Motor disturbances, tremor, asterixis, myoclonus	Dialysis Seizure treatment: phenytoin, sodium valproate or carbamazepine
Carpal tunnel syndrome	5–30 % of patients with CKD	Hand paraesthesia and numbness; weak thumb abduction	Most effective: splinting; local steroid injection; surgical decompression
Myopathy	~50 % of patients with CKD	Proximal weakness of the lower limbs	Most effective: adequate dialysis; exercise programme; adequate nutrition Other options: erythropoietin; l-carnitine

Source: Adapted from Krishnan and Kiernan [1]
Abbreviation: *CKD* chronic kidney disease

Box 26.1. Relevant Guidelines

1. K/DOQI clinical practice guidelines for chronic kidney disease: evaluation, classification and stratification. Part 6. Association of level of GFR with complications in adults. Am J Kidney Dis. 2002;39:S111–69 [4]
2. Kidney Disease: Improving Global Outcomes (KDIGO) CKD Work Group. KDIGO 2012 clinical practice guideline for the evaluation and management of chronic kidney disease. Kidney Int Suppl. 2013;3:1–150. Available from: http://www.kdigo.org/clinical_practice_guidelines/CKD.php [6]

of the big toe, may provide clues to early motor involvement. While damage to large motor and sensory fibres is typical of uremic neuropathy, small fibre neuropathy may also occur. In diabetic patients, small fibre symptoms may dominate with patients experiencing severe burning and shooting pain and altered temperature and pain perception [2].

26.1.1.3 Diagnostic Investigations

Clinical diagnosis of uremic neuropathy requires careful exclusion of alternate causes of neuropathy, including glucose dysmetabolism and connective tissue disease. The presence of glucose dysmetabolism is a critical factor given the likelihood of pre-existing neuropathy and greater severity of neuropathy seen in diabetic CKD

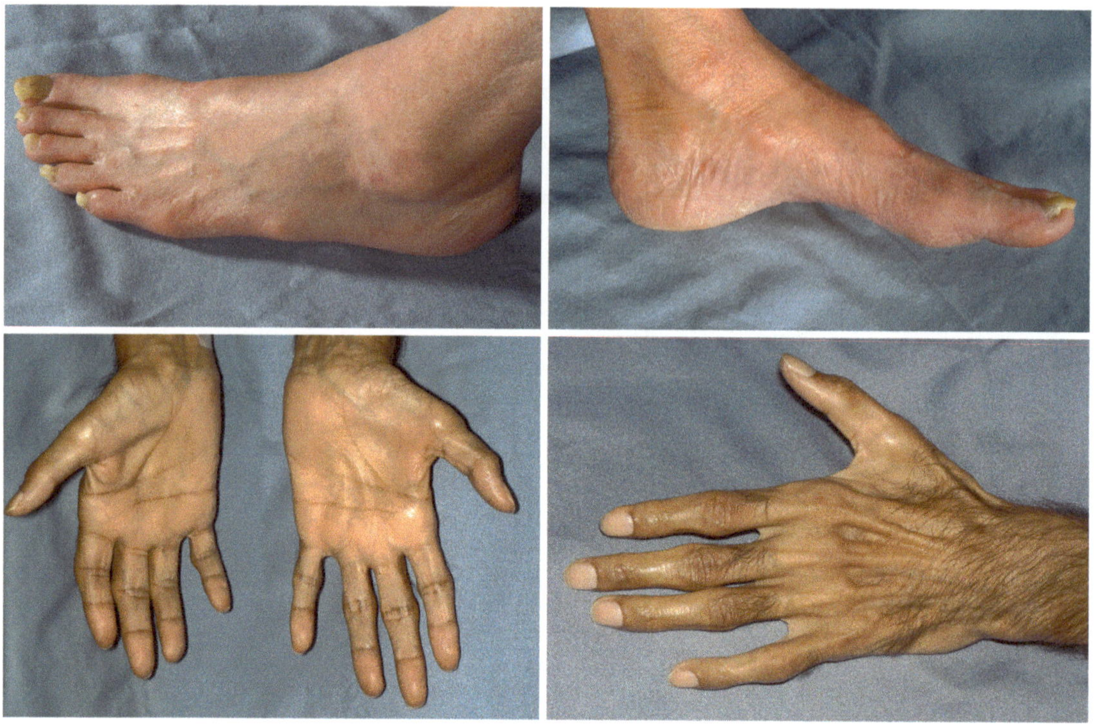

Fig. 26.2 Wasting of the intrinsic distal muscles in two patients with uremic neuropathy. In addition to weakness, the patients complained of numbness and had impaired joint position sense (Reprinted from Krishnan [9])

patients. Connective tissue disorders may be associated with a rapidly progressive neuropathy due to peripheral nerve vasculitis. Other causes of rapidly progressive neuropathy in CKD include inflammatory demyelinating neuropathies, such as chronic inflammatory demyelinating polyneuropathy, which have been described in the context of CKD due to glomerulonephritis [1]. Unlike typical length-dependent uremic neuropathy which presents with sensory features, inflammatory neuropathies are often characterised by marked motor involvement even at the onset of the disease. Demyelinating neuropathies require early recognition, as prompt treatment with immunotherapy may lead to clinical improvement [1].

Nerve conduction studies are the gold standard for the diagnosis of neuropathy. Nerve conduction studies in CKD patients with neuropathy reveal reduced sensory amplitudes and to a lesser extent motor amplitudes with relative preservation of motor and sensory conduction velocities, findings consistent with a generalised neuropathy of the axonal type [9] (Fig. 26.3). In contrast to axonal neuropathies, demyelinating neuropathies demonstrate significant reductions in nerve conduction velocities, often with relatively preserved motor and sensory amplitudes.

26.1.1.4 Management

The presence and progression of severe neuropathy may be an important indicator of the need to initiate dialysis [4]. Routine dialysis treatment may halt the progression of neuropathy but rarely results in clinical improvement. Recent studies suggest that enhanced dialysis strategies such as high flux dialysis and hemodiafiltration may result in improved outcomes. Renal transplantation is the only treatment recognised to enable clinical improvement in peripheral neuropathy. However, in advanced cases of neuropathy, clinical recovery may not occur, emphasising the need for prevention [1]. Recent studies have demonstrated that hyperkalaemia has a detrimental effect

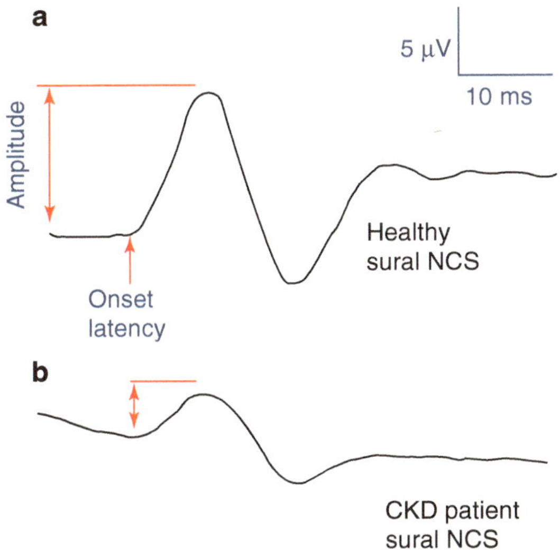

Fig. 26.3 Sensory nerve conduction results of the sural nerve, a lower limb sensory nerve, for a healthy control subject (**a**) and a chronic kidney disease patient (**b**). Results in the chronic kidney disease patient demonstrate a reduction in amplitude of the sensory nerve amplitude consistent with a sensory neuropathy

on nerve function in CKD and emphasise the importance of achieving normokalaemia in CKD patients [1, 7]. Additionally, glycemic control remains an important preventative strategy in patients with diabetic CKD. Attention to foot care is an integral part of managing neuropathy in both CKD and diabetes [8]. Reducing the risk of foot ulcers and infective complications requires assessment of predisposing factors such as ill-fitting shoes which may require the involvement of a podiatrist [8, 9]. Exercise programmes may indirectly prove beneficial to neuropathy by improving muscle strength, cardiorespiratory function and glycemic control [10].

Painful neuropathy may be managed with use of membrane-stabilising neuropathic pain treatments, including a range of tricyclic antidepressants (e.g. amitriptyline) and anticonvulsants (e.g. sodium valproate, carbamazepine, pregabalin and gabapentin) [2]. However, these medications have a constellation of potential side effects, and anticonvulsants typically require dosing restrictions for patients with CKD [2]. Tricyclic antidepressants are often used as first-line treatment for painful neuropathic symptoms due to ease of once-daily dosing which may help improve compliance [1, 2]. However, treatment with these agents may be poorly tolerated by older patients, and these agents are therefore used with caution in patients with cardiac arrhythmias, congestive heart failure, orthostatic hypotension and urinary retention [2]. Alternative treatments include anticonvulsant medications such as pregabalin or gabapentin, although both have dosing restrictions in patients according to creatinine clearance [1, 2]. Symptoms of neuropathic pain in CKD may also be reduced by vitamin supplementation with pyridoxine and methylcobalamin [1].

Demyelinating neuropathies are typically treated with intravenous immunoglobulin; however, the risk of nephrotoxicity with this treatment must be carefully considered in patients who have some degree of residual kidney function [1]. Potential alternative treatments include plasma exchange or steroid treatment.

26.1.2 Autonomic Neuropathy

26.1.2.1 Definition

Autonomic dysfunction is a highly prevalent complication of CKD with potentially life-threatening consequences such as cardiac arrhythmia, silent myocardial ischaemia and sudden cardiac death [1, 2]. Autonomic dysfunction occurs in up to 60 % of patients with stage 5 CKD [4]. Studies of diabetic CKD patients who have CKD of moderate severity have demonstrated prevalence rates of 50 %, underscoring the possibility that autonomic impairment may potentially occur prior to the initiation of renal replacement therapy [4].

26.1.2.2 Clinical Presentation

The most common symptom of autonomic neuropathy is impotence which develops in the majority of male patients [1]. Other clinical manifestations may include bladder and bowel dysfunction and evidence of altered sudomotor function manifesting as dry skin and impaired sweating. Cardiovascular autonomic dysfunction may present with orthostatic intolerance, reduced exercise tolerance, palpitations and loss of consciousness due to cardiac arrhythmia.

26.1.2.3 Diagnostic Investigations

Clinical assessment of autonomic function may be undertaken using a variety of techniques such as assessment of cardiac and pupillary reflexes, sweating and blood pressure control [9]. Assessment of cardiac autonomic neuropathy requires a battery of tests including heart rate variability, Valsalva manoeuvre and changes in heart rate with standing [2].

26.1.2.4 Management

As has been previously discussed in the case of peripheral neuropathy, renal transplantation improves autonomic function, while dialysis treatment rarely results in substantial change [1]. With the commencement of dialysis, intradialytic hypotension may become problematic for patients with autonomic neuropathy. In these cases treatment with midodrine administered 15–30 min prior to dialysis may improve symptoms. Erectile dysfunction responds to treatment with phosphodiesterase type 5 inhibitors such as sildenafil, which is well tolerated [1]. The optimal management for cardiac autonomic neuropathy remains unclear. While some evidence has suggested that angiotensin-converting enzyme inhibitors may be helpful in reducing heart rate variability, other evidence has demonstrated either no benefit or a potentially deleterious effect of these medications [2]. The use of beta blockers in CKD patients has been limited due to concerns for potentially higher rates of adverse effects, including hyperkalaemia and glycaemic abnormalities [2]. However, recent studies have shown that beta blockers may provide cardiovascular protection in patients with advanced CKD. The combined alpha-/beta-blocker carvedilol is metabolically neutral and may provide the beneficial effects of beta blockade on cardiovascular events with a better side-effect profile [2]. In patients with diabetic CKD, adequate glycemic control remains an important step in preventing the progression of both autonomic and peripheral neuropathy [2].

26.2 Carpal Tunnel Syndrome

26.2.1 Definition and Clinical Importance

Carpal tunnel syndrome (CTS) is the result of compression of the median nerve at the wrist. CTS is the most common mononeuropathy in CKD affecting up to 30 % of dialysis patients [9]. The prevalence of CTS in CKD can be attributed to various factors. The presence of fistulae has been implicated in the development of CTS, as the prevalence of CTS in limbs with fistulae is ~30 % compared to ~12 % on the contralateral side [11]. The presence of amyloidosis or poor clearance of β2microglobulin may lead to localised deposition of amyloid in soft tissues leading to compression. Patients with CTS experience sensory symptoms in the hands including paraesthesia, numbness and pain with a characteristic feature of nocturnal exacerbation [9]. Symptoms are often more severe in the dominant hand and are not always confined to median nerve territory. Symptoms may involve any part of the hand and in some cases extend to more proximal regions of the arm. Long-standing disease can result in motor involvement causing weakness and wasting of muscles innervated by the median nerve, particularly abductor pollicis brevis.

26.2.2 Diagnosis

Diagnosis of CTS is made on clinical grounds, and exclusion of other pathologies, such as cervical spondylosis or generalised neuropathy, is important. Neurological examination may demonstrate a reduction in sensation in the median nerve territory or weakness of median-innervated muscles. Phalen's test may also aid in diagnosis. This test is conducted by placing the wrist into end-of-range palmar flexion for 1 min and aims to increase intratunnel pressure and thereby reproduce symptoms [9].

26.2.3 Management

Most patients with CTS should receive a trial of conservative treatment, with splinting of the wrist or a subcutaneous corticosteroid injection at the wrist. Injection of steroids should be avoided where CTS develops in the fistula arm. In patients who are refractory to conservative treatment or those in whom there is significant loss of muscle power or severe abnormalities of median nerve conduction, referral to a hand surgeon may be appropriate for endoscopic decompression of the nerve. While clinical improvement typically occurs with surgical decompression, outcomes are less favourable if the patient had fixed motor and sensory deficits prior to surgery [7]. In cases where amyloid deposition is suspected, biopsy specimens from the flexor retinaculum should be obtained during surgery.

26.3 Myopathy

26.3.1 Definition and Clinical Importance

Myopathy in CKD affects ~50 % of stage 5 CKD patients and is characterised by proximal muscle weakness and wasting, predominantly affecting the lower limbs. In addition, reduced exercise capacity, limited endurance and motor fatigue are prominent features resulting in substantial functional limitations and morbidity. The pathophysiology of uremic myopathy remains unclear though it typically appears with glomerular filtration rates less than 25 mL/min and progression tends to parallel decline of kidney function [12]. Possible aetiologies include hyperparathyroidism, metabolic bone disease with vitamin D deficiency, impaired potassium regulation, accumulation of uremic toxins and carnitine deficiency [1]. A clear association between malnutrition, specifically protein deficiency, and uremic myopathy has been demonstrated in elderly patients [12]. Furthermore, rates of uremic myopathy are higher in patients with diabetic CKD leading to a suggested role for insulin resistance in the development of this condition.

26.3.2 Diagnosis

Diagnosis of uremic myopathy is based on the demonstration of weakness in proximal hip girdle muscles [12]. There are no specific tests for uremic myopathy and electromyography, and creatine kinase levels are typically normal. Muscle biopsy reveals nonspecific features such as type II fibre atrophy and fibre splitting, although the procedure is not undertaken routinely due to its invasive nature and should be considered only after neurological referral.

26.3.3 Management

While no specific treatment exists for uremic myopathy, management requires treatment of potential contributing factors. Adequate management of hyperparathyroidism and vitamin D deficiency must be achieved. Nutritional supplementation, anaemia correction with erythropoietin and exercise programmes have been shown to improve exercise tolerance and neuromuscular function [12].

26.4 Cognitive Dysfunction and Dementia

26.4.1 Definition and Clinical Importance

Cognitive impairment is defined as a new deficit in two or more areas of cognitive function. Mild cognitive impairment is detectable by clinical assessment but does not impact daily functioning, while dementia is characterised by cognitive impairment and behavioural disturbance that interferes with independence and daily functioning [13]. CKD is an independent risk factor for progressive cognitive impairment and dementia. Cognitive impairment is present across the spectrum of CKD with both the prevalence and rate of progression inversely associated with level of kidney function [14]. As such, approximately 70 % of stage 5 CKD patients demonstrate moderate to severe cognitive impairment, with greatest dysfunction reported in the domains of memory and executive function [1, 14].

The underlying cause of cognitive impairment has often been attributed to the various comorbidities and vascular complications that may be present in this patient cohort. There is a high prevalence of cardiovascular risk factors that lead to large and small vessel vascular disease in CKD such as hypertension, diabetes, age and smoking status [13]. A vascular aetiology for cognitive impairment is further supported by association between clinically silent cerebrovascular disease and degree of kidney impairment [1]. Additionally, patients in whom vascular nephropathy is the cause of CKD have a heightened risk of silent white matter disease. However, recent studies have shown that CKD is a risk factor of cognitive impairment independent of vascular and demographic variables [14]. Consideration should be given to secondary hyperparathyroidism and anaemia as potential risk factors for cognitive impairment in CKD. Excess parathyroid hormone levels in patients with CKD are postulated to interfere with neurotransmission in the CNS by increasing brain calcium content. Correction of anaemia has been demonstrated to improve measures of cognition. Dementia is a more powerful predictor of mortality than heart failure or stroke in stage 5 CKD patients and thus presents an important clinical complication [14]. Though moderate to severe cognitive dysfunction has been reported in ~40 % of dialysis patients, less than 3 % of the cohort had cognitive impairment documented as a comorbid condition in medical records, highlighting that the condition is under-recognised in routine clinical practice. There are no specific treatments for cognitive dysfunction in CKD aside renal transplantation [15].

26.4.2 Diagnosis

The mini-mental state examination (MMSE) is the most widely used method of assessment for cognitive impairment [13]. While a score of less than 24 on the MMSE indicates cognitive impairment, the instrument has low sensitivity for mild cognitive dysfunction [13]. Moreover, the MMSE is focused largely on the assessment of memory and attention at the expense of other cognitive domains such as executive function. Scores gained on the MMSE may also be influenced by a subject's educational and cultural background. In patients in whom MMSE is normal but where clinical suspicion for cognitive impairment is high, referral to a neuropsychology service is recommended for more intensive cognitive assessment. In all patients, cerebral imaging with computerised tomography scans (CT) or magnetic resonance imaging (MRI) is also recommended to exclude space-occupying lesions that may represent a treatable cause of cognitive impairment. Screening blood tests are also recommended to exclude other causes of cognitive impairment, including B12 deficiency and hypothyroidism.

26.4.3 Management

Recognition and documentation are crucial first steps in managing CKD patients with cognitive dysfunction or dementia. In patients with dementia, prompt initiation of conservative interventions, including patient and family education and non-pharmacological support plans, should be implemented. Pharmacological interventions are not widely recommended in CKD patients with dementia. Currently available pharmacological interventions for Alzheimer's disease (i.e. acetylcholinesterase inhibitors) have not been trialled in a CKD population [13].

26.5 Encephalopathy, Delirium and Seizures

26.5.1 Definition and Clinical Importance

Encephalopathy refers to diffuse alteration of brain function or structure, which manifests clinically as an altered level of consciousness. Aside

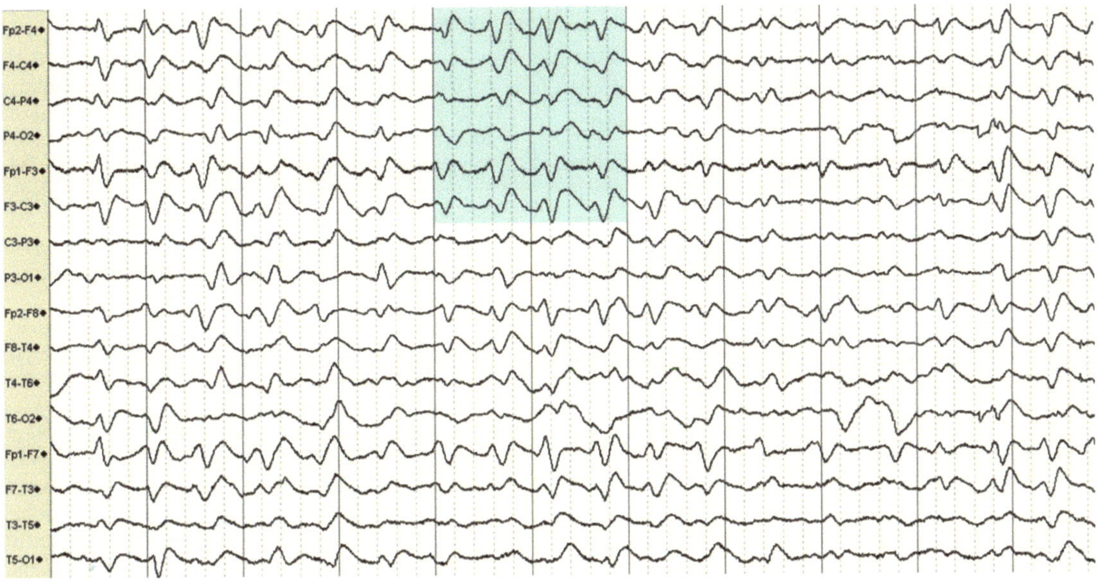

Fig. 26.4 Electroencephalograph for a chronic kidney disease patient who presented with drowsiness and confusion. Findings demonstrate a generalised slowing of the normal background with an excess of delta and theta waves, and abnormal triphasic waves (*blue highlighted section*), consistent with uremic encephalopathy

from renal impairment and the associated accumulation of toxins, other factors that have been implicated in the development of encephalopathy in CKD patients include thiamine deficiency, hypertension, fluid and electrolyte disturbances, drug toxicity, dialysis and transplant rejection [3, 16]. Features of uremic encephalopathy may have insidious onset and may present as a complex of non-specific symptoms related to altered mental functioning and/or motor disturbances, ranging from sensorial clouding to delirium and coma [3]. Early features can include fatigue, apathy, irritability and impaired concentration, while later features are more severe including confusion, disorientation, delirium, hallucinations, coma and seizures [5, 17]. Motor disturbances can accompany alterations in mental status and include tremor, fasciculations, asterixis and seizures, which may be generalised or focal [17]. Prompt recognition and diagnosis are important as encephalopathies may be reversible with treatment [17]. However, the rate of kidney failure seems to have an effect as symptoms are more pronounced and progress more rapidly in acute kidney disease [3, 5, 17].

26.5.2 Diagnosis

Laboratory blood tests should include a complete blood count, electrolyte panel, glucose, urea, creatinine, liver enzymes and ammonia [17]. Though no laboratory values or measures of kidney function correlate with symptoms of uremic encephalopathy, results may be beneficial to investigate cognitive disturbance due to changes in electrolyte or glucose levels. If the patient is febrile, a lumbar puncture may be necessary to investigate the possibility of meningitis or encephalitis [5, 17]. All patients should undergo cerebral imaging with CT or MRI to exclude a space-occupying lesion, haemorrhage or ischaemic stroke [1, 17]. Electroencephalography (EEG) should be undertaken in all patients and may demonstrate a generalised slowing of the normal background with excess delta and theta waves [5]. Triphasic sharp waves on EEG are considered a specific feature of metabolic encephalopathy (Fig. 26.4).

Management – The management of encephalopathy is focused on identification and treatment of the underlying cause. In all patients with CKD, the first step in treatment of uremic encephalopathy is to correct any underlying metabolic disturbance. Symptoms are usually alleviated by dialysis treatment in patients with severe kidney failure, though mental status changes may take 1–2 days to improve [17]. However, rapid shifts in electrolyte concentrations, particularly sodium, may exacerbate symptoms and should be avoided. Anticonvulsants should not be prescribed prophylactically but in those patients who have developed seizures, treatment with anticonvulsants is required. Preferred medications in this setting include phenytoin, sodium valproate and carbamazepine [18].

Before You Finish: Practice Pearls for the Clinician

- Uremic neuropathy manifests in almost all patients with stage 5 CKD and is likely to be present at much earlier stages in patients with diabetic CKD. Painful symptoms may respond to treatment with gabapentin, while dietary potassium restriction, glycemic control and exercise strategies may be beneficial.
- Proximal weakness and exercise intolerance caused by uremic myopathy may respond to exercise programmes, adequate nutritional intake and treatment with erythropoietin.
- For CKD patients with carpal tunnel syndrome, wrist splints or corticosteriod injections may provide benefit.
- Patients with autonomic neuropathy may respond to sildenafil for impotence.
- Cognitive dysfunction and dementia are under-recognised and can be assessed using the mini-mental state examination or formal neuropsychological testing.
- Patients who have developed seizures require treatment with anticonvulsant medications. Preferred options include phenytoin, sodium valproate and carbamazepine.

References

1. Krishnan AV, Kiernan MC. Neurological complications of chronic kidney disease. Nat Rev Neurol. 2009;5:542–51.
2. Pop-Busui R, Roberts L, Pennathur S, Kretzler M, Brosius FC, Feldman EL. The management of diabetic neuropathy in CKD. Am J Kidney Dis. 2010;55:365–85.
3. Brouns R, De Deyn PP. Neurological complications in renal failure: a review. Clin Neurol Neurosurg. 2004;107:1–16.
4. K/DOQI clinical practice guidelines for chronic kidney disease: evaluation, classification and stratification. Part 6. Association of level of GFR with complications in adults. Am J Kidney Dis. 2002;39:S111–69.
5. Burn DJ, Bates D. Neurology and the kidney. J Neurol Neurosurg Psychiatry. 1998;65:810–21.
6. Kidney Disease: Improving Global Outcomes (KDIGO) CKD Work Group. KDIGO 2012 clinical practice guideline for the evaluation and management of chronic kidney disease. Kidney Int Suppl. 2013;3:1–150. Available from: http://www.kdigo.org/clinical_practice_guidelines/CKD.php.
7. Krishnan AV, Kiernan MC. Uremic neuropathy: clinical features and new pathophysiological insights. Muscle Nerve. 2007;35:273–90.
8. Schomig M, Ritz E, Standl E, Allenberg J. The diabetic foot in the dialyzed patient. J Am Soc Nephrol. 2000;11:1153–9.
9. Krishnan AV, Pussell BA, Kiernan MC. Neuromuscular disease in the dialysis patient: an update for the nephrologist. Semin Dial. 2009;22:267–78.
10. Koufaki P, Kouidi E. Current best evidence recommendations on measurement and interpretation of physical function in patients with chronic kidney disease. Sports Med. 2010;40:1055–74.
11. Gousheh J, Iranpour A. Association between carpel tunnel syndrome and arteriovenous fistula in hemodialysis patients. Plast Reconstr Surg. 2005;116:508–13.
12. Campistol JM. Uremic myopathy. Kidney Int. 2002;62:1901–13.
13. Madero M, Gul A, Sarnak MJ. Cognitive function in chronic kidney disease. Semin Dial. 2008;21:29–37.
14. McQuillan R, Jassal SV. Neuropsychiatric complications of chronic kidney disease. Nat Rev Nephrol. 2010;6:471–9.
15. Griva K, Thompson D, Jayasena D, Davenport A, Harrison M, Newman SP. Cognitive functioning pre- to post-kidney transplantation–a prospective study. Nephrol Dial Transplant. 2006;21:3275–82.
16. Seifter JL, Samuels MA. Uremic encephalopathy and other brain disorders associated with renal failure. Semin Neurol. 2011;31:139–43.
17. Van Dijck A, Van Daele W, De Deyn PP. Uremic encephalopathy. In: Miscellanea on encephalopathies – a second look. InTech; 2012. p. 23–38.
18. Israni RK, Kasbekar N, Haynes K, Berns JS. Use of antiepileptic drugs in patients with kidney disease. Semin Dial. 2006;19:408–16.

Part V

Chronic Kidney Disease: Special Conditions

Drug Prescription in Chronic Kidney Disease

27

Jan T. Kielstein

Before You Start: Facts You Need to Know

- Less is more – the lower the pill count, the higher the adherence and the smaller the likelihood of dosing errors and interactions.
- Every drug has potential side effects; thus, the indication for every prescription has to be based on an individual benefit/risk ratio.
- Chronic pharmacotherapy has to be reassessed on a regular basis considering the current risk/benefit ratio, the persistence of indications, and current kidney (and hepatic) function.
- Physicians should educate patients and caregivers about potentially severe adverse events, like hyperkalemia in case of diarrhea under double blockade of the renin-angiotensin-aldosterone system.
- Renal replacement therapy comes in different modes (peritoneal dialysis, hemodialysis), treatment intensities, and accompanying effects (e.g., hypotension) – all have to be considered for adequate timing and drug dose.
- There is little evidence from randomized controlled trials to guide the decisions mentioned above, let alone considering age, comorbidities, and other therapies.

27.1 *Scio Nescio*[1] Paucity of Dosing Studies in CKD

The determination of kidney function is one cornerstone of dosing drugs in CKD patients. Chapter 2 summarizes details to this task. Frequently this alone is of little help as corresponding pharmacokinetic and pharmacodynamic studies of drugs that would allow converting a specific GFR in a specific dose or dosing interval are missing. Based on the linear relationship between the overall drug elimination rate constant and the GFR, individual drug elimination in patients with renal impairment can be estimated from the patient's GFR.

[1]*Scio Nescio* = I know that I know nothing (Socrates)

J.T. Kielstein, MD
Department of Nephrology and Hypertension, Hannover Medical School, Carl-Neuberg-Str. 1, Hannover 30625, Germany

Abteilung für Nieren- und Hochdruckerkrankungen, Medizinische Hochschule Hannover, Carl-Neuberg-Strasse 1, Hannover 30625, Germany
e-mail: kielstein@yahoo.com

M. Arici (ed.), *Management of Chronic Kidney Disease*,
DOI 10.1007/978-3-642-54637-2_27, © Springer-Verlag Berlin Heidelberg 2014

Dettli did this for the first time by means of a simple nomogram according to which either a dose reduction or an increase in the dosing interval has to occur [1]. This can however not be routinely done at the bedside, where dosing is frequently based on package inserts of the manufacturer. Occasionally this information in the official US Food and Drug Administration (FDA) or European Medicines Agency (EMA) product labeling which can also be found in some yearly reissued but not updated pocket books is in sharp conflict with the recommendations derived from post-marketing studies [2]. Why is there insufficient evidence to guide dosing on many commonly used drugs? For decades the industry had neither guidance nor pressure from the regulatory agencies to deal with this matter. Not until 1998 did the FDA (2004 EMA) provide frameworks to help companies decide when to conduct pharmacokinetic and pharmacodynamic studies in CKD patients (Box 27.1). Since the publication of both documents, there are now for the first time explicit recommendations for study design, data analysis, and interpretation of the study results in product labeling.

The following chapter highlights problems with frequently used drugs and gives a general advice how to approach drug dosing in CKD patients (Box 27.2). For a detailed discussion of particular drugs, the reader is referred to reference books [3]. This chapter does not address the dosing of drugs in AKI.

Box 27.1. Recommended Online Resources

1. KDIGO Drug Prescribing in Kidney Disease: Initiative for Improved Dosing. Available from: www.kdigo.org/home/conferences/drug-prescribing-in-kidney-disease-initiative-for-improved-dosing-2010/
2. US Food and Drug Administration Drug Guidances. Available from: http://www.fda.gov/%20Drugs/GuidanceComplianceRegulatoryInformation/Guidances/default.html
3. European Medicines Agency. Evaluation of medicines for human use. Available from: www.ema.europa.eu/docs/en_GB/document_library/Scientific_guideline/2009/09/WC500003123.pdf
4. Dosing – Tool for drug application and security. Department of Clinical Pharmacology and Pharmacoepidemiology, University Hospital Heidelberg. Available from: www.dosing.de

Box 27.2. What the Guidelines Say You Should Do: Drug Dosing Consideration in Patients with Acute and CKD: A Clinical Update from Kidney Disease, Improving Global Outcomes (KDIGO)

Stepwise approach to adjust drug dosage regimens for patients with CKD

Step 1 *Obtain history and relevant demographic/clinical information.* Assess demographic information, past medical history including history of renal disease, and current clinical and laboratory information, including DNA polymorphisms to ascertain drug therapy needs.

Step 2 *Estimate GFR.* Use most appropriate tool to assess eGFR or creatinine clearance for the patient based on age, body size, ethnicity, and concomitant disease states.

Step 3 *Review current medications.* Identify drugs for which individualization of the treatment regimen will be necessary.

Step 4 *Calculate individualized treatment regimen.* Determine treatment and calculate dosage regimen based on pharmacokinetic characteristics of the drug and the patient's volume status and eGFR.

Step 5 *Monitor.* Monitor parameters of drug response and toxicity; monitor drug levels if available/applicable.

Step 6 *Revise regimen.* Adjust regimen based on drug response or change in patient status (including renal function) as warranted.

27.2 Many Roads Lead to Therapeutic Success: Some Are Not Complicated by CKD

The best way to prevent dosing problems in CKD patients is to avoid potentially problematic and unnecessary drugs. Physicians are encouraged to question every pharmacological intervention in the individual patient they aim to treat, such as the use of proton pump inhibitors in virtually every patient. Common sense should prevail but frequently it is not understood that, e.g., hyperphosphatemia is not the key problem for a dialysis patient with incurable plasmacytoma and should therefore not be treated. If indeed a new drug is indicated, there are alternatives for renally excreted drugs; some of those are listed in Table 27.1. Some drugs that should not be used in patients with a GFR <60 ml/min are methotrexate, enoxaparin, lithium, and metformin. But already for the last one, metformin, the books are not closed as a meta-analysis suggests that the risk of lactic acidosis is lower than previously assumed [5]. Some authors suggest that metformin therapy down to a GFR of 27 ml/min can be considered illustrating the fact that views on indications and contraindications for drugs can change over time. A frequently used drug in which dose reduction is of importance is allopurinol, whose metabolite, oxipurinol, accumulates with decreasing GFR and can lead to detrimental adverse events [6], a fact that is being ignored by high-profile trials. But also for this drug which can delay progression of CKD and lower proteinuria, there is an alternative with the same positive effect on GFR and proteinuria [7] for which no dose reduction is necessary down

Table 27.1 Drugs in which dose adaption to kidney function is required and alternatives that do not require dose adjustment

Group	Dependent on GFR	Independent from GFR
Analgesics	Morphine (M6-glucuronide), pethidine (norpethidine)	Fentanyl, levomethadone
Antiarrhythmics	Sotalol	Amiodarone
Antibiotics	Ciprofloxacin, levofloxacin	Moxifloxacin
Oral antidiabetics	Glibenclamide, glimepiride (hydroxymetabolite)	Gliquidone, gliclazide
	Nateglinide	Pioglitazone
	Sitagliptin	
Antiepileptic drugs	Gabapentin, pregabalin, lamotrigine, levetiracetam	Carbamazepine, phenytoin, valproate
ß-blockers	Atenolol	Bisoprolol, carvedilol, metoprolol, propranolol
Cholesterol-lowering drugs	Bezafibrate, fenofibrate	Simvastatin, niacin
Uric acid-lowering drugs	Allopurinol (metabolite oxipurinol)	Colchicine, hydroxychloroquine, leflunomide, febuxostat
Antirheumatic medication	Methotrexate	
Heart failure drugs	Digoxin	Digitoxin
Psychiatric drugs	Lithium, mirtazapine	Amitriptyline, citalopram (metabolite), haloperidol, risperidone
Cytostatic agents	Actinomycin D, bleomycin, capecitabine, carboplatin, cisplatin, cyclophosphamide, doxorubicin, epirubicin, etoposide, gemcitabine (dFdU), ifosfamide, irinotecan, melphalan, methotrexate, oxaliplatin, topotecan	Anastrozole, docetaxel, doxorubicin-peg-liposomal, erlotinib, fluorouracil, gefitinib, leuprorelin, megestrol, paclitaxel, tamoxifene, terozol, vincristine, trastuzumab

Source: Adapted from Kielstein and Keller [4], with kind permission of Springer Science+Business Media

Table 27.2 Antidiabetics in CKD

	GFR < 60 ml/min	GFR < 30 ml/min	GFR < 15 ml/min
Metformin	N	N	N
Sulfonylurea	Dose reduction	N	N
Gliquidone	Y	Y	Y
Repaglinide	Y	Y	Dose reduction
Nateglinide	Y	Y	Dose reduction
Acarbose	Y	N	N
Pioglitazone	Y	Y	N
Vildagliptin	Y	Y	↑ Dosing interval
Saxagliptin	Y	Y	N
Exenatide	Dose reduction	N	N
Liraglutide	Y	Y	Y
Insulin	Y	Dose reduction	Dose reduction

Y – Yes – can be used without dose reduction
N – Do not use

Table 27.3 Anticoagulants in CKD

	GFR < 60 ml/min	GFR < 30 ml/min	GFR < 15 ml/min
Phenprocoumon and warfarin	Y	Y	Y
Unfractionated heparin	Y	Y	Y
Low molecular weight heparins (LMWH)	Dose reduction	Scarce data	Scarce data
Enoxaparin	N	N	N
Dabigatran (*)	Dose reduction	N	N
Rivaroxaban	Y	Dose reduction	N
Apixaban	Y	Y	Dose reduction

(*) can be removed by hemodialysis
Y – Yes – can be used without dose reduction
N – Do not use

to a GFR of 30 ml/min. Tables 27.2 and 27.3 give an overview about the dose adjustment and contraindications of antidiabetics and anticoagulants.

27.3 Start Low Go Slow

For many diseases we treat, there are readily available biological effects like blood sugar, blood pressure, or heart rate that can help to guide dosing. For drugs that have an effect on the central nervous system, we should follow the "start low – go slow" rule of Jerry Gurwitz [8]. This is especially important for opioids and antihistamines which are associated with a substantially higher risk for cognitive impairment in CKD patients [9].

27.4 Hit Hard and Early in Infections and Tumor Therapy

Some clinical conditions, however, merit adherence to Paul Ehrlich's advice to "frapper vite et frapper forte" or "hit hard and early" (Box 27.3). This is the appropriate rule to follow every time the target effect needs to be obtained as soon as possible, as for bacterial or fungal infections, hyperkalemia or hypercalcemia, and anticancer therapy.

Given the high rate of malignancies in which according to the USRDS approaches 20 % in patients with a GFR <30 ml/min, cytostatic drugs and their dosing become increasingly important. There are many cytostatic drugs that are not dependent on kidney function. Cytostatic agents that are

Box 27.3. Antibiotics in CKD

- Prompt initiation of therapy!
- The first dose has to be a full dose! (i.e., the dose you would give a patient without CKD).
- No "one size fits all" strategy! Adjust the dose to the body size of the patients (like the pediatricians do).
- If the patient is not on dialysis or has substantial residual diuresis, check whether there is a less nephrotoxic alternative – even the most expensive antibiotic is cheaper than chronic dialysis.
- No fixed treatment durations (with exception of endocarditis). Duration of therapy should be guided by clinical success and laboratory parameters (procalcitonin).

mainly renally excreted have to be reduced by 40–80 % [10]. For dialysis patients the effect of dialysis has to be taken into account additionally. Gemcitabine and cyclophosphamide do not have to be reduced if a hemodialysis session is performed 1–12 h after the administration of the drug. In case of carboplatin and cisplatin, a hemodialysis session has to be started 60–120 min after the infusion to be effective. Etoposide and epirubicin cannot be removed by dialysis. In contrast to other reports [11], gemcitabine should be considered to be dependent on kidney function as the active metabolite dFdU is renally excreted (Table 27.1). Due to the small therapeutic range, cytostatic agents, dose, timing of administration, and the use of hemodialysis should be tailored to the individual need of the patient by a team of oncologists, nephrologists, and pharmacists (see also Chap. 31).

Infection-related hospitalizations contribute substantially to excess morbidity and mortality in patients with CKD5D, and infection is the second leading cause of death in this population. But also patients with mild and moderate CKD seem to be at higher risk for infection compared to a matched population without CKD. Dosing of anti-infective drugs should be based on the concentration-time relationship and the pharmacodynamics. For meropenem, a carbapenem, maximum killing of bacteria is obtained by optimizing the time of exposure of the drug to the bacteria so that the concentrations remain above the MIC as long as possible. In this case the reduction of dose and not the prolongation of the dosing interval are necessary. In contrast, for antibiotics which kill bacteria by a high peak concentration such as aminoglycosides and quinolones, an increase of the dosing interval and not the decrease of dose is necessary [12]. Aside from these general considerations, a recent study illustrated that interactions of drugs can create problems that do not occur by the use of the single substance. A small, but significant, increased risk of acute kidney injury occurred among men with the use of oral fluoroquinolones, as well as a significant interaction between the concomitant use of fluoroquinolones and renin-angiotensin-system blockers [13].

27.5 The Importance and Peculiarities of ACE Inhibitors and ARBs in CKD

ACE inhibitors and ARBs present the mainstay of therapy in CKD patients with hypertension and heart failure as they exhibit several other effects above and beyond renoprotection, such as inhibition of fibrosis and enhancement of vascular and cardiac remodeling. Although ACE inhibitors are mainly renally excreted, this should not be regarded as a major obstacle in finding the appropriate dose as the biological effect, i.e., blood pressure or proteinuria will guide dosing. The same holds true for ARBs which are mostly excreted by the liver. The current KDIGO guidelines recommend that an ARB or ACE inhibitor be used in diabetic and nondiabetic adults with CKD stage I–IV and urine albumin excretion >300 mg/day in whom treatment with blood pressure-lowering drugs is indicated [14]. Even in patients with proteinuria <300 mg/day, both ACE inhibitor and ARB are the drugs of choice. The important peculiarities of both drug classes are summarized in Box 27.4. Even at a GFR of 26 ml/min, a randomized controlled trial found that start of an ACE inhibitor can retard loss in GFR and reduce proteinuria [15]. At a lower baseline

Box 27.4. ACE Inhibitors/ARBs

- Cause vasodilatation of the efferent > afferent glomerular arterioles → ⇓ intra-glomerular pressure/reduction of GFR and urine albumin excretion.
- Initiation of therapy causes a drop in GFR of up to 30 % which is regarded as reasonably attributable to this physiological mechanism.
- Current evidence does not support the discontinuing ACE inhibitors and ARBs in patients with advanced CKD in an effort to preserve residual kidney function.
- Clinically significant hyperkalemia and hypotension are both reasons for dose reduction/discontinuation of ACE inhibitors and ARBs.
- In case of clinically relevant hyperkalemia, give dietary advice, reduce the dose, or add a loop diuretic.

GFR of 16 ml/min, a small observational trial suggested that the start of renal replacement therapy can be delayed by discontinuation of ACE inhibitor/ARB. Of utter importance is the potential development of hyperkalemia [16]. To avoid this deadly risk, spironolactone should be prescribed in patients with a GFR <30 ml/min at dose of no more than 25 mg/day. Moreover *patients should be advised to stop medication with all drugs inhibiting the renin-angiotensin-aldosterone system in case of dehydration (vomiting, diarrhea)*. In hemodialysis patients, especially those with heart failure, the current literature suggests that spironolactone or eplerenone may be safely used [17].

27.6 Potential Side Effects of Drugs Mainly Used in CKD Patients

Commonly used drugs in CKD patients are only poorly investigated in their potential to affect other drugs concomitantly used. A few examples might help to visualize the problem. A single dose of sevelamer reduces the C_{max} and the AUC of mycophenolate mofetil (MMF). Proton pump inhibitors (PPI) are used in about 80 % of nursing home patients, in 2/3 without the presence of an established indication [18]. A significant interaction exists between PPI and MMF secondary to reduced dissolution of mycophenolate mofetil in higher pH environments. This is important not only for renal transplant recipients but for all patients depending on the immunosuppressive potency of this drug. The total AUC of MMF showed a 37 % reduction in patients using PPI as compared to those treated with no PPI. Long-term PPI therapy, particularly at high doses, is associated with an increased risk of hip fracture.

27.7 Avoid "Nephrex Extra Strength": Combination of Nephrotoxic Drugs

Very often a combination of drugs and interventions, each prescribed for a good reason may have detrimental effects under certain clinical conditions. Reduced intravascular volume in combination with NSAIDs, COX-2 inhibitors make it very likely that the application of contrast media will lead to acute kidney injury.

27.8 Special Indications That Justify Exceptions from the Rule

One clinical important exception is to increase the dose of a drug above the maximum recommended dose as in the nonspecific reduction of proteinuria in nephrotic patients. Two prospective randomized trials indicated an additive antiproteinuric effect of ultrahigh dose of the angiotensin receptor blocker candesartan compared with standard dose. Serum potassium levels should be monitored during such a treatment.

27.9 The Patient on Chronic Hemodialysis

As soon as the patient undergoes "dialysis treatment," the dosing of renally eliminated drugs becomes even more complex (Box 27.5). The main reason is that "dialysis" comes in different modalities (hemodialysis, peritoneal dialysis) and intensities (thrice weekly, daily short dialysis or nocturnal dialysis). Another variable is the type of membrane used. This can be illustrated by the fact that modern polysulfone membranes eliminate about 50 % of the administered vancomycin while old cuprophane membrane only eliminate less than 10 %. This dosing error would be obvious if therapeutic drug monitoring would be conducted on a regular basis, but some institutions avoid the expense on this important laboratory workup.

27.10 Therapeutic Drug Monitoring (TDM)

Therapeutic drug monitoring is important to guide the dosing of drugs with a narrow therapeutic range. Unfortunately this is frequently limited to vancomycin and aminoglycosides as well as calcineurin inhibitors. TDM will however be integral part in the treatment of patients under circumstances where a readily available biological readout (e.g., blood pressure or blood glucose) is not available. Several tertiary care centers started to provide routine measurement of quinolones, carbapenems, and other antibiotics. This is important as the effect of extracorporeal therapy is difficult to standardize.

Box 27.5. Dosing of Drugs in CKD5D (i.e., Patients on Dialysis)

- Not all dialysis are created equal! They vary in mode (peritoneal dialysis, hemodialysis), intensity (blood and dialysate flow, filter type, treatment time, exchange volume, transporter type of the peritoneal membrane).
- If there is a measurable effect of the drug (like blood pressure), tailor the dose to the effect.
- If patients are prone to hypotension toward the end of hemodialysis, reduce/pause blood pressure medication before dialysis.
- Use inpatient dialysis sessions for the administration of important drugs like EPO, iron, and vitamin D.

27.11 Tempora mutantur et nos mutamur in illis?[2]

While dosing errors in drugs that had been licensed a decade or more ago are rather infrequent, new drugs are associated with a high frequency of dosing errors. Among those are newer antiepileptic drugs (Table 27.1) like gabapentin, pregabalin, lamotrigine, and levetiracetam where 50 % or less of the normal dose are sufficient [19]. The same holds true for new oral antidiabetics (Table 27.2) and anticoagulants (Table 27.3). So curb your enthusiasm even if high-profile trials in patients without CKD report incredible results – these can rarely be duplicated in the CKD population.

Before You Finish: Practice Pearls for the Clinician

- First question: Does the patient really need the drug you are about to prescribe?
- Individualize drug choices and therapy targets according to life expectancy, age, comorbidities, risk of progression of CKD, and presence and tolerance of treatment/possible side effects.
- The CKD patient should only have one prescriber! Multiple prescribers put patients at risk for interactions and side effects, increase pill count, and decrease adherence.

[2]The times are changed and we too are changed in them.

References

1. Dettli L. Drug dosage in renal disease. Clin Pharmacokinet. 1976;1(2):126–34.
2. Matzke GR, Aronoff GR, Atkinson Jr AJ, Bennett WM, Decker BS, Eckardt KU, et al. Drug dosing consideration in patients with acute and chronic kidney disease-a clinical update from Kidney Disease: Improving Global Outcomes (KDIGO). Kidney Int. 2011;80(11):1122–37.
3. Seyffart G. Seyffart's directory of drug dosage in kidney disease. 1st ed. Oberhaching: Dustri-Verlag Dr. Karl Feistle GmbH & Co. KG; 2011.
4. Kielstein JT, Keller F. Pharmacotherapy in patients suffering from chronic kidney disease. Internist (Berl). 2012;53(7):802–9.
5. Salpeter SR, Greyber E, Pasternak GA, Salpeter Posthumous EE. Risk of fatal and nonfatal lactic acidosis with metformin use in type 2 diabetes mellitus. Cochrane Database Syst Rev. 2010;(1):CD002967.
6. Hande KR, Noone RM, Stone WJ. Severe allopurinol toxicity. Description and guidelines for prevention in patients with renal insufficiency. Am J Med. 1984;76(1):47–56.
7. Whelton A, MacDonald PA, Chefo S, Gunawardhana L. Preservation of renal function during gout treatment with febuxostat: a quantitative study. Postgrad Med. 2013;125(1):106–14.
8. Gurwitz JH. Start low and go slow: dosing of antipsychotic medications in elderly patients with dementia. Arch Intern Med. 1995;155(18):2017–8.
9. Kurella TM, Larive B, Unruh ML, Stokes JB, Nissenson A, Mehta RL, et al. Prevalence and correlates of cognitive impairment in hemodialysis patients: the Frequent Hemodialysis Network trials. Clin J Am Soc Nephrol. 2010;5(8):1429–38.
10. Boesler B, Czock D, Keller F, Griesshammer M, Seufferlein T, Karges W, et al. Clinical course of haemodialysis patients with malignancies and dose-adjusted chemotherapy. Nephrol Dial Transplant. 2005;20(6):1187–91.
11. Li YF, Fu S, Hu W, Liu JH, Finkel KW, Gershenson DM, et al. Systemic anticancer therapy in gynecological cancer patients with renal dysfunction. Int J Gynecol Cancer. 2007;17(4):739–63.
12. Eyler RF, Mueller BA. Antibiotic pharmacokinetic and pharmacodynamic considerations in patients with kidney disease. Adv Chronic Kidney Dis. 2010; 17(5):392–403.
13. Bird ST, Etminan M, Brophy JM, Hartzema AG, Delaney JA. Risk of acute kidney injury associated with the use of fluoroquinolones. CMAJ. 2013; 185(10):E475–82.
14. Kidney Disease: Improving Global Outcomes (KDIGO) Blood Pressure Work Group. KDIGO clinical practice guideline for the management of blood pressure in chronic kidney disease. Kidney Int Suppl. 2012;20(2):337–414.
15. Hou FF, Zhang X, Zhang GH, Xie D, Chen PY, Zhang WR, et al. Efficacy and safety of benazepril for advanced chronic renal insufficiency. N Engl J Med. 2006;354(2):131–40.
16. Juurlink DN, Mamdani MM, Lee DS, Kopp A, Austin PC, Laupacis A, et al. Rates of hyperkalemia after publication of the Randomized Aldactone Evaluation Study. N Engl J Med. 2004;351(6): 543–51.
17. Baker WL, White WB. Safety of mineralocorticoid receptor antagonists in patients receiving hemodialysis. Ann Pharmacother. 2012;46(6):889–94.
18. Patterson BD, Flores HC, Krueger J, Garretson S, Gorbien MJ, Iacch A, et al. Use of proton pump inhibitors with lack of diagnostic indications in 22 Midwestern US skilled nursing facilities. J Am Med Dir Assoc. 2013;14(6):429–32.
19. Israni RK, Kasbekar N, Haynes K, Berns JS. Use of antiepileptic drugs in patients with kidney disease. Semin Dial. 2006;19(5):408–16.

Pregnancy and Chronic Kidney Disease

28

Sarah Winfield and John M. Davison

Before You Start: Facts You Need to Know

- CKD stages 1 and 2 affect up to 3 % of women of childbearing age and CKD stages 3–5 affect about 1 in 150 women.
- Over 95 % of the women with CKD becoming pregnant will be CKD stages 1 and 2.
- CKD stages 3–5 complicate about 1 in 750 pregnancies.
- Fertility declines with CKD progression over time.
- All women with CKD are at increased risk of pregnancy complications and adverse maternal and fetal outcomes which are related to the severity of prepregnancy kidney dysfunction, increasing further with hypertension and proteinuria and in systemic diseases, such as diabetes and SLE.
- Risk of accelerated decline and irreversible loss of kidney function during pregnancy or immediately afterwards is higher with more severe degrees of kidney dysfunction and with poorly controlled hypertension.
- Progressive hypertension with proteinuria and/or renal deterioration in late pregnancy may be difficult to distinguish from preeclampsia.
- The historically dismal maternal and fetal outcomes are improving with advances in obstetric, nephrological and neonatal care.

The provision of care for women with chronic kidney disease (CKD) contemplating pregnancy or already pregnant must involve clinicians working in a multidisciplinary team (MDT) in a tertiary centre [1, 2]. They must have an up-to-date knowledge of the changes in kidney that occur in normal pregnancy and the potential adverse effects of kidney impairment, an awareness of risks and complications with CKD, experience of modern antenatal and fetal surveillance and an ability to handle delivery care and afterwards. This chapter is based on some of the older literature, the limited evidence-based guidelines that are available, recently reported case series and personal experience [2–10]. The care of women on dialysis or with a kidney transplant will not be dealt with in this chapter.

S. Winfield, BSc, MBBS, MRCOG
Department of Obstetrics and Gynaecology, Leeds Teaching Hospitals NHS Trust, Leeds General Infirmary, Great George Street, Leeds, West Yorkshire LS1 3EX, UK
e-mail: sarah.winfield@leedsth.nhs.uk

J.M. Davison, MSc, MD, FRCPE, FRCOG (✉)
Institute of Cellular Medicine, Royal Victoria Infirmary and Newcastle University, 3rd Floor Leech Building, Medical School, Framlington Place, Newcastle upon Tyne, Tyne & Wear NE2 4HH, UK
e-mail: j.m.davison@ncl.ac.uk

M. Arici (ed.), *Management of Chronic Kidney Disease*,
DOI 10.1007/978-3-642-54637-2_28, © Springer-Verlag Berlin Heidelberg 2014

28.1 Prepregnancy Assessment

The basic components should be establishment of baseline parameters, analysis of risks as well as provision of health education and advice, plus any interventions that might be considered helpful, all 'cemented together' by that much used word 'counselling' (Boxes 28.1 and 28.2). Often a woman (and her partner) may bypass some important questions such as 'should I get pregnant?' and move straight into 'will my pregnancy be alright?' and 'will I have a live, healthy baby?' and possibly 'will I be alright after my pregnancy?' So the MDT must somehow ensure that all the relevant information is passed on, based on fact, not anecdote, covering the 'unasked questions' as well. Even if some of the answers are not favourable, many women will choose to go ahead for a pregnancy (or with the pregnancy) in an effort to re-establish a normal life in the face of chronic illness [7–10]. In some cases, this may cause a breakdown in communication with the MDT, and indeed, some women may not seek advice until already pregnant. This may lead to ethical dilemmas regarding clinicians' duties of care towards women who ignore advice. Attempts are being made to differentiate 'healthy' and 'pathological' levels of assumed risk and to understand the psychology of women who pursue parenthood despite substantial risk to their own health and that of their unborn child.

Thus, in the ideal world, a planned pregnancy is one that is desired before conception, occurs when contraception is discontinued in order to get pregnant and where the woman does try to achieve optimal health beforehand.

Box 28.1. Organisation of Care in CKD

- Before pregnancy, all women of child-bearing age with CKD should be made aware of its implications for their reproductive health and careers.
- Women need input on contraception, modification of remedial risk factors and optimisation of and/or alterations to medication for their CKD and any associated comorbidities (such as hypertension, diabetes or SLE) in addition to explanations about the risks and rates of pregnancy complications, adverse maternal and fetal outcomes and possible impacts on long-term renal prognosis.
- The MDT must work in partnership with these women to tailor personalised prepregnancy, antenatal, delivery and postnatal care, in a centre with all the necessary facilities for dealing with high-risk patients and their babies.
- This 'active preparation for pregnancy' should involve the woman's partner.
- Some women may not seek advice until already pregnant.
- Undiagnosed CKD may be suspected/diagnosed for the first time during pregnancy when a complication or an adverse event occurs.

Box 28.2. Prepregnancy CKD Assessment Criteria

- Cause of CKD (±systemic disease such as SLE or diabetes).
- Stage of CKD (eGFR).
- Presence or absence of significant proteinuria (≥300 mg/24 h).
- Normotension or 'well-controlled hypertension' with diastolic BP ≤80 mmHg.
- Past obstetric history.
- Genetic counselling may be required for familial CKD.
- Assessment of diet, BMI, nicotine and alcohol intake.
- Some advise counselling for CKD 1 and 2 only if there are adverse risk factors.

28.2 Normal Pregnancy

The renal tract undergoes marked anatomical, haemodynamic, tubular and endocrine changes as part of the systemic upheaval of maternal adaptation to pregnancy. The kidneys enlarge because both vascular volume and interstitial space increase but there is no accelerated renal growth nor morphological alterations akin to compensatory renal hypertrophy. The calyces, renal pelves and ureters dilate markedly, invariably more prominent on the right side, seen in 90 % of women, mimicking outflow obstruction. The relevant functional changes are listed in Box 28.3.

28.3 CKD and the Prospects for Pregnancy

A woman may lose up to 50 % of her kidney function and still maintain S_{cr} below 125 μmol/L (1.4 mg/dL), because of hyperfiltration by the remaining nephrons; however, if kidney function is more severely compromised, then further small decreases in GFR will cause S_{cr} to increase markedly. In women with CKD, whilst the pathology may be both biochemically and clinically silent, the internal milieu may already be disrupted. Most individuals remain symptom-free until GFR declines to less than 25 % of normal, and many serum constituents are frequently normal until a late stage of disease. However, degrees of functional impairment that do not appear to disrupt homeostasis in nonpregnant individuals can jeopardise pregnancy (Box 28.4).

The traditional approach [7], with CKD defined as *mild*, *moderate* and *severe*, based on S_{cr} has been replaced by a system based on the current CKD classification that is part of the US National Kidney Foundation (NKF) K/DOQI clinical practice guidelines, endorsed by the UK National Service Framework for Renal Services, and now widely adopted. Estimated GFR (eGFR) is estimated from the Modification of Diet in Renal Disease (MDRD) formula and its refinement CKD-EPI formula. Prepregnancy eGFR has a better sensitivity in detecting

Box 28.3. Normal Pregnancy and Renal Physiology

- Normal cardiovascular function and healthy renal system, with optimal adaptation to increasing demands of pregnancy, are prerequisites for successful obstetric outcome.
- Glomerular filtration rate (GFR) increases to 50 % above prepregnancy values, primarily due to increased renal blood flow (RBF) rather than a rise in intraglomerular pressure, so there is unlikely to be hyperfiltration sclerosis.
- Serum creatinine (S_{cr}) in the 1st, 2nd and 3rd trimesters averages 60, 54 and 64 μmol/L (0.66, 0.59 and 0.70 mg/dL), respectively, with measured creatinine clearances (C_{cr}) of 151, 154 and 129 mL/min, respectively, with return to S_{cr} baseline (70 μmol/L/0.75 mg/dL) by 3 months postpartum. As well as gestational age-specific values, some units now use ethnicity-specific normal ranges as, for example, nonpregnant Afro-Caribbean women have higher S_{cr} levels than Caucasians.
- Serum urea (S_{urea}) averages 3 mmol/L (7 mg/dL) throughout pregnancy, a fall from the nonpregnant value of 5 mmol/L (12 mg/dL).
- Values of S_{cr} of 80 μmol/L (0.9 mg/dL) and S_{urea} of 6 mmol/L (14 mg/dL), which are acceptable in the nonpregnant state, are definitely suspect in pregnancy.
- 24-h urinary total protein excretion (TPE) increases throughout the trimesters in normal pregnancy and up to 300 mg per 24 h can be regarded as normal.
- Serum albumin (S_{alb}) decreases progressively from mean of 38 g/L at 12 weeks gestation to 32 g/L by 36 weeks. Corresponding cholesterol levels are 4.5 mmol/L and 6.6 mmol/L, respectively. Occasionally, S_{alb} may decrease by up to 10 g/L and with bigger increments than usual in serum cholesterol, plus oedema, usually in late pregnancy; nephrotic syndrome may be simulated.

Source: Data from Refs. [2, 7, 10–14]

Box 28.4. CKD and Physiological Adaptation to Pregnancy

- Women with CKD have impaired ability to make physiological adaptations during pregnancy.
- Pregnancy GFR increments may be blunted, even absent, especially in CKD stages 3–5, with the likelihood of further GFR decline as pregnancy progresses.
- Failure of S_{cr} to decrease in the first trimester is suggestive of future complications.
- CKD may be associated with inability to boost renal hormones, leading to normochromic normocytic anaemia, reduced plasma volume expansion and vitamin D deficiency.
- In CKD, so-called significant proteinuria (TPE > 300 mg per 24 h) may correlate with a protein concentration of 30 mg/dL in a 'spot' urine sample, but given the problems with dipstick testing, a 24-h or some timed quantification may be preferred and/or use of 'spot' protein/creatinine ratio, with 30 mg/μmol (0.3 mg/mg) or more being significant.
- Increased TPE up to 3 g/24 h can occur in CKD patients; an exaggeration of the physiological increase in healthy women and even the cessation of renoprotection from antiproteinuric drugs alone rarely indicate functional deterioration.
- Early in pregnancy BP can decrease and in CKD may mask mild hypertension that has been present but undiagnosed before pregnancy.

Source: Data from Refs. [2, 7, 9–11, 13–15]

subclinical renal dysfunction and its influence on pregnancy outcome (if not CKD progression) as compared to S_{cr} alone [5, 9, 10]. The literature is still primarily retrospective. No attempt has yet been made to revisit the older literature on *mild*, *moderate* and *severe* dysfunction and to assess whether or not conversion of those data to CKD staging is even possible from a practical point of view; however, S_{cr} values <125, >125 and >180 μmol/L (<1.4, >1.4 and >2.0 mg/dL) – *mild*, *moderate* and *severe* impairment – respectively, correspond approximately to CKD stages 1, 2 and 3A, 3B, and 4 and 5, respectively. In the longer term, confirmation of outcomes and prognoses and even development of guidelines require adequate prospective trials [6, 7].

28.4 Pregnancy in Women with CKD

Assessment of the CKD patient presents two basic and often conflicting issues: fetal prognosis (the effect of CKD on pregnancy) and the maternal prognosis, both during pregnancy and in the long term [11, 15]. Across the spectrum of CKD, there is a stepwise increase in the likelihood of complications and adverse outcomes such as hypertension, preeclampsia, deteriorating maternal renal function (often persistent), proteinuria, anaemia, urinary infections, fetal growth restriction and fetal loss. Aside from these obvious unfavourable outcomes, there are increases in 'surrogate' outcomes too (compared to normal pregnancy) including preterm delivery, caesarean section and the need for neonatal intensive care unit access, clearly evident between CKD stages 1 and 2, underlining the importance of even minor decreases in kidney function [6, 10, 16] (Box 28.5 and Table 28.1).

CKD Stages 1 and 2 Normotensive women with intact or only mildly decreased but stable kidney function generally do very well, with more than 97 % live births, about 75 % of which are appropriate for gestational age. There is an increased incidence of superimposed preeclampsia or late-pregnancy hypertension as well as increased proteinuria exceeding the nephrotic range (3 g per 24 h) in 50 % of women in the second half of pregnancy. Pregnancy does not appear to adversely affect the course of the CKD [6, 7].

There are exceptions as certain types of CKD appear more sensitive to pregnancy, including lupus nephropathy [15, 20] and perhaps membranoproliferative glomerulonephritis. In addition, women with scleroderma and periarteritis nodosa do poorly (especially when there is marked kidney involvement and associated hypertension) and thus should be counselled to avoid pregnancy. Furthermore, there is some disagreement about whether pregnancy adversely influences the natural history of IgA nephropathy, focal segmental glomerulosclerosis and reflux nephropathy [7]. It seems likely that prognosis with these renal lesions is actually similar to that of women with mild impairment in general, provided prepregnancy function is preserved and high blood pressure absent.

Box 28.5. Influences on Maternal and Fetal Outcomes in CKD

- Level of prepregnancy kidney impairment: CKD stage (eGFR).
- Satisfactory prepregnancy BP: spontaneous or therapeutically achieved normotension and its optimal control throughout pregnancy. Relative risk of fetal death is 10 times higher when prepregnancy mean arterial pressure (MAP) ≥105 mmHg, compared with normotension. Absence of hypertension, almost regardless of kidney impairment, predicts best outcomes.
- Degree of proteinuria.
- Cause of CKD and the presence of a systemic disease/comorbidities.
- In addition, CKD itself has independent and significant effects on fetal outcome.
- Adverse past obstetric history.

Source: Data from Refs. [3, 7, 8, 11, 14, 15]

CKD Stages 3 and 4 Prognoses are poor but live births still approach 90 %. Preeclampsia, fetal growth restriction and/or preterm delivery occur in well over 50 %. Many women experience renal functional loss more rapidly than would be expected from the natural course of their CKD, and poorly controlled hypertension is a harbinger of poor outcome. Best overall outcomes occur when prepregnancy eGFR is 40–60 mL/min and TPE ≤1 g/24 h. Poor outcomes are associated with eGFR <40 mL/min and TPE > 1 g/24 h, this combination resulting in worse outcomes than either feature alone [4].

CKD Stage 5 (But Not on Dialysis) Although there is a paucity of data for analysis, it is obvious that the outlook is markedly curtailed. Preeclampsia/hypertension is common by term

Table 28.1 Prepregnancy CKD stage and estimates of obstetric complications/outcomes and renal prognosis

							Loss of >25 % RF		
CKD stage	Prepregnancy eGFR	S_{cr} (μmol/L)	FGR	Preterm delivery	PE	Perinatal death	During pregnancy	6 months PP	ESRF 1–2 year PP
Normal 1	≥90	<110	14	28	13	2	2	0	0
Mild 2	60–89 (<90)		30	35	40				
Mod 3	30–59 (<60)	>110	40	65	55	5	35	15	2
Severe 4	15–29 (<30)	>180	65	90	60	8	65	50	30
Estab RF 5	<15 (but not on dialysis)	>250	>80	95	>70	15	90	60	45

Estimates are based on Refs. [4–10, 13, 14, 17–19] and from 62 women/93 pregnancies which attained at least 24 weeks gestation (Davison, unpublished data from 1993–2006)

Aim is to provide 'at a glance' information to facilitate counselling and management, whilst not belittling much more detailed coverage and analyses (with their own inherent weaknesses too) in those publications utilised

All estimates expressed as a percentage

FGR fetal growth restriction, S_{cr} serum creatinine, *PE* preeclampsia, *RF* renal function, *PP* postpartum, *ESRF* end-stage renal failure, *eGFR* estimated glomerular filtration rate (mL/min/1.73 m^2)

(>70 %) as is significant proteinuria (60 %), as well as deterioration in kidney function, which is at times, rapid, substantial and irreversible. Although infant survival rates are good (>80 %), rates of preterm delivery (95 %) and fetal growth restriction (FGR) (>80 %) underscore the very high potential for obstetric complications in these women. Many of these women are amenorrhoeic and subfertile but keep trying for a pregnancy since kidney function will keep on declining with time and dialysis is not necessarily 'going to help' and a kidney transplant may involve a many year wait. Furthermore, some women may even seek assisted conception in the face of their infertility.

28.5 Antenatal Strategy and Decision-Making

These patients must be seen as early as possible [1, 2, 21]. Thereafter assessments should be at 2–4 week intervals until 32 weeks' gestation and then every 1–2 weeks, depending on the clinical circumstances. In most cases, the basic principle is to manage the associated clinical features rather than the type of CKD.

1. Assessment of kidney function by S_{cr} or timed C_{cr} and by protein excretion, either as 24-h excretion or a spot protein/creatinine ratio. *The use of eGFR from MDRD or CKD-EPI formulae is not valid in pregnancy, as actual GFR is underestimated* [5]. If eGFR is used, it might erroneously signal to the clinician an exaggerated deterioration in kidney function and might prompt unnecessary delivery. *Cystatin C as a GFR marker is of no use because there is placental production of Cystatin C, especially prominent in the third trimester.*
2. Careful blood pressure monitoring for early detection of hypertension (and assessment of its severity) and preeclampsia. There are debates about so-called tight control, the accuracy of automated devices and the role of ambulatory blood pressure measurements.
3. Early detection and treatment of anaemia, usually by oral/intravenous iron therapy. Some recommend use of recombinant human erythropoietin if haematocrit is 20 % or less, but caution is needed as hypertension can be caused or aggravated. Blood transfusion may need to be considered.
4. From early pregnancy prophylactic low-dose aspirin is advisable. Definitive thromboprophylaxis will be required when proteinuria exceeds 3 g/24 h or S_{alb} <25 g/L, the dose of low molecular weight heparin depending on the level of kidney impairment [11, 15, 22].
5. Early detection of covert bacteriuria or confirmation of urinary tract infection (UTI) and prompt treatment; if there are recurrent UTIs, then antibiotic prophylaxis should be given throughout pregnancy.
6. Biophysical/ultrasound surveillance of fetal size, growth, development and well-being is mandatory, with timing of the scans and decision-making depending on the evolving clinical situation. Doppler studies can be used to assess placental function as well as helping to predict potential complications such as preeclampsia and fetal distress. Not all women, however, with abnormal uterine artery Dopplers will develop complications, and such tests must not be used in isolation.

The clinical 'watchpoints' associated with specific types of CKD are summarised in Table 28.2.

The following guidelines apply to all CKD patients:

28.5.1 Kidney Function

If there is significant deterioration at any stage of pregnancy, then think in terms of 'prerenal, renal or post-renal' and of reversible or remediable causes such as UTI, diarrhoea, over-strict water and salt restriction, subtle dehydration or electrolyte imbalance (occasionally precipitated by inadvertent diuretic therapy), temporary renal tract obstruction or nephrotoxic drugs. Near term, as in normal pregnancy, a decrease in function of 15–20 %, which affects S_{cr} minimally, is permissible. Failure to detect a reversible cause of a significant decrement is grounds to end the pregnancy by elective delivery.

Table 28.2 CKD and pregnancy

CKD	Clinical watchpoints
Chronic glomerulonephritis and focal glomerular sclerosis (FGS)	Can be high blood pressure late in pregnancy but usually no adverse effect if renal function is preserved and hypertension absent before pregnancy. Some disagree, believing coagulation changes in pregnancy exacerbate disease, especially IgA nephropathy, membranoproliferative glomerulonephritis and FGS
IgA nephropathy	Some cite risks of sudden escalating or uncontrolled hypertension and renal deterioration. Most note good outcome when kidney function is preserved
Chronic pyelonephritis (infectious tubulointerstitial disease)	Bacteriuria in pregnancy and may lead to exacerbation
Reflux nephropathy	Some have emphasised risks of sudden escalating hypertension and worsening of kidney function. Consensus now is that results are satisfactory when prepregnancy function is only mildly affected and hypertension is absent. Vigilance for urinary tract infections is necessary. Screening of baby as soon as possible after birth, if not already detected in utero
Urolithiasis	Ureteral dilatation and stasis do not seem to affect natural history, but infections can be more frequent. Stents have been successfully placed and sonographically controlled uterostomy has been performed during gestation
Systemic lupus erythematosus (SLE)	See Boxes 28.6 and 28.7
Diabetic nephropathy	No adverse effect on the renal lesion. Increased frequency of infections, oedema or preeclampsia. Advanced nephropathy can be a problem
Human immunodeficiency virus with associate nephropathy (HIVAN)	Renal component can be nephrotic syndrome or severe impairment. Scanty literature. Should be considered when nephrotic proteinuria occurs suddenly, especially in immunocompromised patients
Adult PCKD	This autosomal dominant disorder is the most common single-gene genetic disease of humans with an incidence of 1 in 400–1,000. May request DNA probe screening of fetus. Functional impairment and hypertension are usually minimal in childbearing years. Most do not have clinical manifestation until fourth or fifth decade; only 17 % diagnosed by age of 25. Patients do well if renal impairment is minimal. One in four has late-pregnancy hypertension
Periarteritis nodosa Scleroderma	Fetal prognosis is poor. Maternal death can occur. Therapeutic abortion should be considered if disease onset during pregnancy shows rapid overall deterioration. Reactivation of quiescent scleroderma can occur during pregnancy and after delivery
Previous urologic surgery	Depending on original reason for surgery, there may be other malformations of the urogenital tract. Urinary tract infection is common during pregnancy and renal function may undergo reversible decrease. No significant obstructive problem, but Caesarean section might be necessary for abnormal presentation or to avoid disruption of the continence mechanism if artificial sphincters or neourethras are present
After nephrectomy, solitary and pelvic kidneys	Pregnancy is well tolerated. Might be associated with other malformations of the urogenital tract. Dystocia rarely occurs with a pelvic kidney

Source: Modified from Davison and Lindheimer [7]

Do not allow acute kidney injury (AKI) to accelerate to such an extent that not even terminating the pregnancy will reverse the decline [2, 23]. When proteinuria occurs and persists, but blood pressure is normal and renal function preserved, pregnancy can be allowed to continue under closer scrutiny. Thus, increased proteinuria in isolation is not used to time delivery.

28.5.2 Temporary Dialysis

This may be judged necessary during pregnancy especially when S_{urea} is much in excess of 20 mmol/L (48 mg/dL), when intrauterine fetal death is more likely [2]. Refractory hyperkalaemia, severe metabolic acidosis, pulmonary oedema responding poorly to diuretics and danger of volume overload with heart failure may also prompt consideration of dialysis.

It is essential to watch for dialysis-induced uterine contractions, and tocolytic agents can be used with care if indicated. Dialysis-induced hypotension must be avoided too, and also remember that, in the supine position, the patient's enlarged uterus may reduce venous return and aggravate the situation. Even when volume fluctuations are minimised, however, umbilical artery Doppler velocimetry still indicates that haemodialysis temporarily causes considerable fetal haemodynamic alterations.

Dialysis may increase the chance of successful outcome by 'buying time' for fetal maturation, but it does not arrest the inexorable decline in kidney function, ultimately to end-stage failure. In trying to avoid extreme prematurity in this way, it has to be asked whether such potential life-threatening effects on the mother's renal prognosis can be justified.

28.5.3 Blood Pressure

The conventional dividing line for obstetric hypertension is 140/90 mmHg and the aim should be to keep it between 120/70 and 140/90 [11, 12, 15, 17, 21, 24–26]. Inappropriately low blood pressure is associated with fetal growth restriction (FGR) and high blood pressure with renovascular damage. Most of the specific risks of hypertension appear to be related to superimposed preeclampsia in women with CKD but the diagnosis cannot be made with certainty on clinical grounds alone as hypertension and proteinuria may be manifestations of the underlying CKD. Also, chronic hypertension alone has an increased preeclampsia risk fourfold that of normotensive pregnant women. Treatment of mild hypertension (diastolic blood pressure less than 95 mmHg in the second trimester or less than 100 mmHg in the third) is not necessary during normal pregnancy, but many treat women with CKD more aggressively, believing that this preserves kidney function [7].

Medications such as methyldopa, calcium channel blockers, labetalol and hydralazine are safe in pregnancy [24, 25]. Angiotensin-converting enzyme (ACE) inhibitors and angiotensin receptor blockers should not be prescribed *during* pregnancy. When patients are taking either of these before pregnancy, however, because of the significant renoprotection effect, there is a view emerging that changing to a safer drug or drugs can wait until the patient becomes pregnant.

28.5.4 Role of Kidney Biopsy in Pregnancy

Experience with kidney biopsy in pregnancy is limited, mainly because clinical circumstances rarely justify the risk of the possible complications, which are much higher in pregnancy than postpartum, 7 and 1 %, respectively, the latter akin to the rate in nonpregnant subjects [27]. Thus, kidney biopsy is usually deferred until after delivery, provided hypertension is well controlled and coagulation indices are normal.

Whilst pregnancy is considered by most to be a relative contraindication, there are a few generally agreed indications such as when severe nephrotic syndrome develops in early pregnancy or when the suspicion is of a rapidly progressive glomerular disease, for example, SLE in the second trimester, severe enough to warrant specific treatment [16].

28.5.5 Timing of Delivery

Decisions need to be individualised and involve the MDT [1], taking into account gestational age, current fetal and maternal well-being and prognosis as well as the risks of neonatal consequences of early delivery against the risks of complications of continuing the pregnancy [17, 26]. Indeed, if complications do arise, the judicious moment for intervention will inevitably take into account fetal status and perhaps a decision about the use of maternal corticosteroids for fetal lung maturation. In the absence of maternal and/or fetal deterioration, delivery should be at or near term (>37 weeks gestation). Planned preterm delivery may be necessary if there is impending warning of intrauterine fetal death, if kidney function deteriorates substantially, if uncontrollable hypertension supervenes or eclampsia occurs [17, 23, 25, 26]. Obstetric considerations should be the main determinant for delivery by caesarean section. There is certainly an increased risk of emergency caesarean section in labour, spontaneous or induced, for either maternal or fetal complications.

During labour, kidney function and BP must be assessed frequently as well as undertaking continuous monitoring of the fetus. Strict fluid balance must be maintained. If appropriate, prophylaxis with magnesium sulphate to prevent eclampsia must be considered. During active management of the third stage of labour, use oxytocin not syntometrine. Where there is a prerenal insult such as haemorrhage, HELLP or acute fatty liver of pregnancy (AFLP), on top of worsening CKD and/or preeclampsia, which can further acutely threaten maternal kidney function, nephrotoxic drugs must be avoided and the maternal circulation restored with careful fluid management as such patients are prone to fluid overload [17, 26, 28, 29].

28.6 Postpartum Care

Immediately after delivery, there is potential for instability in BP control and fluid balance as well as further deterioration in maternal kidney function, so close surveillance is still needed [1, 17, 26, 28, 29]. Be vigilant in avoiding NSAIDs for postdelivery analgesia because in many units these are routinely prescribed, with patient self-administration.

Decisions will be needed about changing back to prepregnancy medication(s), especially renoprotective drugs, if required, but this may be delayed if mother wishes to breastfeed, dependent on any contraindications [24, 25]. With nephrotic syndrome, prophylactic heparin should be continued for 6 weeks after delivery [11].

If required, renal ultrasound should be arranged for the baby. Remember to arrange a postnatal review appointment with the MDT, both to reassess the patient and to debrief her and her partner about their pregnancy experience (which may have been complicated and worrying), their obstetric and renal future as well as contraception [2].

28.7 Systemic Lupus Erythematosus (SLE)

SLE is worthy of special mention because, even in a multidisciplinary setting, the physician and the obstetrician really must have proper experience with SLE and awareness of the extensive literature [2, 15, 16, 18]. SLE may be present with or without other connective tissue diseases (the overlap syndrome) and the complex clinical problems are due to its profound immunological disturbances, its multi-organ involvement and the complicated immunology of pregnancy itself. Prepregnancy assessment and the clinical 'watch-points' for pregnancy management and afterwards are outlined in Boxes 28.6 and 28.7.

28.7.1 SLE and the Fetus

As well as miscarriage and FGR, SLE confers other big risks on the fetus [16]. Congenital heart block (CHB) is associated with maternal anti Ro and anti La autoantibodies and occurs in up to 4 % of the fetuses in these women, with a 15 % recurrence risk in subsequent pregnancies. It develops between 18 and 20 weeks gestation, so if suspected (from a fixed fetal heart rate of 80 bpm), then fetal echocardiography is essential. Sometimes, hydrops fetalis may develop in utero, occasionally severe, and even those babies born unscathed, half will need pacing in the first year of their lives. Neonatal lupus rash, usually on the scalp and face, and classically akin to adult subcutaneous SLE lesions, can occur soon after delivery and up to 6 months thereafter. These very rarely coexist with CHB and may take several months to subside.

Box 28.6. Prepregnancy SLE Assessment and Counselling

- Prediction of good outcome is related to disease activity and remission, as well as optimal and stable medication(s) in preceding 6 months. Degree of renal impairment, level of hypertension, if any, and low complement levels are also important.
- As well as lupus nephritis, the presence of other comorbidities, such as antiphospholipid syndrome (APS), must be considered.
- Pulmonary hypertension is an absolute contraindication to pregnancy.
- Thromboprophylaxis must be carefully reviewed if considering a past history of thrombosis, nephrotic syndrome and/or preeclampsia.
- Past obstetric history has also to be considered for any other adverse features.
- SLE increases the risk of spontaneous miscarriage, which can be as high as 30 %.
- Four out of five pregnancies will be successful when SLE is in complete remission, even if originally there were severe histopathological changes on biopsy and heavy proteinuria.
- Maternal death rate is 20-fold higher than the normal population.

Source: Data from Refs. [2, 7, 15, 16, 18]

Box 28.7. Pregnancy in SLE Patients

- Complications are common: extrarenal flare (25 %), renal flare (most commonly after delivery) (10 %), FGR (at least 30 %), preterm delivery (50 %) and preeclampsia (at least 10 %).
- In pregnancy up to 20 % of patients have GFR decrements, progressive in 8 %.
- Preeclampsia occurs earlier and more frequently in women with lupus nephritis, even compared to women with similar impairment due to a different CKD.
- Presence of lupus anticoagulant strongly associated with development of preeclampsia.
- Lupus nephritis classes III and IV are more likely to be associated with preeclampsia than classes II and V.
- In a known SLE patient, preeclampsia may be difficult to distinguish from a renal 'flare' (even postpartum), but decreasing complement levels, urinary sediment analysis and increasing anti-dsDNA levels may be helpful as well as evidence of increased lupus disease activity in other organs.
- The most reliable arbiter for distinguishing preeclampsia from lupus nephritis is kidney biopsy, but it is rarely undertaken in pregnancy. It may be considered appropriate in 2nd trimester, if felt that result will tailor/alter management, in relation to 'buying time'.
- SLE has a predilection for the childbearing age group, and if SLE nephropathy becomes manifest for the first time in pregnancy, it may be mistaken for preeclampsia.
- Extrarenal 'flares' occur predominantly in the second half of pregnancy, with renal 'flares' more common in puerperium, a time of increased vigilance as SLE medication(s) (if any) may need adjusting as well as those for ongoing management of hypertension and for thrombosis, in line with breastfeeding considerations.

Source: Data from Refs. [2, 7, 15, 16, 18, 25]

28.8 Suspicion and/or Diagnosis of De Novo CKD During Pregnancy

For some women, pregnancy may be their first major contact with health-care services and represents a valuable opportunity to detect chronic medical conditions, including CKD. If this possibility is raised, it is essential to try and establish a diagnosis as well as a course of management that will be helpful to both mother and fetus [7]. When a patient presents with hypertension, proteinuria and/or abnormal kidney function, it is difficult to distinguish parenchymal CKD from preeclampsia [12–14, 19]. A previous history of kidney disorders, abnormal urine analysis, a family history of CKD or a history of systemic illness known to involve the kidneys is obviously very helpful, but even so CKD and preeclampsia may coexist. In 10–20 % of patients where preeclampsia is severe, of early onset and especially with heavy proteinuria, this may in fact be the first clinical presentation, indeed unmasking rather than development, of asymptomatic/undiagnosed CKD from prepregnancy, more so if the woman is multiparous [13, 14, 19].

Proteinuria alone, in the absence of urinary infection, can be an indication of kidney dysfunction. If TPE is consistently ≥500 mg/24 h, then renal impairment will be present in about half, 40 % will go on to develop hypertension, 25 % will have low birth weight babies and 50 % will deliver preterm. Some of these women may have been labelled preeclamptic in previous pregnancies, but remember that undetected CKD is very likely [7, 13, 30].

In women suspected of having CKD, their assessment and subsequent blood testing are similar to those of nonpregnant patients but the definitive diagnosis has to wait until after delivery [14, 30]. Their pregnancies should be allowed to continue if kidney function and blood pressure remain stable. Nephrology follow-up after delivery is essential for continued assessment and perhaps final diagnosis, with the aim of reducing progressive deterioration and concurrent escalation of cardiovascular and metabolic risks. Intervention with lifestyle changes and then timely pharmacological intervention with the first indication of sequelae is particularly important if there was preeclampsia, as it is a marker for remote cardiovascular, cerebrovascular, metabolic and renal problems [30–32].

28.9 Loss of Kidney Function in Pregnancy and Afterwards in Women with CKD

Pregnancy does not cause or otherwise affect the rate of progression beyond what might be expected in the nonpregnant state, provided that before the pregnancy, kidney impairment was minimal and hypertension absent or very well controlled (Box 28.8). During pregnancy of course, there is a hypercoagulable state, with an augmented coagulation cascade and decreased fibrinolytic activity which even if only slightly augmented in CKD patients, could mediate insidious AKI with thrombotic glomerular injury. Prolonged periods of protein trafficking are nephrotoxic too, with induction of proinflammatory and inflammatory cytokines causing glomerular injury along with tubulointerstitial damage. In the long-term prognosis, however, an important factor could be the sclerotic effect that prolonged, gestational renal vasodilation might have in the residual (intact) glomeruli of the kidneys of these women, especially if contributed to by an increased intraglomerular pressure. The situation may be worse in a single diseased kidney, where more sclerosis has usually occurred within the few (intact) glomeruli. Although the evidence in healthy women and those with mild kidney disease argues against hyperfiltration-induced damage in pregnancy, or any increase in intraglomerular pressure, there is little doubt that in some women with moderate, and certainly severe dysfunction, unpredicted, accelerated and irreversible renal decline does occur in pregnancy and/or afterwards [2, 6, 7, 10, 13].

Box 28.8. Worsening CKD During Pregnancy and Afterwards

- Rate of CKD progression and gradual erosion of kidney function usually relates to the level of BP control, degree of proteinuria, underlying CKD and previous rate of GFR decline.
- In pregnancy there may be accelerated and irreversible decline greater than that predicted based on previous course.
- Renal insufficiency and hypertension, especially where poorly controlled, are the major risk factors for permanent exacerbations of underlying CKD.
- Risk of decline is highest when renal insufficiency is greatest.
- Cause of CKD, other than lupus nephritis, is probably not a major determinant of worsening CKD if factored for pre-existing renal insufficiency and hypertension.
- With preeclampsia, kidney function often declines further, mimicking CKD deterioration.
- Sequential S_{cr} measurements showing escalating concentrations may be evidence of preeclampsia in absence of any other renal diagnoses.
- Addition of a prerenal insult may further reduce kidney function, such as antepartum haemorrhage (APH) and/or postpartum haemorrhage (PPH). Regular use of NSAIDs can acutely and additionally threaten maternal kidney function, as can HELLP, preeclampsia, HUS, acute fatty liver of pregnancy (AFLP) or thrombotic microangiopathies.

Source: Data from Refs. [2, 4–7, 9–12, 16, 22–24, 29]

28.10 Preeclampsia: Diagnosis, Significance and Prognosis (Boxes 28.9 and 28.10)

Preeclampsia remains a major cause of maternal and perinatal morbidity and mortality. Interestingly, it is the commonest cause of glomerular disease worldwide. The diagnosis of preeclampsia, with the ability for appropriate intervention is based on traditional but often unreliable and nonspecific criteria of hypertension and proteinuria [12, 13, 21, 25, 26]. Evidence of involvement of one or more other organs with liver function abnormalities, thrombocytopenia, DIC and/or patient-reported symptomatology may help to establish the diagnosis. In addition, marked rises in S_{cr} (without any other explanation), ever-increasing BP and/or escalating antihypertensive requirements may imply superimposed preeclampsia. Nevertheless, preeclampsia cannot be diagnosed clinically with certainty in women with CKD [2, 12–14, 17, 19].

By elucidating the pathophysiology of preeclampsia and identifying some of the many underlying factors, their measurement might then be used as an aid in predicting preeclampsia in 'at-risk' women, like those with CKD, and/or in diagnosing preeclampsia when the diagnosis is suspected. Ideally, it might be possible to distinguish between preeclampsia and the progressive hypertension, proteinuria and renal deterioration of AKI in CKD patients. Said otherwise, there may be a clinically useful 'marker' of preeclampsia, and if presymptomatic biomarker profiling is possible, then prevention or even modification of risk might be feasible, let alone treatment [30, 31, 33, 35].

In preeclampsia the balance between proangiogenic and antiangiogenic factors is altered [13, 14, 30, 35]. This is due to disturbances in the vascular development of the placenta with underperfusion and ischaemia such that the hypoxic trophoblast secretes a wide range of antiangiogenic factors into the maternal circulation. These include placental growth factor (PlGF) as well as soluble fms-like tyrosine kinase-1 (sFlt-1) (a soluble decoy receptor for vascular endothelial growth factor (VEGF)) and soluble endoglin (sEng), both of which block VEGF-mediated signalling, which is important for normal endothelial function.

Box 28.9. Preeclampsia and CKD

- During pregnancy in CKD patients, hypertension worsens or develops in 30 %, proteinuria increases in over 50 % and decline in kidney function can often occur.
- If preeclampsia develops in CKD patients, then maternal kidney function often deteriorates further.
- In CKD, hypertension and proteinuria are not necessarily due to preeclampsia, as exacerbation of CKD can mimic preeclampsia and/or the two may coexist.
- The uncertainty of clinical diagnosis leads to difficulty in differentiating preeclampsia from not only exacerbation of CKD but also HUS, AFLP and thrombotic microangiopathies.
- Risk of developing preeclampsia in CKD is higher with more severe degrees of renal impairment (from 10 % up to 80 %), higher still in the presence of hypertension.
- Preeclampsia is the most common cause of nephrotic syndrome in pregnancy, but it may also be secondary to underlying CKD, or both.
- Clinically useful circulating 'markers' for preeclampsia are being identified and tested to assist not only with diagnosis but also with presymptomatic prediction of risk and/or complications with the potential for therapeutic intervention(s).

Source: Data from Refs. [2–4, 6, 8, 9, 12–14, 17, 19, 20, 22–24, 30, 33, 34]

Box 28.10. Prognosis After Preeclampsia

- No longer assume that preeclampsia is a condition cured by delivery.
- Although renal changes in general are believed to resolve completely after delivery ('delivery cures the disease'), there is evidence that preeclampsia may leave permanent renal impairment or add further to the deficit of already damaged kidneys.
- Damage may be direct or indirect via hypertension and/or widespread endothelial dysfunction.
- After preeclampsia there is a three- to eightfold increased risk of cardiovascular disease (including ischaemic heart disease, hypertension and stroke) as well as obesity, dyslipidaemia and end-stage renal disease.
- Preeclampsia and cardiovascular disease share risk factors such as hypertension, obesity, diabetes and hypercholesterolaemia, so preeclampsia is certainly a marker for cardiovascular risk.
- Not yet definitely known whether preeclampsia per se adds to the risk; if so, then preeclampsia would be an independent risk factor and not just a marker.
- These remote risks are greatest in those who also had preterm births, FGR and/or recurrent preeclampsia, all frequently seen in CKD women anyway.
- Preeclampsia will add to the already unfavourable cardiovascular and metabolic profile of CKD patients, as CKD patients already carry risk factors.
- Offspring of preeclamptic mothers are more likely to have a higher BP from childhood and a stroke in later life.
- There is a need to elucidate the underlying biological factors that underpin the association between preeclampsia and disease later in life.

Source: Data from Refs. [2, 7, 8, 13, 14, 19, 20, 30–32]

Thus, there is widespread endothelial disruption, microangiopathy and a disturbed inflammatory response, potentially creating a favourable setting for autoimmunity, and the glomerulus is afflicted as part of all this, with disruption of podocyte and endothelial symbiosis. Podocyturia as well as markers of endothelial injury, such as von Willebrand factor,

Box 28.11. Relevant Guidelines

1. *American College of Obstetrics and Gynecology (ACOG) guideline*:

   Hypertension in pregnancy. Report of the American College of Obstetricians and Gynecologists' Task Force in Pregnancy. Obstet Gynecol 2013;122: 1122–31. [26]
2. *American College of Rheumatology guideline*:

   American College of Rheumatology Guidelines for screening, treatment and management of lupus nephritis. Arthritis Care Res. 2012;64:797–808. [18]
3. *Centre for Maternal and Child Enquiries (CMACE)*. Saving mothers' lives: reviewing maternal deaths to make motherhood safer: 2006–2008. BJOG. 2011;118(Suppl 1). [http://onlinelibrary.wiley.com/doi/10.1111/bjo.2011.118.issue-s1/issuetoc] [1]
4. *International Society for the Study of Hypertension in Pregnancy (ISSHP) guideline*:

   The definition of severe and early-onset preeclampsia: statements from ISSHP. Pregnancy Hypertens. 2014;4: 97–104. [12]
5. *National Institute for Health and Clinical Excellence (NICE) guidelines*:

   Clinical Guideline 34. Hypertension: management of hypertension in adults in primary care 2006. [www.nice.org.uk/guidance/index.jsp?action=byID&0=10986=byID&0=10986] [24]

   Clinical Guideline 73. Early identification and management of CKD 2008. [http://guidance.nice.org.uk/CG73/Guidance/pdf/English] [20]

   Clinical Guideline 107. Hypertension in Pregnancy. The management of hypertensive disorders in pregnancy 2010. [21] [www.nice.org.uk/nicemedia/live/13098/50418/50418.pdf]

   Clinical Guideline: 169. Acute kidney injury. Prevention, detection and management of acute kidney injury up to the point of renal replacement therapy 2013. [http://guidance.nice.org.uk/CG169/Guidance/pdf/English] [23]
6. *Royal College of Anaesthetists (RCA)*. Providing equity of critical and maternity care for critically ill pregnant or recently pregnant women. 2011. [http://www.rcoa.ac.uk/document-store/providing-equity-of-critical-and-maternity-care-the-critically-ill-pregnant-or] [28]
7. *Royal College of Obstetricians & Gynaecologists (RCOG) Guidelines*:

   Green Top Guideline 37a. Reducing the risk of thrombosis and embolism during pregnancy and the puerperium 2009. [22] [www.rcog.org.uk/files/rcog-corp/GTG37aReducingRiskThrombosis.pdf]

   Green Top Guideline 10(A). Management of severe preeclampsia and eclampsia 2006, reviewed 2010. [http://www.rcog.org.uk/womens-health/clinical-guidance/management-severe-pre-eclampsiaeclampsia-green-top-10a] [17]

   Green Top Clinical Guideline 56. Maternal collapse in pregnancy and the puerperium. 2011. [http://www.rcog.org.uk/files/rcog-corp/GTG56.pdf] [29]

   54th RCOG Study Group: Renal disease in pregnancy 2008. RCOG Press, London, 273 p [2]
8. *Society of Obstetrics & Gynecology of Canada (SOGC) Guidelines*:

   Clinical Practice Guideline 206. Diagnosis, evaluation and management of the hypertensive disorders of pregnancy. Pregnancy Hypertens. 2014;4:105–45 [25] fibronectin and osteopontin, are yet to be proven clinically useful [13, 14, 19, 30].

Pathogenic agonistic autoantibodies, although not specific, are highly prevalent in preeclampsia, one of which (AT_1-AA) can activate the major angiotensin II type 1 receptor (AT_1R) [13, 30, 35]. There then can follow hypertension, hypercoagulation and glomerular dysfunction as well as FGR, secondary to AT_1-AA-induced placental damage and ischaemia and yet a further increase in sFlt-1 and sEng. Antibody titres correlate with the severity of disease and thus may be useful as a presymptomatic biomarker and their blockage and/or removal may potentially be a treatment option [35]. As sFlt-1 and PlGF reflect underlying placental and endothelial pathophysiology, their measurement may also be useful, but sensitivity and specificity issues need assessment, as does the evaluation of many new candidate biomarkers. Even though measurement of PlGF is becoming an integral component of clinical care for the diagnosis and management of suspected preeclampsia, it seems likely that a clinically useful predictive model will also need to include elements of maternal history, demographic information, standard biochemical investigations and ultrasound biophysical assessment as well as biomarkers, in order to achieve useful stratification of risk [31, 33–35].

There is little doubt that women diagnosed with preeclampsia have a substantially increased risk of cardiovascular disease, cerebrovascular disease, end-stage renal disease and metabolic problems in later life and this risk may also be associated with conditions that coexist with preeclampsia, including CKD [30–33]. Lifestyle interventions after preeclampsia may decrease the cardiovascular risks, but information is now needed about the interplay between genetic, proteomic and environmental factors so as to understand the clinical implications [31].

Before You Finish: Practice Pearls for the Clinician

- Prepregnancy assessment/counselling is a crucial yet neglected approach for best management, providing the ideal opportunity to establish baselines, to achieve optimal use of medication(s) and health education and to discuss all aspects of pregnancy.
- Once a CKD patient, always a CKD patient, and important determinants are prepregnancy renal status (CKD stage), the absence or presence of hypertension (and its management) as well as first-class fetal surveillance, timely delivery and appropriate neonatal care.
- All women with CKD are at increased risk of pregnancy complications with overall at least a two- to fourfold higher risk of adverse fetal outcome, even those with CKD Stage 1.
- Absence of severe hypertension or renal dysfunction prepregnancy is favourable for pregnancy and renal prognosis. If dysfunction is severe, there is still a fair chance that pregnancy will succeed, but risks are much greater, including AKI and its aftermath.
- Type of renal disease probably does not influence outcome but the collagen disorders, IgA and reflux nephropathies and certainly SLE need special consideration.
- Proteinuria is common during pregnancy (up to 3 g/24 h) but little is known about the longer-term implications of the increased protein trafficking within the kidney.
- Severe hypertension is a much greater adverse feature than low but stable kidney function. ‘Controlling a sign’ does not modify the basic pathophysiology underlying clinical deterioration. Preeclampsia cannot be diagnosed clinically with certainty.
- Rapidly deteriorating kidney function, however, even without hypertension, can be ominous.
- Postnatal assessment and debriefing are very important.

References

1. Centre for Maternal and Child Enquiries (CMACE). Saving mothers' lives: reviewing maternal deaths to make motherhood safer: 2006–2008. BJOG. 2011;118 Suppl 1:1–203.
2. Davison JM, Nelson-Piercy C, Kehoe S, Baker P, editors. Royal College of Obstetricians and Gynaecologists. 54th Study Group. Renal disease in pregnancy. London: RCOG Press; 2008. 273 p.
3. Fischer MJ. Chronic kidney disease and pregnancy: maternal and fetal outcomes. Adv Chronic Kidney Dis. 2007;14(2):132–45.
4. Imbasciati E, Gregorinin G, Cabiddu G, Gammaro I. Pegnancy in CKD stages 3 to 5: fetal and maternal outcomes. Am J Kindey Dis. 2007;49:753–62.
5. Piccoli GB, Attini R, Vasario E, Conijn A, Biolcati M, D'Amico F, et al. Pregnancy and chronic kidney disease: a challenge in all CKD stages. Clin J Am Soc Nephrol. 2010;5(5):844–55.
6. Alsuwaida A, Mousa D, Al-Harbi A, Alghonaim M, Ghareeb S, Alrukhaimi MN. Impacts of early chronic kidney disease on maternal and fetal outcome of pregnancy. J Matern Fetal Neonatal Med. 2011;24: 1432–6.
7. Davison JM, Lindheimer MD. Pregnancy and chronic kidney disease. Semin Nephrol. 2011;31:86–99.
8. Nevis IF, Reitsma A, Dominic A, McDonald S, Thabane L, Aki EA, et al. Pregnancy outcomes in women with chronic kidney disease: a systematic review. Clin J Am Soc Nephrol. 2011;6(11):2587–98.
9. Piccoli GB, Conijn A, Attini R, Biocalti M, Bossotti C, Consiglio V, et al. Pregnancy in chronic kidney disease: need for a common language. J Nephrol. 2011;24(3):282–99.
10. Picolli GB, Fassio F, Attini R, Parisi S, Biolcati M, Ferraresi M, et al. Pregnancy in CKD: whom should we follow and why? Nephrol Dial Transplant. 2012;27 suppl 3:iii111–8.
11. Coté AM, Sauvé N. The management challenges of non-preeclampsia-related nephrotic syndrome in pregnancy. Obstet Med. 2011;4:133–9.
12. Tranquilli AL, Dekker G, Magee L, Roberts J, Sibai BM, Steyn W, et al. The classification, diagnosis and management of the hypertensive disorders of pregnancy: A revised statement from ISSHP. Pregnancy Hypertens. 2014;4:97–104.
13. Masujama H, Nobumoto E, Okimoto N, Inone S, Segawa T, Hiramatsu Y. Superimposed preeclampsia in women with chronic kidney disease. Gynecol Obstet Invest. 2012;74:274–81.
14. Hennessy A, Makkris A. Preeclamptic nephropathy. Nephrology. 2011;16:134–43.
15. Bramham K, Lightstone L. Pre-pregnancy counseling for women with chronic kidney disease. J Nephrol. 2012;25:450–9.
16. Cauldwell M, Nelson-Piercy C. Maternal and fetal complications of systemic lupus erythematosis. Obstet Gynaecol. 2012;14:167–74.
17. Royal College of Obstetricians and Gynaecologists Green Top Clinical Guideline 10(A). Management of severe preeclampsia and eclampsia. 2006, reviewed 2010.
18. American College of Rheumatology Guideline. American College of Rheumatology Guidelines for screening, treatment and management of lupus nephritis. Arthritis Care Res. 2012;64:797–808.
19. Marciotti GM, Sarno L, Napolitano R, Mazzarelli LL, Quaglia F, Capone A, et al. Preeclampsia in women with chronic kidney disease. J Matern Fetal Neonatal Med. 2012;25:1367–9.
20. National Institute for Health and Clinical Excellence (NICE) Clinical Guideline: 73. Early identification and management of CKD.
21. National Institute for Health and Clinical Excellence (NICE). Hypertension in pregnancy. The management of hypertensive disorders in pregnancy, Clinical Guideline: 107. London: National Institute for Health and Clinical Excellence (NICE); 2010.
22. Royal College of Obstetricians and Gynaecologists Green Top Clinical Guideline 37a. Reducing the risk of thrombosis and embolism during pregnancy and the puerperium 2009.
23. National Institute for Health and Clinical Excellence (NICE) Clinical Guideline: 169. Acute kidney injury. Prevention, detection and management of acute kidney injury up to the point of renal replacement therapy 2013.
24. National Institute for Health and Clinical Excellence (NICE) Clinical Guideline 34. Hypertension: management of hypertension in adults in primary care 2006.
25. Magee LA, Pels A, Helewa A, Rey E, von Dadelszen P. Diagnosis, evaluation, and management of the hypertensive disorders of pregnancy. Pregnancy Hypertens. 2014;4:105–45.
26. American College of Obstetrics and Gynecology (ACOG) guideline. Hypertension in pregnancy. Report of the American College of Obstetricians and Gynecologists' Task Force in Pregnancy. Obstet Gynecol 2013;122:1122–31.
27. Picolli GB, Daidola G, Attini R, Parisi S, Fassio F, Naretto C, et al. Kidney biopsy in pregnancy: evidence for counselling? A systematic narrative review. BJOG. 2013;120:412–27.
28. Royal College of Anaesthetists (RCA). Providing equity of critical and maternity care for critically ill pregnant or recently pregnant women. 2011.
29. Royal College of Obstetricians and Gynaecologists Green Top Clinical Guideline 56. Maternal collapse in pregnancy and the puerperium. 2011.
30. Munkhaugen J, Vikse BE. New aspects of preeclampsia: lessons for nephrologists. Nephrol Dial Transplant. 2009;24:2964–7.
31. Ananth CV, Cleary KM. Preeclampsia and cardiovascular disease: more questions than answers? BJOG. 2013;120:920–3.
32. Männistö T, Mendola P, Vääräsmäki M, Järvelin M-R, Hartikainen A-L, Pouta A, Suvanto E. Elevated

blood pressure in pregnancy and subsequent chronic disease risk. Circulation. 2013;127:681–90.
33. Hyde C, Thornton S. Does screening for preeclampsia make sense? BJOG. 2013;120:1168–70.
34. Chappell LC, Duckworth S, Seed PT, Griffin M, Myers J, MacKillop L, et al. Diagnostic accuracy of placental growth factor in women with suspected preeclampsia: a prospective multicenter study. Circulation. 2013;128:2121–31.
35. Xia Y, Kellens RE. Angiotensin receptor agonistic autoantibodies and hypertension: preeclampsia and beyond. Circ Res. 2013;113:78–87.

29 Surgery and Chronic Kidney Disease

Caroline West and Andrew Ferguson

Before You Start: Facts You Need to Know

- CKD is an independent risk factor for perioperative morbidity and mortality in both noncardiac and cardiac surgeries, with increased incidence of stroke, infection, and cardiovascular complications, as well as prolonged hospital stay.
- Comorbidities and complications of CKD must be screened for and optimized prior to surgery.
- Pulmonary hypertension and aortic sclerosis are underappreciated indicators of higher risk.
- Cardiopulmonary "fitness" is a key indicator of perioperative risk in major surgery.
- Drug handling is altered in CKD, and opioids such as morphine should be used with caution.
- Safe perioperative care requires careful attention to hemodynamics and fluid balance and postoperative step-down or ICU care for high-risk patients.

C. West, MBChB, MRCP, FCARCSI • A. Ferguson, MB, BCh, BAO, MEd, FRCA, FFICM (✉)
Department of Anaesthetics, Craigavon Area Hospital, 68 Lurgan Road, Portadown, Co. Armagh BT63 5QQ, UK
e-mail: cbcprice@yahoo.com; a_ferguson@me.com

29.1 Setting Out the Context for Surgery in the CKD Patient

29.1.1 Prevalence

CKD is a multisystem disorder which continues to increase in prevalence as the prevalence of the primary etiological factors, diabetes and hypertension, increases. In the USA, it has been estimated that 26 million people are living with some degree of CKD [1]. The prevalence of ESRD is 1,752 per million people in the USA [2], and the number of patients with CKD stages 1–4 likely exceeds the number of patients with ESRD by a factor of 50 [3]. Requirements for surgical care increase with age and levels of comorbidity, and this applies to the CKD population as much as to those with normal kidney function. CKD patients also have much higher rates of coronary artery and vascular disease which may also require surgical management, and those approaching CKD stage 5 disease may present for vascular access or fistula preparation or for management of access complications.

29.1.2 What Impact Does CKD and Comorbidity Have on Perioperative Outcomes?

CKD is an independent risk factor for perioperative morbidity and mortality, and this finding is consistent across a range of surgical specialties

M. Arici (ed.), *Management of Chronic Kidney Disease*,
DOI 10.1007/978-3-642-54637-2_29, © Springer-Verlag Berlin Heidelberg 2014

Box 29.1. Examples of Impact of CKD on Perioperative Outcome

Coronary artery bypass grafting (CABG): CKD patients have higher mortality (1.8 % in CKD2, 9.3 % in CKD4) and higher incidence of stroke, reoperation, sternal wound infection, duration of postoperative mechanical ventilation, postoperative atrial fibrillation, and length of hospital stay [4].

Colorectal surgery: Patients with CKD3-4 have a greater risk of postoperative infection and AKI [5].

Orthopedic surgery: CKD patients following joint replacement surgery have greater pulmonary, infectious, cardiovascular, renal, and neurological morbidity at day 5 and suffer more pain, and their hospital stay is up to 4 days longer [6].

Transcatheter aortic valve implantation (TAVI): CKD patients have an increased risk of a composite outcome of stroke, bleeding or 30-day all-cause mortality, and a lower 1-year survival than patients with normal renal function [7].

including cardiac surgery, vascular surgery, colorectal surgery, and orthopedics [4–7] (see Box 29.1). There are a number of factors that play into these findings, not least the recognition of CKD as a multisystem disorder with a significant contribution from baseline comorbidities (including hypertension, heart failure, stroke, ischemic heart disease, diabetes, metabolic syndrome, pulmonary hypertension, and peripheral vascular disease) which not only are considerably more prevalent in the CKD population but also have a higher mortality rate in CKD patients [2, 8].

Pulmonary hypertension is probably the least appreciated comorbidity. Although generally mild to moderate in severity, it can have significant implications for perioperative management and outcome. Unfortunately, data on non-dialysis-dependent CKD patients is sparse. In non-dialysis-dependent stage 5 CKD (NDD-CKD5), the prevalence has been quoted at 9–39 %, which is up to eight times the prevalence in the general population [9]. However, in CKD 4–5 patients with dyspnea where no other cause has been found, pulmonary hypertension is a frequent finding, being present in up to 71 % of patients in one series.

The CKD kidney is also much more vulnerable to insult and interference in the perioperative period. The contributions of tissue damage, renal hypoperfusion, drug toxicity, contrast nephrotoxicity, fluid overload, mechanical ventilation, etc., lead to a higher risk of perioperative acute kidney injury (AKI) in these CKD patients, a complication that has an independent impact on outcome and also has the potential to significantly change for the worse the trajectory of the patient's existing CKD. CKD patients are less likely than patients with previously normal kidney function to regain independence from dialysis after an episode of AKI.

29.2 Preoperative Evaluation and Optimization

Preoperative evaluation or assessment is the critical point in the patient's journey when a detailed overview of their CKD and the status of their comorbidities can be achieved, appropriate investigations ordered, and interventions aimed at optimizing medical status commenced. The outcome of this evaluation feeds into the process of informed consent, decisions on surgical and anesthesia techniques, prognostication, and planning for perioperative care including the need for critical care support. This process is made much more challenging in the emergency setting when time does not permit full investigation and optimization. Practice should be informed by reference to relevant guidelines (Box 29.2).

Effective preoperative evaluation comprises a number of core components, some of which we will look at in more detail:

- Establishing the etiology and stage of the CKD
- Appropriate baseline investigations and tests

Box 29.2. Relevant Guidelines

1. *KDIGO Guidelines*
   KDIGO Clinical Practice Guideline for the Evaluation and Management of Chronic Kidney Disease Chapter 1: Definition and classification of CKD. Kidney Inter 2013;Suppl 3:19–62 [10]
2. *The Renal Association*
   Cardiovascular Disease in CKD. Final version (6 August 2010). Available at: http://www.renal.org/Clinical/GuidelinesSection/CardiovascularDiseaseInCKD.aspx [11]
3. *American Society of Regional Anesthesia and Pain Medicine*
   Regional anesthesia in the patient receiving antithrombotic or thrombolytic therapy: American Society of Regional Anesthesia and Pain Medicine Evidence-Based Guidelines (Third Edition). Reg Anesth Pain Med. 2010;35(1):64–101. Available at: http://journals.lww.com/rapm/Fulltext/2010/01000/Regional_Anesthesia_in_the_Patient_Receiving.13.aspx [12]
4. *American College of Cardiology/American Heart Association Task Force*
   2009 ACCF/AHA focused update on perioperative beta blockade incorporated into the ACC/AHA 2007 guidelines on perioperative cardiovascular evaluation and care for noncardiac surgery. J Am Coll Cardiol. 2009;54(22):e13. Available at: http://circ.ahajournals.org/content/120/21/e169 [13]
5. *European Society of Cardiology/European Society of Anaesthesiology*
   Guidelines for pre-operative cardiac risk assessment and perioperative cardiac management in non-cardiac surgery. Eur Heart J. 2009;30:2769–812. Available at: http://www.escardio.org/guidelines-surveys/esc-guidelines/Pages/perioperative-cardiac-care.aspx [14]

- Establishing the severity of comorbidity and assessing cardiopulmonary "fitness"
- Optimizing medical comorbidities
- Assessing and managing nutritional status
- Case planning (surgery, anesthesia, critical care, nephrology) and goal setting
- Determining perioperative protective strategies – for example, medication management, drug dosing schedules, hemodynamic targets, prevention of contrast nephropathy, and need for preemptive renal replacement therapy

29.2.1 Establishing the Etiology and Stage of CKD

CKD may be identified for the first time on the basis of testing carried out prior to surgery. In this setting, it is important to determine the likely etiology of the kidney disease as well as staging the severity. There may be time for referral to the nephrology service or for additional renal investigations in patients with stage CKD 3–4. Assign GFR category [10] on the basis of a laboratory eGFR calculation using the serum creatinine level adjusted for gender, age, and African-American or African-European descent or using the CKD-EPI or Modification of Diet in Renal Disease (MDRD) equations. Creatinine-based techniques are generally considered accurate down to eGFR of 20 ml/min/1.73 m^2. Importantly, they assume steady-state creatinine kinetics and do not integrate any adjustment for depleted (or excessive) muscle mass. Alternatives to creatinine-based techniques include the use of biomarkers such as cystatin C. This is a cysteine protease inhibitor produced at a constant rate by all nucleated cells and freely filtered by the kidney. Although less influenced by race, gender, and muscle mass than creatinine, cystatin C levels may be impacted by smoking, some cancers, thyroid dysfunction, and significant changes in basal metabolic rate. Cystatin C is useful in confirming CKD in patients with creatinine-based eGFR of 45–59 ml/min/1.73 m^2 but who do not have markers of kidney damage.

29.2.2 What Initial Investigations Should Be Performed?

The aim is to facilitate "staging" of chronic comorbid diseases and operative case planning. The need for more advanced investigations will be determined by the stage of CKD, the degree of comorbidities, and the physiological impact of the surgery (see below):

- *Weight, height, and BMI*:
- *Laboratory testing*:
  - *Complete blood count (CBC)* focusing on hemoglobin, MCV, and platelet count – set Hb goals for surgery.
  - Iron studies and possibly *B12 and folate* in anemic patients (depending on MCV).
  - *Serum biochemistry* for CKD stage and electrolyte derangements including potassium, magnesium, calcium, and phosphate concentrations.
  - In diabetic patients, *blood glucose and glycosylated hemoglobin* levels.
  - In patients with weight loss or malnutrition, check *albumin or prealbumin.*
  - Brain natriuretic peptide (*BNP*) or N-terminal-pro-BNP (*NT-proBNP*) to assess status and trajectory of cardiac dysfunction.
- *Urinalysis*: Especially important on first presentation of CKD, but also look for changes in albuminuria status, and exclude active urinary tract infection.
- *12-lead ECG*: Look for changes from previous or rhythm disturbances that will impact on anesthesia.
- *Chest x-ray*: In patients with functional impairment, long-standing hypertension, ischemic heart disease, or heart failure, look for evidence of cardiomegaly, pleural effusion, pulmonary hypertension, or interstitial edema. The yield from chest x-ray in asymptomatic patients with CKD stages 1–3 is unlikely to be high enough to warrant routine testing.
- *Echocardiogram*: For patients with poor functional status or new murmurs, specifically request assessment of right-sided pressures, right ventricular function, and LV diastolic function in addition to the basics. *Heart failure with preserved ejection fraction* is a contributor to postoperative cardiac events and puts patients at risk of pulmonary edema at lower end-diastolic volumes (preload). *Remember that aortic sclerosis is not innocent* – it is an independent predictor of higher risk and worse outcome in major surgery.

29.2.3 Detailed Assessment of Cardiopulmonary "Fitness"

The general approach to cardiac evaluation prior to major noncardiac surgery is clearly set out in the updated ACC/AHA guidelines [13] and is summarized in Fig. 29.1.

The inability of the cardiopulmonary system to increase oxygen delivery in response to increased demands is a key indicator of risk. To cope well with surgery, a patient must be able to match the demand set up by the stress and inflammatory response that lasts for several days after major surgery. The primary means of matching oxygen delivery to demand is stroke volume augmentation. Changes in hemoglobin content and oxygen saturation are less significant, except at extremes of anemia or hypoxemia. Dissolved oxygen plays little role at normal pressures. Simplified then, we have:

$$O_2 \text{ delivery} = [1.39 \times \text{Hb} \times \text{SaO}_2] \times \text{stroke volume} \times \text{heart rate}$$

Although various functional status questionnaires have been validated (e.g., the Duke Activity Status Index, Table 29.1) and can provide guidance as to the likely peak oxygen uptake, the correlation with outcomes from shuttle walk tests is not always good, and these in turn do not correlate well with formal integrated cardiopulmonary exercise testing (known as CPET or CPEX). CPET offers greater information on the nature of the limiting factors (cardiac vs. respiratory) and

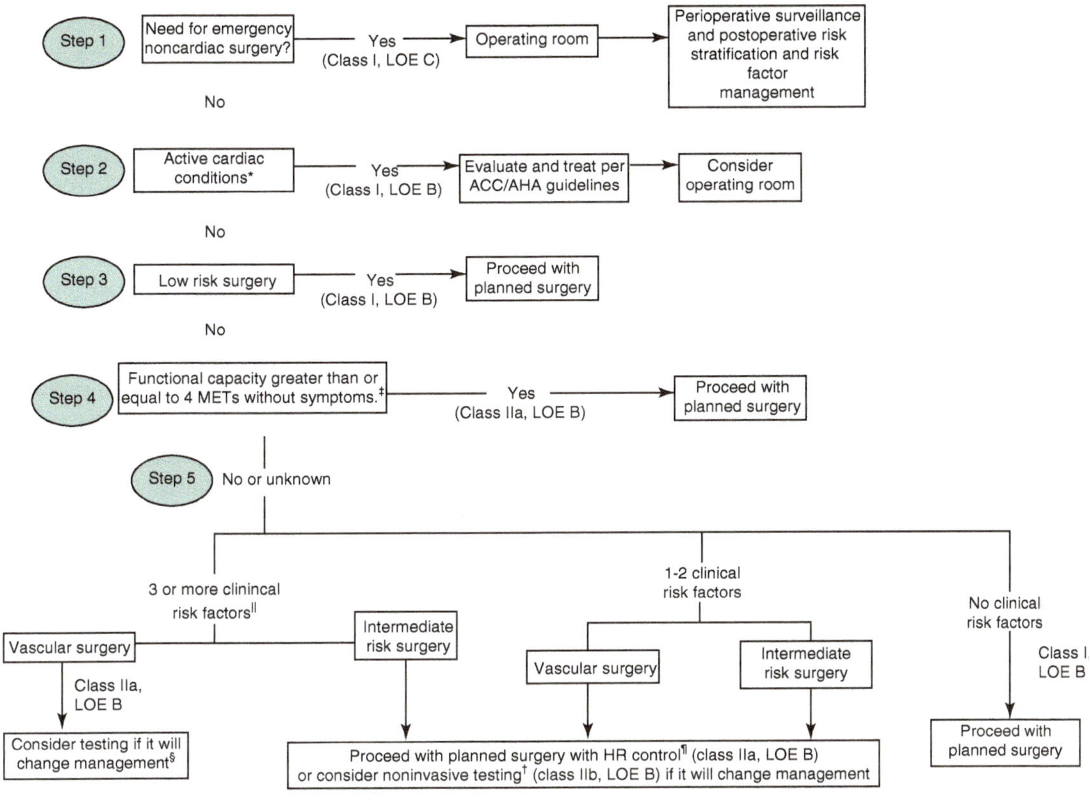

Fig. 29.1 Algorithm for cardiac workup prior to noncardiac surgery. *Active cardiac conditions = unstable angina or recent MI, decompensated heart failure, significant arrhythmias, severe valvular disease. † Noninvasive stress testing is not useful in patients without clinical risk factors undergoing intermediate-risk noncardiac surgery and is not useful for patients undergoing low-risk noncardiac surgery. ‡ See Table 29.1 for estimated MET level equivalent. §Noninvasive testing may be considered before surgery in specific patients with risk factors if it will change management. ||Clinical risk factors include ischemic heart disease, compensated or prior heart failure, diabetes mellitus, renal insufficiency, and cerebrovascular disease. ¶ Perioperative beta-blockade should be considered for populations where this reduces cardiac events; *HR* heart rate, *LOE* level of evidence, *MET* metabolic equivalent (Reprinted from Fleisher et al. [13] Copyright 2009, with permission from Elsevier)

Table 29.1 Duke Activity Status Index

	Activity – can you…	Weight
1	Take care of yourself, that is, eating, dressing, bathing, or using the toilet?	2.75
2	Walk indoors, such as around your house?	1.75
3	Walk a block or 2 on level ground?	2.75
4	Climb a flight of stairs or walk up a hill?	5.50
5	Run a short distance?	8.00
6	Do light work around the house like dusting or washing dishes?	2.70
7	Do moderate work around the house like vacuuming, sweeping floors, or carrying in groceries?	3.50
8	Do heavy work around the house like scrubbing floors or lifting or moving heavy furniture?	8.00
9	Do yard work like raking leaves, weeding, or pushing a power mower?	4.50
10	Have sexual relations?	5.25
11	Participate in moderate recreational activities like golf, bowling, dancing, doubles tennis, or throwing a baseball or football?	6.00
12	Participate in strenuous sports like swimming, singles tennis, football, basketball, or skiing?	7.50

Source: Reprinted from Hltaky et al. [15]. Copyright 1989, with permission from Elsevier
Duke Activity Status Index (DASI) = sum of scores for each question.
Estimated peak oxygen uptake (ml/min) = (0.43 × DASI) + 9.6

also the point during exercise (heart rate, level of oxygen consumption, and delivery) at which decompensation occurs. Detailed discussion of CPET technique is beyond the remit of this chapter and has been well reviewed elsewhere [16].

There are some key parameters that provide the basis for risk stratification. The most commonly used are peak oxygen uptake, ventilatory equivalent for CO_2 (pulmonary ventilation divided by CO_2 production), and the so-called anaerobic threshold (the point at which oxygen delivery is insufficient to meet aerobic metabolic demands).

Patients with a peak oxygen uptake of <14 ml/kg/min or an anaerobic threshold of <11 ml/min/kg in the absence of cardiac ischemia, or 11–14 ml/kg/min with cardiac ischemia, are at increased risk of postoperative cardiopulmonary complications and should receive careful perioperative management after major surgery, ideally in a high-care or critical care area.

Remember the impact of chemotherapy on functional status and the implications for interpretation of CPET results. CPET carried out prior to chemotherapy may give a different (better) result from post-chemotherapy CPET.

29.2.4 Optimizing Medical Comorbidities and Preoperative Condition

Preoperative optimization of medical conditions plays a dual role. Firstly, these conditions are often triggers for renal decline, and their optimal management provides the best hope of minimizing the rate of progression and preventing new insults. Secondly, these conditions are the main contributors to perioperative adverse outcomes:

29.2.4.1 Blood Pressure and Heart Failure Therapy

Arterial pressure control and blockade of the renin-angiotensin system are considered vital in slowing progression of both diabetic and non-diabetic CKD. KDIGO advises a blood pressure target of <140/90 in adults with CKD with a urine albumin excretion of <30 mg/24 h, and <130/80 is advised if the urine albumin excretion is ≥30 mg/24 h [17]. It is worth remembering that drugs such as angiotensin converting enzyme inhibitors (ACEIs), angiotensin receptor blocking drugs (ARBs), and loop diuretics are often omitted on the day of surgery to minimize hemodynamic instability under anesthesia, and reintroduction may be delayed in the postoperative period in cases of major upper gastrointestinal surgery. If control is suboptimal, hypertension and pulmonary congestion may become a problem postoperatively. Patients should also be screened for postural hypotension and for diastolic hypotension which is an underappreciated risk factor for adverse cardiovascular outcomes.

29.2.4.2 Blood Glucose Control

Where elevations in glycosylated hemoglobin suggest less than optimal glucose control, an endocrine consult may be indicated. Perioperative stress, catecholamine medication, etc., will contribute to hyperglycemia and increased insulin requirements, and perioperative hyperglycemia contributes to increased risk of infection. Hospitals often have protocols for discontinuation of oral hypoglycemic agents prior to surgery, and CKD patients are at higher risk of fasting hypoglycemia if the timing of discontinuation is not appropriate.

29.2.4.3 Phosphate and Parathyroid Hormone

Vitamin D deficiency and resultant bone demineralization and hyperphosphatemia are associated with increased risk of mortality. Patients with more advanced CKD may already be taking phosphate binders and vitamin D analogs, and the effectiveness of these regimens should be reviewed preoperatively. Patients with NDD-CKD5, and some patients with CKD4, may have undergone parathyroidectomy and are at risk of "hungry-bone syndrome" with attendant significant hypocalcemia issues. Calcium and phosphate levels should be carefully monitored around the time of surgery when oral therapy may be withheld because of fasting or slow return of gastrointestinal function.

29.2.4.4 Fluid and Electrolyte Status

Surgery and anesthesia are associated with increased insensible losses and also loss of voluntary control of intake. In contrast to the "traditional" opinion that extracellular fluid volume is maintained near normal until CKD5, there is now evidence of fluid accumulation at an earlier stage. Patients with higher stages of CKD are also at risk of hyperkalemia, hyperchloremia, and dysnatremia in the perioperative period, and this risk is amplified by surgical tissue trauma, catabolism, fluid shifts, and changes in eGFR and urine concentrating ability. Perioperative fluid plans should recognize the impact of saline administration on the development of hyperchloremic acidosis and the effect that this might have on renal blood flow, cardiac contractility, and eGFR. It is important that electrolyte levels are carefully managed in the run-up to surgery, and in patients at risk of fluid overload (e.g., heart failure), fluid accumulation must be minimized according to edema and weight while also limiting the incidence of overt dehydration which can lead to profound hypotension under anesthesia. Significant edema reduces wound and gut perfusion and increases risk of poor wound healing and infection. Electrolyte stability, even if not a problem preoperatively, can become a significant problem following surgery. In advanced CKD, loss of potassium through the gastrointestinal tract can become an important part of regulation and that this may be diminished or lost when the integrity of the gastrointestinal tract is compromised. Other perioperative contributors to altered potassium handling, such as insulin administration, acidemia, beta-receptor-active drugs, etc., should be anticipated.

29.2.4.5 Nutritional Status

CKD is a chronic inflammatory disease, and in stage 4 and 5 disease altered blood chemistry can induce anorexia and alter bowel function. Given the impact of hypoalbuminemia on drug carriage and edema formation, significant malnutrition must be addressed prior to elective surgery. In patients with CKD and heart failure, poor gut perfusion can have an additive effect on nutritional status, while edema maintains weight despite altered body composition. There are a number of relatively simple and noninvasive tools to assess body composition, and a nutritional assessment is a worthwhile preoperative consult. In severe cases, supplemental enteral or parenteral nutrition solutions may be needed (see Chap. 17).

29.2.4.6 Anemia Management

In general, anemia secondary to CKD does not become a major issue before late stage 3 disease. In the absence of treatment, hemoglobin concentrations may well fall to below 80 g/l (8.0 g/dl) with hematocrit in the 25–27 % range. This level of anemia has a number of deleterious effects, not least of which is a decline in oxygen delivery and aerobic capacity. This effect will be amplified by disorders such as ischemic heart disease and heart failure and has a serious effect on quality of life. Replacement therapy with erythropoiesis-stimulating agents (ESAs) and iron is used with a goal hemoglobin level of 110–120 g/l (11.0–12.0 g/dl) and a hematocrit of 33–36 % [18]. This is an acceptable level for the vast majority of patients and operative interventions. ESAs are not an option for acutely increasing hemoglobin levels or responding to perioperative blood loss, and blood transfusion should be used as indicated, watching for complications such as fluid overload and hyperkalemia.

29.2.4.7 Bleeding Risk

Chronic exposure to uremic toxins in advanced CKD has significant effects on bleeding time through alterations in platelet function (both activation and aggregation) and von Willebrand factor (vWF) levels (reducing platelet adhesion). This effect is not linearly related to eGFR or urea or creatinine levels and should be considered as a potential problem in CKD3–5 patients. This risk is amplified by the use of antiplatelet drugs, for example, aspirin and clopidogrel. Aspirin is often continued perioperatively in patients without CKD, and a decision to do the same in the CKD patient requires a careful risk/benefit analysis. Drugs such as clopidogrel should be discontinued where possible at least 7 days prior to major surgery. In addition to abnormalities of platelet

Table 29.2 Pharmacological options for correcting bleeding time in uremia

Drug	Dose	Comments
Desmopressin (DDAVP)	0.3 μg/kg iv	Increases factor VIII/vWF release from endothelium Effect starts 1–4 h post dose and lasts 4–12 h. Tachyphylaxis on repeat dosing
Conjugated estrogens	0.6 mg/kg oral or iv daily for 5 days preoperative	Effect starts after 6 h and peaks at day 5–7, lasting 14–21 days
Cryoprecipitate	10 bags American Red Cross prepared over 30 min	Onset 1 h, lasts 4–12 h
rhEPO	40–150 U/kg iv three times weekly aiming for hematocrit > 30 %	Increases platelet margination, aggregation, and reticulation. Not an option for surgery within 4 weeks

Source: Adapted by permission from Macmillan Publishers Ltd: Hedges et al. [19]. Copyright 2007

function, anemia has effects on blood rheology and reduces physiological platelet margination to the periphery of blood vessels (where they can do most good in clot formation). In cases where perioperative bleeding risk is high, consideration should be given to increasing the hematocrit prior to surgery if this is significantly below the conventional goal of 33 %. There are also a number of pharmacological options for improving bleeding time in uremic patients (see Table 29.2) in preparation for surgery. Preemptive dialysis will also act to improve platelet function (remembering to minimize the use of anticoagulation in the preoperative period). The preoperative period is also an appropriate time to consider the impact of agents used as prophylaxis against deep venous thrombosis on bleeding. This is particularly the case for low-molecular-weight heparins which (1) are not easily reversed and (2) have the potential to accumulate in CKD patients. It may be appropriate to measure anti-Xa activity as a means of optimizing dosage and minimizing bleeding risk.

29.2.4.8 Pre-habilitation

This refers to a preemptive preoperative regimen of aerobic exercise aimed at demonstrating improvements in functional and aerobic capacity. In deconditioned patients (and this includes patients suffering from the effects of chemotherapy), as little as 3–4 sessions of this exercise in the run-up to surgery can produce moderate effects on aerobic performance.

29.2.4.9 Preemptive Dialysis

For patients with advanced CKD and, for example, serum creatinine >.5 mg/dl undergoing cardiac surgery, it has been suggested on the basis of small case series that complication rates might be lower if the patients were electively dialyzed pre- and postoperatively. This approach seeks to optimize fluid status and minimize uremic and electrolyte complications that may accompany worsening of renal function in the postoperative period. The jury is still out on the benefit of this technique.

29.3 Anesthesia in CKD

29.3.1 Drug Choices

CKD is associated with alterations to some of the major pharmacological determinants of drug handling such as volume of distribution, protein binding, drug metabolism, and drug excretion:

29.3.1.1 Induction Agents

The effects of intravenous induction agents are terminated not by elimination of the drug from the body but by redistribution of drug out of brain into other tissues. All commonly used induction agents (propofol, etomidate, thiopental, ketamine, midazolam) can be used in CKD patients, provided account is taken of their hemodynamic effects – CKD is not a contraindication, but drug choice should be determined by the comorbidities present.

29.3.1.2 Inhaled Anesthetics

The volatile anesthetic gases are widely used for the maintenance of general anesthesia and also for the gaseous induction of anesthesia in the pediatric population. The most commonly used agents are sevoflurane, isoflurane, and desflurane. Despite metabolism of sevoflurane to release potentially nephrotoxic inorganic fluoride ions, renal toxicity is not observed in humans. Sevoflurane also reacts with some carbon dioxide absorbents during low-flow anesthesia to release a substance called compound A. Although nephrotoxic in rats, extrapolation to humans suggests a nephrotoxic threshold of 150–200 ppm, a level that is not reached even at extremely low gas flows for prolonged periods, for example, after 5 h at 0.25 l/h, the level of compound A peaks at less than 20 ppm. *Sevoflurane and the other inhalational anesthetic gases in common use are considered safe for use in all stages of chronic kidney disease.*

29.3.1.3 Neuromuscular Blocking Drugs and Reversal Agents

Long-acting neuromuscular blocking agents (NMBAs), or those with significant renal excretion, should ideally be avoided in CKD. Neuromuscular function monitoring should be used. Atracurium and its stereoisomer cis-atracurium both undergo a spontaneous degradation process at body temperature and pH known as Hofmann elimination, independent of kidney and hepatic functions. They are often used in CKD patients for this reason. The aminosteroid NMBAs vecuronium and rocuronium both undergo significant renal excretion, and their duration of action is prolonged in patients with severe kidney disease. They may still be used (in particular, because of its rapid onset of action, rocuronium) provided patients are monitored appropriately. Pancuronium is a long-acting non-depolarizing muscle relaxant. It has a reduced clearance and prolonged half-life in CKD, and it also has an active metabolite which is half as potent as pancuronium itself. For this reason, it should only be used (and then with caution) if other agents are not suitable.

Plasma cholinesterase levels are reduced in CKD, and this can prolong the action of the depolarizing muscle relaxant suxamethonium (succinylcholine) and also the non-depolarizing muscle relaxant mivacurium. There has been concern over the use of suxamethonium in kidney disease due to the risk of hyperkalemia; however, it has been proven to be safe for use provided the preoperative potassium level is not raised.

Reversal of non-depolarizing NMBA action is normally performed using neostigmine. Clearance is reduced and half-life prolonged in CKD. Neostigmine is usually administered alongside atropine or glycopyrrolate to balance out its parasympathomimetic effects (bradycardia and AV block). Atropine is shorter acting and may wear off before the neostigmine in CKD. Glycopyrrolate is a better choice. An alternative is the new cyclodextrin drug called sugammadex which reverses the effects of *aminosteroid* muscle relaxants by selectively binding the NMBA. A key feature is that it can be used at deep level of block where traditional acetylcholinesterase inhibitors would be ineffective. The sugammadex-NMBA complex is normally excreted unchanged by the kidney. Although clearance of this complex is reduced, it is not required for drug effect, and the standard dose of sugammadex appears to be effective in kidney disease.

29.3.1.4 Analgesics

Acetaminophen (paracetamol) is safe to use in CKD patients in the perioperative period at the standard dose and frequency. The use of nonsteroidal anti-inflammatory drugs (NSAIDs) for analgesia in the perioperative period is not recommended as the adverse effects are likely to significantly outweigh the benefits. They are potentially nephrotoxic drugs which can produce an acute drop in GFR and may also precipitate acute interstitial nephritis in a patient population already high risk for acute kidney injury. NSAIDs are also associated with an increase in the risk of cardiovascular complications, gastrointestinal bleeding and edema, hypernatremia, and hyperkalemia.

Opioid analgesics (see Table 29.3) are not directly nephrotoxic; however, they may trigger urinary retention and have an antidiuretic effect. Although they are a mainstay of postoperative analgesia after moderate and major surgery,

Table 29.3 Opioids and their metabolites in CKD

Opioid	Metabolism and active metabolites	Excretion	Accumulates in kidney failure	Dialyzed	Safety profile in CKD 4–5
Morphine	Hepatic to morphine-6-glucuronide (M-6-G)	Renal	Yes	Yes	Reduce dose. Increase interval. Caution required
Fentanyl	Hepatic – none active	Renal	Parent compound	No	Safe – reduce dose
Alfentanil	Hepatic – none active	Renal	No	No	Safe – reduce dose (increased free fraction)
Remifentanil	Esterases – none active	Renal	No	No	Safe
Codeine	Hepatic with polymorphism to morphine and M-6-G	Renal	Yes	?	Avoid
Oxycodone	Hepatic with polymorphism to oxymorphone	Renal	Yes	?	Avoid if possible. Extreme caution if used in advanced CKD
Tramadol	Hepatic to O-dimethyl tramadol	Renal	Yes	Yes	Avoid – lowered seizure threshold and altered mental status
Meperidine	Hepatic to normeperidine	Renal	Normeperidine accumulates	No	Avoid – normeperidine leads to seizures
Methadone	Hepatic	Renal/fecal	–	No	Appears safe
Hydromorphone	Hepatic to hydromorphone-3-glucuronide	Renal	Yes	Yes	Avoid if possible. H-3-G causes neuro-excitation. Use lower dose and/or longer interval

Source: Adapted from Trainor et al. [20] © 2011, with permission from John Wiley and Sons

caution is required as many opioids, or their active metabolites, are excreted by the kidney. Morphine, for example, has the active metabolite morphine-6-glucuronide (M6G), and in advanced kidney failure, the half-life of M6G is prolonged from 2 to 27 h. Fentanyl and alfentanil are relatively safe in renal failure although the required dose may be reduced (they have no active metabolites). Drugs such as oxycodone, codeine, tramadol, and meperidine are best avoided in patients with CKD 4–5 and if used in earlier stages of CKD require dose adjustment and caution.

29.3.2 Regional and Neuraxial Anesthesia as an Option in CKD

The most feared complications of neuraxial (spinal and epidural) analgesia and anesthesia are bleeding and infection resulting in neurological complications. These concerns are justified given the impact of uremic toxins on platelet and leukocyte function. Although study data is limited (given the low frequency of these complications, a very large trial would be needed to definitely answer this question), epidural anesthesia has been successfully reported in patients with stage 3–5 CKD in several surgical settings including orthopedics, obstetrics, post-renal transplant, and abdominal and thoracic surgery. Clearly, if clinicians have reason to suspect significant problems with coagulation, then this technique is not suitable, but CKD per se is not a contraindication.

Upper limb nerve blocks have been used to provide anesthesia for the formation of arteriovenous fistulae in CKD5 patients, and peripheral neural blockade is safe in CKD provided standard contraindications are absent. It should be noted that block onset may be delayed and duration reduced in the setting of low bicarbonate level.

With the increasing emphasis on enhanced recovery techniques (minimizing opioid usage, optimizing postoperative mobility, and return of gastrointestinal function), alternative techniques for analgesia in abdominal surgery are popular. These include the transversus abdominis plane (TAP) block and the rectus sheath block. Both techniques are appropriate in CKD patients in the absence of overt coagulopathy. With all regional anesthesia techniques, suitability should be assessed on a case-by-case basis, taking into account the anticipated benefits and the risks. Drugs such as clopidogrel should be stopped 7 days prior to major neuraxial blocks, and low-molecular-weight heparin should not be administered within the 12 h preceding the block, and platelet counts and coagulation testing carried out. This area is well covered in guidelines from the American Society of Regional Anesthesia [12].

29.4 The CKD Patient in the Operating Room

29.4.1 Monitoring

More advanced ECG monitoring with 5-lead systems capable of ST-segment analysis is valuable. Placement of an arterial cannula will allow beat-to-beat blood pressure measurement during the process of induction of anesthesia when hypotension is a significant risk. For patients undergoing major surgery, insertion of a central venous catheter should be considered to facilitate monitoring and administration of inotropes or vasopressors. Subclavian vein access is associated with a lower risk of infection but has a higher risk of venous stenosis with prolonged use than the internal jugular approach.

29.4.2 Hemodynamic and Fluid Status Optimization

High-risk patients include those with anaerobic threshold <11 ml/kg/min or revised cardiac risk index ≥3 or predicted perioperative mortality >5 % undergoing major surgery. There are two main approaches to advanced hemodynamic management. They share the goal of optimizing oxygen delivery through optimizing preload and hence stroke volume and cardiac output.

29.4.2.1 Conventional Approaches Using Static Parameters

The first approach is the use of additional "traditional" static measures including central venous pressure monitoring via central venous catheter (CVC) or pulmonary artery wedge pressure (PAWP) monitoring via a Swan-Ganz right heart catheter for preload estimation. There are significant limitations in using CVP and PAWP to assess intravascular volume status, as the correlation between these measures and response to a fluid challenge is poor. In the absence of cardiac output or stroke volume monitoring, this approach also emphasizes fluid administration and blood pressure control at the expense of optimizing flow, that is, perfusion. The use of predominantly vasopressor agents to reverse hypotension in these patients (e.g., phenylephrine and metaraminol) will sustain blood pressure but diminish forward flow and tissue perfusion, as well as increasing left ventricular afterload. A falsely reassuring picture of adequate mean arterial pressure may be obtained. Cardiac output monitoring helps to maintain a more balanced hemodynamic approach, but if used it should be commenced prior to anesthesia to set a baseline level.

29.4.2.2 Goal-Directed Approaches Using Dynamic Parameters

The second approach is a more formal "goal-directed" dynamic approach aimed at optimizing stroke volume with fluid boluses before adding inotropic or pressor support and also keeping an adequate perfusion pressure target (generally maintaining systolic BP within 25–30 % of baseline and keeping mean arterial pressure above 70 mmHg in normotensive patients and 75–80 mmHg in patients with hypertension). At the extremes of this approach, prespecified cardiac index targets may be chased. This can be done using a pulmonary artery (PA) catheter, but increasingly this has given way to techniques such as esophageal Doppler that make use of a CVC and arterial catheter and are based around thermodilution or indicator dilution-based calibration of stroke volume followed by continuous monitoring based on the shape of the pulse waveform. These techniques involve complex algorithms automated within proprietary monitors and provide information on stroke volume variation (SVV) or pulse pressure variation (PPV) that is used to assess volume status and need for fluid. Techniques such as transpulmonary thermodilution are also able to describe the amount of lung edema (extravascular lung water) and intrathoracic blood volume.

There is still debate around these dynamic approaches, although there are some very positive studies and meta-analyses suggesting beneficial effects on short-term outcome, organ impairments, and hospital length of stay after major abdominal surgery. Studies have not specifically focused on the CKD population. Goal-directed approaches inevitably result in more positive fluid balances, since these techniques are based on the premise of giving fluid until the heart no longer responds with an increase in stroke volume. This is a controversial area, and it could be rationally argued that this approach by definition aims to touch the hem of cardiac failure.

29.4.3 Inotropic Support in Heart Failure

Inotropic support should be considered at an earlier stage in patients with ventricular dysfunction. Drug choices include conventional agents such as norepinephrine and epinephrine, accepting that these agents can significantly increase myocardial oxygen demand and cardiac afterload. Alternative agents such as phosphodiesterase inhibitors (e.g., milrinone) may be more appropriate in the cardiac surgical setting, and while increasing cardiac output, they may result in a drop in arterial pressure through reduction in systemic vascular resistance. An interesting choice is the novel calcium-sensitizing inotrope levosimendan. This agent improves contractility and produces an increase in cardiac output without increasing myocardial oxygen demand. It has not yet achieved widespread use but has been used successfully in both cardiac and noncardiac settings.

29.4.4 Transesophageal Echocardiography (TEE)

TEE should be considered in the cardiac surgical setting and also in very-high-risk patients undergoing major noncardiac surgery. TEE allows for direct visualization and quantification of the cardiac response to fluid, inotropes, and mechanical ventilation. Usage is restricted by the availability of equipment and trained personnel, particularly in the noncardiac surgical setting. However, the availability of single-use probes and dedicated lower-cost equipment, specifically designed for perioperative and ICU usage, will increase the uptake of this technique.

29.4.5 Monitoring Tissue Oxygenation

Given the prevalence of microvascular and endothelial dysfunction in the CKD population, superimposed on macrovascular arterial disease, maintaining tissue oxygenation of vital organs in the perioperative period is a critical goal of care. Measures such as arterial lactate level (goal <2 mmol/l) or central venous oxygen saturation (goal > 65–70 %) are global indices of perfusion, and normal values do not exclude significant regional tissue hypoxia. Cerebral perfusion is a particular concern in both cardiac and noncardiac surgeries. Alterations in perfusion pressure, cardiac output, and carbon dioxide level can all influence cerebral perfusion. The use of cerebral oximetry techniques can detect otherwise silent episodes of cerebral desaturation and allow for attempts to correct them. Cerebral desaturation during surgery is associated with an increased incidence of postoperative cognitive deficit and should be minimized.

29.4.6 Fluid Choices

Where fluids are given perioperatively, recent data from the critical care arena suggest that hydroxyethyl starch solutions are not as benign as they were thought to be, and as potential nephrotoxins these agents should be avoided where possible. It is hard to argue that colloid use provides a significant patient benefit, and balanced crystalloid solutions are the mainstay of perioperative fluids. Many anesthesiologists use solutions such as Ringer's lactate (also known as compound sodium lactate or Hartmann's solution) which contains less sodium and chloride than 0.9 % saline and has lactate which is converted to bicarbonate by the liver. These solutions are less likely to induce hyperchloremia and hypernatremia, but they do contain potassium, and this requires close monitoring if used in significant volumes. Although there is no data demonstrating superiority as a resuscitative fluid, the use of human albumin in the perioperative period is justified in patients with significant hypoalbuminemia (<25 g/l) to assist with drug carriage and to maintain colloid pressure.

29.4.7 Perioperative Renal Protection

The CKD kidney is vulnerable to additional insult and may never get back to where it started if AKI occurs. Approaches to kidney protection can be divided into non-pharmacological and pharmacological [21]. The most important aspect of kidney protection is to do the basics well:

- Avoid hypovolemia or hypervolemia.
- Maintain adequate perfusion pressure but also flow.
- Avoid nephrotoxins where possible.
- Control blood glucose (goal blood glucose levels less than 180 mg/dl).
- Avoid sepsis.
- Aggressively manage postoperative complications.
- Avoid intra-abdominal hypertension.

It is critical to avoid getting into the spiral of repeated fluid challenges and aggressive fluid administration for oliguria or hypotension that does not respond more than transiently to fluid. *Fluid overload is nephrotoxic*. It leads to diminished filtration pressure through increased venous pressures, it raises the prospect of intra-abdominal hypertension which reduces renal perfusion, and it leads to renal interstitial edema. As an encapsulated organ, parenchymal swelling inevitably leads to renal hypoperfusion and hypofiltration. A knee-jerk response of giving yet more fluid will make matters worse, and in this scenario fluid removal may improve renal injury and function.

Potential strategies that have been studied are shown in Table 29.4.

Table 29.4 Summary of status of potential kidney protection strategies

Strategy	Comments
Perioperative statins	Pleiotropic anti-inflammatory effects. Do not appear to have any impact on AKI in noncardiac surgery although studies not focused on prevention in CKD patients. Some work showing cardiac surgical patients who were continued on satins had lower AKI risk
Loop diuretics	No clinical benefit in prevention of perioperative AKI in CKD patients
Mannitol	No clinical benefit in prevention of perioperative AKI in CKD patients in noncardiac surgery. Opinion divided on benefit in cardiac surgery
Dopamine	No preventive effect on AKI development in CKD and carries risk of arrhythmia and cardiac ischemia. There is no place for prophylactic dopamine infusion for renal support. May be considered as a vasopressor
Fenoldopam	Promising agent, however trials demonstrating a reduced incidence of AKI failed to demonstrate reductions in RRT requirement or better mortality
Natriuretic peptides	Studies (albeit small) have demonstrated attenuation of creatinine rise and reductions in AKI incidence in cardiac surgery, but again no clear impact on RRT-free days or mortality
N-acetyl cysteine	Protective for contrast exposure. No effect seen in perioperative use
Off-pump CABG	Reduced incidence of AKI, but no outcome difference for death, myocardial infarction, need for dialysis, or stroke

29.5 Postoperative Care

Disposition: Patients with significant comorbidity who have undergone major surgery are very likely to require monitoring and intervention that is beyond the general ward or floor environment.

Fluid management: Monitor fluid balance closely and where possible aim for neutral balance for the perioperative period by 48 h after surgery. Fluid overload should be strenuously avoided, and this may require the earlier use of vasopressor agents. Maintenance intravenous fluids, if administered, should be given in low volumes depending on urine output and insensible loss, for example, modern enhanced recovery programs tend to use a restrictive maintenance regimen of 0.5–0.66 ml/kg/h assuming normal urine output. Bolus doses of balanced crystalloid can be used to maintain stability or deal with acute losses when blood is not required. There is no clear utility to monitoring central venous pressure or PAWP as these bear little relation to fluid responsiveness. However, CVP is still a commonly used measure and may be more useful as a warning of venous congestion.

Cardiovascular goals: Blood pressure should be maintained within 25 % of baseline values, and ECG monitoring should be continued in high-risk patients for at least the first 72 h.

Laboratory testing: Arterial blood gases, CBC, urea (BUN), creatinine, and electrolytes should be followed to maintain an adequate pH and hematocrit and to enable correction of dysnatremia and dyskalemia. pH should be maintained above 7.3, taking into account the potential for mild respiratory acidosis from the effects of pain or analgesics.

Analgesia: A multimodal analgesic regimen is recommended, including the use of local anesthesia (nerve blocks or infiltration techniques), acetaminophen, and judicious opioid for severe pain that is limiting mobilization and return of function.

Nutrition: This should be recommenced as soon as possible after surgery, ideally via the gut as opposed to parenteral nutrition. Even small volumes of enteral feeding have a trophic effect on gut mucosa and help maintain gut-associated lymphoid tissue.

Medications: Patients should recommence their normal anti-ischemia, antihypertensive, and heart failure medications as soon as their hemodynamic status, kidney function, and fluid losses are suitable for this. This is often done as a staged reintroduction of drug classes.

Before You Finish: Practice Pearls for the Clinician

- Identify and stage patients with chronic kidney disease presenting for surgery and assess their comorbidities.
- Look for areas where general medical status can be optimized prior to surgery.
- Consider all CKD patients to be at risk of cardiovascular complications and acute kidney injury in the perioperative period and patients with ≥ stage 3 CKD to be at high risk for morbidity and mortality.
- Consider cardiopulmonary exercise testing (CPET) for high-risk patients to assess functional capacity, oxygen demand, and delivery. Patients with anaerobic threshold < 11 ml/kg/min are high risk.
- Use additional hemodynamic monitoring and management in a step-down or ICU setting for high-risk cases.
- Avoid the use of nephrotoxic drugs where possible, and use opioids with caution.
- Avoid the temptation to repeatedly give intravenous fluids for hypotension if this is not effective or the effects are very temporary – fluid overload is nephrotoxic!
- There is no magic bullet for renal protection – careful attention to the basics of oxygenation, hydration, and perfusion is the key.

References

1. Snyder JJ, Foley RN, Collins AJ. Prevalence of CKD in the United States: a sensitivity analysis using the National Health and Nutrition Examination Survey (NHANES) 1999–2004. Am J Kidney Dis. 2009;53:218–28.
2. U S Renal Data System. USRDS 2012 annual data report: atlas of chronic kidney disease and end-stage renal disease in the United States. Bethesda: National Institutes of Health, National Institute of Diabetes and Digestive and Kidney Diseases; 2012.
3. Craig RG, Hunter JM. Recent developments in the perioperative management of adult patients with chronic kidney disease. Br J Anaesth. 2008;101: 296–310.
4. Charytan DM, Yang SS, McGurk S, Rawn J. Long and short-term outcomes following coronary artery bypass grafting in patients with and without chronic kidney disease. Nephrol Dial Transplant. 2010;25:3654–63.
5. Canedo J, Ricciardi K, DaSilva G, Rosen L, Weiss EG, Wexner SD. Are postoperative complications more common following colon and rectal surgery in patients with chronic kidney disease? Colorectal Dis. 2013;15:85–90.
6. Ackland GA, Moran N, Cone S, Grocott MPW, Mythen MG. Chronic kidney disease and postoperative morbidity after elective orthopedic surgery. Anesth Analg. 2011;112:1375–81.
7. Dumonteil N, van der Boon RMA, Tchetche D, Chieffo A, Van Mieghem NM, Marcheix B, et al. Impact of preoperative chronic kidney disease on short- and long-term outcomes after transcatheter aortic valve implantation: a Pooled-RotterdAm-Milano-Toulouse In Collaboration Plus (PRAGMATIC-Plus) initiative substudy. Am Heart J. 2013;165(5):752–60. doi:10.1016/j.ahj.2012.12.013.
8. Stevinkel P. Chronic kidney disease: a public health priority and harbinger of premature cardiovascular disease. J Intern Med. 2010;268:456–67.
9. Bolignano D, Rastelli S, Agarwal R, Fliser D, Massy Z, Ortiz A, et al. Pulmonary hypertension in CKD. Am J Kidney Dis. 2013;61:612–22.
10. KDIGO Clinical Practice Guideline for the Evaluation and Management of Chronic Kidney Disease. Chapter 1: Definition and classification of CKD. Kidney Int Suppl. 2013;Suppl 3:19–62.
11. Cardiovascular disease in CKD [Internet]. London: The Renal Association; 2010 [Updated 2010 August 6; cited 2013 April 4]. Available from: http://www.renal.org/Clinical/GuidelinesSection/CardiovascularDiseaseInCKD.aspx.
12. Horlocker TT, Wedel DJ, Rowlingson JC, Enneking FK, Kopp SL, Benzon HT, et al. Regional anesthesia in the patient receiving antithrombotic or thrombolytic therapy: American Society of Regional Anesthesia and Pain Medicine evidence-based guidelines. 3rd Ed. Reg Anesth Pain Med. 2010;35:64–101.
13. American College of Cardiology Foundation/American Heart Association Task Force on Practice Guidelines, Fleisher LA, Beckman JA, Brown KA, Calkins H, Chaikof EL, Fleischmann KE, et al. 2009 ACCF/AHA focused update on perioperative beta blockade incorporated into the ACC/AHA 2007 guidelines on perioperative cardiovascular evaluation and care for noncardiac surgery. J Am Coll Cardiol. 2009;54:e13.
14. The Task Force for Preoperative Cardiac Risk Assessment and Perioperative Cardiac Management in Non-cardiac Surgery of the European Society of Cardiology (ESC) and endorsed by the European Society of Anaesthesiology (ESA), Poldermans D, Bax JJ, Boersma E, De Hert S, et al. Pre-operative cardiac risk assessment and perioperative cardiac management in non-cardiac surgery. Eur Heart J. 2009;30:2769–812. Available from: http://www.escardio.org/guidelines-surveys/esc-guidelines/Pages/perioperative-cardiac-care.aspx.
15. Hltaky MA, Boineau RE, Higginbotham MB, Lee KI, Mark DB, Califf RM, et al. A brief self-administered questionnaire to determine functional capacity (The Duke Activity Status Index). Am J Cardiol. 1989;64:651–4.
16. Guazzi M, Adams V, Conraads V, Halle M, Mezzani A, Vanhees L, et al., European Association for Cardiovascular Prevention & Rehabilitation; American Heart Association. EACPR/AHA Scientific Statement. Clinical recommendations for cardiopulmonary exercise testing data assessment in specific patient populations. Circulation. 2012;126:2261–74.
17. Kidney Disease: Improving Global Outcomes (KDIGO) Blood Pressure Work Group. KDIGO clinical practice guideline for the management of blood pressure in chronic kidney disease. Kidney Int Suppl. 2012;2:337–414.
18. Kidney Disease: Improving Global Outcomes (KDIGO) Anemia Work Group. KDIGO clinical practice guideline for anemia in chronic kidney disease. Kidney Int Suppl. 2012;2:279–335.
19. Hedges SJ, Dehoney SB, Hooper JS, Amanzadeh J, Busti AJ. Evidence-based treatment recommendations for uremic bleeding. Nat Clin Pract Nephrol. 2007;3:138–53.
20. Trainor D, Borthwick E, Ferguson A. Perioperative management of the hemodialysis patient. Semin Dial. 2011;24:314–26.
21. Alsabbagh MA, Asmar A, Ejazc NI, Aiyer RK, Kambhampati G, Ejaz AA. Update on clinical trials for the prevention of acute kidney injury in patients undergoing cardiac surgery. Am J Surg. 2013;206(1):86–95. doi:10.1016/j.amjsurg.2012.08.007.

Chronic Kidney Disease in the Elderly

30

Kai Ming Chow and Philip Kam-tao Li

Before You Start: Facts You Need to Know

- The prevalence of chronic kidney disease increases with the population age.
- Greater longevity and the aging population might contribute to the higher disease burden of chronic kidney disease and potentially higher prevalence of end-stage renal disease.
- Age-related decline in many physiologic systems results in susceptibility to sudden health status changes triggered by minor stressor events, including the increased risk of acute kidney injury and the propensity to developing chronic kidney disease.
- Age-specific cut-points for kidney function and/or chronic kidney disease staging are still debatable, but equations to estimate glomerular filtration rate in the elderly might have to be modified.

30.1 Aging and Chronic Kidney Disease

A rapidly aging population has been observed worldwide, from 461 million people older than 65 years in 2004 to an estimated two billion people by 2050 [1]. By that day, we believe that the number of persons older than 65 years will exceed that of children under the age of 15 years. Population surveys worldwide have repeatedly shown a positive association between increased age and the prevalence of chronic kidney disease. In a cross-sectional survey of a nationally representative sample of 47,204 Chinese adults, the overall prevalence of chronic kidney disease was 10.8 %, whereas the odds ratio for estimated glomerular filtration rate less than 60 ml/min/1.73 m^2 was 1.74 for each individual 10 years older [2]. It becomes apparent that such aging population has profound implication for nephrologists who are seeing more elderly with chronic kidney disease. The continued expansion of end-stage renal disease prevalence is to be expected with greater longevity of the population.

The elderly is notable for their diminishing physiologic reserves available to meet challenges to homeostasis. This concept is known as *homeostenosis*, referring to the increased vulnerability to disease from maturity to senescence. An additional concept, known as *frailty*, refers to the state when physiologic reserves are maximally invoked just to maintain homeostasis and any challenges or minor stressor events will cross

K.M. Chow, MBChB, FRCP
Division of Nephrology, Department of Medicine and Therapeutics, Prince of Wales Hospital, Chinese University of Hong Kong, Shatin, Hong Kong
e-mail: chow_kai_ming@alumni.cuhk.net

P.K.-t. Li, MD, FRCP, FACP (✉)
Department of Medicine and Therapeutics, Prince of Wales Hospital, Chinese University of Hong Kong, Shatin, Hong Kong
e-mail: philipli@cuhk.edu.hk

M. Arici (ed.), *Management of Chronic Kidney Disease*,
DOI 10.1007/978-3-642-54637-2_30, © Springer-Verlag Berlin Heidelberg 2014

some threshold and thus susceptibility to sudden health status changes [1]. The concept of frailty provides a good explanation for the frequent observation that age older than 65 is a risk factor for nonrecovery from acute kidney injury and even progression to severe chronic kidney disease.

It is important to take precaution and keep in mind the renal changes with aging. On the basis of the available evidence, our practice is to consider the changes in terms of anatomic and functional changes (Box 30.1). Proposed anatomic changes of the kidneys with aging are decrease in renal mass, the loss of renal mass primarily being the cortical area and up to 40 % in patients in their eighties. Although there is no standard reference table for normal kidney size or pole-to-pole kidney length according to age, the general consensus is that a normal kidney size for a 40-year-old man can differ from that of a 70-year-old man. Cross-sectional computed tomography studies of patients without evidence of renal disease reported an age-related renal parenchymal thickness loss of 10 % per decade of increasing age in both men and women. The loss of the functional renal parenchyma appears to start from the fifth decade and is often compensated by an increase in peripelvic fat.

A series of pathologic studies have documented a reduced number of functioning glomeruli and an increased number of sclerotic glomeruli with age. A philosophical but pertinent question is how much of histologic abnormalities are normal aging process and how much of them represent disease processes. One of the important studies, based on the core-needle renal biopsy of over 1,000 healthy adult living kidney donors [3], provided a unique opportunity to evaluate the renal histology findings in relation to the age. The prevalence of nephrosclerosis, as defined by the presence of two or more different histology abnormalities (global glomerulosclerosis, tubular atrophy, interstitial fibrosis, arteriosclerosis) increased linearly with age. The prevalence was reported at 55 % among patients aged 60–69 years and up to 75 % among those older than 70 years. Such abnormalities, on the other hand, occur in only 3 % of donors 18–29 years old [3]. *The average age-related decline in glomerular filtration rate has been reported as 6 ml/min/1.73 m^2 with each age decade.* Most interestingly, there was a lack of association between the age-related decline in glomerular filtration rate and nephrosclerosis. Further studies are awaited to determine whether age-specific glomerular filtration rate classification is appropriate. For the time being, data are insufficient to support the idea of lower age-specific glomerular filtration rate cutoffs for chronic kidney disease staging. In particular, a large collaborative meta-analysis by the Chronic Kidney Disease Prognosis Consortium [4] has addressed

Box 30.1. The Aging Kidney: Anatomic and Functional Changes

Anatomic Changes: Age-Related Changes in the Kidney

- Decrease in renal size, with thickness of renal parenchyma
- Increase in renal fat and fibrosis
- Increase in number of sclerotic glomeruli

Functional Changes: Age-Related Changes in the Kidney

- Decrease in renal blood flow
- Decrease in glomerular filtration rate (linear relationship with age)
- Decrease in maximal urine concentrating and diluting capacity (explaining the higher rate of nocturia and predisposition to dehydration, respectively)
- Decrease in functional reserve (explaining the increased risk of acute kidney injury)
- Impaired recovery after renal insults
- Increased dependence on renal prostaglandins to maintain intrarenal perfusion
- Increased susceptibility to nephrotoxicity related to medications or intravenous contrast
- Decrease in plasma renin activity and plasma aldosterone level

this question after combining data from over two million participants across 46 cohorts in 40 countries. Analysis of individual-level data, with a mean follow-up of 5.8 years, showed that lower glomerular filtration rate was associated with higher risk of mortality and kidney failure in every age category. Although the relative risks for mortality were attenuated with older age, the absolute risks were higher in the older age groups [4].

While the kidney is one of the organs that age fastest, our understanding of the aging kidney has recently made similarly fast advance. New insight has been provided about pathways and mediators of aging and renal senescence. Critical telomere shortening, increased cell-cycle inhibition, inflammation with accelerated apoptosis, oxidative stress, intrarenal vessel reduction and simplification and mitochondrial injury have been implicated. In particular, renal sirtuins may be essential in protecting the kidneys from aging and promoting longevity.

30.2 Estimating GFR in the Elderly

If there are multiple effects of aging on the kidneys, the question that follows is whether a special equation to estimate glomerular filtration rate or kidney function in the elderly would have been necessary.

Accurate assessment of renal function remains difficult in the elderly because creatinine production decreases with age. Net reabsorption of creatinine in the renal tubules has been reported in healthy elderly persons, and this might in turn underestimate the glomerular filtration rate. Although most of the commonly used equations listed in Chap. 2 factor age into the estimation of glomerular filtration rate, elderly subjects are underrepresented ins the data sets originally used to derive the equation. The presence of sarcopenia affects the accuracy of creatinine to estimate glomerular filtration rate because the creatinine-based equations correct for body surface area only and do not adjust for muscle mass. The need for a new equation for this unique population of older adults has been advocated and mostly for those older than 65 years. Most of the validated equations are listed in Table 30.1 [5–9], including those incorporating cystatin C in the preferred equations. In part, these results are consistent with the findings from the previous community-based Cardiovascular Health Study, in which cystatin C was a stronger predictor of the risk of cardiovascular events and death than creatinine among adults older than 65 years [10].

30.3 Management of CKD in the Elderly

Priorities in the management of chronic kidney disease in the elderly are similar to those of younger patients: careful assessment of the stage of disease, elimination of factors for acute deterioration, evaluation of any complication or comorbidity and monitoring of the kidney disease. Few important exceptions exist, however.

Safety and efficacy of many medications are often extrapolated from key studies that implicitly or explicitly exclude participants who are older than 70. Results of trials which have enrolled older adults, if any, often conflict with those involving younger low-risk populations. Caution should therefore be exercised when prescribing medications in the elderly. A notable example is angiotensin-converting enzyme (ACE) inhibitor or angiotensin II receptor blocker. Although targeting the renin-angiotensin-aldosterone system is a well-recognised and logical therapeutic approach in chronic kidney disease, elderly patients treated with this class of antihypertensive therapy need more frequent laboratory monitoring. Excessive kidney adverse events after renin-angiotensin-aldosterone system blockade in the elderly are driven by many factors (Box 30.2). Special attention should be given to patient education: the elderly should be informed to avoid concurrent use of nonsteroidal anti-inflammatory drug (NSAID) so as to minimise the risk of acute kidney injury. Recently, increased risk of acute kidney injury has been suggested in patients with concurrent use of triple therapy consisting of diuretics with ACE inhibitor (or angiotensin receptor blocker) and NSAID. Elderly patients might have an even higher risk because of their predisposition to a

Table 30.1 Characteristics of glomerular filtration rate (GFR) estimation methods in the elderly

Diagnostic test study	Number and characteristics of subjects	Reference method to measure GFR	Equations	Comments
Schaeffner et al. [5]	610 participants of a large insurance company (community-based population living in Berlin), aged 70 years or older (mean age 78.5 years)	Iohexol plasma clearance measurement	BIS2 (Berlin Initiative Study) equation for GFR (ml/min/1.73 m^2) = 767 × cystatin C (mg/l)$^{-0.61}$ × creatinine (mg/dl)$^{-0.40}$ × age$^{-0.57}$ × 0.87 (if female) BIS1 (Berlin Initiative Study) equation for GFR (ml/min/1.73 m^2) = 3736 × creatinine (mg/dl)$^{-0.87}$ × age$^{-0.95}$ × 0.82 (if female)	BIS2 equation has the smallest bias (followed by BIS1 and Cockcroft-Gault equations), whereas MDRD study equation considerably overestimated GFR Lowest total misclassification rate for BIS2 equation using the criterion of GFR less than 60 ml/min/1.73 m^2 Subsequent validation in cohorts of 332 Chinese patients, 224 white patients, and 609 patients in France
Kilbride et al. [7]	364 participants recruited from the nephrology clinic and the community in East Kent (Southern England), aged 74 years or older (median age 80 years)	Iohexol plasma clearance measurement	CKD-EPI$_{cr}$ equation for GFR (ml/min/1.73 m^2)	CKD-EPI$_{cr}$ equation less biased and more accurate than the MDRD study equation (particularly at GFR ≥ 60 ml/min/1.73 m^2) Limited to European ancestry population
Shastri et al. [6]	1,028 participants from a large longitudinal study of community-dwelling adults (the Cardiovascular Health Study All Stars), aged 65 years or older (mean age 86 years)	None	One-variable cystatin C equation (eGFR$_{CYS1var}$) for GFR (ml/min/1.73 m^2) = 76.7 × cystatin C (mg/l)$^{-1.19}$	One-variable cystatin C equation yielded the lowest prevalence of chronic kidney disease (than the CKD-EPI and cystatin C three-variable equations) but the strongest association with prevalent cardiovascular disease No direct measurement of glomerular filtration rate
Bevc et al. [9]	317 participants from a referral cohort for ^{51}Cr-EDTA clearance, aged 65 or older (mean age 72.7 years)	^{51}Cr-EDTA clearance measurement	CKD-EPI creatinine and cystatin formula for GFR (ml/min/1.73 m^2) = 177.6 × cystatin C (mg/l)$^{-0.57}$ × creatinine (mg/dl)$^{-0.65}$ × age$^{-0.2}$ × 0.82 (if female)	

Abbreviation: *CKD-EPI* chronic kidney disease epidemiology collaboration, *GFR* glomerular filtration rate, *MDRD* modification of diet in renal disease, *cr* serum creatinine expressed in mg/dl

drastic hypovolaemia exerted by diuretics, which is further exacerbated by the vasoconstrictive effect of NSAID. In another scenario, an elderly can be encountered in the hospital after poor oral intake and community-acquired pneumonia if the elderly is accustomed to taking an ACE inhibitor for hypertension. The appropriate treatment in this situation would be withholding the ACE inhibitor and resuming drug treatment only after the infection has been treated and the extracellular fluid volume has been restored. Moreover, combination therapy with angiotensin-converting enzyme inhibitor and angiotensin II receptor blocker is not advised in the elderly. A legitimate question, on the other hand, is whether an ACE inhibitor (or angiotensin II receptor blocker) is the best option for an elderly with chronic kidney disease. Treatment decision becomes more

Box 30.2. Why Do We Have Safety Concerns with Renin-Angiotensin-Aldosterone System Blockade in the Elderly?

Physiologic changes	Decrease in renal blood flow
	Impairment of renal autoregulation or myogenic reflex to have vasodilatation (hyaline arteriosclerosis and myointimal hyperplasia)
	Decrease in renal tubular function
Hormonal changes	Decrease in plasma renin activity and plasma aldosterone level
	Reduction in nitric oxide production
Vascular changes	Increase prevalence of renal artery stenosis
	Increase in glomerular sclerosis and interstitial fibrosis
Comorbidity	Propensity to volume depletion
	Increase prevalence of diabetes, frequent use of nonsteroidal anti-inflammatory drugs

complex when there are competing health priorities (such as difficult pain control of arthritis without NSAID) and a social situation (such as caregiver burnout from bringing a demented octogenarian repeatedly to the clinic for laboratory testing for serum creatinine and potassium levels after ACE inhibitor treatment). In the setting of elderly patients with chronic kidney disease, the prevalence of low glomerular filtration rate is more common than that of albuminuria. Because the body of evidence supporting the use of ACE inhibitor or angiotensin II receptor blocker is most applicable in proteinuric kidney disease, the indication to choose this class of medication might be relatively less pressing among elderly patients. In fact, the last decade has seen a switch in treatment paradigm for managing geriatric population; clinicians are led to rethink if the traditional disease-based approach should be refined to favour an individualised patient-centred care approach [11]. Efforts have been made to directly address geriatric syndromes in older adults with chronic kidney disease. An individualised patient-centred care approach, as summarised in Table 30.2, appears

Table 30.2 Characteristics of disease-based versus individualised patient-centred approaches in managing elderly patients with chronic kidney disease

	Disease-based approach	Individualised patient-centred approach
Rationale	Most appropriate to provide a simple framework applicable to target well-defined population (versus individual level) with chronic kidney disease	More applicable to older individuals with heterogeneity in health status, multiple different comorbid conditions
	Single disease process	More than one disease processes (complexity)
Clinical decision-making	Focus on prevention, diagnosis and treatment of chronic kidney disease process	Focus on the priorities and preferences of individual patients
	Priorities include nephrology follow-up and blood pressure control to slow down kidney disease progression	Priority list depends on exploring concerns and preferences of the elderly patient and/or caregivers
Treatment goal	Focus on clinical outcomes most relevant to the underlying kidney disease process	Focus on clinical outcomes that matter most to the patient
	Survival is often considered to be the most important outcome	Quality of life, functional status, pain control and independence can take precedence over patient survival outcome
	Blood pressure control, proteinuria reduction and preservation of kidney function, cardiovascular risk reduction often emphasised	Can be modified and negotiable: example of blood pressure and kidney function trade-offs after taking NSAID to alleviate pain, allowing freedom to lead a more active life
Implication	Standardised	Dynamic
	Outcome assessment and performance easily measured	Less easy to teach and quantify

to be more relevant in addressing the complex interplay of pathologic processes, aging, social and psychological factors. As we learn more about the frailty of geriatric patients, the role of individualised patient-centred care approach is now being recognised to be appropriate for those with more comorbidities and functional impairments.

Similar concerns may apply to other aspects of the treatment goal in elderly patients. Special consideration is often necessary for blood pressure and glucose control in the elderly. As a general rule, antihypertensive medication should not be withheld simply because the patient is very elderly. A randomised controlled trial, involving 3,845 patients older than 85 years with systolic hypertension, confirmed the benefit of active treatment with a 30 % reduction in fatal and non-fatal stroke, as well as a 21 % reduction in all-cause mortality [12]. Despite the proven benefits of antihypertensive medication in the elderly, clinicians and health-care providers should consider dietary lifestyle intervention (including reduced sodium intake and weight loss). This has been shown to reduce the need for antihypertensive medication (number and dosage) in older patients. The effect of dietary sodium restriction and weight loss (to <20 % above ideal body weight for height) is well established and should be advised in the elderly patients. This is especially important in older patients who have high potential for medication-related adverse effects. There are also concerns with age-related alteration in drug distribution and metabolism and quality-of-life issues. When drug treatment is needed, timing of taking antihypertensive medication warrants consideration. As previously tested in adult patients with chronic kidney disease (not exclusive to elderly patients), taking at least one antihypertensive medication at bedtime reduces cardiovascular events compared with taking all medications in the morning [13]. The Kidney Disease: Improving Global Outcomes Clinical Practice Guideline for management of blood pressure in chronic kidney disease [14] did not grade the recommendation in elderly patients with chronic kidney disease, but acknowledged the concept of increased hazards of trying to achieve target blood pressure in these patients. Individualised treatment is the key, with close attention to adverse events, orthostatic hypotension and drug side effects [14]. Orthostatic hypotension should be watched out in older adults taking antihypertensive medication and is defined as a systolic blood pressure decrease of 20 mmHg or more or a diastolic blood pressure decrease of 10 mmHg or more, within 3 min of assuming an erect posture. Combination therapy appears to be superior to treatment with high-dose ACE inhibitor or high-dose angiotensin II receptor blocker among elderly chronic kidney disease patients. A recent multicentre study randomised elderly Japanese patients (65–84 years) to high-dose angiotensin II receptor blocker alone or standard dose angiotensin II receptor blocker in combination with a calcium-channel blocker [15]. Significantly more cardiovascular events, non-cardiovascular deaths and cerebrovascular and heart failure events occurred in the high-dose angiotensin II receptor blocker treatment group [15]. It should be noted that such differences were not found among patients without chronic kidney disease. In other words, elderly patients who have chronic kidney disease deserve special attention to the way how blood pressure control is controlled; better protection against cardiovascular events can be achieved by drug combination than a strategy of high-dose of angiotensin II receptor blockade alone. Given the previously discussed concerns with renin-angiotensin-aldosterone system blockade in the elderly (Box 30.2), a tablet combining the second drug is probably more desirable than escalating the dose of ACE inhibitor or angiotensin II receptor blocker when target blood pressure is not achieved.

Elderly patients with diabetes mellitus and stages 3–4 chronic kidney disease, for instance, have particular needs that differ significantly from those of younger patients. The assumption that the same treatment approaches for the younger age groups can be uniformly applied to the elderly has been called into question. Since frail elderly patients have high hypoglycaemic risk, it is reasonable to target a less stringent glycosylated haemoglobin level in elderly patients with chronic kidney disease. No randomised, controlled trials have been performed to assess the impact of strict glucose control on primary cardiovascular disease prevention for elderly patients with diabetes (whereas this effect is not even demonstrated in young adults). The beneficial effects of lipid-lowering therapy can be evident as early as 6 months to 2 years and should be considered appropriate even in elderly subjects. In fact, the relative reduction of cardiovascular disease with serum low density lipoprotein cholesterol reduction has been shown to be comparable between elderly and younger patients. Statins are the drug of choice, and their safety profile is similar for younger and older patients. As advised by the latest American College of Cardiology / American Heart Association guideline on treatment of blood cholesterol, patients older than 75 years with clinical atherosclerotic cardiovascular disease) should be offered moderate-intensity statin therapy (whereas high-intensity statin are more appropriate for age <75). On the other hand, fibrates are preferably avoided in elderly patients with chronic kidney disease because new prescription of fibrates has been associated with increases in serum creatinine level and increases in hospitalisations and nephrologist consultation in a population-based cohort of community-dwelling subjects aged 66 years or older [16].

The management of elderly patients with advanced or stage 4 chronic kidney disease deserves special consideration. Another important concern in the management of chronic kidney disease is the rate of progression of kidney function among elderly patients. Information of their glomerular filtration rate decline is best sought from prospective longitudinal study in this population. Elderly patients and their families should be reassured that according to a large community-based cohort of over 10,000 elderly older than 66 years, the majority of them had minimal or no progression of kidney disease over a median follow-up of 2 years. The study reported a relatively slow rate of decline in estimated glomerular filtration rate for elderly women and men without diabetes mellitus: 0.8 and 1.4 ml/min/1.73 m^2, respectively [17]. To aid clinical decision and better inform the treatment planning, such as identifying older adults at low risk of developing end-stage renal disease within 1 year, new models with good predictive ability have been proposed and validated [18].

Overall, among chronic kidney disease patients, the outcome event of end-stage renal disease is far less common than death and cardiovascular events. And this observation is of particular relevance for older patients with chronic kidney disease. In other words, the relative risk of progression to end-stage renal disease among patients with chronic kidney disease decreases with age. It is important to keep in mind that older persons with moderate chronic kidney disease are more likely to die (and less likely to reach end-stage renal disease) compared with their younger counterparts. Although age itself is not a contraindication for transplantation, the access to transplantation for the elderly is often limited by the allocation system, patient eligibility and other comorbidities. Other options for the elderly with advanced chronic kidney disease include dialysis and conservative management. To put the epidemiological results into clinical perspective, the clinicians and caring team should take into consideration the patient's life expectancy (and overall quality of life) before referring an elderly patient with glomerular filtration rate between 15 and 20 ml/min/1.73 m^2 for surgical creation of a vascular access. For example, a US study had previously showed that among 85–100-year-olds with an estimated glomerular filtration rate lower than 15 ml/min/1.73 m^2, only one in four patients started dialysis within 6 months, and one in three started dialysis within a year [19]. Trade-off in early fistula creation is unnecessary and a costly surgical procedure. *If we advocate routine referral for access at a glomerular filtration rate threshold of 15 ml/min/1.73 m^2 among elderly chronic kidney disease patients with a 6-month survival, three accesses would have to be created for every access used.* Besides haemodialysis, peritoneal dialysis can be another option for renal replacement therapy for the elderly. Advantages include its nature of home-based treatment and avoidance of the haemodynamic changes. Avoiding the need for travel to the haemodialysis units might be more attractive for the frail elderly. Assisted peritoneal dialysis, defined as peritoneal dialysis performed at the patients' home with the assistance of a health-care technician, a community nurse, a family member or a partner, is another option for those elderly incapable of performing peritoneal dialysis exchanges.

In addition to the judicious vascular access planning and the choice of peritoneal dialysis, the importance of discussing the risks and benefits of dialysis in the elderly is supported by the finding that increasing age represents a significant risk factor for dialysis withdrawal. As many as 35 % of elderly patients in the United States discontinue dialysis according to the US Renal Data System (USRDS) annual data reports. Compared with nondialytic conservative management, elderly patients who undergo dialysis can expect to spend more of their remaining life years in dialysis units or in the hospital and are two to three times more likely to die in the hospital [18]. Since accumulating data suggest an association between chronic kidney disease and increased risk for cognitive decline and dementia, detailed assessment of the functional status such as the elderly's ability to walk, bath, dress and use the toilet should be made. The decision to initiate dialysis in frail elderly patients is complex and should be a joint decision (between patients and care team) after full disclosure of the pros and cons. Before initiation of dialysis, elderly patients and family should be informed about its modest benefit in this age group and the possibility of palliative care that does not involve dialysis. A contemporary study in the United States [20] confirmed that nursing home residents who were beginning to undergo dialysis showed a marked decline in functional status around the period of initiating dialysis and by 1 year after the start, only one of eight residents had functional capacity that was maintained at the predialysis level. The majority of them continued to show functional decline despite the initiation of dialysis [20].

In summary, we must define the coexistence of chronic conditions before we can effectively care for elderly subjects with chronic kidney disease. The treatment priority may differ substantially from those of younger, healthier patients with chronic kidney disease. The answer to treating chronic kidney disease in the elderly mandates the integration of geriatrics and nephrology (Box 30.3).

Box 30.3. What the Guidelines Say You Should Do

- Take into consideration age, comorbidities and other therapies, as recommended by the KDIGO Clinical Practice Guideline, and have gradual escalation of treatment of blood pressure in elderly patients with chronic kidney disease. Pay attention to treatment-related adverse events including orthostatic hypotension and electrolyte disorders.
- Inquire about postural dizziness and check for orthostatic hypotension regularly when treating elderly chronic kidney disease patients with antihypertensive drugs.
- The threshold to initiate drug therapy for patients older than 60 is 150/90 mmHg, as recommended by the Eighth Joint National Committee (JNC 8) guideline.
- In elderly chronic kidney disease patients with comorbidities or limited life expectancy and risk of hypoglycaemia, extend target HbA1c above 7.0 % (53 mmol/mol).

Source: KDIGO Blood Pressure Work Group [21], JNC 8 [22]

Before You Finish: Practice Pearls for the Clinician

- Complex comorbid conditions are more common at old age. An individualised patient-centred approach is more appropriate in managing the elderly with chronic kidney disease, in order to address the heterogeneity in their life expectancy, functional status and treatment preference.
- The safety and efficacy of recommended drug intervention are often unknown in older adults.
- Octogenarians with stage 4 chronic kidney disease are more likely to die of associated comorbidity than to require dialysis. Nephrologists should take into consideration the relatively slow decline of kidney function in the nondiabetic elderly with chronic kidney disease, instead of pursuing multiple unnecessary vascular access surgery or peritoneal dialysis catheter insertion.
- Nondialysis treatment of advanced chronic kidney disease may be a positive treatment option for elderly patients in whom dialysis is unlikely to prolong or improve quality of life.

References

1. Clegg A, Young J, Iliffe S, Rikkert MO, Rockwood K. Frailty in elderly people. Lancet. 2013;381:752–62.
2. Zhang L, Wang F, Wang L, Wang W, Liu B, Liu J, et al. Prevalence of chronic kidney disease in China: a cross-sectional survey. Lancet. 2012;379:815–22.
3. Rule AD, Arner H, Cornell LD, Taler SJ, Cosio FG, Kremers WK, et al. The association between age and nephrosclerosis on renal biopsy among healthy adults. Ann Intern Med. 2010;152:561–7.
4. Hallan SI, Matsushita K, Sang Y, et al. Age and association of kidney measures with mortality and end-stage renal disease. JAMA. 2012;308:1–12.
5. Schaeffner ES, Ebert N, Delanaye P, et al. Two novel equations to estimate kidney function in persons aged 70 years or older. Ann Intern Med. 2012;157:471–81.
6. Shastri S, Tighiouart H, Katz R, et al. Chronic kidney disease in octogenarians. Clin J Am Soc Nephrol. 2011;6:1410–7.
7. Kilbride HS, Stevens PE, Eaglestone G, et al. Accuracy of the MDRD (modification of diet in renal disease) study and CKD-EPI (CKD epidemiology collaboration) equations for estimation of GFR in the elderly. Am J Kidney Dis. 2013;61:57–66.
8. Levey AS, Stevens LA, Schmid CH, et al. A new equation to estimate glomerular filtration rate. Ann Intern Med. 2009;150:604–12.
9. Bevc S, Hojs R, Ekart R, Gorenjak M, Puklavec L. Simple cystatin C formula compared to sophisticated CKD-EPI formulas for estimation of glomerular filtration rate in the elderly. Ther Apher Dial. 2011;15:261–8.
10. Shlipak MG, Sarnak MJ, Katz R, Fried LF, Seliger SL, Newman AB, et al. Cystatin C and the risk of death and cardiovascular events among elderly persons. N Engl J Med. 2005;352:2049–60.
11. Bowling CB, O'Hare AM. Managing older adults with CKD: individualized versus disease-based approaches. Am J Kidney Dis. 2012;59:293–302.
12. Beckett NS, Peters R, Fletcher AE, Staessen JA, Liu L, Dumitrascu D, et al. Treatment of hypertension in patients 80 years of age or older. N Engl J Med. 2008;358:1887–98.
13. Hermida RC, Ayala DE, Mojón A, Fernández JR. Bedtime dosing of antihypertensive medications reduces cardiovascular risk in CKD. J Am Soc Nephrol. 2011;22:2313–21.
14. Wheeler DC, Becker GJ. Summary of KDIGO guideline. What do we really know about management of blood pressure in patients with chronic kidney disease? Kidney Int. 2013;83:377–83.
15. Kim-Mitsuyama S, Ogawa H, Matsui K, Jinnouchi T, Jinnouchi H, Arakawa K, OSCAR Study Group. An angiotensin II receptor blocker-calcium channel blocker combination prevents cardiovascular events in elderly high-risk hypertensive patients with chronic kidney disease better than high-dose angiotensin II receptor blockade alone. Kidney Int. 2013;83:167–76.
16. Zhao YY, Weir MA, Manno M, Cordy P, Gomes T, Hackam DG, et al. New fibrate use and acute renal outcomes in elderly adults: a population-based study. Ann Intern Med. 2012;156:560–9.
17. Hemmelgam BR, Zhang J, Manns BJ, Tonelli M, Larsen E, Ghali WA, et al. Progression of kidney dysfunction in the community-dwelling elderly. Kidney Int. 2006;69:2155–61.

18. Drawz PE, Goswami P, Azern R, Babineau DC, Rahman M. A simple tool to predict end-stage renal disease within 1 year in elderly adults with advanced chronic kidney disease. J Am Geriatr Soc. 2013;61:762–8.
19. O'Hare AM, Bertenthal D, Walter LC, Garg AX, Covinsky K, Kaufman JS, et al. When to refer patients with chronic kidney disease for vascular access surgery: should age be a consideration? Kidney Int. 2007;71:555–61.
20. Kurella Tamura M, Covinsky KE, Chertow GM, Yaffe K, Landefeld CS, McCulloch CE. Functional status of elderly adults before and after initiation of dialysis. N Engl J Med. 2009;361:1539–47.
21. KDIGO Blood Pressure Work Group. KDIGO clinical practice guideline for the management of blood pressure in chronic kidney disease. Kidney Int. 2012;2(Suppl):337–414.
22. James PA, Oparil S, Carter BL, et al. Evidence-based guideline for the management of high blood pressure in adults: report from the panel members appointed to the Eighth Joint National Committee (JNC 8). JAMA. 2014;311:507–20.

Chronic Kidney Disease and Cancer

31

Vincent Launay-Vacher

Before You Start: Facts You Need to Know

- Chronic kidney disease (CKD) is highly prevalent in the general population and also in cancer patients.
- Cancer prevalence is higher in the CKD population, for a number of tumors. Cancer screening in the CKD population is key, but appropriate screening tools and protocols remain to be defined.
- Measuring the actual glomerular filtration rate (GFR) of a patient (isotopic methods) is the gold standard method, but cannot be routinely performed.
- Estimating the GFR by calculations from serum creatinine can be performed.
- There are specific rules and processes to manage drugs, and especially anticancer drugs, in patients with CKD.
- Nephrotoxic drugs should be avoided, whenever possible, in patients presenting with preexisting renal impairment. In some cases, for a similar expected efficacy, several drugs may be used, among which the less nephrotoxic should be chosen. This applies, for instance and in some circumstances, to platinum salts (cisplatin being more nephrotoxic than carboplatin which is more nephrotoxic than oxalipatin) and intravenous bisphosphonates (zoledronate being more nephrotoxic than pamidronate which is more nephrotoxic than ibandronate).

31.1 Introduction

Screening for chronic kidney disease (CKD) in cancer patients is an emerging question, and this is crucial for several reasons. The first reason is the direct consequence of the better oncological care delivered to those patients which has now made cancer a chronic disease, at least for some solid tumors for which the increasing efficacy of treatments and the increasing number of treatments available, and thus the multiplication of treatment lines, allow significant survival rates for patients. In those patients, early diagnosis of CKD is a priority so that they can benefit from the advances in nephrology care. Such advances can slow the progression in the reduction of kidney function, i.e., the glomerular filtration rate (GFR), thus sparing the need for dialysis in a number of patients who will not reach the terminal stage of CKD. Furthermore, it has been clearly demonstrated that CKD is an independent risk factor for cardiovascular disease and

V. Launay-Vacher, PharmD
Service ICAR – Department of Nephrology,
Pitie-Salpetriere University Hospital,
83 Boulevard de l'Hospital, Paris 75013, France
e-mail: vincent.launay-vacher@psl.aphp.fr

M. Arici (ed.), *Management of Chronic Kidney Disease*,
DOI 10.1007/978-3-642-54637-2_31, © Springer-Verlag Berlin Heidelberg 2014

cardiovascular mortality. With the increasing survival of cancer patients, the prevention of cardiovascular morbidity and mortality has become an issue, and this requires early diagnosis of CKD. In addition, some anticancer treatments, such as anthracyclines, may also exhibit a cardiac toxicity, which may be more preoccupating in patients already at risk for cardiovascular events. The second reason is pharmacological. In patients with reduced GFR, the pharmacokinetics of drugs are modified. Adjusting drug doses to renal function is mandatory to avoid overdose and overdose-induced side effects. The pharmacokinetics and tolerance profiles for anticancer drugs are often modified in patients with CKD. In those cases, screening for abnormal GFR and adjusting anticancer drug doses allow better tolerance with maintained efficacy (see Chap. 27).

31.2 Screening for CKD in Cancer Patients

31.2.1 Evaluation of Kidney Function in Cancer Patients

Routinely measuring the actual GFR with a gold standard method such as ^{51}Cr-EDTA in all cancer patients is unrealistic. As a result, such as in the general population, it is recommended to calculate GFR from serum creatinine (SCr), with recommended formulae (see Chap. 2). In this purpose, only considering the raw value of SCr is misleading. In fact, the same SCr value may reflect totally different GFR depending on the production rate of creatinine in a particular patient, essentially from muscle catabolism. Calculating GFR (or creatinine clearance (CrCl) which is assumed to be an acceptable estimate of the GFR) with the two formulae recommended allows an appropriate evaluation of kidney function. The Cockcroft-Gault formula [1] still is the most used formula to calculate CrCl. A more recently released formula is the Modification of Diet in Renal Disease (MDRD) study formula [2].

Both formulae do not present with the same performance in terms of precision in estimating the GFR, as compared to a measured GFR, with a gold standard method. In particular, there are some special populations of patients in whom the Cockcroft-Gault formula may result in false estimates and should not be used. Those populations include patients older than 65 and patients with a body mass index greater than 30, i.e., the obese. Contrarily, the MDRD formula allows a precise estimation of the kidney function of the patient. Furthermore, in some recent studies specifically conducted in patients with cancer, the MDRD formula confirmed its better precision as compared to Cockcroft-Gault in those patients [3, 4], and it has been recommended to estimate cancer patients' kidney function with this formula, even in elderly cancer patients [5].

Once the estimation of kidney function has been performed, CKD should be defined by its stage (1–5) even in cancer patients rather than with the "ancient" terminology using terms such as "moderate" or "severe."

Particular attention should be paid to the units of the results in GFR estimates, especially when attempting to compare the performances of different formulae. On one hand, the MDRD formula gives an estimate of the GFR in mL/min/1.73 m^2. On the other hand, Cockcroft-Gault and other formulae give results in mL/min. As a result, any comparison between formulae requires prior conversion of the raw results of calculations into the same units. There are, unfortunately, a number of published studies in which such conversions were not made. Their results and conclusions can thus not be considered.

In clinical practice, estimates in both units are needed for a particular patient. The estimate in mL/min/1.73 m^2 is mandatory to diagnose CKD and stratify its stage since the international definition is based on GFR estimates expressed in this unit. The estimate expressed in mL/min is also needed to determine the precise level of kidney function (i.e., value of the GFR) to determine the adjusted dose of medications the patient will be administered. This is of a particular importance for anticancer drug management, which requires a precise dose: neither too high nor too low.

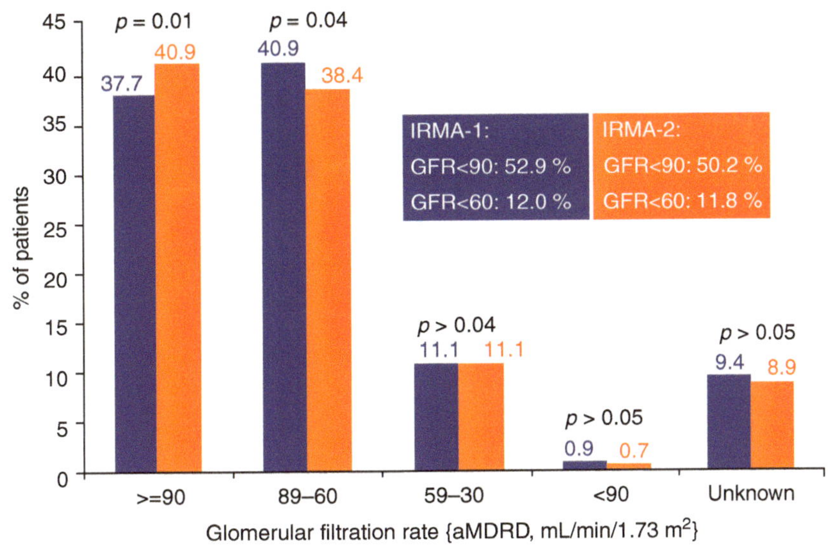

Fig. 31.1 Prevalence of kidney disease in cancer patients: IRMA-1 and IRMA-2 results

31.2.2 Prevalence of Kidney Disease in Cancer Patients

In France, two studies have recently been conducted in order to evaluate the prevalence of CKD in cancer patients, only with solid tumors, excluding patients on dialysis. Those studies called "IRMA" (Insuffisance Rénale et Médicaments Anticancéreux – Renal Insufficiency and Anticancer Medications) both demonstrated the high prevalence of CKD in those two cohorts of about 5,000 patients each [6, 7] (Fig. 31.1).

Adult patients, not on dialysis, and with a diagnosis of cancer were included in the studies. Demographical, biological, clinical, and pharmacological data were collected. Patients' kidney function was estimated with the MDRD formula. The average age of the patients was 58.1 and 59.4 years, respectively, in IRMA-1 and IRMA-2. Patients presented with different types of tumors, mainly breast, colorectal, and lung, and approximately half of them were nonmetastatic at the time of inclusion.

The prevalence of an elevated serum creatinine (SCr) value was low, and strictly the same in both studies: 7.2 % of the patients had a SCr greater than or equal to 110 μmol/L (around 1.25 md/dL). However, when the kidney function of those patients was estimated with the MDRD formula, 52.9 and 50.2 % of the patients in IRMA-1 and IRMA-2 respectively, had in fact a reduced GFR (lower than 90 mL/min/1.73 m^2) and 12.0 and 11.8 % had stage 3 or more CKD (lower than 60 mL/min/1.73 m^2) (Fig. 31.2).

In patients with kidney cancer, the study of Huang et al. is particularly interesting. The authors reported a prevalence of abnormal kidney function (lower than 90 mL/min/1.73 m^2) of 87 % in a cohort of 662 patients with a renal cortical tumor (<4 cm) and awaiting partial or radical nephrectomy. The prevalence of a GFR lower than 60 mL/min/1.73 m^2 was also high, higher than the one we reported in the IRMA studies, with 26 % of the patients with a stage 3–4 kidney disease [8]. The authors then further demonstrated that, in addition to this high prevalence of abnormal renal dysfunction prior nephrectomy, the GFR at baseline was highly predictive of developing CKD after the nephrectomy had been performed. For these reasons, evaluating kidney function with the MDRD formula is mandatory in every cancer patient, and also in kidney cancer patients.

Other studies also retrieved high prevalences of CKD in cancer patients, in Belgium [9], the United States [10], and Japan [11]. In these studies, the prevalence of a GFR lower than 60 mL/min/1.73 m^2 ranged from 16.1 to 25.0 % of patients presenting with a variety of solid tumors.

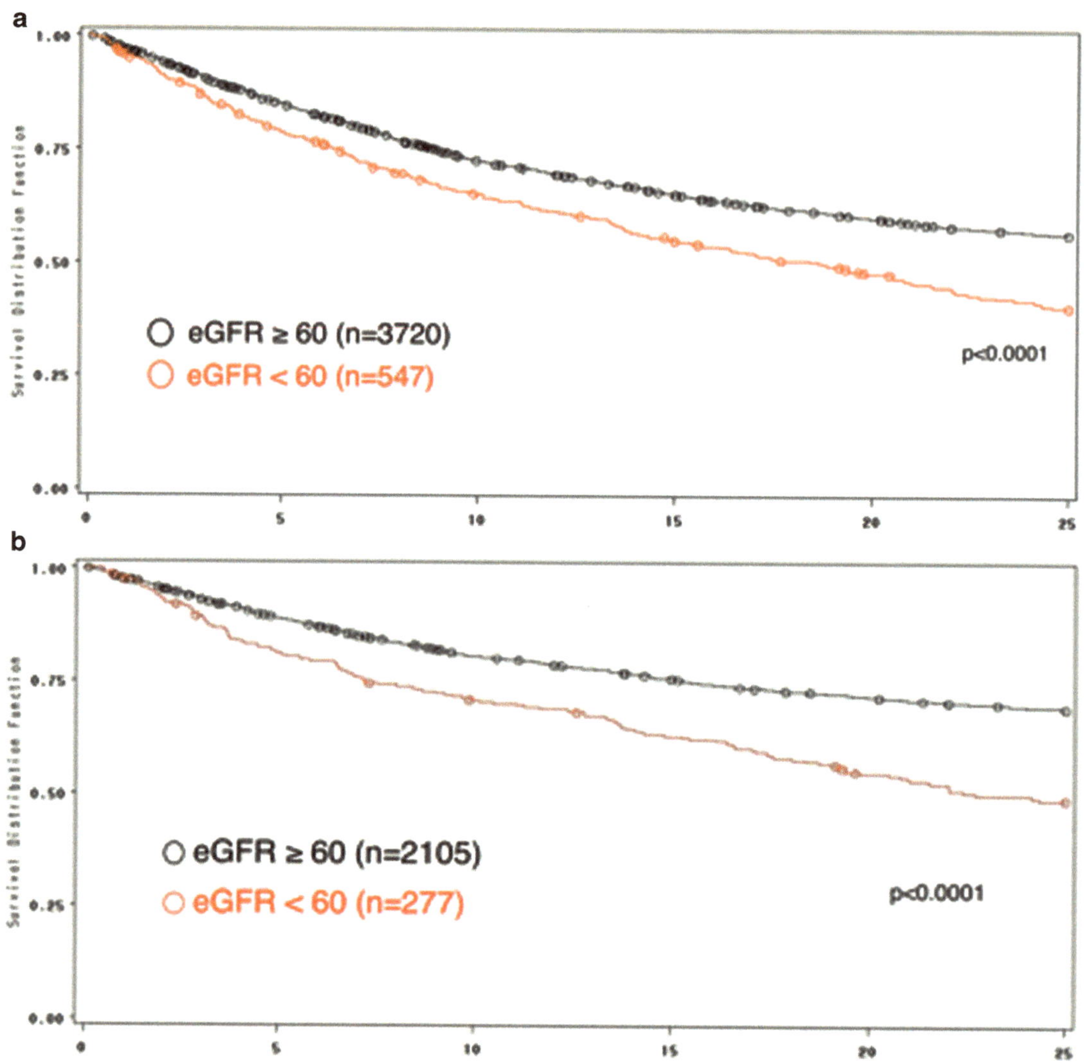

Fig. 31.2 Survival rate in IRMA-2 patients with cancer according to baseline GFR at inclusion. (**a**) All patients ($n=4267$) and (**b**) nonmetastatic patients ($n=2382$)

31.3 Consequences of Kidney Disease in Cancer Patients

31.3.1 Impact on Patient Survival

In the IRMA-2 study, the potential impact of CKD on patient survival has been assessed on a 2-year follow-up of the patients. The results showed that patients with a GFR lower than 60 mL/min/1.73 m^2 at time of inclusion in the study had a lower survival rate as compared to patients with a GFR greater than or equal to 60 mL/min/1.73 m^2 [12] (Fig. 31.3). In fact, multivariate analysis adjusted for several factors, including the age, showed that patients with a GFR lower than 60 mL/min/1.73 m^2 had a mean survival of 16.4 months as compared to 25.0 months for patients with a GFR greater than or equal to 60 mL/min/1.73 m^2 among the whole cohort of patients, whatever the type of tumor and the stage of the cancer disease ($N=4{,}267$). Considering the 2,382 patients who had a non-metastatic disease, the impact of CKD on survival was still significant with survivals of 21.0 vs. 25.0 months for patients with a GFR lower than or greater than or equal to 60 mL/min/1.73 m^2,

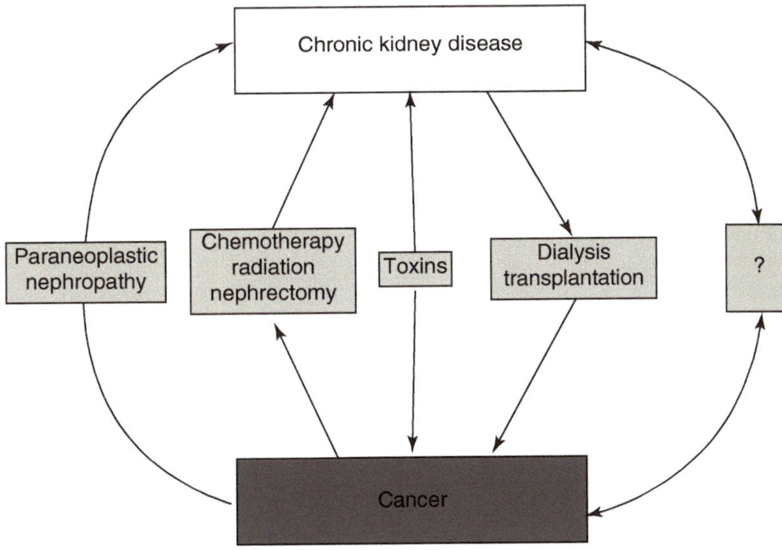

Fig. 31.3 Various pathways linking chronic kidney disease and cancer

Table 31.1 Multivariate analysis on the risk of death according to the level of renal function at inclusion in the IRMA-2 study

Population	Median survival (months)		Hazard ratio [CI 95 %] (Cox model)
	GFR ≥ 60	GFR < 60	
All patients (n=4,267)	25.0*	16.4*	1.27** [1.12–1.44]
Nonmetastatic patients (n=2,382)	25.0*	21.0*	1.42*** [1.17–1.72]

IRMA Insuffisance Rénale et Médicaments Anticancéreux *(Renal Insufficiency and Anticancer Medications)*, *GFR* glomerular filtration rate, *CI* confidence interval
*$p<0.0001$; **$p<0.0002$; ***$p<0.0003$

respectively. Hazard ratios [95 % confidence interval] were 1.27 [1.12–1.44] (p=0.0002) and 1.43 [1.17–1.72] (p=0.0003) for the whole population and the nonmetastatic population only, respectively (Table 31.1).

In Japan [11] and Korea [13], other authors reported a significantly reduced survival rate in patients with CKD. In the Korean study, the authors demonstrated that CKD was an independent predictor of cancer-specific mortality, with hazard ratios for death of 1.12 (p=0.04) and 1.75 (p<0.001) for patients with a GFR within 30 and 60 mL/min/1.73 m^2 and below 30 mL/min/1.73 m^2, respectively.

31.4 Incidence of Cancer in Kidney Disease Patients

There are multiple pathways which may link cancer and CKD [14], and the other side of the coin is the potentially higher incidence of cancers in patients with kidney disease. Wong et al. [15] demonstrated that, over a cohort of 3,654 participants, men, but not women, with at least stage 3 CKD had a significantly increased risk for cancer (test of interaction for gender p=0.004). The higher risk began at 55 mL/min/1.73 m^2, and the risk of cancer (mostly lung and urinary tract, not prostate) was increased by 29 % for each 10-mL decline in eGFR (MDRD formula).

A Danish registry study conducted over 16 years (1993–2008) reported on the incidence and prevalence of cancer in 823 patients with autosomal dominant polycystic kidney disease (APKD) and end-stage renal disease (ESRD). The authors analyze the data over two 8-year periods of time: 1993–2000 and 2001–2008. The incidence of cancer per year of risk did not change significantly: 3.1 % (95 % CI 1.8–5.4) in 1993–2000 vs. 2.6 % (95 % CI 2.1–3.3) in 2001–2008 (p=0.4). However, the average percentage in cancer prevalence gradually increased, from 10.4 % (95 % CI

Table 31.2 Unadjusted death rates from the primary causes of death in Danish patients with ADPKD and ESRD

	Time periods		
	1993–2000	2001–2008	*P*
Cardiovascular disease	40.3	26.4	<0.01
Cerebrovascular disease	17.1	4.8	<0.001
Infections	12.1	16.8	NS
Cancer	8.1	12.3	NS

Source: Reprinted from Orskov et al. [16] by permission of Oxford University Press

APKD autosomal dominant polycystic kidney disease, *ESRD* end-stage renal disease, *NS* not significant

8.1–13.3) in 1993–2000 to 14.0 % (95 % CI 12.8–15.4) in 2001–2008, resulting in a rise of 35 % ($p=0.0002$). Considering yearly prevalences, it almost doubled, from around 8.5 in 1993 to 15 in 2008 [16]. The primary causes of death among the 431 patients who died over the whole period changed when ranked according to the death rates/1,000 years on renal replacement therapy (Table 31.2). Death rates for cancer and infections did not significantly change between the two periods while deaths from cardiovascular and cerebrovascular diseases significantly decreased, by 1.5 and 3.6, respectively. This made cancer the third cause of death during the second period (2001–2008). The most frequent cancers in this population were basal cell carcinoma, squamous cell carcinoma of the skin, breast cancer, cancer of cervix uteri, melanoma, and cancers of the colon, respiratory tract, bladder, prostate, and kidney, by descending order of frequency.

Other sources suggest a number of factors which may account for increased cancer risk in CKD patients, such as defects in immunological functions secondary to uremic state, carcinogenic uremic toxins (nitrosodimethylamine), impaired antioxidant defenses, vitamin D deficiency, use of erythropoiesis-stimulating agents, cumulative immunosuppression, and risk of acquired cystic kidney disease [17]. The interpretation of usual tumor markers screening tests in ESRD patients appears to be tricky due to a high incidence of false-positive results. Tumor markers such as cancer antigen 125 (CA 125), carcinoembryonic antigen (CEA), squamous cell carcinoma antigen (SCC), or neuron-specific enolase (NSE) are glycoproteins with a relatively moderate-to-high molecular weight. They are not effectively removed by renal replacement therapies such as hemodialysis or peritoneal dialysis, and they thus may accumulate and be falsely elevated. On the opposite, alpha-fetoprotein, beta-human chorionic gonadotropin (HCG), and prostate-specific antigen (PSA) seem to be reliable. Stool occult blood testing is also altered by the high incidence of mucosal bleed and gastric and colonic angiodysplasia in patients on dialysis, and the rate of false-positive is also high. In practice, cancer screening protocols need to be modified/adjusted for ESRD patients since they may not be useful as such in these patients.

Finally, in polypathological patients, there is evidence that patients may be at increased risk for cancer, due to sequential and parallel mechanisms, e.g., diabetes. Diabetic patients are known to be at risk for developing CKD. As a result, the prevalence and the incidence of CKD in these patients are higher than in nondiabetic. Other evidence showed that these patients also present with a higher risk for cancer, especially for liver, pancreas, and endometrial cancers but also for breast, colon, kidney, and bladder cancers, of which incidences may be increased by 20–50 % as compared to nondiabetics [18].

This also emphasizes why evaluating and monitoring kidney function is also important to identify potential at-risk patients for cancer.

31.4.1 Practical Consequences on Anticancer Drugs' Handling

In patients with reduced GFR, the pharmacokinetics of drugs is most often modified. Not only the urinary route of elimination is impaired but also the other phases of the pharmacokinetics. These modifications may require dosage adjustments of anticancer medications in patients with CKD and cancer. Most often, these consist of a reduction of the administered dose in order to reduce saccumulation, overdosage, and dose-dependent side effects. However, the dose must not be too much reduced to maintain efficacy. Most often in patients whose GFR is greater than 60 mL/min, there is no need for dose adjustment and the usual dosage can be and must be used. Reducing the dose in these patients will lead to a loss in efficacy. In patients whose GFR is lower than 60, approximately 50 % of anticancer drugs require dosage reductions. Taxanes and anthracyclines usually do not require any dose modification in CKD. In contrast, platinum salts cisplatin and carboplatin require dosage adjustment, while it is not the case for oxaliplatin. Cyclophosphamide and ifosfamide may require dose reductions, but only in patients with a GFR lower than 15 mL/min. Capecitabine will require a reduction in the dose as early as the GFR is lower than 60 mL/min.

31.5 Handling of Targeted Therapies in Patients with CKD

In a recent study on the pharmacokinetics of sunitinib in patients with renal insufficiency, the authors observed a lower exposure to sunitinib in CKD patients as compared to patients with normal kidney function, suggesting a lower absorption of sunitinib from the gastrointestinal tract in patients with CKD, and thus a risk for lower exposure and lower efficacy [19].

Vandetanib is a recently approved tyrosine kinase inhibitor indicated in the treatment of aggressive and symptomatic medullary thyroid cancer. It acts on the vascular endothelial growth factor receptor 2 (VEGFR-2), the epidermal growth factor receptor (EGFR), and the RET tyrosine kinase. The drug has been shown to be eliminated via hepatic metabolism and biliary excretion as its major route of elimination, with minor urinary excretion, accounting for less than 25 % of the total elimination of the drug. However, the pharmacokinetics of vandetanib was not altered in patients with moderate-to-severe hepatic impairment, whereas significant modifications were reported in patients with renal impairment [20]. These modifications resulted in a nearly doubled exposure to vandetanib in patients with severe renal impairment as compared to patients with normal kidney function. As mentioned in the summary of product characteristics (SmPC) of the drug, total body clearance may be reduced by 30 % and area under the concentration-time curve (AUC) may be increased by 1.5–2-fold in case of renal impairment, thus requiring dose adjustment in patients with a GFR within 30–60 mL/min, to avoid overdose and toxicity. So far, no recommendation has been made for patients with a lower GFR.

Furthermore, for drugs that are almost completely degraded by the liver, the potential activity and toxicity of the metabolites have to be considered, those latter often being secondarily excreted in the urine. This is the case for the majority of tyrosine kinase inhibitors, for instance, sunitinib, sorafenib, erlotinib, and lapatinib. However, data are lacking on their pharmacokinetics, parent drug and metabolites, in patients with CKD. It is important to note that, according to available data, the pharmacokinetics of therapeutic monoclonal antibodies (rituximab, bevacizumab, trastuzumab, denosumab, cetuximab, panitumumab, etc.) are not significantly modified in patients with CKD. They thus can be used at their usual dose, whatever the level of the GFR.

This is a crucial issue in oncology. The IRMA studies demonstrated the high prevalence of CKD in patients with cancer. They further demonstrated that, in "real life," most patients received anticancer drugs that necessitated dose adjustment in case of CKD. Indeed, in the IRMA-1 study, patients were treated with a total number of 7,181 prescriptions of 75 different anticancer agents. 79.9 % of the patients received at least one drug which dose must be adjusted in case of CKD, and 80.1 % of the patients received at least one anticancer drug which may be toxic to the kidneys, which are highly vulnerable in case of preexisting CKD.

Conclusion

In cancer patients, estimating renal function with an appropriate and validated method (like MDRD) is mandatory in order to diagnose kidney disease. In patients with a reduced

GFR, specific attention should be paid to the cardiovascular system, with baseline and periodic evaluations, especially in case of anticancer treatments with potential cardiac toxicities, such as anthracyclines. Anticancer drugs' handling in those patients also requires specific evaluation. In all patients with a GFR lower than 60 mL/min, dose adjustment must be considered. Reliable and updated sources of information should be used. These latter should be evidence-based since official informations provided in drugs' SmPCs often lack precision and clarity regarding this specific topic (Box 31.1).

Box 31.1. Drug Dose Adjustment in CKD Patients: A Practical Approach

Service ICAR (Information Conseil Adaptation Rénale) is a medical advisory service offered to French nephrologists, hematologists, and oncologists, among other specialties, developed in France in 1999 as part of the Department of Nephrology of Pitié-Salpêtrière University Hospital in Paris. Physicians and clinical pharmacists of Service ICAR are available on call to help retrieve information on drug dose adjustment in patients with CKD and determine the appropriate dose of a drug, for a particular patient, based on an exhaustive literature analysis. A website has been developed in 2010 (SiteGPR® – ww.sitegpr.com) which provides healthcare professionals with evidence-based recommendations on drug dose adjustment. Recommendations are available in French and English languages.

Before You Finish: Practice Pearls for the Clinician

- A GFR estimate must be calculated with the MDRD equation in all cancer patients to screen for kidney disease.
- CKD patients are at a higher risk for a number of cancers. Usual screening protocols may need to be modified in CKD patients since there is a higher frequency of false-positive for several tumor markers.
- A GFR estimate lower than 60:
  - Is an independent risk factor for reduced survival
  - Requires drug dose adjustments to limit the risk of overdose and toxicity
- Even drugs with a major non-urinary elimination route may require dose reductions in case of reduced GFR.

References

1. Cockcroft DW, Gault MH. Prediction of creatinine clearance from serum creatinine. Nephron. 1976;16(1):31–41.
2. Levey AS, Bosch JP, Lewis JB, Greene T, Rogers N, Roth D. A more accurate method to estimate glomerular filtration rate from serum creatinine: a new prediction equation. Modification of Diet in Renal Disease Study Group. Ann Intern Med. 1999;130(6):461–70.
3. Holweger K, Lipp HP, Dietz K, Hartmann JT, Bokemeyer C. Novel algorithm for more accurate calculation of renal function in adults with cancer. Ann Pharmacother. 2008;42(12):1749–57.
4. Faluyi OO, Masinghe SP, Hayward RL, Clive S. Accuracy of GFR estimation by the Cockcroft and Gault, MDRD, and Wright equations in Oncology patients with renal impairment. Med Oncol. 2012;29(2):755–60.
5. Launay-Vacher V, Chatelut E, Lichtman SM, Wildiers H, Steer C, Aapro M. International Society of Geriatric Oncology. Renal insufficiency in elderly cancer patients: International Society of Geriatric Oncology clinical practice recommendations. Ann Oncol. 2007;18(8):1314–21.

6. Launay-Vacher V, Oudard S, Janus N, Gligorov J, Pourrat X, Rixe O, Renal Insufficiency and Cancer Medications (IRMA) Study Group, et al. Prevalence of Renal Insufficiency in cancer patients and implications for anticancer drug management: the renal insufficiency and anticancer medications (IRMA) study. Cancer. 2007;110(6):1376–84.
7. Janus N, Oudard S, Beuzeboc P, Gligorov J, Ray-Coquard I, Morere J, et al. Prevalence of renal insufficiency in cancer patients: data from the IRMA-2 study. J Clin Oncol. 2009;27:15s. suppl; abstr 9559.
8. Huang WC, Levey AS, Serio AM, Snyder M, Vickers AJ, Raj GV, et al. Chronic kidney disease after nephrectomy in patients with renal cortical tumors: a retrospective cohort study. Lancet Oncol. 2006; 7(9):735–40.
9. Janus N, Launay-Vacher V, Byloos E, Machiels JP, Duck L, Kerger J, et al. Cancer and renal insufficiency results of the BIRMA study. Br J Cancer. 2010;103(12):1815–21.
10. Canter D, Kutikov A, Sirohi M, Street R, Viterbo R, Chen DY, et al. Prevalence of baseline chronic kidney disease in patients presenting with solid renal tumors. Urology. 2011;77(4):781–5.
11. Nakamura Y, Tsuchiya K, Nitta K, Ando M. Prevalence of anemia and chronic kidney disease in cancer patients: clinical significance for 1-year mortality. Nihon Jinzo Gakkai Shi. 2011;53(1):38–45.
12. Launay-Vacher V, Janus N, Spano J, Gligorov J, Ray-Coquard I, Beuzeboc P, et al. Impact of renal insufficiency on cancer survival: results of the IRMA-2 study. J Clin Oncol. 2009;27:15s (suppl; abstr 9585).
13. Na SY, Sung JY, Chang JH, Kim S, Lee HH, Park YH, et al. Chronic kidney disease in cancer patients: an independent predictor of cancer-specific mortality. Am J Nephrol. 2011;33(2):121–30.
14. Stengel B. Chronic kidney disease and cancer: a troubling connection. J Nephrol. 2010;23(3):253–62.
15. Wong G, Hayen A, Chapman JR, Webster AC, Wang JJ, Mitchell P, et al. Association of CKD and cancer risk in older people. J Am Soc Nephrol. 2009;20(6):1341–50.
16. Orskov B, Sørensen VR, Feldt-Rasmussen B, Strandgaard S. Changes in causes of death and risk of cancer in Danish patients with autosomal dominant polycystic kidney disease and end-stage renal disease. Nephrol Dial Transplant. 2012;27(4):1607–13.
17. Nayak-Rao S. Cancer screening in end-stage renal disease. Saudi J Kidney Dis Transpl. 2009;20(5):737–40.
18. Hartmann A, Jenssen T, Holdaas H. Diabetes, chronic kidney disease and cancer risk. Nephrol Dial Transplant. 2012;27:3018–20.
19. Khosravan R, Toh M, Garrett M, La Fargue J, Ni G, Marbury TC, et al. Pharmacokinetics and safety of sunitinib malate in subjects with impaired renal function. J Clin Pharmacol. 2010;50(4):472–81.
20. Weil A, Martin P, Smith R, Oliver S, Langmuir P, Read J, et al. Pharmacokinetics of vandetanib in subjects with renal or hepatic impairment. Clin Pharmacokinet. 2010;49(9):607–18.

Chronic Kidney Disease in the Intensive Care Unit

32

Pedro Fidalgo and Sean M. Bagshaw

Before You Start: Facts You Need to Know

- CKD patients have a high prevalence of comorbid disease compared to non-CKD patients; however, CKD patients have reasonable short-term outcomes following ICU admission compared to non-CKD patients.
- The most common diagnoses contributing to ICU admission in CKD patients are sepsis and septic shock and decompensated cardiovascular disease.
- AKI is a common complication of critical illness, most often precipitated by sepsis, and remains a strong negative modifier of short- and long-term survival.
- CKD is an important and independent non-modifiable risk factor for development of AKI and long-term accelerated loss of kidney function among CKD survivor of critical illness.
- While numerous factors influence the decision to start renal replacement therapy, the most common initial modality prescribed after ICU admission worldwide remains continuous renal replacement therapy, particularly for hemodynamically unstable patients, and this may be associated with higher likelihood of recovery of renal function and dialysis independence.

32.1 Introduction

The worldwide prevalence and incidence of chronic kidney disease (CKD) and end-stage renal disease (ESRD) are increasing substantially, largely attributable to an aging population coupled with large increases in the rates of hypertension, type 2 diabetes mellitus, and obesity.

CKD patients are characterized by a higher burden of comorbid illness, including coronary artery disease, heart failure, diabetes mellitus, hypertension, and cerebrovascular disease, and generally have higher health services utilization, including rates of hospitalization, when compared to non-CKD critically ill patients. Moreover, CKD patients, in particular for the subset with

P. Fidalgo, MD
Division of Critical Care Medicine, Faculty of Medicine and Dentistry, University of Alberta, 2-124E Clinical Sciences Building, 8440-122 Street, Edmonton, AB T6G2B7, Canada

S.M. Bagshaw, MD, MSc, FRCPC (✉)
Division of Critical Care Medicine, Faculty of Medicine and Dentistry, University of Alberta, 2-124E Clinical Sciences Building, 8440-122 Street, Edmonton, AB T6G2B7, Canada

Alberta Innovates, Edmonton, AB, Canada
e-mail: bagshaw@ualberta.ca

M. Arici (ed.), *Management of Chronic Kidney Disease*,
DOI 10.1007/978-3-642-54637-2_32, © Springer-Verlag Berlin Heidelberg 2014

ESRD, have a several-fold higher risk of developing critical illness. When considering these features, coupled with rising prevalence rates, the demand for intensive care unit (ICU) support for CKD patients is expected to increase. This will likely present challenges for clinicians working in resource-limited settings regarding decision-making for ICU support for CKD patients.

32.1.1 Epidemiology of CKD and ESRD in ICU

There is limited data available on the prevalence of CKD among all critically ill patients supported in ICU settings, and most studies have focused on the subset of dialysis-dependent patients with ESRD [1]. Available data would suggest the proportion of patients admitted to ICU with ESRD ranges between 1 and 9 %. The reported variability in ESRD admissions across studies is likely accounted for by differences in practice patterns, availability of ICU resources, patient case-mix, and study design. ESRD patients have consistently been shown to have an estimated 25–30-fold higher annual likelihood of admission to ICU when compared with the non-ESRD general population.

ESRD patients admitted to ICU have several notable differences in baseline characteristics when compared with non-ESRD patients. ESRD patients are generally younger, have more comorbid disease, more likely medical (i.e., nonoperative admissions), and have higher illness severity scores compared with non-ESRD patients. However, these observations may be susceptible to selection bias. Available epidemiologic surveys of ESRD patients admitted to ICU are limited by not accounting for those patients referred and refused ICU admission.

32.1.2 Precipitants for Critical Illness in CKD and ESKD

The most common precipitants of critical illness prompting ICU admission among ESRD patients are sepsis/septic shock and decompensated cardiovascular disease including cardiogenic shock, myocardial ischemia/infarction, arrhythmic complications, and heart failure/pulmonary edema. Cardiac arrest and cardiopulmonary resuscitation (CPR) are more common events occurring among ESRD patients compared with non-ESRD prior to ICU admission. This may relate to several factors including a higher prevalence of comorbid cardiovascular disease and diminished cardiopulmonary reserve, a higher incidence of primarily arrhythmic complications, and the unique pathophysiologic stress of dialysis (i.e., rapid fluid-/electrolyte-related shifts).

32.1.3 Outcomes for CKD and ESRD in ICU

Surprisingly, the early mortality for critically ill ESRD patients is lower than for those with acute kidney injury (AKI), suggesting that the prognosis is driven largely by acute illness severity rather than baseline comorbidities. However, ESRD patients have consistently higher short-term mortality rates (9–44 %) when compared to non-AKI critically ill patients and an age- and sex-matched general population. Factors that have been shown to be associated with ICU mortality in ESRD patients are older age, higher illness severity score (i.e., APACHE II or SAPS II), burden of nonrenal organ dysfunction/failure, medical or nonsurgical admission type, and provision and duration of life-sustaining technologies (i.e., mechanical ventilation, vasopressor therapy).

Studies reporting long-term survival among ESRD patients show a trend for an increased mortality rate within the first 6 months after ICU discharge, with a relatively stable but increased risk for mortality thereafter. At 2 years after ICU admission, survival is generally poor. Observational studies estimate only 1/3 of ESRD patients admitted to ICU were still alive. Although long-term mortality in ESRD patients is several times higher when compared to the general population, the presence of ESRD does not appear to independently predict long-term mortality, suggesting short-term prognosis is more related to the acute illness severity rather than CKD and dialysis dependence.

It has been increasingly recognized that CKD influences the risk of developing AKI and that AKI per se contributes to CKD progression and incidence of ESRD. Around 50 % of patients who survive an episode of AKI requiring RRT show significant loss of glomerular filtration rate (GFR) resulting in dialysis dependence after hospital discharge in approximately 10 % of patients. The most important risk factor for incident ESRD and dialysis dependence among survivors of critical illness is prior CKD. This would suggest continued surveillance of kidney function among survivors of critical illness is vital.

Data on changes to functional status and health-related quality of life (HRQL) for ESRD patients surviving an episode of critical illness are currently lacking. However, in non-ESRD critically ill patients surviving critical illness, in particular for those with severe AKI requiring acute RRT, long-term reductions in HRQL and impaired functional status are common. These data coupled with the reduced HRQL for ESRD patients imply this may be a significant issue for survivors of critical illness.

CKD, in particular ESRD patients, consume more health resources in association with admission to ICU compared with non-CKD patients. These patients have longer durations of ICU stay, longer duration of hospitalization, and higher rates of short-term rehospitalization. Moreover, these patients often remain chronically ill following ICU discharge due to issues related to cardiovascular comorbidity, malnutrition, and deconditioning. These likely reflect diminished physiologic reserve and increased vulnerability to further adverse events.

32.1.4 Prognostic Scoring for CKD and ESRD in ICU

ICU prognostication using ICU-specific illness severity or organ failure scores (i.e., APAHCE II, SAPS III, SOFA) can be challenging among patients with ESRD. Most scoring systems have not been specifically validated for ESRD patients, and their performance routinely overestimates the risk of death [1]. This may contribute to the perceived lack of benefit of ICU support for CKD/ESRD patients referred for ICU support.

32.2 ICU Support of the Patient with Chronic Kidney Disease

The pathological changes accompanying CKD, although frequently not clinically evident until later stages of kidney disease, can present unique challenges for CKD patients presenting with critical illness. Details of some of the unique challenges in the acute management of CKD patients in the ICU are detailed in Table 32.1.

There is a paucity of data with respect to the specificity of the management of CKD patients in the ICU especially in the early stages of the disease. CKD patients should receive the same standard of care as the general population while accounting for some of the unique challenges that patients with CKD/ESRD may pose to ICU management.

32.2.1 Hemodynamic Monitoring and Mechanical Ventilation Support

The general principles for support and management of critically ill patient in the ICU focus on advanced hemodynamic and physiologic monitoring and multimodal organ support to guide restoration of tissue perfusion and oxygen delivery (Table 32.2).

The majority of patients have intravascular placement of arterial catheter for continuous blood pressure monitoring, due either to the presence of hemodynamic instability or to monitoring resuscitation (i.e., fluid therapy or titration of vasoactive therapy) or need for frequent blood sampling. Arterial catheters display systolic, diastolic, and mean arterial pressure readings along with a continuous waveform. Analysis of the pressure waveform may provide useful information regarding a patient's clinical status. Variability on pulse contours is related to the

Table 32.1 Selected challenges to the ICU management of critically ill patients with CKD and ESRD

Parameter	Issue	Consequence
Comorbid disease	High prevalence of DM, hypertension, CVD, frequent exclusion from RCT of ICU-specific interventions	Increased susceptibility to poor wound healing, compromised perfusion to vital organs/organ dysfunction, low-quality evidence base for many aspects of management
Volume homeostasis	Reduced GFR and relative oliguria	Fluid accumulation, diuretic resistance, susceptibility to fluid overload complications
Dry weight evaluation	Unmeasured fluid losses and muscle wasting	Inaccurate estimation for determined fluid removal targets for RRT
Electrolyte homeostasis	Reduced GFR, reduced capacity to excrete free water and K^+, PO_4^{3-}, Mg^+, and other electrolytes	Increased susceptibility to hyponatremia, hyperkalemia, and other electrolyte abnormalities
Hemostasis	Alternations in vWF complex, platelet activation/aggregation, and NO metabolism	Increased susceptibility to bleeding
Anemia	Relative EPO deficiency, functional iron deficiency, reduced RBC lifespan, anemia chronic disease	Increased incidence of anemia, greater susceptibility to transfusion
Immunology/ inflammatory response	Impaired T-cell activity, deficient antibody production, altered opsonization/ phagocytosis, chronic increased production of inflammatory cytokines/mediators	Increased susceptibility to infection, blunted response to infection
Antimicrobial therapy	Altered pharmacokinetics (reduced clearance, altered Vd, extracorporeal clearance), multiple prior antimicrobial exposures	Increased prevalence/susceptibility to ARO, increased susceptibility to treatment failure/ toxicity
Vascular access	Vascular calcification, PD or CVC present, multiple prior central venous catheters	Difficulty obtaining arterial and venous access, susceptibility to catheter-related infection, risk of vessel stenosis

Abbreviations: *DM* diabetes mellitus, *CVD* cardiovascular disease, *GFR* glomerular filtration rate, *NO* nitric oxide, *Vd* volume of distribution, *ARO* antimicrobial-resistant organisms, *RCT* randomized controlled trial, *ICU* intensive care unit, *PD* peritoneal dialysis, *CVC* central venous catheter, *vWF* von Willebrand factor, *RBC* red blood cells, *NO* nitric oxide

elasticity, amplification, and distortion of smaller peripheral arterioles. CKD patients with significant peripheral vascular disease and/or arteriolar calcification may have reduced vessel elasticity (i.e., arterial stiffness) and exacerbated amplification that results in relative increases in systolic pressure and low diastolic pressure with rapid diastolic runoff (i.e., widened pulse pressure). ESRD patients with a fistula or graft will have accelerated diastolic runoff and as a consequence lower diastolic and mean arterial pressure. In addition, given the prevalence of comorbid conditions in CKD such as cardiac valvular disease, ventricular hypertrophy (LVH), or pulmonary hypertension, arterial catheters may have misleading instantaneous accuracy, though likely have preserved trending [2].

Additional static hemodynamic measures, such as central venous pressure (CVP) and pulmonary artery occlusion pressure (PAOP), have focused on providing an estimate of left ventricular preload to guide fluid resuscitation. The challenge with these fixed pressure-derived measures is their lack of predictability to determine whether a patient will positively response to a fluid challenge (i.e., show improvement in cardiac output and performance associated with a fluid bolus). These measures are confounded by alterations in ventricular wall compliance (i.e., LVH in ESRD). Both CVP and PAOP lack precision in individual patients and should not be used in isolation to guide resuscitation. This may contribute to excessive and inappropriate fluid prescription. The central venous oxygenation ($ScVO_2$) is generally accepted surrogate for the venous oxygen saturation (S_vO2) and reflects the adequacy of global cardiac output and oxygen delivery.

Functional dynamic metrics that utilize the observed variability in left ventricular filling

Table 32.2 Methods for monitoring and support of organ failure in critically ill patients

Organ system	Monitoring	Support
Circulatory	Indwelling arterial catheter, central venous catheter, pulmonary artery catheter, respiratory variation in pulse pressure or stroke volume (LiDCO, PiCCO, FloTrac/Vigileo), echocardiography, impedance cardiography, cardiac-specific troponin, b-type natriuretic peptide	Fluid therapy, vasoactive therapy (inotropes, vasopressors), pacemaker, indwelling mechanical support (intra-aortic balloon pump, Impella, ventricular assist device), extracorporeal support (venoarterial extracorporeal membrane oxygenation)
Respiratory	Pulse oximetry, arterial blood gas, end-tidal CO_2, flow-volume loops on mechanical ventilator, chest radiography	Noninvasive mechanical ventilation (nasal, mask, helmet CPAP, or BIPAP), conventional mechanical ventilator, oscillator, extracorporeal support (venovenous extracorporeal membrane oxygenation)
Renal	Routine blood/urine biochemistry, urine microscopy, urine output, fluid balance, novel urine or plasma kidney damage-specific biomarkers (NGAL, KIM-1, IL-18, L-FABP, NAG), renal ultrasound, renal Doppler resistive index	Renal replacement therapy (CRRT, SLED, IRRT)
Gastrointestinal	Feeding tolerance, diarrhea, routine blood biochemistry, abdominal radiography	Enteric nutrition, parenteral nutrition, glycemic control, micronutrient supplementation
Liver	Routine blood biochemistry (liver enzymes, lactate, glucose, ammonia)	Molecular adsorbent circulation system
Hematologic/ inflammatory	Clinical examination, complete blood count/ smear, C-reactive protein, procalcitonin	Blood transfusion, early/broad-spectrum antimicrobials, extracorporeal blood purification
Neurologic	Neurologic examination, CSF examination, brain radiology (CT, MRI, angiography), EEG, brain damage-specific biomarkers (neuron-specific enolase, S100β, myelin basic protein), invasive ICP monitoring, cerebral microdialysis	Sedation, antiepileptic therapy, intracranial hypertension management, intraventricular drain

Abbreviations: *CO_2* carbon dioxide, *CPAP* continuous positive airway pressure, *BIPAP* bilevel positive airway pressure, *NGAL* neutrophil-associated lipocalin, *KIM-1* kidney injury molecule-1, *IL-18* interleukin-18, *FABP* fatty acid binding protein, *MARS* molecular adsorbent circulation system, *NAG* N-acetyl-β-D-glucosaminidase, *CRRT* continuous renal replacement therapy, *SLED* sustained low-efficiency dialysis, *IRRT* intermittent renal replacement therapy, *ICP* intracranial pressure

across the respiratory cycle, measured as the variation in pulse pressure (PPV) or stroke volume (SVV), have been shown to better predict fluid responsiveness in mechanically ventilated critically ill patients (Box 32.1). The premise is that variations in systolic blood pressure and stroke volume are greater in hypovolemic states due to the increase collapsibility of the vena cava, increased transmural effect on the right atrium, and the relationship between stroke volume and preload being on the steep portion of the Frank–Starling curve. Large variation in SVV or PPV (>12 %) indicates fluid administration will translate into improved cardiac output. There are important limitations to the use of PPV/SVV and measures are susceptible to errors in states where patients are not adapted to controlled mechanical ventilation (i.e., breathing spontaneously, variable tidal volume [Vt]) or are not in sinus rhythm (i.e., atrial fibrillation). Variation in the inferior vena cava diameter during respiration as seen by echocardiography is additional functional dynamic measure of fluid responsiveness. In spontaneously breathing patients, only passive leg raising (PLR) has been shown to reliably predict fluid responsiveness. PLR involves transient elevation of the lower extremities above the heart of a recumbent patient, mimicking the effect of a large fluid bolus on the central circulation.

Box 32.1. Definitions of Functional Hemodynamic Metrics

Pulse pressure variation (PPV): Defined as the maximum pulse pressure minus the minimum pulse pressure, divided by the average of these two pressures over a mechanically delivered breath. PPV is based on the premise of pulsus paradoxus, the changes in arterial pressure during inspiration and expiration. PPV is not a true measure of preload or volume status, but an indicator of the position of the Frank–Starling relationship curve between stroke volume and preload to predict fluid responsiveness:

$$PPV(\%) = \left(PP_{max} - PP_{min} / \left[\left(PP_{max} + PP_{min}\right)/2\right]\right) \times 100$$

Stroke volume variation (SVV): Defined as the percentage of change between the maximum and minimum stroke volumes over a certain interval. Similar to PPV, SVV is not a true measure of volume status or preload but rather an assessment of response to fluid resuscitation:

$$SVV = (SV\ maximum - SV\ minimum) / \left[(SV\ maximum + SV\ minimum)/2\right]$$

Table 32.3 Common modes of invasive mechanical ventilation in the ICU

Mode	Description	Advantages	Disadvantages
VCV	Machine delivered, patient triggered, flow targeted, frequency equal to minimum set rate; present Vd (volume limited)	Ensures the delivery of a minimum Vt and total ventilation	May be uncomfortable if high inspiratory flow needed by patient, may predispose to dynamic hyperinflation (auto-PEEP), may predispose to VILI
PCV	Machine delivered, patient triggered, pressure targeted, frequency equal to minimum set rate; breath terminated by present Ti (pressure limited)	Pressure limited; control of plateau/mean airway pressure; better patient comfort	Vt variable; does not ensure delivery of minimum ventilation
PSV	Patient triggered and pressure targeted Vt; breath terminated by present inspiratory flow rate; patient determined Vt, Ti, and frequency	Better patient–ventilator synchrony; augments patients' breather; better patient comfort; used commonly to wean	Vt, Ti, frequency variable; does not ensure delivery of minimum ventilation; unsuitable for patients with impaired respiratory drive
SIMV	Machine-delivered synchronized breaths at present Vt, flow or pressure targeted; preset minimum rate; patient can breathe spontaneously with PSV between machine-delivered breaths	Ensures the delivery of a minimum Vt and total ventilation, allows some spontaneous breathing	May be uncomfortable, may increase work of breathing, may prolong weaning
CPAP	Machine set PEEP; patient triggered; patient determined Vt, Ti, and frequency	Augments spontaneous breathing; reduced inspiratory work; patient comfort; used commonly to wean	Vt, Ti, frequency variable; does not ensure delivery of minimum ventilation; may increase work of breathing

Abbreviations: *VCV* volume-controlled ventilation, *PCV* pressure-controlled ventilation, *PSV* pressure support ventilation, *SIMV* synchronized intermittent mandatory ventilation, *Vt* tidal volume, *PEEP* positive end-expiratory pressure, *VILI* ventilator-induced lung injury, *Ti* inspiratory time

Mechanical ventilation is a core life-sustaining technology that largely defined the modern practice of critical care. Most critically ill patients require mechanical ventilation, whether for lung-specific indications (i.e., acute lung injury), systemic indications (i.e., shock), or postoperative support. A summary of the most common modes of mechanical ventilation provided in the context of critical illness is shown in Table 32.3. Epidemiologic data have shown an increased utilization of mechanical ventilation for critically ill patients in recent years. These patients are generally burdened with a high prevalence of comorbid disease, in particular CKD, representing up to one quarter of all mechanically ventilated patients.

Kidney disease, both acute and chronic, can present unique challenges with respect to respiratory physiology, lung–kidney interaction, and mechanical ventilation support [3]. First, CKD/ESRD patients often have high prevalence of comorbid respiratory illness such as restrictive or obstructive defects, pleural disease, pulmonary calcification, sleep apnea, or dialysis-associated hypoxemia. Patients receiving PD have chronically elevated intra-abdominal pressure and diminished functional residual capacity. These factors predispose to limited pulmonary reserve. Second, CKD/ESRD patients often have diminished cardiac reserve and all have compromised capacity to excrete solute and water. Acute cardiac events and/or fluid accumulation (i.e., noncompliance with diet, inappropriate dry weight prescription, missed dialysis) can predispose to acute cardiorenal syndrome and pulmonary edema. Third, the development of acute injury to the kidney can induce a systemic inflammatory response with distant pathophysiologic effects in the lung (i.e., alterations in alveolar permeability and aquaporin expression). Fourth, the positive pressure applied during mechanical ventilation acts to increase intrathoracic, intrapleural, and intra-abdominal pressures both during inspiration and for the duration of the respiratory cycle (i.e., PEEP) with the aim to improve and maintain adequate gas exchange. This can stimulate an array of hemodynamic, neural, and hormonal responses that can negatively impact kidney perfusion and further inhibit excretory function. This is observed as immediate and reversible declines in urine output and fluid retention, contributing to worsening fluid accumulation. Finally, mechanical ventilation may provoke ventilator-induced lung injury (VILI) leading to an exacerbating cascade of systemic inflammation that may have distant injurious effects on the kidney [3]. Data have also shown the development of AKI may delay weaning from mechanical ventilation [4]. This is likely multifactorial and related to greater difficulties with volume and acid–base homeostasis in AKI. By extension, CKD/ESRD patients are similarly likely to encounter prolonged weaning from mechanical ventilation.

The most severe form of respiratory failure is acute respiratory distress syndrome (ARDS), defined as rapid-onset (1 week) respiratory symptoms and hypoxemia associated with bilateral opacities resulting in respiratory failure not fully explained by cardiac failure or fluid overload. The incidence of milder forms of ARDS is 78.9/100,000 person-years while more severe ARDS occurs at a rate of 58.7/100,000 person-years. The most common predisposing factor is pulmonary and non-pulmonary sepsis. The mortality remains significant, in the range of 35–40 %, and long-term morbidity among survivors remains severely burdensome. The development of AKI or worsening kidney function in the setting of ARDS is common, occurring in excess of 35 %, and has an important modifying impact on increasing mortality risk (60–80 %) [4]. It is believed part of the attributable mortality in ARDS has been related to the development of secondary harm associated with the mechanical ventilator (i.e., VILI). Accordingly, a number of "lung protective" strategies for improving outcome in ARDS have been evaluated (Table 32.4). The advent of open lung low tidal volume ventilation to prevent alveolar overdistension, cyclic collapse, and barotrauma may be associated with iatrogenic alveolar hypoventilation and hypercarbic respiratory acidosis. This may be poorly tolerated in patients with AKI or CKD/ESRD with loss of renal compensation and inability to buffer the accumulated CO_2. These patients are likely to require early initiation of RRT to mitigate severe acidemia and excessive fluid accumulation.

32.2.2 Fluid, Electrolyte, and Acid–Base Management

Patients with CKD/ESRD are more susceptible to fluid and metabolic complications due to impaired fluid, electrolyte, and acid–base homeostasis.

Table 32.4 Ventilation and other supportive therapies in ARDS

Strategy	Description	Comment
Lung protective ventilation	Target tidal volume 4–6 mL/kg ideal body weight; set positive end-expiratory pressure (PEEP) to avoid alveolar collapse; maintain plateau pressure <30 cm H_2O; may precipitate permissive hypercapnia	The "low tidal" volume and "open" lung ventilatory strategy are aimed at minimizing iatrogenic injury from mechanical ventilation (i.e., ventilator-induced lung injury [VILI]). VILI is induced by volutrauma, barotrauma, atelectrauma, and biotrauma. Level I evidence has shown utilizing lung protective ventilation has shown reductions in mortality, durations of ventilation, and durations in ICU
Recruitment maneuvers (RM)	The rationale for utilizing RM in ARDS is to improve alveolar recruitment and gas exchange. RM are generally a series of continuously applied (20–40 s) high levels of PEEP (30–40 cm H_2O)	RM can improve oxygenation in suitable ARDS candidates with recruitment of alveolar segments; however, it can be associated with hemodynamic instability. No level I evidence
Neuromuscular blockade (NMB)	Early short-term use of continuous NMB (<48 h) in severe ARDS may improve gas exchange and reduce VILI	Recent level I evidence found lower 28-day and hospital mortality associated with a strategy of early short-term continuous infusion of NMB in severe ARDS and no increase in the rate of ICU-acquired weakness
Daily sedation interruption	A strategy of daily interruption or minimal sedation has been advocated to reduce duration of ventilation, duration of ICU stay, and the incidence of delirium	These patients did not necessarily have ARDS. Recent level I evidence did not show evidence of reduced duration of ventilation or delirium associated with daily sedation interruption among ventilated patients receiving a sedation protocol
Conservative versus liberal fluid therapy strategy	The rationale for a conservative fluid management strategy is based on the premise of minimizing nonessential fluid and active removal of excess fluid once physiologic stability was achieved	Recent level I evidence found that a conservative fluid strategy, compared with a liberal fluid strategy, resulted in a nonsignificant reduction in mortality and significant shorter durations of mechanical ventilation, ICU stay, and trends for lower utilization of RRT. These findings were similar for the subgroup with AKI
Prone positioning	ARDS is often a heterogeneous syndrome with worse air space consolidation in basal (dependent) lung segments. The rationale for prone positioning is to improve V/Q matching and reduce VILI by having patients in prone position for 12–16 h per day	Prior trials have found prone positioning improves oxygenation; and recent level I evidence found a strategy of early prone positioning was associated with improved survival at 28 and 90 days. Prone positioning should be protocolized
Inhaled vasodilators (iNO, prostacyclin)	The rationale for inhaled vasodilators, by reducing PVR and improving V/Q matching in ARDS, can improve oxygenation	Meta-analyses of small randomized trials have found no improvement in mortality with inhaled vasodilators for ARDS; however, it was associated with transient improvements in oxygenation and increased risk of AKI. Inhaled vasodilators are a reasonable salvage therapy for refractory hypoxemia
High-frequency oscillatory ventilation (HFOV)	The premise for HFOV is to utilize sub-anatomical tidal volumes, high mean airway pressures, and high respiratory rates to maintain open lung ventilation, minimize the risk of VILI, and allow lungs injury to recover	Recent level I evidence found early utilization of HFOV, compared with standard lung protective ventilation, was associated with increased in-hospital mortality, greater use of sedation, neuromuscular blockade, and vasoactive therapy. HFOV should be reserved for salvage therapy in those with refractory hypoxemia
Extracorporeal membrane oxygenation (ECMO)	Candidates should have potentially reversible respiratory failure, severe hypoxemia (Murray score >3.0), ideally venovenous circuit via dual-lumen catheter, early referral to experienced centers	ECMO has generally been reserved as salvage therapy for adult patients; however, recent level I evidence from randomized trials and observational data during the pH1N1 pandemic found reasonable survival

Table 32.4 (continued)

Strategy	Description	Comment
Ineffective or harmful interventions	Surfactant, antioxidants/glutamine supplementation, N-acetylcysteine, ibuprofen, ketoconazole	Numerous high-quality randomized trials in adults have no clear evidence of benefit for these therapies

Abbreviations: *AKI* acute kidney injury, *ARDS* acute respiratory distress syndrome, *ECMO* extracorporeal membrane oxygenation, *HFOV* high-frequency oscillatory ventilation, *iNO* inhaled nitric oxide, *NMB* neuromuscular blockade, *PVR* pulmonary vascular resistance, *RM* recruitment maneuvers, *VILI* ventilator-induced lung injury

Fluid therapy is perhaps the most common intervention received by critically ill patients. The key concept for dosing fluid therapy in critically ill patients is to actively address ongoing losses coupled with constant reassessment of need for further hemodynamic support. While the optimal endpoints for fluid therapy during resuscitation remain controversial, increasing evidence suggests that resuscitation needs to be individualized and that the integration of functional hemodynamic measures to guide fluid responsiveness are superior to static measures of volume status.

Fluid therapy also represents a central cornerstone for the prevention and/or the management of AKI. Of the numerous strategies evaluated to date for prevention of AKI, only fluid therapy has been shown to be consistently effective. Importantly, however, *there is no evidence that fluid therapy will reverse AKI once established.* Reduced urine output is common and often precedes overt AKI; however, it lacks specificity. Oliguria in the absence of clear hypovolemia or fluid responsiveness is not necessarily an indication for a fluid challenge. The distinction is important. In the context of hypovolemia and/or reduced arterial filling, fluid therapy would appear appropriate. However, there is no evidence to support a fluid challenge in the resuscitated patient with oliguric AKI. While such a fluid challenge may be intended to promote diuresis, dilute tubular toxins, and attenuate tubular obstruction from casts, there is no data to suggest it attenuates the severity of AKI or improves clinical outcome. Instead, the liberal use of fluid therapy in these circumstances may exacerbate fluid overload and lead to harm. Fluid accumulation can also mask the presence and severity of AKI by increasing the total body water and hemodiluting creatinine. Recent evidence suggests that classifying AKI after correcting creatinine concentration for the volume of fluid administered improves the ability to classify AKI and predict mortality. Unnecessary fluid accumulation and overload are associated with clear increases in morbidity, including worsening AKI and delayed renal recovery, and mortality, in particular in patients with compromised kidney function across a range of clinical settings [5]. Diuretic therapy should be reserved for mitigating fluid overload in responsive patients rather than for preventing AKI or promoting recovery of kidney function. In patients whose fluid balance cannot be managed adequately with conservative fluid administration or diuretic therapy, RRT should be considered. In addition, the routine practice of providing "maintenance" of unmeasured fluid deficits such as "third space losses" for the majority of critically ill patients is questionable, in particular for those with CKD/ESRD, and often contributes unnecessary fluid accumulation.

In addition, the types of fluid administrated are increasingly recognized as having dose-dependent qualitative toxic effects. Colloids are commonly used for acute resuscitation in critically ill patients. Synthetic colloids, such as hydroxyethyl starch (HES), have appeal for resuscitation fluids based on the premise that they attenuate the inflammatory response, mitigate endothelial barrier dysfunction, improve microcirculatory flow, and contribute to more rapid hemodynamic stabilization; however, accumulated data have now suggested use of these fluids in critical illness is associated with dose-dependent risk for severe AKI requiring RRT, bleeding complications, and death (Box 32.2). In addition, these solutions are prohibitively more expensive when compared with crystalloids. Albumin is routinely used for resuscitation in liver failure patients with spontaneous bacterial peritonitis for prevention of hepatorenal syndrome and limited clinical data suggest albumin may improve outcome in severe sepsis.

Resuscitation with high chloride concentration solutions (i.e., 0.9 % saline – strong ion difference: 0 mEq/L) can directly contribute to iatrogenic hyperchloremic metabolic acidosis. The physiologic stress with large volume resuscitation of chloride-rich solutions may be less tolerated in CKD patients. Recent data have compared resuscitation with saline (0.9 %) to balanced crystalloid solutions (i.e., Ringer's lactate, Plasma-Lyte). Preferential use of these balanced solutions with a lower "chloride load" that more closely mimic the chloride content and strong ion difference of plasma has been associated with fewer metabolic complications (i.e., metabolic acidosis, hyperkalemia, hypernatremia), reduced blood product utilization, reduced AKI, and need for RRT and cost savings [6] (Box 32.3).

There is uncertain benefit for supplemental intravenous bicarbonate therapy for treatment of metabolic acidosis. Bicarbonate is commonly used in critical illness when confronted by severe metabolic acidosis (i.e., pH <7.15); however, its use is guided by limited clinical evidence. Bicarbonate supplementation intended to treat loss of bicarbonate from the buffer pool (i.e., renal tubular acidosis) would appear logical; however, its use to treat acidosis due to elevated lactate has been associated with increased mortality. Bicarbonate administration (1–2 mEq/kg) can transiently increase serum pH and serum bicarbonate; however, it may precipitate untoward adverse effects including worsening intracellular acidosis, extracellular accumulation of CO_2,

Box 32.2. What the Guidelines Say You Should Do: Fluid Resuscitation in Critically Ill Patients

- Do not use HES in patients with severe sepsis or at risk of AKI.
- Gelatin should not be used in patients at risk for AKI.
- Do not use HES or gelatin in organ donors.
- Do not use synthetic colloids in patients with head injury or intracranial bleeding.
- Albumin may be used for resuscitation in severe sepsis.
- Do not use albumin in patients with head injury.
- Hyperoncotic solutions should not be used for fluid resuscitation.
- New colloid should be introduced into clinical practice only after patient safety parameters are established.

Source: Reproduced with kind permission from Springer Science and Business Media: Reinhart et al. [7]

Box 32.3. Definition and Calculation of the Strong Ion Difference

The strong ion difference is the difference between the sums of concentrations of the strong cations and strong anions dissolved in plasma. In normal plasma with preserved serum protein content, the SID is approximately 40 mEq/L.

Strong ion difference (SID): $[Na^+]+[K^+]+[Ca^+]+[Mg^+]-[Cl^-]-$ [other strong anions]

Solution	$[Cl^-]$ (mEq/L)	SID (mEq/L)
Plasma	95–105	40
0.9 % Saline	154	0
Plasma-Lyte	98	50

Chloride is the predominant strong anion capable of modifying serum pH. Increases in serum chloride concentration (0.9 % saline administration) will reduce SID and contribute to metabolic acidosis with normal anion gap.

Accumulation of organic acids (i.e., lactate, keto acids) will increase other strong anions and induce metabolic acidosis by lowering SID with a normal serum chloride concentration and elevated anion gap.

and hypocalcemia. The current Surviving Sepsis Guidelines do not recommend use of bicarbonate for serum pH >7.15 in patients with lactic acidosis associated with severe sepsis. When bicarbonate is administered, consideration should be given for a slow infusion, allowance for adequate CO_2 removal, and correction of hypocalcemia along with reversal of the underlying contributing factor for the acidosis.

32.2.3 Nutritional Support

Malnutrition is an important contributor to increased morbidity and mortality in critical illness. Critically ill patients, in particular those with premorbid comorbid disease such as CKD and those with acute organ dysfunction such as AKI, can often present nutritionally at risk or overtly malnourished at the time of admission. Critical illness is a physiologic state characterized by widespread system inflammation, metabolic derangement, and catabolism. In these circumstances, critically ill patients, in particular those already malnourished, may be unable to adequately absorb or utilize nutrients. This may be further compounded by added clearance of nutrients during RRT.

The goal in critical illness is to provide sufficient nutritional support as to maintain homeostatic and metabolic needs without precipitating complications. Importantly, determination of the optimal caloric intake for critically ill patients ideally should involve the interdisciplinary contributions of a dietician. Dieticians can assist with ensuring optimal nutritional prescription for critically ill patients with AKI or CKD/ESKD as their course and therapies evolve (i.e., resolving organ dysfunction, recovering kidney function, transition from continuous to intermittent RRT). Early nutritional support in critical illness will not be significantly modified by the presence of CKD; however, in patients with advanced CKD or ESRD not supported with RRT, specialized enteric formulas are available that are more caloric dense (2 kcal/mL), low in electrolytes (i.e., K^+, PO_4^-, Mg^+), and fluid restricted. The intent of these specialized formulations is to provide adequate nutritional support while mitigating the development of metabolic complications or unnecessary fluid accumulation in patients with reduced GFR. In patients with AKI, one of the few interventions proven to improve renal recovery is delivery of adequate nutritional support, and therefore, more recent guidelines discourage protein restriction in critically ill patients with AKI and supplement protein further in patients receiving RRT [8].

The preferred method for delivery of nutritional support is by the enteric route. This should be started early after ICU admission (within 24–48 h). The rationale for prioritizing enteric delivery of nutrition (EN) is based on the premise that it will preserve gut mucosal integrity, reduce bacterial and endotoxin translocation, and reduce the risk of gastrointestinal bleeding. However, critical illness, coupled with baseline susceptibilities (i.e., diabetes mellitus), may be associated with enteric feeding intolerance from gut dysmotility (i.e., medications, electrolyte disorders, comorbid disease) and suboptimal absorption (i.e., gut wall edema). Two recent trials in critically ill patients have shown no incremental outcome benefit for a strategy of "trophic" feeds (i.e., 10–25 mL/h) during the first few days of critical illness. Likewise, high-quality evidence to support a strategy of intentional "permissive hypofeeding" (target 60–70 % total caloric intake) is currently lacking and cannot be recommended. Measures to improve the success of enteric nutritional support include use of prokinetic agents (i.e., dose-adjusted metoclopramide, domperidone), advancement of small bowel feeding tubes, elevation of the head of the bed (~30–45°), and not using specified gastric residual thresholds that often result in suboptimal delivery of targeted feeds.

If there remains intolerance to EN and failure to meet nutritional targets with EN, or there are other medical or surgical reasons to avoid EN, current evidence would suggest starting total parenteral nutrition (TPN) after a period of several days.

The optimal amount of protein supplementation in AKI is unknown. Current practice guideline recommendations are to avoid protein restriction in critically ill patients if the intent is to prevent worsening azotemia with the goal of preventing or delaying the initiation of RRT. Indeed, patients with AKI are often catabolic and require protein supplementation, in particular to account for the added clearance of amino acids while receiving RRT.

There is insufficient data to suggest the use of routine micronutrient supplementation [6]. In fact, there is an increased risk of mortality associated with the use of glutamine in patients with multiorgan failure.

The acute stress of critical illness coupled with nutritional support can often precipitate stress-induced hyperglycemia. The avoidance of significant hyperglycemia, hypoglycemia, and variation in glycemic control is associated with improved outcomes. However, recent trials have suggested that tight glycemic control (TGC) with intensive insulin therapy (IIT) (BG 4.4–6.0 mmol/L) may be associated with increased risk for hypoglycemia and worse outcome. Accordingly, current practice guidelines recommend a more pragmatic and less intensive strategy targeting glycemic control between 6.1 and 10.0 mmol/L (110–180 mg/dL) (Box 32.4).

32.2.4 Sepsis

Sepsis is an important precipitant of critical illness and commonly prompts acute hospitalization and admission to ICU. Data from the USRDS suggest infection is the leading cause of death among patients with ESRD. CKD patients may be more susceptible to development of infectious complications and sepsis for a number of reasons including:

- Presence and repeated access to indwelling central venous catheters (CVC) and arteriovenous fistulas (AVP) for dialysis access
- Acquired immunodeficiency related to primary etiology of kidney disease
- Immune dysregulation related to retention of uremic toxins (i.e., defective host responses in phagocytic cells, lymphocytes, and antigen processing, dysbiosis of gut microflora)
- Repeated episodes of systemic inflammation related to altered gut permeability and bacterial/endotoxin translocation during dialysis

This risk is further modified by additional factors such as comorbid disease (i.e., peripheral vascular disease and diabetes mellitus, smoking) and frequent interaction with health-care services (i.e., colonization with antimicrobial-resistant

Box 32.4. What the Guidelines Say You Should Do: Nutritional Support in Critically Ill Patients

- Initiate nutritional support via the enteral over parenteral route.
- Initiate early enteral nutrition (EN) (within 24–48 h).
- If there is intolerance, or inability to meet caloric needs or contraindications with EN, parenteral nutrition (PN) should be started after 5–7 days.
- In critically ill patients, initial caloric and protein targets should be 20–30 kcal/kg/day and 0.6–1.7 g/kg/day adapted to catabolism levels and individual needs.
- Protein restriction is not recommended during the early catabolic phases of critical illness for patients with AKI, CKD, or ESRD. Additional protein supplementation is needed for patients receiving RRT.
- Glycemic control with insulin is recommended for target blood glucose between 6.1 and 10.0 mmol/L (110–180 mg/dL). Hyperglycemia, hypoglycemia, and wide variations in blood glucose should be avoided.
- Do not use glutamine supplementation in patients with severe sepsis or multiorgan dysfunction.
- Indications for PN in AKI/CKD are similar to non-AKI/non-CKD patients.
- Interdisciplinary consultation with critical care dietician is recommended.

Source: Reprinted from Cano et al. [8].

organisms [MRSA, VRE] and frequent exposure to antimicrobials).

The utilization of indwelling access catheters is a significant source of bloodstream infection and sepsis in CKD/ESRD patients, is directly related to the duration of usage, is most commonly caused by gram-positive organism (coagulase-negative staphylococcus, *Staphylococcus aureus*), and is associated with considerably higher risk of morbidity and mortality. The risk is two- to threefold higher for non-tunneled (most commonly inserted in the ICU) compared with tunneled catheters. For ESRD patients receiving dialysis via tunneled catheters, the risk of bloodstream infection, infection-related hospitalization, and infection-related death is further two- to threefold higher than for those receiving hemodialysis via arteriovenous fistulas or grafts. Important morbidity from temporary catheters arises from the risk of development of metastatic foci of infection from highly virulent bacteria, such as *Staphylococcus aureus*, and includes endocarditis, septic arthritis, osteoarthritis, and epidural abscess.

The most common sources of non-dialysis-related infections among CKD/ESRD patients are:

- Upper and lower respiratory tract infections (i.e., community and/or hospital-acquired)
- Genitourinary infections (i.e., pyocystis, pyelonephritis, perinephric infection)
- Cellulitis/osteomyelitis
- Gastrointestinal infections (i.e., *Clostridium difficile*, cholangitis, hepatitis, gastroenteritis, diverticulitis, cholangitis)
- Central nervous systems infections (i.e., mucormycosis)
- Other infections: HIV and tuberculosis

Pneumonia is a common contributor to morbidity and mortality in CKD/ESRD patients. The risk of developing pneumonia is 3–5 times higher among CKD/ESRD patients compared with matched population with normal kidney function and is associated with a higher likelihood of ICU admission and 4–6 times the total duration of hospitalization.

The prevalence of asymptomatic pyuria among CKD/ESKD patients with residual urine production is common (30–40 %) but of undetermined significance, and the diagnosis of genitourinary infection mandates the presence of a positive culture result. Indeed, genitourinary infections may be the most common source of nosocomial infection occurring in hospitalized CKD/ESRD patients due primarily to urinary catheterization. These sources of infection may predispose to bloodstream infection in susceptible CKD/ESRD patients and necessitate ICU referral for resuscitation and hemodynamic support. In anuric ESRD patients, urinary catheterization except for diagnostic indications should be avoided.

Cellulitis is a common precipitant of infection in CKD/ESRD patients often predisposed by poor peripheral circulation (i.e., diabetes mellitus, peripheral vascular disease) coupled with extravascular peripheral edema or infection introduced through repeated puncture of the native vascular access. By extension, suboptimally treated cellulitis may result in osteomyelitis of adjacent bony structures. Severe cellulitis may present with bloodstream infection in susceptible CKD/ESRD patients and prompt ICU admission.

The incidence of common gastrointestinal infections in CKD/ESRD patients is similar to the general population; however, their physiologic reserve to withstand these infections may be severely blunted and further predispose to added morbidity. The exceptions include susceptibility to infectious hepatitis (hepatitis B and C virus), peritonitis among patients receiving peritoneal dialysis, and *Clostridium difficile* colitis due to frequent antimicrobial exposure and interaction with health services.

Sepsis is defined as the presence of infection together with systemic manifestations of inflammation. Severe sepsis is defined as sepsis plus sepsis-induced organ dysfunction or tissue hypoperfusion, and septic shock is defined as severe sepsis plus hypotension not reversed with fluid resuscitation [9]. The diagnostic criteria for sepsis and sepsis-related organ dysfunction are shown in Box 32.5. It is important to recognize that many of these criteria may be modified due to CKD/ESRD and its treatment alone (i.e., dialysis-induced endotoxemia or hypotension) or due to concomitant comorbid disease (i.e., reduced cardiac reserve due to cardiorenal syndrome, autonomic dysfunction due to diabetes mellitus), drug therapy (i.e., β-blockers, Coumadin), or not being applicable (i.e., serum creatinine elevation or oliguria in anuric ESKD).

The general principles and initial management of sepsis in CKD/ESRD patients are similar to the acute resuscitation of patients with suspected sepsis and AKI without kidney disease (Boxes 32.6 and 32.7). Early "bundled" resuscitation coupled with prompt broad-spectrum antimicrobial therapy and source control should be established in accordance with clinical practice guidelines [9]. If there is suspicion that the source of sepsis is a vascular access catheter, this should be promptly removed once further central venous access has been confirmed.

Box 32.5. Diagnostic Criteria for Sepsis Syndrome and Sepsis-Related Organ Dysfunction

Infection (confirmed or suspected) plus some of the following criteria:
General variables
Fever (>38.3 °C) or hypothermia (<36.0 °C)
Heart rate >90/min or more than 2 standard deviations above normal for age
Tachypnea
Altered mental status
Significant edema or positive fluid balance (>20 mL/kg over 24 h)
Hyperglycemia (blood glucose >7.7 mmol/L) in the absence of DM
Inflammatory variables
Leukocytosis (WBC >12,000/μL) or leukopenia (WBC <4,000/μL) or >10 % immature forms
Plasma C-reactive protein more than 2 standard deviations above the normal value
Plasma procalcitonin more than 2 standard deviations above the normal value
Hemodynamic variables
Arterial hypotension (SBP <90 mm Hg, MAP <70 mm Hg, or SBP decrease >40 mm Hg or less than 2 standard deviations below normal for age)
Organ dysfunction variables
Arterial hypoxemia ($PaO_2/FiO_2 < 300$)
Acute oliguria (urine output <0.5 mL/kg for 2 h despite fluid resuscitation)
Creatinine increase (>44.2 μmol/L)
Coagulation abnormalities (INR >1.5, aPTT >60s)
Ileus (absent bowel sounds)
Thrombocytopenia (platelet count <100,000/μL)
Hyperbilirubinemia (plasma bilirubin [total] >70 μmol/L)
Tissue perfusion variables
Hyperlactatemia (>1 mmol/L)
Decrease capillary refill or mottling

Source: Reproduced with kind permission from Springer Science and Business Media: Dellinger et al. [9]

32.2.5 Acute Kidney Injury

Acute kidney injury (AKI) is a common complication encountered in hospitalized patients, particularly in the setting of critical illness, occurring in up to two-thirds of patients [13].

Recently, the KDIGO Clinical Practice Guidelines for Acute Kidney Injury published updated consensus criteria for the diagnosis and staging of AKI [11] (Table 32.5). These criteria do not currently integrate evolving novel diagnostic biomarkers specific for kidney damage (i.e., NGAL, KIM-1, IL-18, L-FABP). Yet, these novel biomarkers show significant promise to improve the capacity for early diagnosis, prognostication, and informed decision-making in AKI by helping to better discriminate etiology of loss of kidney function (i.e., AKI vs. CKD), risk of worsening AKI and need for RRT, and long-term risk of CKD.

Development of AKI portends a worse clinical prognosis in critically ill patients and predicts such adverse outcomes as need for renal replacement therapy (RRT), prolonged ICU and hospital stay, and increased mortality risk [14]. Importantly, for the CKD patients developing acute-on-chronic AKI, the risk of worsened CKD and accelerated decline in function toward ESRD is increased several fold. More severe forms of AKI are also associated with gradient increases in the risk of death and/or non-recovery of kidney function and dialysis dependence [15].

Box 32.6. What the Guidelines Say You Should Do? Surviving Sepsis Campaign Guideline: Sepsis "Bundles"

To be completed within 3 h

- Measure serum lactate.
- Obtain blood cultures prior to administration of antimicrobials.
- Administer broad-spectrum antimicrobials.
- Administer 30 mL/kg crystalloid for hypotension or lactate ≥4 mmol/L.

To be completed within 6 h

- Administer vasopressors (for hypotension not responsive to initial fluid resuscitation) to maintain a mean arterial pressure (MAP) ≥65 mmHg.
- Measure central venous pressure (CVP) and central venous oxygenation ($ScVO_2$) and resuscitate to target CVP ≥8 cmH_2O and $ScVO_2$ ≥70 %.
- Remeasure serum lactate if initial value was elevated and resuscitate to target normalization.

Antimicrobial therapy and source control

- Aim to administer broad-spectrum "effective" intravenous antimicrobial therapy within the first 1 h of recognition of sepsis. Each 1 h delay in administration of appropriate antimicrobials during the first 6 h is associated with an 8 % decrease in survival.
- Initial short-term (3–5 days) administration of empiric combination antimicrobial therapy should be undertaken for severe sepsis/septic shock or difficult-to-treat sources of infection or suspicion of multidrug-resistant organisms.
- Evaluation for a specific anatomical diagnosis of infection should be undertaken for consideration for emergent (within 6–12 h) source control measures (i.e., surgical for septic arthritis, catheter removal for bloodstream infection, chest thoracostomy tube insertion for empyema). Delay to source control when present is also associated with significant decrease in survival.

Source: Reproduced with kind permission from Springer Science and Business Media: Dellinger et al. [9]

Box 32.7. Relevant Clinical Practice Guidelines

1. *Chronic kidney disease:* Kidney Disease: Improving Global Outcomes (KDIGO) Chronic Kidney Disease Working Group. KDIGO 2012 Clinical practice guideline for the evaluation and management of chronic kidney disease. Kidney Int Suppl. 2013;3(1):1–163 [10]. Available at: http://kdigo.org/home/guidelines/ckd-evaluation-management/
2. *Acute kidney injury:* Kidney Disease: Improving Global Outcomes (KDIGO) Acute Kidney Injury Work Group. KDIGO 2012 Clinical practice guideline for acute kidney injury. Kidney Int Suppl. 2012;2:1–141 [11]. Available at: www.kdigo.org/clinical_practice_guidelines/index.php
3. *Sepsis:* Dellinger RP, Levy MM, Rhodes A, Annane D, Gerlach H, Opal SM, et al. Surviving sepsis campaign: international guidelines for management of severe sepsis and septic shock: 2012. Crit Care Med. 2013;41(2):580–637 [9]. Available at: www.survivingsepsis.org/Pages/default.aspx
4. *Fluid therapy:* Reinhart K, Perner A, Sprung CL, Jaeschke R, Schortgen F, Johan Groeneveld AB, Beale R, Hartog CS; European Society of Intensive Care Medicine. Consensus statement of the ESICM task force on colloid volume therapy in critically ill patients. Intensive Care Med. 2012;38(3):368–83 [7].
5. *Nutritional support:* Critical Care Nutrition – Canadian Clinical Practice Guidelines [12]. Available at: www.criticalcarenutrition.com/index.php

AKI is a syndrome with a spectrum of contributing factors. The risk factors for development of AKI are often multidimensional and are related to synergy between premorbid susceptibility (i.e., older age, CKD, diabetes mellitus, hypertension, liver disease) and factors contributing to critical illness (i.e., sepsis, shock states, diagnostic procedures involving contrast media, major surgery) [13, 14]. The diagnostic evaluation of AKI should

Table 32.5 KDIGO diagnostic criteria and severity staging for AKI

AKI is defined as any of the following:		
Increase in serum creatinine ≥26.5 μmol/L (≥0.3 mg/dL) within 48 h		
Increase in serum creatinine to ≥1.5 times baseline, which is known or presumed to have occurred within the prior 7 days		
Urine volume <0.5 mL/kg/h for 6 h		
AKI staging	**Serum creatinine**	**Urine output**
Stage I	Increase of 1.5–1.9 times baseline or ≥26.5 μmol/L (≥0.3 mg/dL)	<0.5 mL/kg/h × 6–12 h
Stage II	Increase of 2.0–2.9 times baseline	<0.5 mL/kg/h × ≥12 h
Stage III	Increase of ≥3.0 times baseline or ≥ 353.6 μmol/L (≥4.0 mg/dL) or start of RRT	<0.3 mL/kg/h × ≥24 h or anuria ≥12 h

Source: Reprinted by permission from Macmillan Publishers Ltd: Kidney Disease: Improving Global Outcomes (KDIGO) Acute Kidney Injury Work Group [11], copyright 2012. Available at: http://www.nature.com/kisup/index.html

integrate routine biochemistry, urinalysis and imaging where indicated to rule out immediately reversible etiologies (i.e., post-obstructive) or those requiring specialized interventions (i.e., vasculitis).

An understanding of the pathophysiology of AKI is important to provide appropriate management for these patients. Our current understanding of the pathophysiologic mechanisms contributing to AKI remains incomplete; however, contrary to the conventional view, recent data argue against ischemia–reperfusion as the predominant pathophysiologic mechanism contributing to AKI. The causal role of alternations in renal blood flow, microcirculation, and endothelial function, immune cell infiltration and activation, immune-mediated toxic injury and apoptosis, and inflammatory mediator-induced organ cross talk is only beginning to be better understood.

The general strategies for prevention and management of AKI are similar for those with and without CKD [16] (Table 32.6). Specific interventions for prevention and treatment of established AKI are few and most have focused on preventing development of contrast-induced AKI in susceptible patients such as those with CKD. Several specific examples of mitigating risk of developing AKI or its complications are outlined in Table 32.7 [11, 16].

32.2.6 Renal Replacement Therapy

Renal replacement therapy (RRT) is a vital, life-sustaining, and organ support technology applied in approximately 4–8 % of all critically ill patients and in approximately 70 % of those with more severe forms of AKI [14].

However, RRT also increases the complexity and health resource use for critically ill patients, and recent data have suggested its utilization may be associated with higher risk of death and dialysis dependence among survivors. These data highlight the existing uncertainty regarding many aspects of the decision to initiate and process of delivery of RRT to critically ill patients.

Current guidelines recommend the utilization of an uncuffed, non-tunneled dialysis catheter for acute RRT in the ICU. The position of these acute catheters should avoid insertion in the subclavian vessels to mitigate the risk of long-term complications such as stenosis/thrombosis. Existing tunneled dialysis catheters may be used if already in situ; however, use of fistulas or grafts in acute critical care settings, in particular for CRRT, should be avoided.

The optimal time to start RRT in critically ill patients with AKI and/or CKD is currently unknown. There is general consensus that RRT should be urgently initiated in the presence of life-threatening complications related to AKI such as severe electrolyte abnormalities (i.e., hyperkalemia), acid–base disturbances (i.e., academia), and fluid balance (i.e., pulmonary edema); however, outside of these indications, the optimal time to start is uncertain [11] (Table 32.8). It is likely more important to

Table 32.6 Summary of strategies for initial resuscitation of critically ill patients with CKD/ESRD and for the prevention and management of AKI

Intervention	Comment
Restore/optimize arterial filling[a]	Responsiveness to a fluid challenge should be assessed using functional hemodynamic monitoring. Isotonic or balance crystalloid solutions should be used for acute resuscitation. Synthetic colloids (i.e., hydroxyethyl starch) and hyperoncotic solutions should be avoided for fluid resuscitation in those at risk for AKI
Restore/optimize cardiac output[a]	The addition of inotropic therapy should be considered for patients with absolute or relative low cardiac output states
Restore/optimize mean arterial pressure[a]	The addition of vasopressor therapy, in conjunction with fluid therapy, should be considered in patients with refractory hypotension
Restore/optimize oxygen-carrying capacity	The consideration for blood transfusion should be given for ICU patients with AKI or CKD patients with severe anemia and evidence of tissue hypoperfusion and hypoxia. No evidence to support increasing the dose of erythropoietin-stimulating agents during acute illness and possible risk of harm (increased risk of thrombosis)
Remove/avoid all nonessential nephrotoxins or perform appropriate therapeutic monitoring/dose adjustment when necessary	Avoid aminoglycosides unless there is no suitable alternative; utilize azole or echinocandin antifungals or lipid formulations of amphotericin if there is no suitable alterative to treat systemic fungal infection
Consider context-specific interventions based on current clinical practice guidelines	For contrast media exposure, hepatorenal syndrome, rhabdomyolysis, sepsis, vasculitis
Monitor for/avoid excess fluid accumulation	AKI and CKD are associated with greater risk for fluid accumulation. Monitor daily fluid intake/output and daily/cumulative fluid balance, recognizing there is some "ebb and flow" to fluid balance in critical illness
Monitor for/avoid complications of overt kidney failure	Monitor AKI and CKD patients for serious complications such as hyperkalemia, acidemia, fluid overload, and drug toxicities and appropriately plan for RRT
Maintain glycemic control	Glycemic control has been associated with reduced incidence of AKI and lower utilization of RRT. The balance of evidence now recommends maintaining glycemic control with a target blood glucose (BG) of 6.1–10.0 mmol/L (110–180 mg/dL) rather than using intensive insulin therapy (IIT) to maintain tight glycemic control, with BG of 4.4–6.0 mmol/L (80–110 mg/dL), due to the increased risk of hypoglycemia

[a]There should be early use of invasive/functional hemodynamic monitoring (i.e., arterial catheter, central venous pressure, echocardiography, pulmonary artery catheter, or methods to measure stroke volume or pulse pressure variation)

evaluate the broad clinical context of critically ill patients' admission diagnosis, illness severity, non-kidney organ dysfunction, the probability of worsening AKI or non-recovery, and additional conditions that may be modified by RRT (i.e., fluid accumulation) rather than reliance on absolute thresholds in conventional biochemical markers such as creatinine or urea. Early initiation of RRT in patients with AKI or advanced CKD has the intuitive appeal of avoiding life-threatening AKI complications while ensuring the adequate delivery of essential medications (i.e., antimicrobials) and nutrition and transfusion support without concern for excessive fluid accumulation. Recent systematic reviews have supported this concept, suggesting earlier RRT initiation may improve survival; however, studies included in these analyses were highly susceptible to bias [17, 18].

The choice of ideal RRT modality for critically ill patients has long been debated. Systematic reviews have not shown a clear survival advantage

Table 32.7 Selected examples of acute physiology and interventions with the potential for negative effects on kidney function

Intervention	Example	Action
Altered systemic hemodynamics		
Reduced arterial filling	Diuretics	Discontinue
Negative inotropic therapy	β-Blockers	Discontinue
Antihypertensive therapy	CCB	Discontinue
Altered renal hemodynamics		
Afferent arteriolar vasoconstrictors	NSAIDs	Discontinue
Efferent arteriolar vasodilators	ACEi/ARB[a]	Discontinue
Altered renal venous pressure		
Elevated intra-abdominal pressure	Excess fluid accumulation	Avoid
Nephrotoxins		
Antibiotics	Aminoglycosides, vancomycin, colistin, sulfamethoxazole, foscarnet	Discontinue, monitor, or dose-adjust
Antifungals	Amphotericin	Discontinue, monitor, or dose-adjust
Antivirals	Acyclovir, HAART	Discontinue, monitor, or dose-adjust
Immunosuppression	Tacrolimus, cyclosporine	Discontinue, monitor, or dose-adjust
Fluid therapy	Dextrans, hydroxyethyl starch	Avoid
Diagnostic imaging	Radiocontrast media	Avoid
Cytotoxic chemotherapy	Cisplatin, methotrexate	Discontinue, monitor, or dose-adjust

Abbreviations: *CCB* calcium channel blockers, *NSAIDs* nonsteroidal anti-inflammatory drugs, *ACE* angiotensin converting enzyme, *ARB* angiotensin receptor blocker, *HAART* highly active antiretroviral therapy, *IAP* intra-abdominal pressure

[a]ACEi and ARB lead to reduction in glomerular blood flow, which has beneficial effects for kidney survival in chronic kidney disease patients but may lead to worsening kidney function in patients with AKI

for one modality, continuous RRT (CRRT), slow low-efficiency dialysis (SLED), or intermittent RRT (IRRT), over another in critically ill patients with AKI [19] (Table 32.9). Ideally, the modality chosen should suit the patient's acute physiology and therapeutic objectives while avoiding treatment-related complications. CRRT is the preferred modality in hemodynamically unstable patients and those with acute brain injury or fulminant hepatic failure and at risk for intracranial hypertension and cerebral edema [11]. CRRT has also been shown superior for maintaining fluid homeostasis and mitigating fluid overload. A recent systematic review suggested that initial therapy with CRRT in critically ill patients is associated with lower rates of dialysis dependence among survivors when compared with IRRT [20]. These data may imply CRRT may be the preferred initial modality for surviving critically ill patients at increased risk for incident or worsening CKD (i.e., those with baseline CKD).

The optimal mode of CRRT to improve outcome remains uncertain. The purported advantages to hemofiltration (CVVH) compared with hemodialysis (CVVHD) are the improved convective clearance of middle molecular weight solutes such as inflammatory and toxic mediators. Recent data have suggested equivalent outcomes in terms of survival and recovery of kidney function; however, CVVH may be associated with short filter lifespan compared with CVVHD [21].

The optimal time to transition from CRRT to either SLED or IRRT is currently unknown; however, it pragmatically will coincide with physiologic stabilization and following weaning from vasoactive support.

The utilization of peritoneal dialysis in critical illness may be impractical and result in insufficient solute clearance in catabolic patients and inadequate fluid removal. These factors may have contributed to the observation of higher mortality for critically ill patients treated with

Table 32.8 Indications for starting RRT in ICU

Indication	Comment
Renal replacement therapy	
Life-threatening indications	These indications have not been evaluated in trials
Hyperkalemia	Evidence of refractory elevated potassium and rapidly rising or cardiac toxicity. RRT is effective for temporarily reducing serum potassium
Acidemia	Evidence of refractory academia and inability to adequately compensate (pH <7.15). RRT can rapidly mitigate metabolic acidosis; however, correction requires targeted treatment of the precipitating disease
Pulmonary edema	Evidence of fluid overload contributing to worsening hypoxemia, contributing to need for ventilatory support or prevention of weaning from ventilatory support. RRT can effectively reduce extravascular lung water in diuretic-resistant states
Uremic complications	Pericarditis, bleeding, encephalopathy. In modern ICU practice, withholding RRT until uremic complications arise would be uncommon
Nonemergent indications	
Azotemic control	Conventional criteria evaluate blood accumulation of urea and creatinine; however, numerous additional metabolites/uremic toxins can also accumulate. Blood concentrations of these metabolites may be confounded by added factors such as nutritional status, catabolism, and volume status
Fluid overload/accumulation	Fluid overload/accumulation that is refractory to diuretics or when there are diuretic-induced electrolyte abnormalities can both be an important determinants for starting RRT
Acid–base/electrolyte abnormalities	Additional factors such as metabolic acidosis and marked electrolyte abnormalities (sodium, magnesium) can be potentially treated with RRT; however, no standardized criteria exist
Renal support	These indications in critical illness may occur separately from patients with either life-threatening complications of AKI or advanced AKI and rather can be viewed as a platform for organ support to prevent complications and facilitate treatment
Volume homeostasis	Fluid accumulation is worse in AKI and is associated with worse outcome. RRT may represent part of a strategy to mitigate excessive fluid accumulation
Nutritional support	RRT can better enable the delivery of full nutritional support (i.e., enteral or parenteral) without the concern for excessive fluid accumulation
Acid–base/electrolyte homeostasis	RRT may represent part of a strategy to enable "permissive hypercapnia" in ICU patients with severe ARDS and AKI/CKD or mitigate adverse effects from anticipated electrolyte disorders (i.e., tumor lysis syndrome)
Immunomodulation	RRT may represent a strategy for modulating and restoring immune function in sepsis and associated severe inflammatory states. Studies are ongoing
Drug delivery	RRT can better enable the delivery of essential drugs (i.e., antimicrobials) without the concern for excessive fluid accumulation

Abbreviations: *ARDS* acute respiratory distress syndrome, *ICU* intensive care unit, *RRT* renal replacement therapy

peritoneal dialysis compared with those treated with hemodialysis.

Determination of the optimal dose intensity for small solute clearance for critically ill patients with AKI has long been a clinical priority. Early randomized trials clearly favored a more intensive strategy; however, recent high-quality data have not shown a benefit with this approach. Two multicenter randomized trials, the Department of Veterans Affairs/National Institutes of Health (VA/NIH) Acute Renal Failure Trial Network (ATN) Study and the Randomized Evaluation of Normal versus Augmented Level (RENAL) Replacement Therapy Study, found no incremental benefit in critically ill patients with AKI from a more intensive (high-dose) RRT compared with a less intensive RRT strategy [22, 23]. The more intensive strategy did not decrease mortality, accelerate recovery of kidney function, or alter the rate of nonrenal organ failure. Importantly, these findings do not imply that the dose of RRT is not important, but rather, the evidence would

Table 32.9 Description of the characteristics and comparisons of RRT modalities used to treat critically ill patients

Characteristics	CRRT	SLED/EDD	IRRT
Duration (h)	20–24 h/day	8–12 h/day	3–6 h/day
Blood flow rate	100–250 mL/h	200–300 mL/h	400–500 mL/h
Dose intensity	20–25 mL/kg/h	Kt/V 1.2–1.4	Kt/V 1.2–1.4
Comparison			
Risk of hemodynamic instability	↓↓	↑/↓	↑↑
Azotemic control	↑↑	↑/↓	↓↓
Electrolyte homeostasis	↑↑	↑/↓	↓↓
Volume control	↑↑	↑/↓	↓↓
Risk of bleeding	↑↑	↑/↓	↓↓
Patient mobilization	↓↓	↑	↑↑
Immunomodulation	↑↑	↓	↓↓
Cost (per day)	↑↑	↑/↓	↓↓
Special circumstances[a]	Most suitable	Not recommended	Not recommended

Abbreviations: *CRRT* continuous renal replacement therapy, *SLED/EDD* slow low-efficiency dialysis/extended daily dialysis

[a]Shock states, severe hyponatremia, elevated intracranial pressure (i.e., traumatic brain injury, fulminant hepatic failure)

suggest there is no need to exceed a CRRT dose of 20–25 mL/kg/h effluent flow rate or IHD three times per week with delivered Kt/V_{urea} 1.2–1.4 per treatment for small solute clearance.

In general, RRT should be discontinued when it is no longer indicated due to either sufficient residual or recovering kidney function or a change in the overall goals of care of the patient. The best predictor for successful weaning from RRT for critically ill patients is the volume of spontaneous urine production in 24 h. Those capable of producing ≥450–500 mL urine per day have a higher likelihood of short-term recovery and dialysis independence. There is no evidence to suggest improved or accelerated recovery and dialysis independence with early forced diuresis with furosemide.

32.2.7 Pharmacotherapy

Drug pharmacokinetics in critical illness and AKI is significantly modified due to alterations in drug bioavailability, reduced protein binding, increased volume of distribution, altered biotransformation, and reduced intrinsic clearance and elimination. Appropriate drug dosing is further complicated by a number of factors, including baseline comorbid disease of patients (i.e., CKD), need for multiple drugs that potentially interact with vital functions, lower thresholds for toxicity, evolving illness severity and organ dysfunction (i.e., changes in GFR), and superimposed extracorporeal drug removal (Table 32.10).

In general, there are several pragmatic steps to help guide drug dosing in critically ill patients with AKI and those receiving RRT [24]. First, the literature should be reviewed for existing data on drug dose guidance for a specific drug [25]. Second, for drugs with primary renal elimination, a bedside estimate of baseline GFR and a dynamic assessment of total creatinine clearance, if applicable, should be undertaken, assuming there is no significant secretion or reabsorption. In particular, consideration should be given to patients receiving RRT who have recovering or residual renal function. Third, particularly for drugs with a narrow therapeutic index and risk of toxicity, therapeutic drug monitoring when possible should be undertaken (i.e., phenytoin, vancomycin, aminoglycosides). Fourth, several drug classes may be administered based on their observed clinical response, such as with sedatives, analgesics, or vasoactive medications. However, selected drugs have potentially toxic

Table 32.10 Summary of factors affecting drug elimination in critically ill patients receiving RRT

Factor	Comment
Drug characteristics	Molecular weight, charge, and nonrenal elimination can impact clearance
Drug availability	
Vd	Increased in critical illness and AKI, generally requires larger loading dose, and reduces drug availability for EC clearance
PB	Only unbound fraction available, reduced in critical illness and AKI, reduces drug availability for EC clearance
[plasma]	Only drug within intravascular compartment available for EC clearance
Extracorporeal therapy	
Dose intensity	Higher dose intensity, such as prescription of HVHF, will increase EC clearance; clearance impacted if large discrepancy between prescribed and delivered dose
BFR	Higher blood flow rate will deliver more drug to filter, only important at either very low or high blood flow or large discrepancy between prescribed and delivered dose
Mode (convention vs. dialysis)	EC clearance dependent on total effluent flow rate and/or dialysate flow rate
Replacement fluid	Prefilter replacement fluid administration will result in hemodilution and lower EC clearance
Filter membrane	Sieving/diffusion coefficient important, whereas surface area has limited impact on EC clearance
Organ recovery	Residual or recovery kidney function can greatly increase overall clearance during extracorporeal therapy

metabolites that can accumulate in patients with reduced kidney function. As examples, the elimination of α1-hydroxymidazolam (main metabolite of midazolam) and glucuronide metabolites of morphine are principally eliminated by the kidneys and thus may accumulate in AKI/CKD. Finally, given the complexity, there is a recognized need for a dedicated ICU pharmacist among the interdisciplinary ICU team, particularly for patients with CKD or AKI.

Conclusions

The prevalence of CKD and ESRD is increasing. These patients are burdened by high comorbid disease, are more likely to interact with critical care services, and have worse short-term and long-term outcomes compared with non-CKD patients. Short-term mortality is predominantly driven by acuity of illness rather than CKD status per se, and CKD status should likely not preclude critical care support. The pathophysiologic changes associated with CKD/ESKD and development of superimposed AKI can present unique challenges for clinicians in the ICU management of these patients.

Before You Finish: Practice Pearls for the Clinician

- CKD and specially ESRD status alone should not exclude consideration for admission in the ICU.
- Prognostic score results should be carefully considered since they routinely overestimate mortality in ESRD patients.
- The principles of management of sepsis should be applied to CKD, fluid overload being an obvious caveat.
- Fluid therapy should be considered a drug therapy and dosed accordingly.
- Long-term kidney function monitoring is mandatory after an AKI episode.
- Consider initiation of RRT ahead of absolute indications. CRRT is the preferred option for the hemodynamically unstable patient.
- Avoid nephrotoxic drugs for patients with CKD and/or at risk for AKI.
- Adjust drug regimens to kidney function, except for the loading dose of antibiotics.

References

1. Arulkumaran N, Annear NM, Singer M. Patients with end-stage renal disease admitted to the intensive care unit: systematic review. Br J Anaesth. 2013;110(1):13–20.
2. Davison DL, Patel K, Chawla LS. Hemodynamic monitoring in the critically ill: spanning the range of kidney function. Am J Kidney Dis. 2012;59(5):715–23.
3. Koyner JL, Murray PT. Mechanical ventilation and the kidney. Blood Purif. 2010;29(1):52–68.
4. Seeley EJ. Updates in the management of acute lung injury: a focus on the overlap between AKI and ARDS. Adv Chronic Kidney Dis. 2013;20(1):14–20.
5. Prowle JR, Echeverri JE, Ligabo EV, Ronco C, Bellomo R. Fluid balance and acute kidney injury. Nat Rev Nephrol. 2010;6(2):107–15.
6. Yunos NM, Bellomo R, Bailey M. Chloride-restrictive fluid administration and incidence of acute kidney injury–reply. JAMA. 2013;309(6):543–4.
7. Reinhart K, Perner A, Sprung CL, et al. Consensus statement of the ESICM task force on colloid volume therapy in critically ill patients. Intensive Care Med. 2012;38(3):368–83.
8. Cano NJ, Aparicio M, Brunori G, et al. ESPEN guidelines on parenteral nutrition: adult renal failure. Clin Nutr. 2009;28(4):401–14.
9. Dellinger RP, Levy MM, Rhodes A, et al. Surviving sepsis campaign: international guidelines for management of severe sepsis and septic shock: 2012. Crit Care Med. 2013;41(2):580–637.
10. Kidney Disease: Improving Global Outcomes (KDIGO) Chronic Kidney Disease Work Group. KDIGO 2012 clinical practice guideline for the evaluation and management of chronic kidney disease. Kidney Int. 2013;3(1):1–163.
11. Kidney Disease: Improving Global Outcomes (KDIGO) Acute Kidney Injury Work Group. KDIGO clinical practice guideline for acute kidney injury. Kidney Int. 2012;Suppl (2):1–138.
12. Critical Care Nutrition. Canadian Clinical Practice Guidelines 2013. 2013;2013.
13. Bellomo R, Kellum JA, Ronco C. Acute kidney injury. Lancet. 2012;380(9843):756–66.
14. Uchino S, Kellum JA, Bellomo R, et al. Acute renal failure in critically ill patients: a multinational, multicenter study. JAMA. 2005;294(7):813–8.
15. Wald R, Quinn RR, Luo J, et al. Chronic dialysis and death among survivors of acute kidney injury requiring dialysis. JAMA. 2009;302(11):1179–85.
16. Joannidis M, Druml W, Forni LG, et al. Prevention of acute kidney injury and protection of renal function in the intensive care unit. Expert opinion of the working group for nephrology, ESICM. Intensive Care Med. 2010;36(3):392–411.
17. Karvellas CJ, Farhat MR, Sajjad I, et al. A comparison of early versus late initiation of renal replacement therapy in critically ill patients with acute kidney injury: a systematic review and meta-analysis. Crit Care. 2011;15(1):R72.
18. Seabra VF, Balk EM, Liangos O, Sosa MA, Cendoroglo M, Jaber BL. Timing of renal replacement therapy initiation in acute renal failure: a meta-analysis. Am J Kidney Dis. 2008;52(2):272–84.
19. Bagshaw SM, Berthiaume LR, Delaney A, Bellomo R. Continuous versus intermittent renal replacement therapy for critically ill patients with acute kidney injury: a meta-analysis. Crit Care Med. 2008;36(2):610–7.
20. Schneider AG, Bellomo R, Bagshaw SM, et al. Choice of renal replacement therapy modality and dialysis dependence after acute kidney injury: a systematic review and meta-analysis. Intensive Care Med. 2013;39(6):987–97.
21. Friedrich JO, Wald R, Bagshaw SM, Burns KE, Adhikari NK. Hemofiltration compared to hemodialysis for acute kidney injury: systematic review and meta-analysis. Crit Care. 2012;16(4):R146.
22. Bellomo R, Cass A, Cole L, et al. Intensity of continuous renal-replacement therapy in critically ill patients. N Engl J Med. 2009;361(17):1627–38.
23. Palevsky PM, Zhang JH, O''Connor TZ, et al. Intensity of renal support in critically ill patients with acute kidney injury. N Engl J Med. 2008;359(1):7–20.
24. Matzke GR, Aronoff GR, Atkinson Jr AJ, et al. Drug dosing consideration in patients with acute and chronic kidney disease-a clinical update from Kidney Disease: Improving Global Outcomes (KDIGO). Kidney Int. 2011;80(11):1122–37.
25. Heintz BH, Matzke GR, Dager WE. Antimicrobial dosing concepts and recommendations for critically ill adult patients receiving continuous renal replacement therapy or intermittent hemodialysis. Pharmacotherapy. 2009;29(5):562–77.

Part VI

Chronic Kidney Disease: Final Path to Renal Replacement Therapy

Chronic Kidney Disease Management Programmes and Patient Education

33

Kevin Harris, Coral Graham, and Susan Sharman

Before You Start: Facts You Need to Know

- The incidence and prevalence of CKD are increasing with a wide spectrum of disease from mild and asymptomatic to those patients requiring renal replacement therapy.
- Successful management programmes address the progression of CKD and the management of CKD-associated complications and help manage comorbidities associated with CKD.
- Management programmes require the integration of care by multidisciplinary teams built around the needs of the patient. They typically span primary and secondary care.
- Tailored patient-focused education aimed at empowering patients is an integral part of chronic disease management in CKD.
- Significant resources may be required to establish an effective CKD management programme. Programmes therefore benefit from national policy guidance on the optimal management of CKD.

K. Harris, MD, MB, BS, FRCP (✉)
John Walls Renal Unit, Leicester General Hospital, University Hospitals of Leicester, Gwendolen Road, Leicester LE5 4PW, UK
e-mail: kevin.harris@uhl-tr.nhs.uk

C. Graham, MSc
School of Nursing and Midwifery, De Montfort University, The Gateway, Leicester LE19BH, UK
e-mail: coral.graham@uhl-tr.nhs.uk

S. Sharman, DiPHE, BA
John Walls Renal Unit – Renal Community Team, Leicester General Hospital, Gwendolen Road, Leicester LE5 4PW, UK
e-mail: susan.sharman@uhl-tr.nhs.uk

33.1 Disease Management in Chronic Kidney Disease

The management of chronic kidney disease (CKD) is one of the most important challenges facing health-care systems. The incidence of CKD is increasing especially amongst the elderly. As a result, CKD now poses a significant public health challenge especially in the Western world. It imposes a substantial burden on patients with loss of productivity and social isolation and results in a significant and disproportional cost to the health-care systems caring for them. CKD is strongly associated with cardiovascular risk and cardiovascular comorbidities including hypertension, cardiovascular disease and diabetes. Many people with CKD survive for a considerable period of time needing ongoing care. Although

M. Arici (ed.), *Management of Chronic Kidney Disease*,
DOI 10.1007/978-3-642-54637-2_33, © Springer-Verlag Berlin Heidelberg 2014

patients with CKD are more likely to die than reach end-stage renal disease, significant decline in kidney function may occur with time, and a minority of patients ultimately require treatment with expensive renal replacement therapy.

In the past decade, chronic disease management programmes for CKD have been introduced in a number of countries in an attempt to improve the management and outlook of patients with the expectation that this will in turn reduce the economic burden of CKD.

There is no universal approach to chronic disease management, and programmes have varied depending on the organisation and resources available within a given health-care system. They may target individuals (e.g. providing education and ensuring care is coordinated so the individual receives the right support at the right time), health-care delivery systems (e.g. development and promotion of evidence-based guidelines with decision support tools) or populations (e.g. health promotion aimed at reducing the incidence of common diseases which cause CKD such as diabetes). Typically, programmes follow a systematic approach, involve coordination of multiple stakeholders and have the specific aim of improving patient outcomes and cost-effectiveness. There is an emphasis on utilising evidence-based practice guidelines and patient empowerment strategies to prevent exacerbations and complications whilst constraining the costs of care. The Kaiser Permanente care triangle can be usefully adapted for the management of the different stages of CKD by:

- Supporting self-care for people with early stages of CKD (typically stages 1–2–3a) who are at low risk of complications and hospitalisation
- Providing proactive disease management for people with more advanced CKD (typically stage 3, especially 3b) with regular routine follow-up to prevent progression of CKD and the development of complications
- Ensuring case management for people with advanced CKD (stages 4–5) who have complex needs and are likely to require secondary care services either routinely or in an unplanned way

Ensuring a focus on optimal CKD management in the community should avoid unnecessary hospitalisations and thus control the major contributor to the cost of care in patients with CKD [1].

The typical elements contained within a CKD chronic disease management programme are shown in Box 33.1.

Box 33.1. The Typical Elements Contained Within a CKD Chronic Disease Management Programme

Proactive identification of patients with CKD
Risk stratification and analysis of patient needs
Development of evidence-based guidelines (a number of international and national societies have produced clinical guidelines for the management of CKD – see Box 2.10 in Chap. 2)
Coordination of primary and secondary care
Delivering evidence-based practice:
- Slowing progression of CKD
- Optimal management of complications

Clinician education programmes
Patient education programmes:
- Patient empowerment
- Smoothing transition to renal replacement therapy

Programme evaluation

33.2 Organisation of CKD Care

The provision of comprehensive clinical care in the setting of a specialised renal clinic has been shown to improve a number of quality parameters including stabilisation of GFR and preparation for dialysis. Such clinics allow integration of nephrological expertise, patient education and comprehensive multidisciplinary team support [2]. However, given the prevalence of CKD, it is neither practical nor desirable for all patients to be seen in a secondary care renal clinic. As a result, the importance of involving primary care colleagues in the management of CKD is now increasingly recognised. As CKD is a relatively new concept for primary care, it is not surprising that primary care practitioners are generally less confident in managing CKD than hypertension or diabetes, despite the fact that these are commonly associated with CKD [3]. Primary care clinicians are less likely to achieve control of hypertension, one of the key measures for improving the care of patients with CKD, when their confidence is low. Thus, improving knowledge and confidence of primary care may provide the key to improving the quality of CKD management, especially for higher-risk patients with diabetes and with proteinuria or associated hypertension. The CKD expertise in secondary care therefore should increasingly be used to support and nurture the institution of management programmes for CKD in primary care. Primary care nurses in particular should have specific training as this clinician group delivers much of the chronic disease management in primary care. A recent study has confirmed the health outcome benefits of a CKD-specific 'audit-based education programme' aimed at primary care [4].

A more cohesive multidisciplinary team (MDT) approach to the management of CKD may help avoid fragmentation of care among nephrologists, primary care clinicians and members of patient education teams [5]. Patients with complex comorbidities and CKD may particularly benefit from this approach. The required composition of MDT-CKD care teams is not well defined, but input from many of the clinicians outlined in Box 33.2 may be required.

Box 33.2. Potential Composition of MDT-CKD Care Teams

Nephrologist
General practitioner (primary care)
Renal nurse
Dietician
Pharmacist
Social worker
Clinical psychologist
Occupational therapist
(Other specialist clinical teams, that is, diabetologist, cardiologist)

The management of patients with CKD relies heavily on the collection and interpretation of biomedical data. Thus, there is the potential to improve the quality of care for these patients with the introduction of remote monitoring and tele-consultation. Using IT resources appropriately should allow care to be provided closer to home and reduce the need for the patient to travel, thereby improving their experience. At the same time, such innovation may allow expensive specialist care resources to be targeted to areas where they have the greatest impact and can deliver the maximum value to patients. Patients can also be encouraged to undertake self-monitoring of their condition with, for example, home blood pressure monitoring. This should improve their empowerment and compliance with medication. To date, however such approaches have not been formally evaluated, and their potential to impact positively on the management of patients with CKD remains unknown.

A number of countries have now included CKD in a national noncommunicable chronic disease programme ensuring that CKD has the necessary strategic profile to allow effective coordination of high-quality care at a national level (see reference [6] for overview). In general, it is also important that the financial incentives within a health-care system are appropriately aligned with the delivery of the desired quality standards. Policymakers have also recognised that traditional methods of reimbursement for care often fail to reward the delivery of high-quality treatment and around the world a number of different 'pay for performance' schemes have been introduced to improve the management of CKD. For example, primary care in the UK is incentivised to improve quality of CKD management through the quality outcome framework with incentives tailored to reward achievement of quality standards as defined by NICE [7].

33.3 Do Chronic Disease Management Programmes Improve Outcomes in CKD?

Planned, proactive care has been shown to result in a better quality of life and improved health outcomes for people with a number of chronic diseases [8]. As such there is a compelling rationale to believe that a similar systematic approach to the management of CKD would be likely to be both an optimal and cost-effective way of reducing the rate of progression of CKD and preventing the development of CKD-associated complications. Disease management programmes for CKD have been introduced in a number of countries in the past few years. Whilst a number of these programmes appear to have improved survival and resulted in slowing progression of CKD, others have not. Evaluation of the programmes has not always been rigorous, and randomised controlled trials demonstrating cost-effectiveness are generally lacking. Thus, although promising, chronic disease management approaches to the management of CKD do require further investigation. This uncertainty and the significant cost of this approach have led to some disease management programmes for CKD being discontinued.

Chronic disease management programmes may contain many different interventions making it difficult to evaluate which element either alone or in combination is effective. In a meta-analysis provider education, patient education, patient reminders and patient financial incentives were associated with improvements in provider adherence to guidelines and improvements in patient outcomes [9]. However, the authors were unable to conclude which interventions were most effective commenting on the irony that whilst disease management programmes are designed to reduce unexplained variations in care, the large and unexplained variations in their design, development and implementation impede their effective evaluation.

33.3.1 Developing, Implementing and Evaluating a CKD Management Programme

A tailored chronic disease management programme for CKD has been examined in a primary care setting in the UK in an observational study that included 483 patients with borderline CKD 3/4, CKD 4 and CKD 5 [10]. The programme was coordinated and delivered by a team of nurses, a dietitian and a social worker, and each patient was provided with ongoing support from a named nurse who provided telephone and face-to-face contact without the need for appointments, plus proactive intervention from the clinical team. The programme had four key components:

- Patient education aimed at empowering patients to become involved in their own care
- Medicine management
- Provision of dietetic advice
- Optimisation of clinical management to achieve clinical targets

The objectives of this study are outlined in Box 33.3. The disease management programme reduced the median fall in eGFR in the 9 months prior to joining the programme from 3.69 (1.49–7.46) ml/min/1.73 m^2 to 0.32 ml/min/1.73 m^2 in the 12 months following entry into the programme. More than 85 % of the patients with CKD stage 4 whose kidney function had deteriorated significantly in the 9 months prior to joining the disease management programme subsequently demonstrated stabilised or improved renal function. Systolic BP fell from 139 to 130 mmHg and diastolic BP from 76 to 71 mmHg, and there was an overall improvement in the lipid profile of the patients. Extrapolating from studies in the general (non-CKD) population, a reduction of blood pressure and lipid levels of this magnitude would be expected to translate into a cardiovascular event reduction (stroke and myocardial infarction) in the region of 30 %. An independent economic evaluation of this programme demonstrated that the detection and rigorous systematic treatment and monitoring in primary care of previously undetected cases of CKD led to a decrease in secondary care costs.

It is not clear which elements of the programme had the most powerful effect, and it is of note that this study focused on a small number of predominantly white individuals with more advanced CKD and was observational rather than randomised. Therefore, it is unclear whether these results can be extrapolated more widely to

Box 33.3. Objectives of a Disease Management Programme [10]

- Institute routine eGFR reporting using the four variable MDRD equations.
- Develop and maintain an automated patient identification system, to increase the recognition of patients with CKD, leading to a reduction in the proportion of patients commencing dialysis as an emergency.
- Change referral patterns to ensure that patients were referred in an appropriate and timely manner.
- Improve patient outcomes against nationally accepted and audited quality criteria, leading to a slowing of progression of renal failure and a reduction in comorbidity.
- Carry out risk stratification of all patients with CKD stages 4 and 5.
- Reduce resource utilisation in terms of outpatient visits and unplanned hospitalisation.
- Deliver a patient education programme to patients with CKD stages 4 and 5.
- Reduce the proportion of patients commencing dialysis without permanent vascular access.
- Improve vaccination uptake, particularly against hepatitis B.

different stages of CKD in different populations. Nonetheless, it provides compelling support for the benefits of such an approach.

In most CKD management programmes, the nephrologist provides leadership for the quality improvement process, but it is vital to recognise the importance of everyone's contribution and the need for effective coordination between primary and secondary care. The nurse has a central role in coordinating care and providing ongoing support to encourage the patient to adhere to the plan of care, and in order to fulfil this role, the nurse should have advanced knowledge and training in nephrology in addition to advanced communication skills. The team should also coordinate the management of the comorbid conditions and complications associated with CKD. A multidisciplinary CKD clinic where all members of the team come together around the patient is an ideal environment.

33.4 Barriers and Challenges to Successful CKD Disease Management Programmes

Disease management programmes for CKD face unique challenges. In any population, identification of the patient with CKD can be difficult, not least because patients with CKD are asymptomatic until the late stages of the disease. Historically, 25–30 % of new renal replacement therapy patients present late to renal services which increases the likelihood of an unplanned start onto dialysis with associated increased morbidity, mortality and excessive costs. Identification of patients with CKD is significantly improved by the introduction of automated reporting of eGFR, and a number of countries including the UK have implemented this at a national level. However, in countries where this is not available, complete case ascertainment of patients with CKD is challenging as the serum creatinine may be normal or only slightly elevated despite a significantly reduced eGFR especially in elderly patients. Identification of patients with CKD is also hampered by the incomplete use of the International Classification of Diseases, Ninth Revision (ICD-9) codes for CKD.

CKD is both common and increasing in incidence, and therefore primary care will need to play an integral role in managing CKD patients especially in the early stages of the disease. Confidence to manage CKD is variable in primary care, and the challenge of educating the primary care team to take on this role cannot be underestimated. Nephrologists, specialist renal nurses and dietitians need to play a central role in educating primary care teams about kidney disease, delaying progression, cardiovascular risk reduction and criteria for referral to kidney services. There is scope to integrate evidence-based guidelines for the management of CKD into existing primary care management systems with which they are more familiar such as diabetes and cardiovascular disease.

The number of staff desired, the complexity of the interventions required to manage the multiple CKD-associated comorbidities and the need for a robust integrated IT platform tend to make the establishment of a CKD disease management programme more costly than disease management programmes for other chronic diseases. Although the health and financial benefits of avoiding the need for renal replacement therapy are self-evident, longer periods of follow-up are often required to demonstrate benefit in a CKD disease management programme than in many other chronic diseases. It is therefore essential that contracts for chronic disease management in CKD are set to reflect this or benefits will not be realised.

33.5 Patient Education in CKD

Enhanced educational interventions are routinely provided as part of chronic disease management programmes to improve adherence and allow the patient to take maximum advantage of available care. A programme of predialysis education is considered an integral part of care for patients diagnosed with CKD [11] and has been endorsed by NICE (see Box 33.4). The aim of education for patients is twofold:

- To empower them to work with their clinicians to slow down the progression of their disease.
- To aid decision-making about treatment options. As dialysis is a long-term therapy, it is essential that patients are supported to make effective choices to maximise their quality of life.

Enhanced educational intervention with an emphasis on empowering patients to self-care by providing knowledge on subjects such as kidney function, diet, pharmacological regimens, nutrition and lifestyle along with regular telephone support from a health educator has been shown to delay time to dialysis [12].

Box 33.4. NICE Recommendations for the Provision of Information and Education in CKD [7]

- Offer people with CKD education and information tailored to the stage and cause of CKD, the associated complications and the risk of progression.
- When developing information or education programmes, involve people with CKD in their treatment planning.
- Offer people with CKD high-quality information or education programmes at appropriate stages of their condition to allow time for them to fully understand and make informed choices about their treatment.
- Health-care professionals providing information and education programmes should ensure they have specialist knowledge about CKD and the necessary skills to facilitate learning.
- Health-care professionals working with people with CKD should take account of the psychological aspects of coping with the condition and offer access to appropriate support.

Educational aims are shown in Box 33.5. Good predialysis education will lead some patients to choose conservative kidney management, avoiding the need for dialysis and offering them a better quality of life and a more appropriate outcome.

33.6 How Should Patient Education Be Done?

Good communication between the health-care professional and patient is essential. It is important that all members of the multidisciplinary team (see Box 33.2) are involved in developing the educational programme and that they provide a consistent message to the patient. The education should be supported by evidenced-based written information tailored to the person's needs

Box 33.5. Educational Aims

Understanding the CKD disease process and how it will affect you

Understanding what you should ask your doctor about CKD

Understanding how you can help manage your condition:
- Importance of good blood pressure management
- Management of diabetes (if applicable)

Understanding of health-related issues:
- Diet
- Weight loss
- Smoking cessation
- Exercise

Medicine management:
- Concordance with prescribed therapies
- Over-the-counter medicines (risks of NSAIDs)

Provision of psychological support

Providing information about renal replacement therapy at the appropriate time

Box 33.6. Explicit and Implied Constructs in the Health Belief Model

1. Perceived susceptibility to the illness: What is the perceived personal risk for developing the condition or worsening the condition?
2. Perceived severity of the illness: How bad can it get, what difficulties would the illness create and what would be the effects on quality of life?
3. Perceived benefits of taking preventative action: Will the new behaviour decrease the risk of either developing the condition or worsening the condition?
4. Perceived barriers to taking preventative action: What are the obstacles in the way of adopting the new behaviour?

and should be culturally appropriate. It should also be accessible to people with additional needs such as physical, sensory or learning disabilities and to people who do not speak or read the official language of the country.

The patient and the clinicians should mutually agree the care plan, setting achievable targets and a review date. Knowledge is a prerequisite for change so people need to understand how their lifestyle habits may be affecting their health and appreciate the positive outcomes of changing their behaviour.

As well as incorporating informational elements to improve patient knowledge, a successful education programme will include psychological methods to empower patients and modify behaviour. For behavioural change to occur, people need to be motivated to take control of their health. However, changes to lifestyle such as taking medications as prescribed, smoking cessation and taking regular exercise can be especially difficult to achieve. Just knowing the health risks associated with their behaviour may not be enough to make people want to change, since they may have psychosocial reasons for continuing with behaviour which is damaging to health (e.g. smoking may give a sense of belonging). The health belief model [13] provides a useful framework for designing health behaviour interventions. The underlying principles of the health belief model are given in Box 33.6.

The patient is more likely to respond to messages about health promotion and change behaviour when the patient believes that:

1. He or she *is* at risk of developing the condition.
2. The risk *is* serious and the consequences are undesirable.
3. The risk *will* be reduced by behavioural change.
4. Any barriers to behavioural change *can* be overcome.

Knowing what aspect of the model the patient accepts or rejects can help the clinician to decide on the most appropriate interventions – for example, if the patient is unaware of the risk factors for disease, teaching should be directed at informing the patient about his or her personal risk factors; alternatively, if the patient understands the risk but feels he or she cannot achieve the behavioural change due to perceived barriers, efforts can be focused on overcoming the barriers. Making small successful changes motivates the individual to attempt further change and is preferable to attempting large changes that are usually unsustainable. Regular support is fundamental to the success of an educational programme. The patient should have access to all of the members of the MDT to provide specific expertise, plus a named key worker usually the renal nurse who can provide ongoing contact and can encourage the patient to adhere to the prescribed plan of care. Nurses are well placed to take the lead in this area because of the unique working relationships they develop with patients and their perceived credibility within health promotion. *Contact may be offered in a variety of forms such as group meetings, face-to-face, telephone conversation or* via *the use of technologies such as Skype and text messaging.*

CKD education must be adjusted to acknowledge the diversity of patients with CKD and provision made for the young, the elderly, those with different ethnic backgrounds and those for whom the official language of the country is not the first language. The programme should also be adjusted to take account of the comorbidities that accompany CKD, inevitably increasing the complexity of the education required.

Traditional patient information is usually provided in a two-dimensional written format, but this is inadequate for making complex decisions about therapy options. The use of multimedia teaching (DVD) may be beneficial in helping patients choose their optimal therapy option, reducing uncertainty and decision regret [14]. This approach allows patients and families to repeatedly access at their own pace the information they require and can reduce the time spent by staff.

Holistic predialysis education should also take account of the views of patient's families as well as those of the patient. Feelings of isolation and alienation are common among patients in the predialysis phase, and it has been shown that a group education setting can be a constructive way of helping patients and their relatives out of their isolation [11]. Families and caregivers should also be provided with the information and support they need and with the patient's consent have the opportunity to be involved in decisions about treatment and care. It may also be appropriate, subject to the patient's permission, to liaise with and educate the patient's employer to ensure that appropriate support can be provided in the work environment to allow the patient to stay in employment through the course of their illness.

Obtaining an understanding of the perceptions of patients in the predialysis phase will inform how they will adjust to and accept their diagnosis of end-stage disease. This allows target interventions aimed at improving patient outcomes. Anticipated benefits of patient education in CKD are shown in Box 33.7.

The increasing prevalence of CKD, the time required to deliver education effectively and increasingly constrained health-care expenditure are challenges to the development of CKD

Box 33.7. Anticipated Benefits of Patient Education in CKD

- Improved concordance with medication
- Better blood pressure control
- Better control of diabetes
- A slower rate of progression of CKD
- Reduction in cardiovascular risk
- Improved bone biochemistry
- Reduction in emotional stress and uncertainty
- Improved self-esteem and interpersonal relationships
- Improved opportunity for ongoing employment
- Engagement with decision-making including facilitating live related pre-emptive renal transplantation or adoption of conservative kidney care if appropriate

education programmes. Programmes need to be targeted to provide maximum value, responsibility for which must be shared between primary and secondary care. In earlier stages of CKD, the focus will be on delaying disease progression and improving cardiovascular outcomes. In latter stages, preparation for renal replacement therapy is essential. Patients and their families are required to adapt to changes in health, lifestyle and attitude towards life. If patients and families fail to engage during the early phase, then a lack of understanding and fear prevail with patients then failing to reach a balanced decision about treatment options. Success requires adequate time to absorb the information, process it and adjust accordingly. Thus, the earlier the patient is involved, then the better the outcome. In general, education should begin in the predialysis stage and continue after the commencement of maintenance dialysis. However, the patient has to be ready to accept the need for information before they can engage more fully with it.

Patients must be able to easily and repetitively access information in a format of their choosing. The availability of online information is growing but should not replace human contact. Information points may be provided in hospitals allowing patients to select information in a supported environment and then email it to themselves at home. Follow-up is essential to improve understanding and compliance, and education should not be viewed as a one-stop opportunity with further intervention seen as a luxury.

Providing education in the home environment usually creates a more relaxed atmosphere where the time pressures are less obvious. This also allows an opportunity to assess the home environment in the event a home-based renal replacement therapy is required. Patients may feel more able to ask questions and discuss difficult subjects more easily in their own home. However, other patients may prefer the hospital setting as they wish to keep their home life and medical matters separate. A 'neutral' territory such as a community centre may be appropriate for some and offer the opportunity for groups of patients to be seen together.

In summary, the provision of timely high-quality education to patients throughout the stages of CKD can offer improved patient outcomes. However, it cannot be overemphasised that an effective CKD education programme requires experienced and well-trained staff, who are themselves encouraged and supported. As such this requires support at a national level with investment in the education of the educators as well as the patients.

Before You Finish: Practice Pearls for the Clinician

- CKD chronic disease management programmes have been shown to improve the quality of care and outcomes for patients with CKD.
- A programme should address the progression of CKD and the management of CKD complications and integrate with the care required for common CKD-associated comorbidities principally hypertension, cardiovascular disease and diabetes.
- Effective coordination of a multidisciplinary team with care built around the needs of the patient is essential.
- Patient education, with a focus on patient empowerment, is a fundamental component of any programme. Education should be tailored to the needs of the patient, and the requirements depend on the stage of CKD.
- Economic benefits are more difficult to demonstrate but are likely to be seen in the longer term.
- Professionals involved in the management of CKD also require ongoing development and support.
- The introduction of CKD management programmes is facilitated by national policy guidance on the management of CKD.

References

1. Rastogi A, Linden A, Nissenson AR. Disease management in chronic kidney disease. Adv Chronic Kidney Dis. 2008;15(1):19–28.
2. Ghossein C, Serrano A, Rammohan M, Batlle D. The role of comprehensive renal clinics in chronic kidney disease stabilization and management: the Northwestern experience. Semin Nephrol. 2002;22:526–32.
3. Tahir MA, Dmitrieva O, de Lusignan S, van Vlymen J, Chan T, Golmohamad R, et al. Confidence and quality in managing CKD compared with other cardiovascular diseases and diabetes mellitus: a linked study of questionnaire and routine primary care data. BMC Fam Pract. 2011;12:83.
4. de Lusignan S, Gallagher H, Jones S, Chan T, van Vlymen J, Tahir A, et al. Audit-based education lowers systolic blood pressure in chronic kidney disease: the Quality Improvement in CKD (QICKD) trial results. Kidney Int. 2013;84(3):609–20. doi:10.1038/ki.2013.96. Epub 27 Mar 2013.
5. Bayliss EA, Bhardwaja B, Ross C, Beck A, Lanese DM. Multidisciplinary team care may slow the rate of decline in renal function. Clin J Am Soc Nephrol. 2011;6(4):704–10.
6. Tonelli M, Agarwal S, Cass A, Garcia GG, Jha V, Naicker S, et al., for the ISN CKD Policy Task Force. How to advocate for the inclusion of chronic kidney disease in a national noncommunicable chronic disease program. Kidney Int. Advance online publication 13 Feb 2013. doi:10.1038/ki.2012.488.
7. National Institute for Health and Clinical Excellence (NICE). Chronic kidney disease. National clinical guideline for early identification and management in adults in primary and secondary care (Clinical Guideline 73). London; NICE, 2008. [Updated 2010 March 30, cited 2013 April 20] Available from: http://www.nice.org.uk/Guidance/CG73/Guidance/pdf/English.
8. Ofman JJ, Badamgarav E, Henning J, Knight K, Gano AD, Levan RK, et al. Does disease management improve clinical and economic outcomes in patients with chronic diseases? A systematic review. Am J Med. 2004;117(3):182–92.
9. Weingarten SR, Henning JM, Badamgarav E, Knight K, Hasselblad V, Gano Jr A, Ofman JJ. Interventions used in disease management programmes for patients with chronic illness which ones work? Meta-analysis of published reports. Br Med J. 2002;325(7370):925.
10. Richards N, Harris K, Whitfield M, O'Donoghue D, Lewis R, Mansell M, et al. Primary care-based disease management of chronic kidney disease (CKD), based on estimated glomerular filtration rate (eGFR) reporting, improves patient outcomes. Nephrol Dial Transplant. 2008;23:549–55.
11. Da Silva GM, Goovaerts T, Elseviers M, Lindley EJ. Information and Counselling for patients approaching end-stage renal failure in selected centres across Europe. EDTNA/ERCA J. 2002;28(1):49–55.
12. Devins G, Mendelssohn DC, Barre PE, Binik Y. Predialysis psychoeducational intervention and coping styles influence time to dialysis in chronic kidney disease. Am J Kidney Dis. 2003;42(4):693–703.
13. Rosenstock IM, Strecher VJ, Becker MH. Social learning theory and the health belief model. Health Educ Behav. 1988;15.2:175–83.
14. Chiou CP, Chung YC. Effectiveness of multimedia interactive patient education on knowledge, uncertainty and decision making in patients with end stage renal failure. J Clin Nurs. 2011;21:1223–31.

Conservative/Palliative Treatment and End-of-Life Care in Chronic Kidney Disease

34

Jean L. Holley and Rebecca J. Schmidt

Before You Start: Facts You Need to Know About End-of-Life Care

Palliative or conservative, non-dialytic care should be offered to all patients with advanced CKD. Prognosis is an inherent issue in transitioning to end-of-life care, but there are few tools to predict outcomes in CKD patients who choose not to begin dialysis. Patient-centered advance care planning is an integral aspect of palliative care and is based on determining a patient's goals for care. Advance care planning should be part of the overall care plan for each CKD patient, and nephrology providers need to initiate advance care planning discussions. Advance directives like identifying a health-care surrogate or proxy decision-maker and do-not-resuscitate preferences should be determined for each patient. Symptom burden is high throughout CKD, including near the end of life, and symptom assessment and management are therefore important aspects of palliative care for CKD patients.

34.1 Conservative or Palliative Care in CKD

The word "palliative" has been defined as that which reduces violence associated with disease or a process of easing burdens associated with disease during the dying process that is not curative in nature. The World Health Organization defines palliative care as "An approach that improves the quality of life of patients and their families facing the problems associated with life-threatening illness, through the prevention and relief of suffering by means of early identification and impeccable assessment and treatment of pain and other problems, physical, psychosocial, and spiritual." Life-sustaining technology such as dialysis may provide palliation of some symptoms although the use of organ sustaining technology might be considered counter to the palliative approach. The term "active non-dialytic management" is increasingly used to describe a program of care that excludes renal replacement therapy but encompasses management of biochemical abnormalities as well as symptoms

J.L. Holley, MD (✉)
Department of Internal Medicine and Nephrology, University of Illinois, Urbana-Champaign and Carle Physician Group, S2S2, 602 West University Avenue, Urbana, IL 61801, USA
e-mail: jholley@illinois.edu; jean.holley@carle.com

R.J. Schmidt, DO
Department of Medicine, Nephrology Section, West Virginia University School of Medicine, One Medical Center Drive, 9165, Morgantown, WV 26506, USA
e-mail: rschmidt@hsc.wvu.edu

M. Arici (ed.), *Management of Chronic Kidney Disease*,
DOI 10.1007/978-3-642-54637-2_34, © Springer-Verlag Berlin Heidelberg 2014

accompanying CKD and, ultimately, the dying process. Importantly, conservative, supportive, or palliative care without dialysis can be proactive and deliberate as directed by patient preferences and values and does not necessarily mean "no care." International interest in conservative or palliative care continues to increase, particularly for the elderly who constitute a large and growing proportion of dialysis patients and for whom the costs of care are formidable. In contrast to the 1980s–1990s and even early years of the last decade when the ability to provide life-prolonging care perhaps promoted a blind eye to the propriety of doing so, the concept that dialysis may not be the best option for every patient is quietly growing in acceptance.

Providing informed consent requires an individualized approach and the presentation of clear expectations. In patients with CKD, the option of dialysis is ideally posed before symptoms develop, and there is need for active intervention to delay death. A patient's decision to pursue or forego dialysis will likely be influenced by clinical information provided about prognosis, the dying process, and the quality of life on dialysis. Sharing one's expectations about the anticipated clinical course for a patient poised to die from complications of kidney failure may be helpful to patients as they contemplate their wishes informed by evidence-based information provided to them by their physicians.

Because older patients and those with poor functional status may not live long enough to need dialysis [1–3], it is reasonable to consider prognosis when deciding whether or not to proceed with dialysis. Tools for predicting outcomes in patients with advanced CKD are available [4] and useful to help patients and families decide on the best course of action. Poor functional status and the presence of frailty suggest shorter survival among older dialysis patients as do older age, poor nutritional status, comorbid conditions (especially dementia, peripheral vascular disease, and ischemic heart disease), and answering "no" to the surprise question ("Would you be surprised if this patient died within the next 6 months?") [5, 6].

Such clinical hallmarks of a poor prognosis are important factors to consider when contemplating dialysis as well as when discussing goals of care. The burdens associated with dialysis are multifaceted (social, financial, medical, and logistic), and some patients may not be willing to accept such burdens, instead favoring quality over quantity of additional life. Thus, identifying patients likely to benefit from palliative, conservative, and non-dialytic management before starting dialysis may save them the traumas accompanying renal replacement therapy. For those choosing to proceed with dialysis, repeated evaluation and ongoing conversations about quality of life and the burdens of dialysis should accompany changes in clinical, physiologic, emotional, and social functioning as such changes may prompt a patient, their family, or their nephrologist to consider withdrawal of dialysis.

34.2 End-of-Life Care in CKD

Although care at the end of life is an integral aspect of total care of an individual with CKD, we know even less about end-of-life (EOL) care in CKD than we do about EOL care in those on dialysis. There are few studies of illness trajectory in CKD patients who choose not to begin dialysis, and, thus, there is little information about dying and EOL care in this population. An understanding of prognosis and engagement in advance care planning are foundations upon which all EOL care depends (Fig. 34.1). In CKD patients choosing not to begin dialysis, principles of decision-making will rely on prognosis, including expected survival and quality of life with and without dialysis. Most of our information about EOL care in CKD comes from the dialysis population and reports of family members of patients who withdrew from dialysis. We also have some information about prognosis in dialysis patients which may be applicable to those with CKD choosing not to begin dialysis. However, more specific information in CKD patients would help our understanding of EOL care issues for these patients and their families. Small studies of elderly patients with CKD who choose conservative management (no dialysis) show a shortened

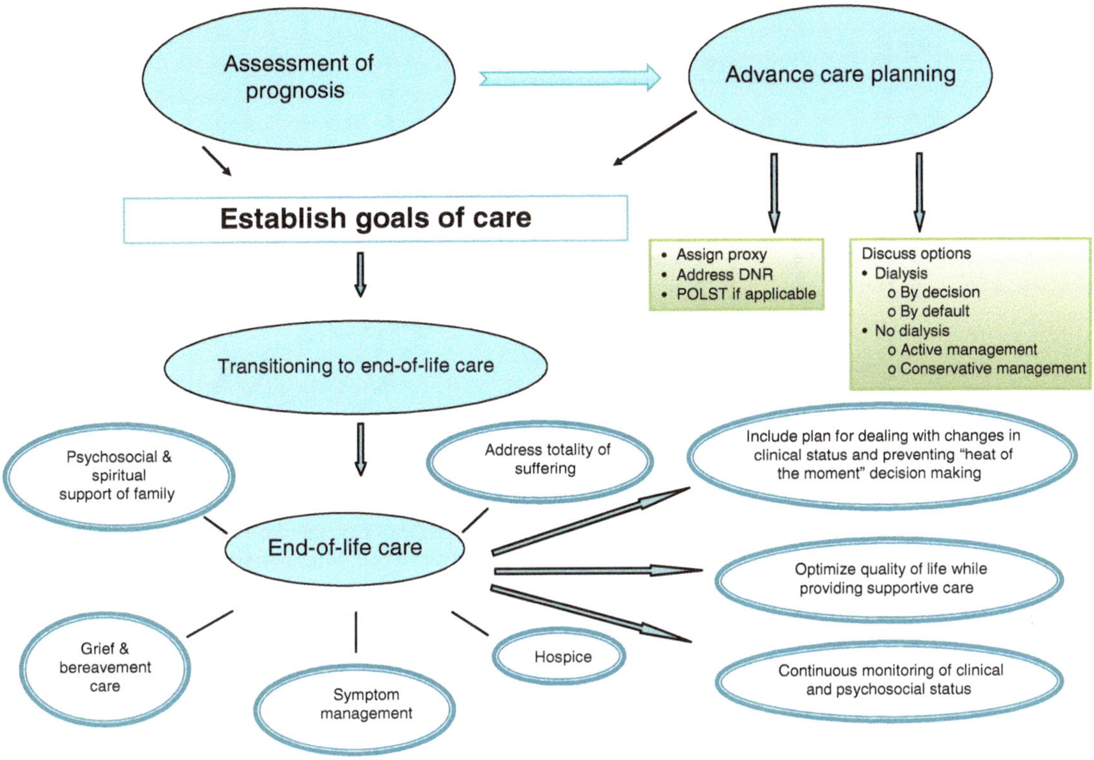

Fig. 34.1 Palliative care in CKD includes advance care planning as well as end-of-life care. This figure depicts an algorithm for palliative care in CKD. *DNR* do not resuscitate, *POLST* Physician Orders for Life-Sustaining Treatment

Table 34.1 Survival in elderly patients with and without dialysis

	N		Survival			
Author	Dialysis	Conservative	Dialysis	Conservative	Age	Est GFR
Carson [7]	173	20	37.8 months	13.9 months	≥70	11[a]
Brunori [8][d]	56	56	84 % 1 year	87 % 1 year	>70	5–7[b]
Murtaugh [9]	52	77	84 % 1 year	68 % 1 year	>75	<15[a]
Joly [10]	107	37	74 % 1 year	29 % 1 year	≥80	<10[c]
DaSilva-Gane [11]	124	30	1,317 days	913 days[e]	33–84	10–17[a]

[a]Modification of Diet in Renal Disease (MDRD) formula
[b]Mean of creatinine clearance and urea clearance in a 24-h urine collection
[c]Cockcroft-Gault formula
[d]Diet intervention
[e]Comorbidity was the primary factor

survival compared with patients beginning dialysis (Table 34.1). In these studies, as in dialysis patients, comorbidity portends a poor prognosis as do age and poor functional status. The typical illness trajectory of patients with solid organ disease (e.g., congestive heart failure or chronic obstructive pulmonary disease) is characterized by a progressive downward slope with intermittent acute episodes or sentinel events from which the patient never returns to his or her baseline status (Fig. 34.2). It is assumed that dialysis patients also follow this pattern of illness with sentinel events represented by hospitalizations, e.g., with a myocardial infarction, limb amputation, or episode of

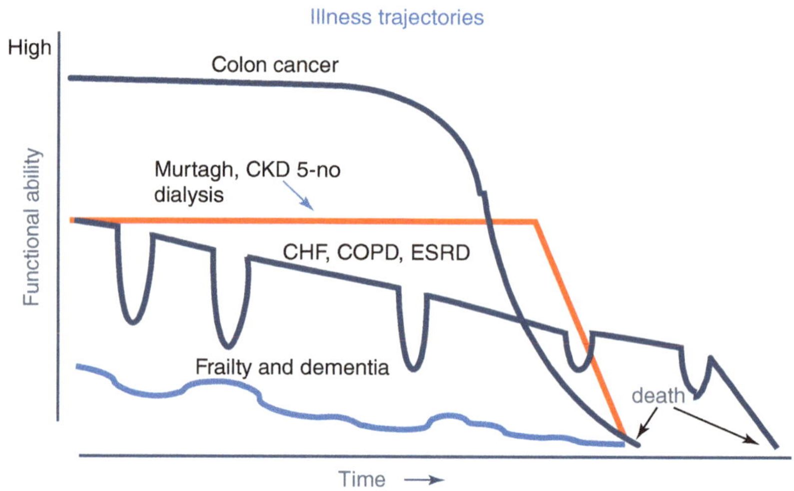

Fig. 34.2 Illness trajectories of various chronic diseases; *CHF* congestive heart failure, *COPD* chronic obstructive pulmonary disease, *ESRD* end-stage renal disease (Reprinted from Holley [12] with permission from the American Society of Nephrology)

access-associated bacteremia. There is only one study of illness trajectory in CKD [13]. A small number of elderly CKD patients managed with palliative or supportive care (no dialysis) demonstrated a fairly well-preserved functional status until shortly before death when an abrupt fall in functional status heralded a rather quick death (Fig. 34.2). Knowing the usual illness trajectory serves multiple purposes including functioning as a guide for addressing and reviewing advance care planning and goals of care, planning for future events and interventions, and completing tasks required before death. Illness trajectories are intimately entwined with illness prognosis and an understanding of each in CKD will facilitate identification of appropriate individuals for decision-making and assist in the transition to EOL care. Additional study of prognostic factors and illness trajectory in CKD is needed.

Transitioning to EOL care requires an honest assessment of prognosis, establishment of goals of care through advance care planning, and educating the patient and family about options for EOL care (Fig. 34.1). As with all other patient populations, ethical and cross-cultural issues will affect decision-making and EOL care in CKD patients. This is most evident during the advance care planning process where a patient and family's values will influence and direct goals of care. Useful questions for addressing values and stimulating discussion during advance care planning are shown in Box 34.1.

Box 34.1. Useful Questions for End-of-Life and Advance Care Planning Discussions

Addressing patient goals

- Given the severity of your illness, what is most important for you to achieve?
- What are your biggest fears?
- What are your most important hopes?
- Is it more important to you to live as long as possible, despite some suffering, or to live without suffering but for a shorter time?

Addressing patient values

- What makes life most worth living for you?
- Are there any circumstances under which you would not find life worth living?
- What do you consider your quality of life to be like now?
- Have you seen or been with someone who had a particularly good (or difficult) death?

34.3 Establishing and Achieving Goals of End-of-Life Care

Assessment of a patient's wishes for EOL care is an important part of comprehensive care irrespective of whether or not a patient chooses to begin dialysis. Many choose to forego dialysis in order to avoid prolongation of the dying process and in an attempt to assure that their desires about treatment remain under their control. Patients and families have taught us that they use advance care planning for a variety of things, to achieve a sense of control, to have treatment choices followed, to relieve burdens on family, to strengthen relationships with loved ones, to avoid inappropriate prolongation of dying, and to be at peace with God [14, 15].

Pertinent issues to address include whether the patient wishes to die at home, in hospital, or elsewhere and specifics about what symptoms are and are not acceptable. Patients who choose to forego or even withdraw from dialysis may be offered the option of reconsidering, an act which may be emotionally helpful to some patients who fear that the dying process will be too unbearable.

Aims of non-dialytic but active and caring management include control of symptoms such as itching, restlessness, dyspnea, confusion, and pain, as well as emotional and spiritual support. Patients choosing the non-dialysis route should be prepared for symptoms arising as a result of renal functional decline. The development of symptoms will vary depending on the degree of remaining kidney function. Patients dying from complications of kidney disease as well as those with other significant comorbidities may develop symptoms of volume overload or biochemical abnormalities of life-threatening magnitude at variable rates, making predicting survival difficult.

Chronic pain has been reported in half of dialysis patients, 82 % of whom have moderate-severe pain [16] (see also Chap. 22). Pain management for patients choosing to forego dialysis requires attention to the reduced renal clearance of many drugs. In addition, the myriad sources of pain in patients with kidney disease also require consideration. The propensity for side effects which may be exacerbated in patients with kidney failure prompted the development of specific recommendations for managing pain and other symptoms in patients on dialysis (Table 34.2). Pain management, irrespective of whether a patient chooses dialysis or the non-dialytic route, is a key component to the care of patients with advanced kidney failure. Plans for treatment should be made in anticipation of symptoms. Neuropathic pain is common and often poorly responsive to opioids, requiring addition of adjuvant medications like tricyclic antidepressants or anticonvulsants. An important part of active non-dialytic management is recognizing evolving symptoms of respiratory distress which may in turn cause anxiety and a patient or family member to question their decision to forego dialysis. Preparing the patient for such events, both emotionally and with specific plans to ameliorate the symptoms, will help avoid patient and family

Table 34.2 Treatment of common EOL symptoms in CKD patients

Symptom	Treatment options
Pruritus	Antihistamines, skin lotion with menthol, dexamethasone
Dyspnea	Relaxation exercises, diuretics, oxygen, morphine
Pain	Opioids ± adjuvants[a]
Dry mouth	Artificial saliva, swabs, good local care
Nausea, vomiting	Haloperidol at 50 % normal dose, Compazine
Constipation	Senokot, stool softeners, lactulose, enemas prn—avoid phosphosoda, magnesium
Respiratory tract secretions	Hyoscyamine 0.125 mg po or SL, scopolamine patch

Source: Data from Davison [16], Douglas [17], and Davison [18]

Adjuvants for neuropathic pain (e.g., gabapentin, pregabalin) require dose adjustments and slow titration of dose; avoid >600 mg daily of gabapentin

[a]If needed for more than 1–2 days, use fentanyl, short-acting hydromorphone although metabolites may accumulate without dialysis. Do not use fentanyl patch in opioid naïve patients. Long-term morphine, meperidine, codeine, propoxyphene contraindicated. Use with caution: oxycodone, tramadol (avoid sustained release form in CKD)—limited data in CKD. Whenever an opioid is prescribed, stool softeners and laxatives also need to be prescribed

anxiety. A plan to address dyspnea, itching, control of pain, and a generalized discussion of what a family might expect is the key to a smooth and acceptable course of conservative care.

Family members of patients choosing conservative management or dialysis withdrawal may need emotional support in addition to guidance in recognizing changes in symptoms that might warrant adjustments in the management program. The logistics of providing care must be considered if families choose not to engage hospice. Just as the acceptance of dialysis infers the acceptance of its associated burdens, the acceptance of the non-dialytic route infers that although death may be imminent and symptoms difficult to control, all efforts to achieve symptom control and a peaceful dying process will be made. Close monitoring of clinical and psychosocial as well as emotional parameters in addition to routine symptom assessment by the health-care providers focusing on new pain, worsening chronic pain, or the development of new symptoms is integral to ongoing care. For CKD patients choosing to proceed with dialysis, establishing goals of care includes plans for dealing with symptoms and changes in clinical status. It is important to continually monitor the patient's response to dialysis, their comorbid conditions, functionality, and quality of life on dialysis. The opportunity for withdrawal from dialysis should be incorporated into the overall plan of care as the patients' desires change or medical status deteriorates.

Advance care planning is best initiated in the early as opposed to late stages of CKD when a plan for EOL care can be established and tailored to a patient's prognosis, values, and preferences (Fig. 34.1). Conservative or palliative care without dialysis can be proactive, deliberate, and directed by individual patient preferences and values and does not mean "no care." Presenting clear expectations, setting contingencies, and incorporating the opportunity for withdrawal for those who choose dialysis may facilitate decision-making in times when clinical events make objectivity difficult. Discussions of prognosis and advance care planning afford patients and families the opportunity to shape the direction of life at its end and, by doing so, provide solace, comfort, and hopefully peace.

34.4 Advance Care Planning

Advance care planning is an important component of palliative care and should be addressed with each CKD patient. The purpose of advance care planning is to establish the goals of care within a care plan consistent with a patient and family's desires [12]. Advance care planning requires the patient's participation and thus his or her ability and interest in the process as well as some perceived benefit and the resources to participate. Completing written advance directives may be an aspect of advance care planning, but because circumstances change and most patients make decisions about desired interventions based on their health status and quality of life (as opposed to the intervention being considered), completing a written advance directive is not the goal of advance care planning. However, some written directives are useful and their completion should be encouraged by all patients. These include designation of a surrogate decision-maker or health-care proxy, completion of a do-not-resuscitate (DNR) form if applicable, and completion of Physician Orders for Life-Sustaining Treatment (POLST) or the equivalent where available (Box 34.2). Various states and regions in the USA have adopted POLST, making them legal documents and therefore not strictly written advance directives. Forms with physician orders for scope of treatment are signed physician orders indicating interventions to be performed or avoided. Orders on the POLST generally include DNR status, preferences for hospitalization, artificial nutrition and hydration including feeding tubes and intravenous fluids, intubation and ventilation, and, in some cases, dialysis. Although discussing advance directives and engaging in the process of advance care planning may be difficult, surveys of various patient groups indicate that patients and families overwhelmingly believe their physicians should raise these issues and initiate the discussions. Focusing on the day-to-day issues raised by medical care can often prevent the setting of goals and exacerbate hopelessness, fear, and uncertainty. Helping CKD patients see future possibilities consistent with their personal values can help maintain hope. Thus, engaging in discussions of prognosis

Box 34.2. Web Resources for Advance Care Planning and End-of-Life Care

1. Coalition for Supportive Care of Kidney patients and website is: (www.kidney-supportivecare.org).
2. The Caring Connections website offers information about advanced care planning and free downloads of state-specific, legal advanced directives (http://www.caringinfo.org/stateaddownload).
3. The Physician Orders for Life-Sustaining Treatment form contains patients' end-of-life wishes in an easily identifiable, portable format with reviewable medical orders. The form honored throughout the health-care system is recognized as a preferred practice by the National Quality Forum in its A National Framework and Preferred Practices for Palliative Care and Hospice Care Quality (http://www.polst.org).
4. Hemodialysis mortality predictor (http://touchcalc.com/calculators/sq).
5. The UK website for end-of-life care (http://www.endoflifecareforadults.nhs.uk/assets/downloads/EndofLifeCareAKD.pdf).

and advance care planning should not be viewed by nephrologists as an act that extinguishes hope for patients and their families. Advance care planning affords patients and their families the opportunity to direct and control their care (Fig. 34.1) and requires physician input.

Once the goals of care are established, plans for EOL care services can be determined. In dialysis patients, we know that EOL care should be discussed whenever conversations involve consideration of prognosis, treatments with low probabilities of success, patients' hopes and fears, and if the physician would not be surprised if the patient died within the next 6–12 months. It seems reasonable to extend this recommendation to those with advanced CKD. Interdisciplinary coordinated care provides opportunities for peaceful dying and "good deaths" by addressing all the domains of suffering (physical, psychological, spiritual, functional, and social) as well as managing symptoms occurring during the end of life (Fig. 34.1).

Figure 34.3 shows the symptoms reported on the Memorial Symptoms Assessment Scale-Short Form during the last 30 days of life in 49 patients with CKD stage 5 managed conservatively and followed prospectively [19]. There are few studies of symptoms experienced at the end of life in any population. Murtagh et al. [19] is the only report of end-of-life symptoms in CKD patients who chose not to begin dialysis. In her study, the mean number of symptoms reported was 16.65 ± 4.04 SD with a range of 6–24; the maximum number of symptoms reportable on the MSAS-SF is 32. Seven additional "renal symptoms" assessed in Murtagh's study included restless legs, muscle cramps, bone/joint pain, dry skin, muscle soreness, chest pain, and headaches [19]. The total number of symptoms possible was therefore 39, and the mean reported number of the 49 studied patients was 20.35 ± 5.20. Similar symptoms have been reported by patients with ESRD who discontinued dialysis with pain, fatigue, dyspnea, and anxiety commonly noted by surviving loved ones [20]. The little information available about symptoms experienced by patients at the end of life suggests that CKD patients have higher symptom distress than cancer patients, especially pruritus, drowsiness, and dyspnea. Constipation, edema, dry mouth, and fatigue were similar among the CKD patients and previous reports of cancer patients during EOL care. There is no information to determine the cause of these symptoms or whether they are due to underlying uremia or comorbid conditions. Clearly, symptoms near the end of life are common among CKD patients, and additional study is needed. End-of-life care for CKD patients foregoing dialysis should include routine symptom assessment with treatment focused on reported symptoms. Table 34.2 illustrates some treatments for commonly reported symptoms. Multidisciplinary care, including hospice and outpatient palliative medicine consultation and follow-up, should be encouraged for all patients in an attempt to alleviate distressing symptoms.

Coordination of EOL care for CKD patients may rest with the patient's primary care provider,

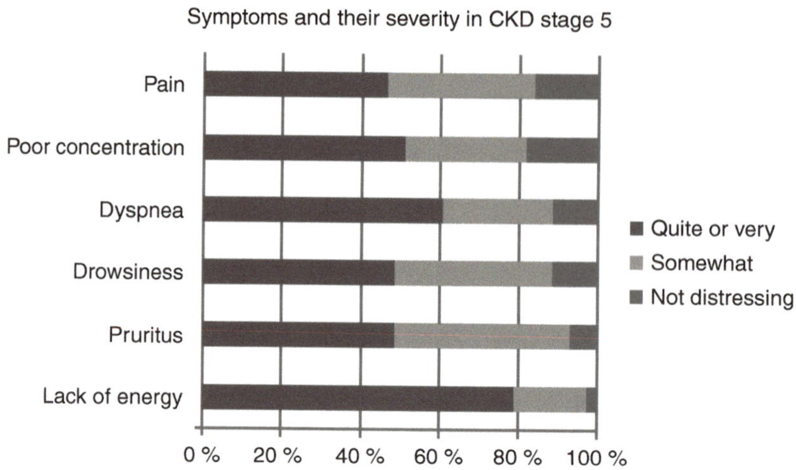

Fig. 34.3 Symptoms reported by CKD stage 5 patients undergoing conservative care (Adapted from Murtagh et al. [19], Copyright 2010, with permission from Elsevier)

nephrologist, or palliative medicine specialist, depending on the availability of services and the patient and family's desires. Hospice care is a Medicare benefit in the US health-care system and requires an anticipated survival of 6 months or less, stipulated by two physicians based on the usual course of the patient's underlying disease. The patient must elect hospice care which requires acknowledgement by the patient and family of the likelihood of death and the relinquishment of attempts at curative therapies. Hospice care includes nurses, aides, clergy, volunteers, and physicians (the patient's own primary provider as well as the hospice director and palliative medicine specialist if available) who work with the family to treat the patient's physical and psychological symptoms and to provide psychosocial and spiritual support to the patient and family. Most hospice care is performed in the home with the family and loved ones acting as the primary caregivers. Hospice care continues after the death of the patient through grief and bereavement care provided to the family and loved ones (Fig. 34.1). This continues for a year following the patient's death.

Although there are multiple guidelines for complications of CKD, there are no specific guidelines for EOL in CKD patients. The Renal Physicians Association clinical practice guideline, *Shared Decision-Making in the Appropriate Initiation of and Withdrawal from Dialysis* (Box 34.3), includes guidelines on establishing a shared decision-making relationship, informing patients about CKD, advance care planning, decisions to withhold or discontinue dialysis, resolving conflicts around dialysis decision-making, providing effective palliative care, and communicating about prognosis, treatment options, and goals of care and is the one guideline focused on aspects of EOL care for CKD and dialysis patients. This guideline also incorporates clinical tools addressing depression and cognitive capacity assessment, functional status, prognosis assessment, and communication skills [2].

Guidelines for comprehensive conservative management for CKD patients are included in the Canadian Guideline for the management of CKD (Box 34.3) but are general (recommending shared decision-making and interdisciplinary care) and, due to lack of controlled trials in this aspect of nephrologic care, are opinions rather than evidence-based recommendations. An EOL care guideline is planned as part of the UK CKD guidelines but is not yet available; general guidelines for EOL care are available in the UK (Box 34.3). Thus, EOL and conservative management of CKD are now recognized as topics of importance to nephrologists and the kind of care they provide. However, we are in the beginning stages of studying and developing evidence-based guidelines for CKD EOL care.

Box 34.3. Relevant Guidelines for EOL Care in CKD

1. Renal Physicians Association Clinical Practice Guideline. Shared decision-making in the appropriate initiation of and withdrawal from dialysis. 2nd ed. Rockville: Renal Physicians Association; 2010 [2]
2. Levin A, Hemmelgarn B, Culleton B, Tobe S, McFarlane P, Ruzicka M, et al. Guidelines for the management of chronic kidney disease. CMAJ. 2008;179:1154–62 [21]
3. Douglas C, Murtagh FEM, Chambers EJ, Howse M, Ellershaw J. Symptom management for the adult patient dying with advanced chronic kidney disease: a review of the literature and development of evidence-based guidelines by a United Kingdom Expert Consensus Group. Pall Med. 2009;23:103–10 [17]

Box 34.4. What the Guidelines Says You Should Do: Key Components of End-of-Life Discussions

- Clarify that palliative care is available irrespective of their decision to pursue or forego dialysis.
- Consider hospice particularly for patients with additional terminal illness.
- Assure decision-making capacity and cognitive capacity for comprehension.
- Determine and agree on the patient's goals for both short- and long-term care.
- Recognize the importance of life experience and tailor the discussion accordingly.
- Engage the patient's family in the decision-making process.
- Distinguish informed consent for the option of dialysis from that associated with the dialysis procedure.
- Present estimate of renal and overall prognosis with and without dialysis.
- Present anticipated changes in functional status with and without dialysis.
- Describe burdens of dialysis, including potential for both intra- and inter-dialytic distress.
- Explain risks of dialysis procedure, including those risks related to dialysis access.
- Make plans for dealing with symptoms that could occur should renal failure progress faster than anticipated and/or faster than other comorbid conditions.
- Discuss desires for acute symptom management and goals to avoid heat of the moment decisions.
- Incorporate the opportunity for withdrawal into practical plan and monitor patient's status accordingly.
- Respect and assure the integrity of the informed consent process.

Source: RPA Clinical Practice Guideline [2]

Although decisions about initiating dialysis are among the most important made by a patient with advanced CKD, until recently, there was little discussion of prognosis and the option of conservative, non-dialytic management of patients with CKD. These discussions are difficult and require an assessment of the patient's goals and values (Fig. 34.1). Such discussions naturally lead to advance care planning, an activity that should be initiated by nephrologists for all patients and families facing advanced CKD. Resources for this aspect of clinical nephrology exist on the web (Box 34.2) and through clinical practice guidelines (Box 34.3) which will undoubtedly expand over the next several years. Figure 34.1 and the available guidelines (Boxes 34.3 and 34.4) focus on key components in EOL discussions which can be addressed whenever a nephrologist initiates a conversation about dialysis. Supportive or conservative care is appropriate for some patients and deserves equal consideration by patients and families. It is only through nephrologist-initiated discussions that this plan of care can be considered.

Before You Finish: Practice Pearls of End-of-Life Care

Initiate advance care planning early in the continuum of chronic kidney disease. Develop a plan for end-of-life care according to the patient's prognosis, values, and preferences and readdress these issues throughout the trajectory of CKD. For patients with advanced kidney disease progressing to dialysis, present the risks and benefits of dialysis as well as those anticipated should the patient choose to forego dialysis. Assure patients that conservative or palliative care without dialysis can be proactive, deliberate, and directed by individual patient preferences and values and does not mean "no care." Patients choosing conservative management and those withdrawing from dialysis should be offered hospice care as interdisciplinary care can assist in the management of symptoms and end-of-life care for patients and families.

References

1. Chandna SM, Da Silva-Gane M, Marshall C, Warwicker P. Survival of elderly patients with stage 5 CKD: comparison between conservative management and renal replacement therapy. Nephrol Dial Transplant. 2011;26:1608–14.
2. Renal Physicians Association Clinical Practice Guideline for shared decision making in the appropriate initiation and withdrawal from dialysis, 2nd ed. Rockville: Renal Physicians Association; 2010.
3. Couchoud C, Labeeuw M, Moranne O, Allot V, Esnault V, Frimat L, et al. A clinical score to predict 6-month prognosis in elderly patients starting dialysis for end-stage renal disease. Nephrol Dial Transplant. 2009;24:1553–61.
4. Conway B, Webster A, Ramsay G, Morgan N, Neary J, Whitworth C, et al. Predicting mortality and uptake of renal replacement therapy in patients with stage 4 chronic kidney disease. Nephrol Dial Transplant. 2009;24:1930–7.
5. Cohen LM, Ruthazer R, Moss AH, Germain MJ. Predicting six-month mortality for patients who are on maintenance hemodialysis. Clin J Am Soc Nephrol. 2010;5:72–9.
6. Kurella TM, Covinsky KE, Chertow GM, Yaffe K, Landefield CS, McCullough CE. Functional status of elderly adults before and after initiation of dialysis. N Engl J Med. 2009;361:1539–47.
7. Carson RC, Juszczak M, Davenport A, Burns A. Is maximum conservative management an equivalent treatment options to dialysis for elderly patients with significant comorbid disease? Clin J Am Soc Nephrol. 2009;4:1611–9.
8. Brunori G, Viola BF, Parrinello G, DeBiase V, Como G, Franco V, et al. Efficacy and safety of a very low protein diet when postponing dialysis in the elderly: a prospective, randomized, multicenter, controlled study. Am J Kidney Dis. 2007;49:569–80.
9. Murtagh FE, Marsh JE, Donohoe P, Ekbal NJ, Sheerin NS, Harris FE. Dialysis or not? A comparative survival study of patients over 75 years with chronic kidney disease stage 5. Nephrol Dial Transplant. 2007;22:1955–62.
10. Joly D, Anglicheau D, Alberti C, Nguyen A-T, Touam M, Grunfeld J-P, et al. Octogenarians reaching end-stage renal disease: cohort study of decision-making and clinical outcomes. J Am Soc Nephrol. 2003;14:1012–21.
11. DaSilva-Gane M, Wellsted D, Greenshields H, Norton S, Chadna SM, Farrington K. Quality of life and survival in patients with advanced kidney failure managed conservatively or by dialysis. Clin J Am Soc Nephrol. 2012;7:2002–9.
12. Holley JL. Advance care planning in CKD/ESRD: an evolving process. Clin J Am Soc Nephrol. 2012;7:1033–8.
13. Murtagh FEM, Sheerin NS, Addington-Hall J, Higginson IJ. Trajectories of illness in stage 5 chronic kidney disease: a longitudinal study of patient symptoms and concerns in the last year of life. Clin J Am Soc Nephrol. 2011;7:1580–90.
14. Singer PA, Martin DK, Kelner M. Quality end-of-life care: patients' perspectives. JAMA. 1999;281:163–8.
15. Steinhauser K, Chastakis NA, Clipp ED, McNeilly M, McIntyre L, Tulsky JA. Factors considered important at the end of life by patients, family, physicians, and other care providers. JAMA. 2000;248:2476–82.
16. Davison SN. The prevalence and management of chronic pain in ESRD. J Palliant Med. 2007;10:1277–87.
17. Douglas C, Murtagh FEM, Chambers EJ, Howse M, Ellershaw J. Symptom management for the adult patient dying with advanced chronic kidney disease:

a review of the literature and development of evidence-based guidelines by a United Kingdom Expert Consensus Group. Palliant Med. 2009;23:103–10.
18. Davison SN. The ethics of end-of-life care for patients with ESRD. Clin J Am Soc Nephrol. 2012;7:2049–57.
19. Murtagh FE, Addington-Hall J, Edmonds P, Donohoe P, Carey I, Jenkins K, et al. Symptoms in the month before death for stage 5 chronic kidney disease patients managed without dialysis. J Pain Symptom Manage. 2010;40:342–52.
20. Cohen LM, Germain MJ, Woods AL, Mirot A, Burleson JA. The family perspective of ESRD deaths. Am J Kidney Dis. 2005;45:154–61.
21. Levin A, Hemmelgarn B, Culleton B, Tobe S, McFarlane P, Ruzicka M, et al. Guidelines for the management of chronic kidney disease. CMAJ. 2008;179:1154–62.

How to Prepare a Chronic Kidney Disease Patient for Transplantation

35

Rahmi Yilmaz and Mustafa Arici

Before You Start: Facts You Need to Know

- Preparing a patient with CKD for transplantation involves careful evaluation for contraindications of transplantation and potential medical and surgical complications.
- A potential renal transplant recipient (RTR) should be evaluated for underlying cause of ESRD, comorbidities such as obesity and diabetes mellitus, malignancies, infectious diseases, gastroenterological evaluation, urologic disorders, hematologic disorders, and cardiovascular status.
- Evaluation of a potential RTR should be initiated with a thorough medical, surgical, and psychosocial history and a detailed physical examination.
- Pretransplantation workup includes a number of serologic tests and radiologic and immunologic studies.
- HLA alloantibody profile of potential RTRs should be assessed to delineate the antigens regarded as unacceptable for transplantation.
- Immunologic evaluation should include the detection and characterization of clinically relevant antibodies.

35.1 Time for Referring to Transplant

Renal transplantation should be recommended to patients with irreversible advanced chronic kidney disease (CKD). The rate of progression in renal injury among patients with CKD is unpredictable because of underlying various kidney diseases and superimposed acute kidney injury attacks. Therefore, for patients not requiring dialysis, time referring to a transplant program remains unclear (Box 35.1). However, referral to a renal transplant program does not imply immediate transplantation. Patients with CKD stage 4 or a glomerular filtration rate (GFR) less than 30 mL/min/1.73 m^2 should be referred to a transplant program [1]. The 2005 Canadian Society of Transplantation consensus guidelines suggest that transplantation should not be performed unless the GFR is less than 20 mL/min and there is evidence of progressive irreversible deterioration over a period of 6–12 months [2]. Patients with a potential contraindication to transplantation

R. Yilmaz, MD (✉)
Department of Nephrology, Hacettepe University Hospital, Medical Faculty of Hacettepe University, Ankara 06100, Turkey
e-mail: ryilmaz@hacettepe.edu.tr; drrahmiy@hotmail.com

M. Arici, MD
Department of Nephrology, Faculty of Medicine, Hacettepe University, Ankara 06100, Turkey
e-mail: aricim@gmail.com

M. Arici (ed.), *Management of Chronic Kidney Disease*,
DOI 10.1007/978-3-642-54637-2_35, © Springer-Verlag Berlin Heidelberg 2014

Box 35.1. What the Guidelines Say You Should Do: Time for Referring to Transplant

- The timing of transplantation should maximize the use of the patient's own kidneys, but avoid the morbidity and expense of access placement and dialysis treatments [1].
- Potential transplant recipients should be referred for evaluation by a transplant program once renal replacement therapy is expected to be required within the next 12 months [2].
- Preemptive kidney transplantation should not proceed unless the measured or calculated glomerular filtration rate is less than 20 mL/min and there is evidence of progressive and irreversible deterioration in renal function over the previous 6–12 months [2].

should be individually discussed with a transplant center to determine candidacy. Several studies have reported improved patient and graft survival when patients receive their first transplant before the need for maintenance dialysis, although this is not the case for patients who are receiving a second transplant; among the latter, a period of dialysis prior to retransplantation is associated with better patient survival [3].

35.2 Evaluation of a Potential Renal Transplant Recipient

Evaluation of a potential renal transplant recipient (RTR) should be initiated with a thorough medical, surgical, and psychosocial history and a detailed physical examination. History of blood transfusion, pregnancies, and previous transplantation should be assessed for potential risks for sensitization. Previous cardiopulmonary diseases and abdominal operations should be carefully evaluated. In addition to history and physical examination, a number of routine laboratory tests are required. After this information is collected, possible contraindications for renal transplantation in each case should be reviewed.

35.2.1 Contraindications to Transplantation

The main contraindications are infections, malignancies, obesity, and cardiovascular diseases (Box 35.2). Serious cardiac dysfunction and untreatable cardiovascular diseases are absolute contraindications for transplantation. Some guidelines listed cardiovascular contraindications as follows: patients who had a myocardial infarct within the last 6 months, patients with a left ventricular ejection fraction less than 35 %, or patients with a stroke or transient ischemic attack within the past 6 months [4, 5]. Despite the lack of long-term data, the benefits of myocardial revascularization procedures before wait-listing are recommended [5]. Diabetes is not contraindicated unless associated with multiple organ failure or significant cardiovascular complications [6]. It is important to note that diabetics gain survival advantage with transplantation as compared to those remaining on dialysis even though long-term survival of diabetic transplant recipients was poor. Guidelines suggested simultaneous pancreas-kidney transplantation for patients with type 1 diabetes [4, 6, 7]. Obesity is associated with more transplant surgery-related complications; however, it is not an absolute contraindication. However, there are some data suggesting that no benefit from kidney transplantation was noted in patients with a BMI greater than 40. In those patients, diet, exercise, and lifestyle changes have to be recommended to achieve a target body mass index (BMI) of <30 kg/m^2 before transplantation [6, 7]. Active cancer is an absolute contraindication for transplantation. Immunosuppression could accelerate progression of the cancer or early recurrence of malignancy associated with high morbidity and mortality. Patients with previous cancer could be eligible for transplantation, but various cancer-free periods are recommended [4, 6, 7]. If possible, acute or chronic infections should be treated before transplantation. However, in some situations infections such as hepatitis B and C and HIV infections are not completely curable. Therefore in those patients, risks and benefits of transplantation must be carefully considered. Guidelines recommended that patients with active HBV, HCV, and HIV infection must be individually assessed, and wait-listing is delayed until completing the treatment [2, 6, 7]. Patients with liver cirrhosis from HBV or HCV infection should be wait-listed for a combined liver and kidney transplantation [1, 2, 6, 7]. There are several comorbidities including some metabolic and severe airway and gastrointestinal diseases which may be contraindications for transplantation. Patients with severe primary oxalosis should be recommended for a liver-kidney transplant [1, 2, 7, 8]. Severe Fabry disease and systemic amyloidosis [2], severe chronic obstructive pulmonary disease or cor pulmonale [2], and acute pancreatitis or active inflammatory bowel disease [2, 7, 8] are contraindications for renal transplantation. Cholecystectomy for gallstones and partial colectomy for colonic diverticulitis are recommended before wait-listing [1, 8]. Surgical interventions and treatment with medication are recommended to patients with genitourinary disorders for appropriate urinary tract drainage before transplantation [1, 9, 10]. Smoking cessation is strongly recommended in some guidelines before wait-listing [6]. Evaluation of psychosocial factors is an important aspect of the transplantation workup. Despite the influence of mental illness on treatment adherence; it is not an absolute indication for elimination from the wait list. However, uncontrolled psychosis or psychiatric disorders and active substance abuse are absolute contraindications for transplantation [7, 8].

Box 35.2. Contraindications to Renal Transplantation [4–7]

Untreatable cardiovascular disease
Obesity (BMI >40 kg/m^2)
Active malignancy
Active infection
Life expectancy <2 years
Severe Fabry disease
Severe systemic amyloidosis
Severe chronic obstructive pulmonary disease and cor pulmonale
Uncontrolled psychosis or psychiatric disorders
Active substance abuse
Immunologic barriers (positive T-cell crossmatch)

35.2.2 Medical Evaluation of a Potential Renal Transplant Recipient

35.2.2.1 Age

Advanced age alone is not a contraindication for renal transplantation but age-related comorbidity is an important limiting factor [7]. Many elderly patients (over 65 years old) have been transplanted successfully and with an acceptable rate of long-term graft function. Additionally, global mortality in elderly patients on the wait list is higher than among elderly RTRs. However, those patients have a greater risk of developing concomitant illnesses or neoplasms and limited life expectancy which reduces the potential benefit of transplantation. Therefore, life expectancy is a more important factor rather than identifying a specific age cutoff. Estimated life expectancy of those patients should be longer than predictable waiting time and enough to reveal the benefits of renal transplantation. A recommended criterion is that the patient would be expected to survive for at least 5 years after transplantation [1, 4].

35.2.2.2 Obesity

Obesity is related with increased posttransplant complications, delayed graft function, surgical wound infection, higher mortality (associated cardiovascular complications), and poorer graft survival. Although upper limit of BMI is controversial, no benefit was noted in patients with BMI greater than or equal to 40 kg/m^2 [7]. Therefore, weight reduction to BMI of 30 kg/m^2 or less should be recommended before the transplantation [1, 4, 6, 7]. In particular, obese patients with cardiovascular disease history should not go through the transplantation before an adequate amount of weight loss has been reached.

35.2.2.3 Diabetes Mellitus

Renal transplantation provides the survival benefit in diabetic patients with ESRD as compared to those diabetics on wait list. Pancreas transplantation provides glycemic control and improves the microvascular or macrovascular complications and quality of life of renal transplant recipients. Therefore, the pancreas transplantation should be considered as an alternative to insulin therapy for ESRD patients

Box 35.3. What the Guidelines Say You Should Do: Diabetes Mellitus

- Simultaneous kidney-pancreas transplantation or living donor renal transplantation is the treatment of choice for patients with type 1 diabetes mellitus who are suitable for renal transplantation [7].

with type 1 diabetes who have undergone, or plan to undergo, renal transplantation (Box 35.3). Patients who have a living kidney donor should consider undergoing renal transplantation before considering subsequent, cadaveric, pancreas transplantation [1, 7]. However, cardiovascular diseases are most frequent in diabetic patients and a thorough evaluation is recommended to exclude silent cardiovascular diseases prior to transplantation [2]. Similarly, as a complication of DM, neurogenic bladder is frequently seen in diabetic patients; therefore, a detailed urologic evaluation is recommended before transplant operation [2, 10].

35.2.2.4 Infections

The clinical preparation of a patient prior to transplantation should include exposure history, cultures for colonization, serologic tests, and administration of vaccines. Exposure to several microorganisms that may be activated by immunosuppressive agents after grafting and current latent infections and colonization should be investigated through a detailed history. Travel history for endemic infections (parasitosis, fungal infections, hepatitis viruses, mycobacterium, etc.); employment and hobbies that expose one to pets, soil, and toxins (psittacosis, endemic fungi, atypical mycobacteria); history of sexually transmitted diseases (especially HIV exposure); vaccinations and childhood illnesses; prior surgery such as splenectomy, portosystemic shunting, or sinus surgery; exposure to mycobacterial infection, especially mycobacterium tuberculosis; BCG vaccination; the results of previous tuberculin skin testing or interferon-gamma release assays; and drug and alcohol use should be questioned in each patient [8]. Transplant candidate vaccination is to be checked for hepatitis A, hepatitis B, pneumococcus, diphtheria, tetanus, pertussis, polio, varicella, measles, mumps, and rubella. Laboratory testing should be performed for past infectious exposures and active or latent infections. However, some tests should be applied to selected patients with high-risk factors. Routine and special tests for potential recipients are presented in Box 35.4. Screening for cytomegalovirus (CMV), hepatitis B virus (HBV), hepatitis C virus (HCV), human immunodeficiency virus (HIV), tuberculosis, *Treponema pallidum*, Epstein-Barr virus (EBV), human T-lymphotropic virus (HTLV), herpes simplex virus (HSV), toxoplasmosis, strongyloides, and varicella-zoster virus (VZV) is recommended for assessing the risk for posttransplant disorders and prophylactic strategies [7, 8]. Patients with HIV and hepatitis B and C should be evaluated by viral load testing. Testing for latent tuberculosis, or tuberculin skin testing (TST), is recommended despite anergy, which is the most common finding in those patients. Additionally, interferon-gamma release assays (IGRAs) may be useful in the detection of latent tuberculosis. X-ray chest films can also be helpful in determining prior exposure to tuberculosis. Transplant candidates,

Box 35.4. Recommended Laboratory Tests to Evaluate a Potential Renal Transplant Recipient [7, 8]

Urinalysis, urine culture
Serologic examination
Hepatitis A, B, and C
Tuberculosis (tuberculin skin testing or interferon-gamma release assays)
HIV
Cytomegalovirus (CMV)
Epstein-Barr virus (EBV)
Herpes simplex virus (HSV)
Varicella-zoster virus (VZV)
Syphilis (Venereal Disease Research Laboratory [VDRL] or rapid plasma reagin [RPR])
Human T-lymphotropic virus (HTLV)-I and HTLV-II
Urine and feces ova examination for parasites (if serology is positive)

Box 35.5. What the Guidelines Say You Should Do: Infections

- All potential transplant recipients should be tested for prior exposure to viral infections [7].
- HIV per se is not a contraindication for kidney transplantation [6].

Box 35.6. What the Guidelines Say You Should Do: Cardiovascular Evaluation

- Noninvasive stress testing may be considered in kidney transplantation candidates with no active cardiac conditions based on the presence of multiple coronary artery disease risk factors regardless of functional status [5].
- Kidney transplantation candidates who have a left ventricular ejection fraction less than 50 %, evidence of ischemic left ventricular dilation, exercise-induced hypotension, angina, or demonstrable ischemia in the distribution of multiple coronary arteries should be referred to a cardiologist for evaluation and long-term management [5].

who have a history of tuberculosis exposure or recent TST conversion or positive IGRA and who have no clinical or radiologic evidence of active disease should receive antituberculosis prophylaxis. If donor has a history of untreated tuberculosis, prophylaxis should be administered to recipients of transplants [7, 8] (Box 35.5).

35.2.3 Pulmonary Evaluation

There is limited information about optimal pretransplant evaluation of patients with pulmonary diseases. However, the evaluation should be similar to that for the general population who undergo other types of surgery. The 2005 Canadian Society of Transplantation consensus guidelines suggest that patients with home oxygen therapy requirement, uncontrolled asthma, and severe chronic obstructive pulmonary disease/pulmonary fibrosis/restrictive disease should not be candidates for transplantation. Predictive value of FEV1 <25 %, PO_2 room air <60 mmHg with exercise desaturation SaO_2 <90 %, >4 lower respiratory tract infections in the last 12 months, and moderate disease with progression are the criteria for severity of pulmonary disease [2]. The pulmonary complications in smoking patients have been reported to be increased over that of nonsmoker patients. Thus, smoking cessation should be strongly recommended to patients who smoke before transplantation [6].

35.2.4 Cardiovascular Diseases

Patients with ESRD have high prevalence of cardiovascular disease. It is important to optimize the cardiovascular status of the transplant recipient before surgery because of high perioperative risk and posttransplant complications. The stress of surgery and anesthetic agents can stimulate various cardiac events. In addition, perioperative cardiac complications may cause delayed graft function [11]. Interventions such as coronary angioplasty/stenting or coronary artery bypass surgery could also affect the allograft. Therefore, transplant recipients should be evaluated for cardiovascular risk and cardiac interventions prior to transplantation [5, 11] (Box 35.6).

A careful history and physical examination are recommended to recognize active cardiac diseases. In addition, a preoperative resting 12-lead ECG is recommended for potential renal transplantation recipients with or without known cardiovascular diseases. Noninvasive stress testing such as exercise testing or thallium perfusion scintigraphy/dobutamine echocardiography for patients with limited mobility should be considered in asymptomatic patients with multiple cardiovascular risk factors including diabetes mellitus, prior cardiovascular disease, more than 1 year on dialysis, left ventricular hypertrophy, age greater than 60 years, smoking, hypertension, and dyslipidemia [5]. Echocardiography may be considered to identify valvular disease, cardiomyopathy, or systolic/diastolic dysfunction and pulmonary hypertension [5]. If initial evaluation reveals that transplant candidates have cardiac failure or exercise-induced angina or hypotension or ischemia, those patients should be referred for further cardiological evaluation. Coronary angiography is recommended in patients with strong evidence of ischemic heart disease [5, 8]. Coronary revascularization by surgery or via angioplasty with stent placement should be considered before transplantation. However, the routine prophylactic coronary revascularization is not recommended for patients with stable coronary artery disease [5, 8].

Transplant candidates should be carefully assessed for peripheral vascular disease which may lead to technical complications during transplant surgery. In addition to physical examination of pulse and evaluation of arterial murmurs, abdominal X-ray study is also recommended. A Doppler ultrasonographic study is indicated for patients with signs of arterial occlusion and vascular calcifications. Angiography may be considered in patients with severe peripheral vascular disease for vascular repair before transplantation [10]. Cerebrovascular disease may also be an important cause of morbidity and mortality in patients after transplantation. If transplant candidates are presented with signs or symptoms or vascular calcifications in X-ray study, Doppler ultrasonographic evaluation of supra-aortic trunk is indicated to complete evaluation. Patients with a history of transient ischemic attack should be referred for further neurological evaluation. If carotid surgery is required, it should be applied before transplantation [10].

35.2.5 Malignancies

Active malignancy is an absolute contraindication to transplantation [6]. This contraindication is linked with short survival and/or progression or de novo development of malignancy by immunosuppressive therapy. For patients with a history of malignancy, close consultation with oncology is essential. Minimum disease-free waiting time is required for almost all cancers before transplantation. Waiting time depends on the type of tumor and changes between 1 and 5 years [4, 8, 10, 12] (Table 35.1). For potential transplant recipients, screening is

Table 35.1 Waiting time for neoplastic diseases before transplantation [4, 8, 11, 12]

Neoplastic disease	Waiting time
Incidental renal cancer	No
Bladder cancer (noninvasive papilloma)	No
In situ cervical carcinoma	No/2 years
Basal cell tumor	No/2 years
Squamous cell carcinoma (skin)	No/2 years
Wilms tumor	2 years
Renal cancer if < 5 cm	2 years
Breast carcinoma (stage 0–2)	2–5years
Melanoma (in situ)	2–5years
Bladder carcinoma (invasive)	2 years
Uterine body cancers	2 years
Testicular cancer	2 years
Thyroid cancer	2 years
Lymphoma	2–5 years
Colorectal carcinoma	
Duke A or B1	2–5 years
Duke C	2–5/>5 years
Duke D	2–5/contraindicated
Invasive cervical carcinoma	>5 years
Renal cell carcinoma if >5 cm	>5 years
Breast carcinoma (stages III–IV)	>5 years/contraindicated
Melanoma invasive	>5 years
Multiple myeloma	Contraindicated

Table 35.2 Screening procedures for cancer before transplantation

Organ	Procedure
Renal	Native renal ultrasound to assess for acquired cystic disease or masses
Lung	Chest X-ray
Hematologic	Complete blood count Leukocyte formula Erythrocyte sedimentation rate Immunofixation electrophoresis (>60 years of age)
Colorectal	Abdominal ultrasonography Colonoscopy if >50 years of age
Prostate	PSA for male >50 years of age
Cervical	Pap smear
Breast	Mammogram for women >40 years of age or with family history of breast cancer

Box 35.7. What the Guidelines Say You Should Do: Malignancies

- Current or active malignancy was absolutely contraindicated for wait-listing in adults and children because of "the risk of dissemination and fatal outcome" with exceptions made for small or superficial skin, prostate, or bladder cancers [4].
- Renal transplantation should only be considered in potential recipients with previous malignancy (excluding non-melanoma skin cancer) if there is no evidence of persistent cancer [7].
- Patients with current or previous cancer should be discussed with an oncologist and considered on a case-by-case basis [6].

recommended for renal, colorectal, prostate, cervical, and breast cancer prior to transplant [8, 10, 11] (Table 35.2) (Box 35.7).

35.2.6 Urologic Disorders

Urinary tract pathologies are observed in up to 25 % of all ESRD patients; therefore all potential renal transplant recipients should be evaluated for the presence of urologic disorders [13]. Congenital or acquired anomalies of urinary system should be treated before transplantation. Detailed clinical history and physical examination, microscopic urine sediment examination, and abdominal ultrasound are basic instruments of urologic evaluation. Additional complementary urodynamic studies may be helpful to assess the recurrent urinary infections, micturition dynamics, and residual diuresis. Augmentation cystoplasty and urinary diversion procedures may be required in some patients with dysfunctional bladder. Similarly, prostate resection before transplantation may be necessary in some male transplant recipients with outflow tract obstruction due to prostate hypertrophy. Pretransplant native nephrectomy is not recommended for all patients with autosomal dominant polycystic kidney disease (ADPKD). Recurrent infection, bleeding and/or intractable pain, and enormously enlarged kidneys may be indications for unilateral or bilateral nephrectomy [10, 13].

35.3 Causes of Kidney Disease

Certain kidney diseases have a chance to recur in the posttransplantation period. Although the incidence of recurrence and graft loss are heterogeneous, the reported recurrence rates of kidney diseases after renal transplantation are presented in Table 35.3 [8, 10, 14]. Despite the high risk for some kidney diseases to recur, recurrence rarely causes early graft loss. Therefore, transplantation is generally not contraindicated; however, a waiting time period is recommended for diseases with a high recurrence risk. In patients with anti-glomerular basement membrane disease, lupus nephritis, vasculitis, and thrombotic microangiopathy, transplantation is recommended after the disease becomes inactive for 6–12 months on minimum or no immunosuppression [6, 7].

35.3.1 Gastrointestinal Disorders

The potential transplant recipients should be evaluated for gastrointestinal disorders prior to transplantation. Peptic ulcer disease may be aggravated after transplantation; therefore candidates with

Table 35.3 Recurrence and graft loss rate of primary renal disease after transplantation [8, 10, 14]

Disease	Recurrence %	Graft loss %
FSGS	20–40	20–50
IgA nephropathy	20–60	45–70
Membranous GN	10–30	10–50
MPGN type I	20–65	15
MPGN type II	50–100	30
Systemic lupus erythematosus	5–54	7
ANCA-associated vasculitis	9–36	7–30
AA amyloidosis	14	Frequent
Anti-GBM disease	Infrequent	Frequent
Cryoglobulinemia	50	Frequent
Fibrillary glomerulonephritis	43	Frequent
Hemolytic uremic syndrome	60	73
Henoch-Schonlein purpura	15–35	11–13

peptic ulcer should be treated until the lesions disappeared by endoscopic examination before transplantation. In addition, H2 receptor antagonists or proton pump inhibitors should be admitted to all candidates for prophylaxis in the posttransplant period [15]. Cholecystitis or diverticulitis may cause serious morbidity and mortality in immunosuppressed patients [8, 10]. Therefore, transplant candidates should be evaluated by ultrasonography and colonoscopy for the presence of cholelithiasis or diverticulosis. If a potential transplant recipient has cholelithiasis, it may be an indication for cholecystectomy. Similarly, presence of diverticulitis history in a transplant candidate with diverticulosis should be considered as an indication for segmental sigmoidectomy prior to transplantation [8, 10].

35.3.2 Hematologic Disorders

Hematologic pretransplantation workup includes complete blood count, measurement of partial thromboplastin time, and international normalized ratio (INR). Coagulation disorders may cause posttransplantation thrombosis, thereby graft loss. If transplant candidates have history of recurrent miscarriage, arteriovenous thrombosis, hemodialysis graft or fistula thrombosis, lupus, and prior graft thrombosis, they should be screened for activated protein C resistance ratio or factor V Leiden mutation, antiphospholipid antibody, lupus anticoagulation, protein C or protein S deficiency, antithrombin III deficiency, and homocysteine levels. Hypercoagulability is not a contraindication for transplantation; however, anticoagulation therapy is recommended for patients in the perioperative period [8, 9].

35.4 Psychiatric/Psychosocial Evaluation

A psychosocial state of transplant candidates should be evaluated by an experienced competent individual before transplantation. Cognitive impairment, mental illness, nonadherence to therapy, and drug or alcohol abuse are potential problems that might adversely affect the outcome of transplantation. Cognitive impairment is not an absolute contraindication to kidney transplantation. Some individuals with irreversible cognitive impairment may be acceptable candidates for transplantation in the presence of a reliable primary support person who will take charge of administering immunosuppressive medications and monitor compliance with medical follow-up. Patient nonadherence to therapy is a contraindication to kidney transplantation. Renal transplantation should be delayed until patients have demonstrated adherence to therapy for at least 6 months. Alcohol and substance abuse can interfere with a patient's ability to adhere to therapy after renal transplantation. Patients with alcohol and/or substance abuse need to be adequately treated before transplantation. Renal transplantation should be delayed until the patient has demonstrated freedom from substance abuse for at least 6 months. Individuals with a significant mood or anxiety disorder, psychosis, substance abuse, or a severe personality disorder should be referred for psychiatric diagnoses, treatment, and follow-up to reduce barriers to transplantation. However, active affective disorders are contraindications to transplantation, depression in ESRD can be readily treated, and case reports also demonstrate the successful transplantation in patients with major psychoses, if adequate support and supervision is provided [1, 2].

35.5 Immunologic Evaluation

Pretransplant immunologic evaluation involves a number of immunologic tests before transplantation (Box 35.8). Besides the blood antigens (ABO), human leukocyte antigens (HLAs) are the strongest transplantation antigens and can stimulate a primary immune response. Antibodies against HLA are found in patients who have been immunized by pregnancy, blood transfusion, or a prior HLA-mismatched allograft. The presence of HLA antibodies is associated with antibody-mediated rejection in the early period of transplantation. Patients with HLA antibodies have increased risk of delayed graft function and rejection in the perioperative period. However, in recent years, patients were successfully transplanted with immunologically incompatible grafts (HLA or ABO incompatible) using various desensitization protocols that reduce the preexisting antibody levels in transplant recipients. An increased degree of HLA antigen mismatching is associated with a greater risk of chronic graft loss and short graft survival, although not early rejection. Therefore, tests for blood and HLA typing and for antibodies to lymphocyte antigens are recommended to potential transplant recipients before transplantation [6, 16–18] (Box 35.9).

Box 35.8. Immunologic Tests Before Transplantation

For Patients on Wait List

- Blood antigens (ABO) typing
- Human leukocyte antigen (HLA) typing
- HLA antibody detection
- PRA
- Donor-specific antibody (DSA) determination by single-antigen bead assays

For Patients with a Known Potential Donor

- Crossmatches by CDC, ELISA, flow cytometry, Luminex

Box 35.9. What the Guidelines Say You Should Do: Immunologic Evaluation

- High immunologic risk is indicated when there are high titers circulating antibodies specific for mismatched donor HLA antigens present at the time of transplantation [18].
- A patient's HLA alloantibody profile must be assessed to delineate the antigens regarded as unacceptable for transplant [18].
- A pretransplant crossmatch should be performed for all patients unless a program exists for identifying those individuals who can confidently be defined as sensitized.
- Patients with no detectable HLA-specific antibodies can be transplanted on the basis of a negative virtual crossmatch (vXM) without waiting for a crossmatch test to be performed [18].
- Serum samples of patients in wait list must be sent to the histocompatibility laboratory no less than three monthly for routine antibody monitoring and also following transfusion of any blood products [18].
- ELISA technology is more sensitive than complement-dependent cytotoxicity (CDC), whereas Luminex bead technologies are more sensitive than both CDC and flow cytometry, enabling the detection of low levels of HLA-specific antibody [17].

Panel-reactive antibody (PRA) defines the presence of HLA antibodies and sensitization against the potential donors. Complement-dependent cytotoxicity (CDC) and the enzyme-linked immunoabsorption (ELISA), flow cytometry, and Luminex-based assays can be used to determine the PRA. When a potential donor is known, a test called crossmatch (XM) which evaluates for any evidence of preformed antibodies with specificity for potential donor is recommended for prevention of hyperacute or acute antibody-mediated rejection. Different techniques included CDC with antihuman globulin (AHG) or dithiothreitol (DTT) and flow cytometry and ELISA and Luminex are available assays which differ in their degree of sensitivity. Recently, a highly sensitive screening technique as single-antigen bead assay has been introduced. This technique can provide virtual crossmatch and immunologic risk assessment for transplant recipients before transplantation. HLA antibody screening and donor-specific antibody (DSA) determination should be regularly performed by PRA tests or single-antigen bead assays especially in highly sensitized patients. CDC T- and B-cell AHG crossmatch are usually recommended for all allograft recipients in many centers. When CDC XM is positive, the process should be repeated with addition of DTT. CDC-positive/DTT-negative test should not prevent transplantation. The result of a CDC-positive/DTT-positive test is a contraindication to transplantation unless donor-specific antibodies (DSAs) can be reduced with desensitization protocols. Flow cytometry can be used as a crossmatch test and is routinely performed in some centers; however, T- and B-cell flow crossmatch are recommended for highly sensitized potential recipients with a history of a positive PRA or with a previous transplant history in others. Despite that the setting of a positive flow crossmatch with negative CDC XM is associated with increased risk for acute antibody-mediated rejection, it is not a contraindication to transplantation. Similarly, if DSA positivity is present in single-antigen bead assay but the CDC XM is negative, this should be interpreted as an increased immunologic risk; however, it is not an absolute contraindication to transplantation especially after elimination of DSA by desensitization [6, 16–18].

35.6 Follow-Up in the Wait List

Transplant candidates on wait list should be ready for transplantation at any time. Therefore, dialysis nephrologists and potential transplant recipients themselves must inform the transplant programs about major developments in the patient's health that could be relevant to their transplant candidacy. Standard health maintenance screening is required, together with the routine updating of serologic and other blood test results that may be relevant to the pre- and/or posttransplant management. Patients considered to be low risk on wait list should be reevaluated at least every 2 years. Annual screening for coronary artery disease (CAD) is required for patients accepted to be at high risk because of previously documented CAD, diabetes mellitus, advanced age, or obesity. Patients with obesity are frequently requested or required to lose weight in order to be listed on the wait list or maintain their active status. Those patients should be also encouraged to engage in frequent physical activity [2, 19]. Patients on wait list may be sensitized by the development of antibodies against histocompatibility antigens as a result of blood transfusion, pregnancy, and prior failed transplants. A patient's HLA alloantibody profile must be assessed to delineate the antigens regarded as unacceptable. Therefore, pretransplant samples should be obtained and tested at three monthly intervals and after known sensitizing events [18] (Box 35.10).

Box 35.10. Relevant Guidelines

1. *American Society of Transplantation Guideline*: The evaluation of renal transplantation candidates: clinical practice guidelines. Am J Transplant. 2001;suppl 1:5–95 [1]. https://www.unitedhealthcareonline.com
2. *Canadian Society of Transplantation Guideline*: Consensus guidelines on eligibility for kidney transplantation. CMAJ. 2005;173:S1 [2]. https://www.cst-transplant.ca
3. *UK Renal Association Guideline*: Clinical practice guideline on the assessment of the potential kidney transplant recipient. Nephron Clin Pract. 2011;118:c209 [7]. https://www.renal.org/guidelines
4. *American Heart Association/The American College of Cardiology Foundation Guideline*: Cardiac Disease Evaluation and Management Among Kidney and Liver Transplantation Candidates. Journal of the American College of Cardiology 2012;60(5):434–80 [5].
5. *British Society for Histocompatibility & Immunogenetics and British Transplantation Society Guideline*: The detection and characterization of clinically relevant antibodies in allotransplantation. Int J Immunogenet. 2010;37(6):435–7 [18]. https://www.bts.org.uk
6. *Deutsche Gesellschaft für Immungenetik (G.O., C.S., and N.L.), The European Federation for Immunogenetics (F.H.J.C. and S.V.F.), and the British Society for Histocompatibility and Immunogenetics Association (C.J.T.) Consensus Report*: Consensus Guidelines on the Testing and Clinical Management Issues Associated With HLA and Non-HLA Antibodies in transplantation. Transplantation 2013; 95(1):19–47 [17]. https://www.efiweb.eu
7. *The European Renal Best Practice (ERBP) Guideline*: Management of donor and recipient of kidney transplant in the peri-operative phase (including preparation and acceptance of living donors). Nephrol Dial Transplant 2013;28: ii1–71[6]. https://www.european-renal-best-practice.org

Before You Finish: Practice Pearls for the Clinician

- Advanced age is not a contraindication to transplantation.
- Kidney transplantation is not beneficial in potential RTR with BMI greater than or equal to 41 kg/m^2.
- Renal or combined kidney-pancreas transplantation provides significant survival advantage to diabetic patients.
- Cardiac interventions such as coronary angioplasty/stenting or coronary artery bypass surgery to transplant recipients with coronary artery disease should be performed before transplantation.
- Regardless of no clinical or radiologic evidence of active tuberculosis, potential RTRs, who have a history of tuberculosis exposure or recent TST conversion or positive IGRA, should receive antituberculosis prophylaxis.
- Minimum disease-free waiting time is required for almost all cancers before transplantation.
- Pretransplant native nephrectomy is not recommended for all patients with autosomal dominant polycystic kidney disease.
- Despite the high risk for some kidney disease to recur, recurrence rarely causes early graft loss.
- Hypercoagulability is not a contraindication for transplantation; however, anticoagulation therapy is recommended for patients in perioperative period.
- The result of a CDC-positive/DTT-positive test is a *contraindication* to transplantation unless donor-specific antibodies (DSAs) can be reduced with desensitization protocols.

References

1. Kasiske BL, Cangro CB, Hariharan S, Hricik DE, Kerman RH, Roth D, et al. The evaluation of renal transplantation candidates: clinical practice guidelines. Am J Transplant. 2001;1:3.
2. Knoll G, Cockfield S, Blydt-Hansen T, Baran D, Kiberd B, Landsberg D, et al. Canadian Society of transplantation: consensus guidelines on eligibility for kidney transplantation. CMAJ. 2005;173:S1.
3. Kasiske BL, Snyder JJ, Matas AJ, Ellison MD, Gill JS, Kausz AT. Pre-emptive kidney transplantation: the advantage and the advantaged. J Am Soc Nephrol. 2002;13:1358–64.
4. Batabyal P, Chapman JR, Wong G, Craig JC, Tong A. Clinical practice guidelines on wait-listing for kidney transplantation: consistent and equitable? Transplantation. 2012;94:703–13.
5. Lentine KL, Costa SP, Weir MR, Robb JF, Fleisher LA, Kasiske BL, et al. Cardiac disease evaluation and management among kidney and liver transplantation candidates. J Am Coll Cardiol. 2012;60(5): 434–80.
6. Abramowicz D, Cochat P, Claas F, Dudley C, Harden P, Heeman U, et al. The ERBP guideline on management of donor and recipient of kidney transplant in the peri-operative phase (including preparation and acceptance of living donors). Nephrol Dial Transplant. 2013;28:ii1–71.
7. Dudley C, Harden P. Renal Association clinical practice guideline on the assessment of the potential kidney transplant recipient. Nephron Clin Pract. 2011;118:c209.
8. Pham PT, Pham PA, Pham PC, Parikh S, Danovitch G. Evaluation of adult kidney transplant candidates. Semin Dial. 2010;23(6):595–605.
9. Kälble T, Alcaraz A, Budde K, Humke U, Karam G, Lucan M, Nicita G, Süsal C. Kidney recipient. Guidelines on renal transplantation. Arnhem, the Netherlands: European Association of Urology (EAU); 2009 Mar. p. 29–43.
10. Benavente RC, Dorado CQ, Martin LL, Rodriguez CS, Gonima PC, Enguita CG. The candidate for renal transplantation work up: medical, urological and oncological evaluation. Arch Esp Urol. 2011;64(5): 441–60.
11. Bunnapradist S, Danovitch GM. Evaluation of adult kidney transplant candidates. Am J Kidney Dis. 2007; 50:890–8.
12. Girndt M, Köhler H. Waiting time for patients with history of malignant disease before listing for organ transplantation. Transplantation. 2005;80 Suppl 1:S167–70.
13. Power E, Hickey DP, Little DM. Urological evaluation prior to renal transplantation. Transplant Proc. 2004;36:2962–7.
14. Canaud G, Audard V, Kofman T, Lang P, Legendre C, Grimbert P. Recurrence from primary and secondary glomerulopathy after renal transplant. Transpl Int. 2012;25:812–24.
15. Khedmat H, Ahmadzad-Asl M, Amini M, Lessan-Pezeshki M, Einollahi B, Pourfarziani V, et al. Gastro-Duodenal lesions and Helicobacter pylori infection in uremic patients and renal transplant recipients. Transplant Proc. 2007;39:1003–7.
16. Lee PC, Ozawa M, Hung CJ, Lin YJ, Chang SS, Chou TC. Reappraisal of HLA antibody analysis and crossmatching in kidney transplantation. Transplant Proc. 2009;41:95–8.
17. Tait BD, Süsal C, Gebel HM, Nickerson PW, Zachary AA, Claas FH, et al. Consensus guidelines on the testing and clinical management issues associated with HLA and non-HLA antibodies in transplantation. Transplantation. 2013;95(1):19–47.
18. Howell WM, Harmer A, Briggs D, Dyer P, Fuggle SV, Martin S, et al. British Society for Histocompatibility & Immunogenetics. British Transplantation Society British Society for Histocompatibility & Immunogenetics and British Transplantation Society guidelines for the detection and characterisation of clinically relevant antibodies in allotransplantation. Int J Immunogenet. 2010;37(6):435–7.
19. Danovitch GM, Hariharan S, Pirsch JD, Rush D, Roth D, Ramos E, et al. Management of the waiting list for cadaveric kidney transplants: report of a survey and recommendations by the clinical practice guidelines committee of the American Society of Transplantation. J Am Soc Nephrol. 2002;13:528–35.

36 How to Prepare a Chronic Kidney Disease Patient for Dialysis

Ricardo Correa-Rotter and Juan C. Ramírez-Sandoval

Before You Start: Facts You Need to Know

- Preparation for dialysis must be patient centered.
- The goals of preparation include an informed selection of dialysis modality, preemptive transplant when possible, timely placement of appropriate dialysis access, timely initiation of dialysis, reduction of morbidity, and optimal survival.
- Dialysis access should be placed early to preclude the need for temporal venous catheters.
- The decision of when to start dialysis should be individualized based on symptoms and/or the appearance of complications yet should not be delayed until patient reaches a specific value of estimated eGFR or becomes too symptomatic.

R. Correa-Rotter, MD (✉)
J.C. Ramírez-Sandoval, MD
Department of Nephrology and Mineral Metabolism, Instituto Nacional de Ciencias Médicas y Nutrición Salvador Zubirán, Vasco de Quiroga 15, Delegación Tlalpan, Mexico City, DF 14000, Mexico
e-mail: correarotter@prodigy.net.mx; juancarlosramirezsandoval@yahoo.com

36.1 The Importance of Preparation Before Dialysis Initiation

Careful planning before dialysis is required and may prevent many medical and social problems associated with advanced end-stage renal disease (ESRD). Patients with ESRD have exceedingly high morbidity and mortality rates, particularly in the first year after dialysis initiation, when annual mortality rate may exceed 25 %. All-cause mortality peaks in the second to third months on hemodialysis (HD) and then falls significantly and even more after the first year. For example, incident HD patients in 2009 had an all-cause mortality of 435 deaths per 1,000 patient years at risk in month 2 and then fell to 206 at month 12; cardiovascular mortality peaked at 169 at month 2 and decreased to 78 at month 12. Mortality due to infection peaks at months 2 and 3 with 40–43 per 1,000 patient deaths [1]. In some reports nearly 35 % of HD patients died within the first 90 days. A retrospective cohort study using data from the Dialysis Outcomes and Practice Patterns Study (DOPPS; 1996 through 2004) found a mortality risk highest during the first 120 days after HD initiation (27.5 deaths per 100 person-years) compared with risk from days 121 to 365 after initiation (21.9 deaths per 100 person-years; *p*: 0.002) [2]. All these studies suggest that inadequate predialysis nephrology care may be strongly associated with mortality, highlighting the potential benefits of a careful preparation plan before dialysis.

M. Arici (ed.), *Management of Chronic Kidney Disease*,
DOI 10.1007/978-3-642-54637-2_36, © Springer-Verlag Berlin Heidelberg 2014

Table 36.1 Adjusted hazard ratios (AHR) and 95 % confidence interval between patients' characteristics and death <120 days after initiation of HD among incident HD patients ($n = 4{,}802$), DOPPS 1996–2004

Variable	AHR, 95 % CI
Age, per 10 years	
65–74	1.65, 1.22–2.22
≥75	2.49, 1.86–3.31
White race versus nonwhite	1.40, 1.07–1.80
Catheter versus AV fistula or AV graft	1.62, 1.05–2.51
Serum albumin <3.5 g/dl	1.57, 1.18–2.09
Serum phosphorus <3.5 mg/dL	1.47, 1.02–2.10
Comorbid conditions (yes versus no)	
Cancer, other than skin	1.41, 1.07–1.85
Congestive heart failure	1.71, 1.35–2.17
HIV/AIDS	2.85, 1.34–6.06
Lung disease	1.33, 1.04–1.69
Psychiatric disorders	1.35, 1.09–1.68
Nephrology pre-ESRD care (yes versus no)	0.65, 0.51–0.83

Source: Data from Bradbury et al. [2]

Some factors associated with an increased risk of mortality (Table 36.1) at dialysis initiation are not modifiable, including age >75 years, cancer history, lung disease, neurologic disease, HIV/AIDS, or psychiatric disorders, among many others. Nevertheless, there are other patients' features associated with mortality, such as temporary access use at the beginning of HD, serum albumin levels <3.5 g/dl, or serum phosphorus levels <3.5 mg/dl that can be modifiable with clinical care [2]. An optimal preparation for dialysis allows proper patient education, modality selection, and creation of a permanent access.

Adequate preparation for dialysis can improve survival. There is no study that has tested an intervention strategy focused in preparing patients before chronic dialysis; nevertheless, there is strong evidence that a targeted program of medical and teaching intervention at the beginning of HD results in improved morbidity and mortality during the first 90 days, and this improvement is sustained during the following 120 days [3]. A longer duration of predialysis nephrology care is associated with a graded survival benefit, especially when evidence-based KDOQI guidelines goals are accomplished [4]. According to KDIGO guidelines [5], patients with progressive chronic kidney disease (CKD) in whom the risk of kidney failure within 1 year is 10–20 % or higher, as determined by validated risk prediction tools, should be managed in a multidisciplinary care setting. In counterpart, suboptimal HD or peritoneal dialysis (PD) initiation (defined as initiation as an inpatient and/or with a central venous catheter (CVC) in the case of HD) is associated with an increased mortality in the following 6 months [6].

In this chapter, we discuss the goals of an adequate preparation for dialysis and present a practical step-by-step approach to help bridge the gap in care and reduce the high mortality seen in the first few months after initiation.

36.2 Objectives of Adequate Preparation for Dialysis

The goals of an adequate preparation for dialysis are:

- Patients must not require hospitalization for the management of untreated acute or chronic complications of uremia.
- Patients must have a thorough understanding of the different treatment options.
- Patients must have a functioning permanent access for the dialysis therapy decided jointly between the patient and the nephrologist.

36.3 Selection of the Patient

The first step is to properly identify CKD patients who may progress in the near future to a more advanced stage and require renal replacement therapy. It is inappropriate to consider only one element such as an estimated glomerular filtration rate (eGFR) below a certain threshold (v.gr. according to what was agreed in previous reviews you told us it would be e.g. <30 ml/min/1.73 m^2; e*GFR KDOQI Stage 4*) for renal replacement therapy preparation, as specific conditions vary among patients. For example, many elderly individuals with CKD are unlikely to exhibit sufficient progressive renal function decline to require dialysis, or the likelihood of dying prior to initiating dialysis far exceeds the likelihood of starting dialysis therapy. In addition, patients with certain nephropathies, in

Box 36.1. Characteristics Associated with Progression to ESRD

- eGFR <30 ml/min/1.73 m^2 and young age, high blood pressure, underlying renal disease (diabetes, APKD, primary glomerular disease), and development of CKD complications (such as increased serum phosphorus and/or decline in hemoglobin levels)
- Rapid decline in kidney function over time (slope of eGFR against time)
- Persistent albuminuria (albuminuria category 3 KDIGO [A3] = albumin excretion rate >300 mg/day or albumin/creatinine ratio >30 g/g)
- History of acute kidney injury and requirement of transient dialysis

Source: Data from Kidney Disease: Improving Global Outcomes (KDIGO) CKD Work Group [5]

particular tubulointerstitial, display a slower progression pattern, which may justify an individualized delay in the preparation for dialysis.

No single characteristic can reliably identify which individuals and at what rate are to progress to ESRD. In Box 36.1, we focus on at least one additional evaluation tool, associated with a high probability of reaching ESRD, in addition to an isolated low eGFR, which could aid to identify those who would benefit from preparation for future dialysis. The slope of decline of the eGFR against time allows us to recognize those patients whose renal function is deteriorating at a rate that predicts they will require dialysis in the next 1–2 years and who therefore should be referred to the multidisciplinary team. Age alone should not be used as a barrier for referral and treatment; dialysis decision should be made on a composite assessment of the health and functional status of the individual. In every consultation with a patient likely to reach ESRD, the nephrologists must work in the process of information and therefore timely preparation for dialysis. Moreover, all patients with advanced CKD could benefit from education tailored to each individual's probability of need of future dialysis.

36.4 Selection of Dialysis Modality

Preparation for dialysis should begin early enough in the course of CKD to allow time for patients to consider different treatment options and to establish a permanent functioning access for the dialysis modality of choice. Patient education in those with CKD is shown to be highly effective when focused on health promotion, shared decision-making, and discussion of treatment options (Chap. 33). Depending on multiple factors including patients' personal will, style of life, age, presence of comorbidities, and availability of local dialysis facilities, among many others, patient's/physician's choice can include three options: non-dialytic maximum conservative management (Chap. 34), preemptive kidney transplantation (Chap. 35), and dialysis.

36.4.1 Hemodialysis Versus Peritoneal Dialysis

We summarize the general characteristics of two major modalities of renal replacement therapy: HD and PD in Table 36.2. The preferred choice of dialysis modality in patients with ESRD differs between countries, within countries between communities, and due to a multiplicity of reasons: availability of the technologies, economic capabilities of the health system and in some instances of the individuals themselves, economic incentives to provide specific modes of treatment, the experience of the physicians in particular and in general of the dialysis center, the appropriate training of health-care professionals to provide home dialysis therapies, and many others [7].

The available epidemiological evidence of published survival studies is not strong enough to guide patients'/physicians' selection of a specific dialysis modality. Previous studies described that the relative risk of death between the HD and PD appears to change over time after dialysis initiation. Several studies in the last decades indicated that PD is associated with better survival during the first 1–2 years of renal replacement treatment, whereas HD is associated with better survival thereafter. Explanations for this shift have been

Table 36.2 Hemodialysis and peritoneal dialysis

Modality of renal replacement therapy	Hemodialysis	Peritoneal dialysis
Technique	Blood is exposed to dialysate across a semipermeable membrane. Small solutes and electrolytes diffuse down a gradient due to concentration differences	The peritoneum is a semipermeable membrane and is exposed to high intraperitoneal osmotic or oncotic gradients (glucose or glucose polymers)
	Water can be driven through the membrane by hydrostatic force	Small solutes diffuse through small pores and macromolecules diffuse through large pores by convection
Dialysate characteristics	A solution containing predefined concentrations of electrolytes	A solution containing high glucose or glucose polymers and a predefined concentration of electrolytes
Patients' characteristics favored by method	1. Patients' desire of dialysis-free days	1. Infants or very young children
	2. Functional dialysis access	2. Difficult vascular access
	3. Possibility to attend a dialysis center	3. Desire to avoid attending a dialysis center
Advantages	Patients are free of other dialysis responsibilities between sessions	PD may be less expensive in most environments
		PD may allow patients more independence and freedom to travel
Consider	Home HD, performed in some centers (nocturnal or short HD), has shown a relatively better survival as compared with in-center conventional HD	PD may not be the best option for patients who do not have social stability and family support, in particular if elderly

proposed, including a reduced rate of loss of residual renal function in PD patients, and a greater level of comorbidity among HD patients at initiation [8] seems to benefit early PD survival, whereas technique failure due to recurrent peritonitis and loss of ultrafiltration with an increase in peritoneal membrane transport [9] and less frequent monitoring of PD patients by their nephrologists might be factors becoming adversely relevant after the first few years on PD. The other explanation was that patients with little or no predialysis nephrology care invariably started HD with a central venous catheter. In this case, the absence of predialysis nephrology care and of course the use of a hemodialysis catheter instead of a well-planned permanent access were strong factors that made the death risk of HD to appear higher, early in the course of renal replacement treatment.

On the other hand, at present, there is no consistent evidence of higher long-term death risk in PD patients in the USA. The adjusted survival of PD and HD is almost identical in recent studies [10]. Furthermore, the 10-year survival of patients who started treatment with any of the two therapies in 1999 was remarkably similar (HD and PD 12 %) [1]. Conclusion from old studies suggests that these survival differences are not attributable to the dialysis therapy itself. Instead, they either reflect biases arising from where geographically patients were treated with HD and PD or point opportunities for improvements in patient management.

In addition to general differences between treatment modalities, survival is also dependent on other patient-specific influential factors such as age, gender, race, body weight, and educational status. Understanding these subgroup differences and mortality trends is essential for optimizing patient outcomes. In Table 36.3 absolute and relative contraindications to HD and PD are listed. The majority of patients with ESRD are suitable for treatment with either PD or HD.

Patients selected to HD or PD must know and understand the following points:

1. *Preservation of veins and avoidance of unnecessary catheters*. Most patients undergoing HD will require several arteriovenous fistulae

Table 36.3 Contraindications to PD or hemodialysis

	Peritoneal dialysis	Hemodialysis
Absolute	Peritoneal adhesions, fibrosis, or abdominal malignancy which precludes use of the peritoneal cavity	Impossibility to have an appropriate vascular access
	Non-correctable hernia, abdominal wall stoma, or diaphragmatic fluid leak	
Relative	Recent abdominal aortic graft	Coagulopathy
	Ventriculoperitoneal shunt	Difficult vascular access
	Body mass index ≥40 kg/m^2	Needle phobia
	Skin infection	
	Inflammatory bowel disease (e.g., Crohn's, ulcerative colitis)	

or grafts in both upper extremities in particular if they are not subjected to early kidney transplantation. Patients selected to PD also must preserve their veins, considering the potential failure of the PD technique during the course of treatment. Cannulation of veins above the wrist in either upper extremity should be avoided in as much as possible [11]. Every effort should be made to limit phlebotomy and intravenous catheters to veins in the hand. Peripherally inserted central catheters (commonly known as PICC lines) must not be used because they can cause thrombosis of the upper arm veins precluding future vascular access in the entire ipsilateral upper extremity. PICC lines in patients with prior venous thrombosis and use of double-lumen 5-F or triple-lumen 6-F PICCs are risk factors for deep venous thrombosis. If the patient needs a temporary central venous access during surgery or hospitalization, internal jugular access must be the preferable site. Subclavian site for catheter placement should be considered as a last resort given the significant risk of subclavian vein stenosis, which may compromise the construction of a permanent access.

2. *Timely construction of a vascular access.* Sufficient time should be allocated for placement and maturation of a permanent dialysis access. Education about CKD, dialysis therapies, and dialysis access should be initiated in individuals with an eGFR 20–30 ml/min/1.73 m^2. Furthermore, vascular access should be placed in patients with an eGFR 15–20 ml/min/1.73 m^2, in whom progression to ESRD seems likely (Fig. 36.1).

36.4.1.1 Hemodialysis

The first permanent vascular access, either arteriovenous (AV) fistula or arteriovenous vascular (AV) graft, should be placed early enough to allow, if needed, the time to either revise the initial access or second access to be placed, mature, and adequate for cannulation prior to initiation of dialysis. The only justification not to place an AV fistula or an AV graft is the technical or mechanical impossibility to place them; in these cases, a cuffed catheter may be the appropriate vascular access. In Table 36.4 the advantages and disadvantages of vascular accesses, including AV fistulae, AV grafts, and cuffed catheters, are summarized. If the patient is going to be on HD, the first option must always be AV fistula and an AV graft as a second-line option. For new HD patients initiating with an AV fistula, median time to first cannulation varies greatly between countries: Japan and Italy (25 and 27 days), Germany (42 days), Spain and France (80 and 86 days), and the UK and USA (96 and 98 days). Cannulation of an AV fistula within the first 2–3 weeks of creation is associated with reduced long-term fistula survival. AV grafts ideally should be left to mature for at least 14 days before the first cannulation.

36.4.1.2 Peritoneal Dialysis

Peritoneal catheters may be categorized as acute (without subcutaneous cuff) or chronic (with subcutaneous cuff, commonly known as Tenckhoff catheter due to the fact that this model is the one most extensively used). A chronic catheter should be placed initially in all cases, as acute catheters are rigid and imply an increased risk of perforation,

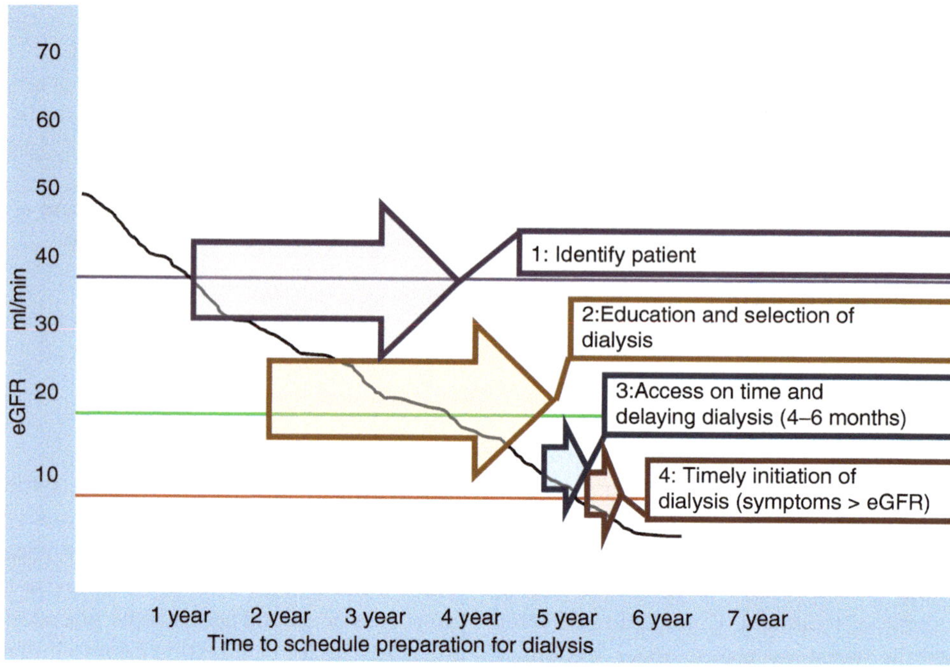

Fig. 36.1 Preparation for dialysis. The figure shows a hypothetical case progressing from CKD stage 3b to ESRD (stage 5) with a relentless and time-dependent decline in kidney function along 6 years of follow-up. In this hypothetical case, the identification of progression from stage 3b to 4 (*purple arrow*) should indicate the right time to start patient education and selection of dialysis modality, when GFR is around 30–20 ml/min/1.73 m^2 (*brown arrow*). Once modality is selected, construction of a vascular access or placing of a peritoneal catheter must be done according to clinical criteria and institutional facilities, months (HD) or weeks (PD) before planned initiation of dialysis (*blue arrow*). The initiation of HD or PD must happen according to clinical judgment, not only by an isolated eGFR value. Almost all patients should start dialysis when eGFR is above 7 ml/min/1.73 m^2. Some authors have suggested that the majority of patients do not show this progressive and predictable decline in kidney function, and this scheme must be adapted according to different clinical scenarios

Table 36.4 Vascular access

Vascular access	Advantages	Disadvantages	Commentary
AV fistula	Can last many years	Early failure (failing to mature)	Preferred vascular access
	Lower frequency of stenosis, thrombosis, and infection, as compared to AV grafts	Longer time to first cannulation than AV graft	
AV Graft	Lower risk of early failure than AV fistula	Requires more frequent intervention for maintaining patency	Useful in elderly patients with limited life expectancy
	Early cannulation		May be selected in patients with history of AV fistula failure to mature
Cuffed venous catheter	No "waiting time" after placement	Patients with catheters develop infections more often, have higher levels of inflammatory markers and higher mortality	Effective flow >350 ml per minute can rarely be obtained, which results in lower dialysis efficiency
	Can be used as a long-term vascular access for patients in whom an AV access cannot be created	High rate of vascular stenosis and potential development of superior vena cava syndrome	Increased recirculation which lowers dialysis efficiency

Source: Data from Saggi et al. [12]

do not have cuffs to protect against bacterial migration from the skin site to the subcutaneous tract so incidence of peritonitis increases beyond 3 days of use, and need to be replaced in short periods of time. In addition, acute catheters commonly present early dysfunction and hernia formation. Acute catheters were extensively employed in the past, yet nowadays there is no justification for their use in clinical practice unless this is the only available option.

In patients who have been selected or chosen to perform PD, the optimal interval between chronic catheter placement and the start of PD is approximately 2 weeks (known as the break-in period), which allows sufficient time for the catheter track to heal and minimizes the chance of a leak when dialysate is instilled in the peritoneal cavity [13]. During the break-in period, at least once per week and preferably up to 3 times per week during the break-in period, heparinized saline or 1.5 % dialysate is infused into the abdomen and drained. When PD has to be started within a week of catheter placement or even immediately after placement, the abdomen is drained and left dry for part of each day, the volume of infusion may be reduced to half of its total usual volume, and patient activity is initially restricted when peritoneal fluid is preset to minimize intraperitoneal pressure increase.

While chronic PD catheters are typically implanted by surgical dissection in the operating room, effective and safe techniques for placement at the bedside or in an ambulatory surgical suite, utilizing guidewire and dilators or peritoneoscopy, also exist. It has often been argued that PD can be used for patients who are referred late, as in most patients PD can be started within 24–96 h of placement of a PD catheter, as long as care is taken to instill low volumes of fluid with the patient lying supine. Implementation of a "PD first" program, as a policy or as a preferable system, has been argued by some as of benefit, yet it is clear that this may depend on local resources and expertise and should also ideally depend on patient's participation on the decision process [14]. In some centers, the use of the embedded PD catheter technique is associated with low rates of surgical, mechanical, and infectious complications. In this technique, the free end of the catheter is embedded in a tunnel under the abdominal subcutaneous fat for a period of 4–6 weeks.

36.5 Timely Initiation of Dialysis

As stated above, among patients with advanced CKD, the decision to start dialysis should not be solely based upon the value of serum creatinine or eGFR. We should not postpone dialysis until the kidney function reaches a prespecified eGFR, especially in patients who develop uremic symptoms, volume overload, hyperkalemia refractory to medical therapy, or significant protein energy wasting syndrome. In the last decade, guidelines recommended that starting dialysis should be considered when a certain eGFR value was reached ($\leq$10 ml/min/1.73 m^2 or even higher in diabetic patients) [11]. One of the problems with this recommendation is that the calculation of eGFR based on serum creatinine may be quite inaccurate when kidney function is extremely reduced. Although a low serum creatinine concentration generally indicates a better GFR, a low creatinine concentration may also be caused by decreased muscle mass due to malnutrition or may be increased by overhydration. Furthermore, there is data that indicates that among patients with advanced CKD, serum creatinine is more dependent on muscle mass than kidney function itself. In the only trial that has consistently explored the outcome of advanced CKD patients in relation to the actual kidney function at which they initiated renal replacement treatment, the IDEAL study [15], there was no difference in survival between patients randomly assigned to begin dialysis early (creatinine clearance of 10–14 ml/min) or late (at a creatinine clearance of 5–7 ml/min). It was remarkable that 76 % of patients randomized to the late start group developed uremic symptoms before creatinine clearance reached 7 ml/min and there was a 6-month separation between the groups in the start time of dialysis. An important conclusion of the study is that waiting to initiate dialysis until signs of uremia appear does not necessarily jeopardize the patient and that starting renal replacement therapy

Box 36.2. What Guidelines Say You Should Do: Timing the Initiation of Dialysis

- Dialysis should be initiated when one or more of the following are present: symptoms or signs attributable to kidney failure, inability to control volume status or blood pressure, a progressive deterioration in nutritional status refractory to dietary intervention, or cognitive impairment. This often but not invariably occurs in the GFR range between 5 and 10 ml/min/1.73 m^2.

Source: Kidney Disease: Improving Global Outcomes (KDIGO) CKD Work Group [5]

on the basis of a predefined estimated GFR value does not improve the outcome (Box 36.2).

Box 36.3. What the Guidelines Say You Should Do: Retarding CKD Progression

- Define CKD progression based on one of more of the following: Decline in GFR category (a certain drop in eGFR is defined as a drop in GFR category accompanied by a 25 % or greater drop in eGFR from baseline).
- Rapid progression is defined as a sustained decline in eGFR of more than 5 ml/min/1.73 m^2/year.
- The confidence in assessing progression is increased with increasing number of serum creatinine measurements and duration of follow-up.

Source: Kidney Disease: Improving Global Outcomes (KDIGO) CKD Work Group [5]

36.6 Retarding Initiation of Dialysis

Preparation for dialysis should begin about 4–12 months prior to the anticipated dialysis need if one takes in consideration 1–6 months of iterative CKD education for patients to accept potential need for dialysis and 3–6 months for placement and maturation of dialysis access [12] (Box 36.3). Of note, CKD progression rates can change over time, making it challenging to precisely anticipate the need for dialysis. Complications of advanced CKD such as fluid overload, anemia, hyperkalemia, and acidosis must be approached and treated according to what is written in other chapters of this book.

In certain patients with advanced CKD, the following strategies can defer dialysis initiation:

1. *Prevent drug-induced nephrotoxicity.* Abrupt onset and irreversible acute kidney injury that precipitates end-stage renal disease can occur with the use of nephrotoxic drugs such as non-steroidal anti-inflammatory drugs (NSAIDs), aminoglycosides, contrast dye, diuretics, or others, especially in patients with risk factors (age > 60 years, CKD, volume depletion, heart failure, or sepsis). Selective cyclooxygenase-2 inhibitors have a similar adverse kidney effect in glomerular autoregulation to other NSAIDs. Acetaminophen can be associated with chronic interstitial nephropathy. CKD patients with chronic pain should use alternate agents for pain and avoid NSAIDs as much as possible [16].
2. *Stop inhibitors of the renin-angiotensin system.* In patients with proteinuria <1 g/g and eGFR <20 ml/min/1.73 m^2, stopping angiotensin-converting enzyme inhibitors (ACEi) and/or angiotensin receptor blockers (ARB) may increase eGFR and postpone dialysis initiation for several months. In some patients, this maneuver may increase eGFR up to >50 % from the value at the time of discontinuation of ACEi/ARB, especially in patients >65 years old or those whose kidney function was declining in spite of ACEi/ARB treatment.
3. *Correction of metabolic acidosis.* Patients with serum bicarbonate 16–20 mmol/l on two consecutive measures and controlled blood pressure (<150/90) must receive oral sodium bicarbonate tablets 600 mg thrice daily increased as necessary to achieve and maintain HCO_3 level ≥23 mmol/l. Absence of a deleterious effect on BP despite increased sodium intake has been observed suggesting that sodium salts other than sodium chloride have a negligible effect on BP [17].
4. *Diet.* The benefits of dietary protein restriction to approximately 0.6–0.8 g/kg per day on the

progression of CKD in humans remain controversial, and there is a lack of controlled and randomized studies to support extensive protein restriction. In addition, the use of nutritional supplements with low amounts of protein, phosphorous, and potassium; ketoanalog-supplemented very-low-protein diets; or vegetarian diet might prove to be useful, yet, there is a lack of scientific validated and controlled information supporting them. Dietary restrictions should be considered on an individual case-by-case basis. 2012 KDIGO guidelines suggest the use of a lower, high-quality protein diet of 0.8 g/kg per day among select predialysis patients who are highly motivated to follow such a diet [5]. Patients who are on a protein-restricted diet should be closely monitored, preferably by a dietitian, with follow-up every 2–3 months for adequate caloric intake and evidence of protein malnutrition, which in itself may provide a deleterious environment and an increased risk at dialysis initiation [18]. Given that it has been strongly demonstrated that initiating dialysis with a poor nutritional status is associated with inflammation and higher mortality, it may be questionable to try to delay progression to ESRD for a few months with excessive protein restriction [19].

36.7 Problems in Preventing Urgent Dialysis

The aim of KDIGO 2012 CKD guidelines is to avoid late referral, defined as referral to specialized services less than 1 year before the start of renal replacement therapy. Late referral to a nephrologist is associated with higher morbidity and higher death risk [20]. However, *early referral to a nephrologist is not synonymous of optimal dialysis initiation*. Many patients still initiate dialysis late or suboptimally prepared, despite early referral and care for >12 months by factors such as patient-related delays, acute-on-chronic kidney disease, surgical delays, and late decision-making, among others (Box 36.4). An important limitation to timely referral for proper preparation of a patient before dialysis is the unpredictable, nonlinear, and rapid progression to ESRD triggered by the occurrence of an AKI episode, when it occurs in patients with CKD. This situation may be common among older patients [21]

Box 36.4. What Guidelines Say You Should Do: Early Referral

- Timely referral for planning renal replacement therapy in people with progressive CKD in whom the risk of kidney failure within 1 year is 10–20 % or higher, as determined by validated risk prediction tools, and avoidance of late referral, defined as referral to specialist less than 1 year before start of RRT.
- Patients with progressive CKD should be managed in a multidisciplinary care setting team that should have access to dietary counseling and education and counseling about different renal replacement treatment modalities, transplant options, vascular access surgery, and ethical, psychological, and social care.

Source: Kidney Disease: Improving Global Outcomes (KDIGO) CKD Work Group [5]

36.8 Myths Associated with Dialysis

First PD, after HD. Due to the differences in early and late survival, some have suggested using a "dual-modality" or "integrative-care" approach with initiation of PD, followed by timely transfer to HD. One study showed a survival advantage in a matched-pair analysis of patients who started on PD and were transferred to HD versus patients who started and remained on HD. Yet, another study reported that initial dialysis modality was not a significant predictor of survival after adjusting for age, sex, and primary renal diagnosis. Thus, in the absence of randomized controlled studies, definite recommendations regarding the dialysis modality based on mortality rates cannot be made, even when some data seem to suggest that starting patients on PD might be beneficial. A non-planned change from PD to HD is associated with an increased risk of hospitalization and mortality.

PD is more appropriate for patients with cardiovascular comorbidities providing hemodynamic stability and avoiding rapid fluid shifts that may be harmful to the cardiovascular system. There is evidence provided by some studies that the risk of death is significantly greater in patients on PD, in particular in elderly patients with diabetes, coronary artery disease, and congestive heart failure. We have to consider that some of the previous results could be due at least in part to biased selection. Another explanation is that fluid control is potentially more difficult in PD and fluid overload may be the main cause of death in some of these reports. Nevertheless, it certainly contradicts the expressed opinion that PD is more appropriate for patients with preexisting significant cardiovascular disease.

PD is the preferred dialysis modality in diabetic patients. Initial reports suggested that PD improve survival in diabetic ESRD patients. At present, most studies have concluded that both HD and PD appear to have similar survival in diabetic patients after adjustment of multiple variables [9]. PD has advantages in diabetic patients such as fewer episodes of hypotension during dialysis, avoidance of vascular access complications, home setting, fewer episodes of blood-borne diseases, and fewer episodes of hemorrhagic retinopathy; nevertheless it also has disadvantages that include an increased risk of fluid overload, gain of weight precipitated by continuous glucose absorption (100–300 g of glucose in a conventional DP), and large insulin requirements when hypertonic solutions are used, among others. The majority of these disadvantages can be overcome by adequate care.

Before You Finish: Practice Pearls for the Clinician

- In each clinical visit, a CKD patient should be assessed for progression and risk of dialysis, in particular looking closely to those with eGFR <30 ml/min/1.73 m^2, high blood pressure, type of underlying renal disease (diabetes, APKD, primary glomerular disease), and development of CKD complications.
- The slope of eGFR against time is useful to predict those CKD patients that require dialysis in the next 1–2 years.
- The decision to start dialysis should also include a careful evaluation of symptoms and signs of uremia and other clinical conditions, and not solely eGFR.
- Patients in preparation for dialysis must preserve their veins, and cannulation of veins above the wrist in either upper extremity should be avoided.
- Vascular access should be placed in patients with an eGFR 15–20 ml/min/1.73 m^2 or before, in whom progression to ESRD seems likely. In HD the first option must be AV fistula created 1–4 months before dialysis; in peritoneal dialysis a chronic catheter should be placed approximately 2 weeks before dialysis.
- Retarding initiation of dialysis while a vascular access is created and, before, may be accomplished with appropriate medical care that would include optimal blood pressure control, avoidance of NSAIDs, and other measures, including discontinuing inhibitors of the renin-angiotensin system, correcting metabolic acidosis, and appropriate diet restrictions.
- In spite of early nephrology referral, many patients are not efficiently prepared for a programmed dialysis initiation as multiple factors such as patient-related delays, acute-on-chronic kidney disease, surgical delays, and late decision-making could take place.
- Once renal replacement is needed, most patients can be treated with either PD or HD. The selection of dialysis modality is influenced by a number of considerations, and results of survival studies between HD and PD should not guide patient/physician selection of dialysis modality.

References

1. U.S. Renal Data System. USRDS 2012 annual data report: atlas of chronic kidney disease and end-stage renal disease in the United States. Bethesda: National Institutes of Health, National Institute of Diabetes and Digestive and Kidney Diseases; 2012.
2. Bradbury BD, Fissell RB, Albert JM, Anthony MS, Critchlow CW, Pisoni RL, et al. Predictors of early mortality among incident US hemodialysis patients in the Dialysis Outcomes and Practice Patterns Study (DOPPS). Clin J Am Soc Nephrol. 2007;2(1):89–99.
3. Wingard RL, Pupim LB, Krishnan M, Shintani A, Ikizler TA, Hakim RM. Early intervention improves mortality and hospitalization rates in incident hemodialysis patients: right start program. Clin J Am Soc Nephrol. 2007;2(6):1170–5.
4. Slinin Y, Guo H, Gilbertson DT, Mau LW, Ensrud K, Rector T, et al. Meeting KDOQI guideline goals at hemodialysis initiation and survival during the first year. Clin J Am Soc Nephrol. 2010;5(9):1574–81.
5. Kidney Disease: Improving Global Outcomes (KDIGO) CKD Work Group. KDIGO 2012 clinical practice guideline for the evaluation and management of chronic kidney disease. Kidney Int Suppl. 2013; 3:1–150.
6. Mendelssohn DC, Curtis B, Yeates K, Langlois S, MacRae JM, Semeniuk LM, et al. Suboptimal initiation of dialysis with and without early referral to a nephrologist. Nephrol Dial Transplant. 2011;26(9):2959–65.
7. Correa-Rotter R. The cost barrier to renal replacement therapy and peritoneal dialysis in the developing world. Perit Dial Int. 2001;21 Suppl 3:S314–7.
8. Collins AJ, Hao W, Xia H, Ebben JP, Everson SE, Constantini EG, et al. Mortality risks of peritoneal dialysis and hemodialysis. Am J Kidney Dis. 1999;34(6):1065–74.
9. Jaar BG, Coresh J, Plantinga LC, Fink NE, Klag MJ, Levey AS, et al. Comparing the risk for death with peritoneal dialysis and hemodialysis in a national cohort of patients with chronic kidney disease. Ann Intern Med. 2005;143(3):174–83.
10. Mehrotra R, Chiu YW, Kalantar-Zadeh K, Bargman J, Vonesh E. Similar outcomes with hemodialysis and peritoneal dialysis in patients with end-stage renal disease. Arch Intern Med. 2011;171(2):110–8.
11. KDOQI. Vascular Access 2006 working group. Clinical practice guidelines for vascular access. Am J Kidney Dis 2006;48(Suppl 1):S176–322.
12. Saggi SJ, Allon M, Bernardini J, Kalantar-Zadeh K, Shaffer R, Mehrotra R, Dialysis Advisory Group of the American Society of Nephrology. Considerations in the optimal preparation of patients for dialysis. Nat Rev Nephrol. 2012;8(7):381–9.
13. Figueiredo A, Goh BL, Jenkins S, Johnson DW, Mactier R, Ramalakshmi S, et al. International Society for Peritoneal Dialysis. Clinical practice guidelines for peritoneal access. Perit Dial Int. 2010; 30(4):424–9.
14. Mehrotra R, Kermah D, Fried L, Kalantar-Zadeh K, Khawar O, Norris K, et al. Chronic peritoneal dialysis in the United States: declining utilization despite improving outcomes. J Am Soc Nephrol. 2007; 18(10):2781–8.
15. Cooper BA, Branley P, Bulfone L, Collins JF, Craig JC, Fraenkel MB, et al. A randomized, controlled trial of early versus late initiation of dialysis. N Engl J Med. 2010;363(7):609–19.
16. Naughton CA. Drug-induced nephrotoxicity. Am Fam Physician. 2008;78(6):743–50.
17. de Brito-Ashurst I, Varagunam M, Raftery MJ, Yaqoob MM. Bicarbonate supplementation slows progression of CKD and improves nutritional status. J Am Soc Nephrol. 2009;20(9):2075–84.
18. Brunori G. Treatment of chronic kidney disease in the elderly: diet or conservative management. J Nephrol. 2012;25 Suppl 19:S28–31.
19. Wang AY, Woo J. Early versus late initiation of dialysis and nutrition: does a transition mean a change in dietary protein intake? J Ren Nutr. 2013;23(3): 228–32.
20. Smart NA, Titus TT. Outcomes of early versus late nephrology referral in chronic kidney disease: a systematic review. Am J Med. 2011;124(11):1073–80.
21. Udayaraj UP, Haynes R, Winearls CG. Late presentation of patients with end-stage renal disease for renal replacement therapy–is it always avoidable? Nephrol Dial Transplant. 2011;26(11):3646–51.

Quality of Life in Chronic Kidney Disease

37

Rachael L. Morton and Angela C. Webster

Before You Start: Facts You Need to Know

- Health-related quality of life (HRQoL) relates to the measurement of how disease or treatments impact on a person's sense of subjective well-being.
- HRQoL is best measured using a validated method or 'tool', commonly self-administered questionnaires.
- Generic tools enable comparison with the general population and other groups but may be insensitive to the impact of disease-specific symptoms. Common generic tools are The Medical Outcomes Study Short Form 36 (SF-36) or the EuroQol 5 dimensions (EQ-5D).
- Disease-specific tools are more sensitive to relevant symptoms but cannot be used for comparison with other populations. Common disease-specific tools include Kidney Disease Quality of Life – short form (KDQOL-SF).
- HRQoL declines as a person's GFR declines. Many dialysis patients report an HRQoL equivalent to people dealing with a terminal malignancy, although HRQoL improves but does not normalise after transplantation. CKD impacts HRQoL more profoundly for younger people compared with older people.

37.1 What Is Quality of Life and What Does It Mean for CKD Patients?

Quality of life is a complex construct for which there is no agreed definition. Terms sometimes used to describe closely related constructs include subjective well-being and life satisfaction. The term 'quality of life' when applied to health refers to the effects of the disease or treatments as perceived and reported by the individuals themselves. In the case of chronic kidney disease (CKD), this includes patients, their families and caregivers. To emphasise the focus on health, it is preferable to use the term health-related quality of life (HRQoL) [1] (Box 37.1).

R.L. Morton, MScMed (Clin Epi)(Hons), PhD
Sydney School of Public Health, University of Sydney, Sydney, NSW 2006, Australia

Nuffield Department of Population Health, Health Economics Research Centre, University of Oxford, Headington, Oxfordshire OX3 7LF, UK
e-mail: rachael.morton@sydney.edu.au

A.C. Webster, MBBS, MM (Clin Epid), PhD (✉)
Sydney School of Public Health, University of Sydney, Sydney, NSW 2006, Australia

Centre for Transplant and Renal Research, Westmead Hospital, Sydney, NSW Australia
e-mail: angela.webster@sydney.edu.au

M. Arici (ed.), *Management of Chronic Kidney Disease*,
DOI 10.1007/978-3-642-54637-2_37,

Box 37.1. Glossary of Important HRQoL Terminology

Caregiver	Informal or unpaid family member or close person who provides care for the individual with chronic kidney disease
Domain	A dimension of quality of life, for example, mobility
HRQoL	Health-related quality of life
Instrument	A survey tool or questionnaire for measuring quality of life
Proxy	Someone other than the individual reporting on the individual's quality of life, for example, a doctor or family member
QALY	Quality adjusted life year
QoL	Quality of life
Tool	A survey, questionnaire or technique for measuring quality of life
Utility	A quality of life weighting between 0 (death) and 1 (full health)
Validation	The process by which a data collection instrument is assessed for its dependability. That is, does the instrument produce data that are reliable and true?

A patient's HRQoL is influenced by their lived experience of illness across a broad range of dimensions. These dimensions, often called domains, may include symptoms of CKD and other coexisting illnesses; side effects from treatment; a person's physical functioning, their role; psychological, social, sexual and cognitive functioning; satisfaction with care or unmet needs for information and support services; financial demands; and spiritual well-being (Fig. 37.1).

CKD can affect a patient's HRQoL in many ways. The CKD diagnosis may cause fear, anxiety and depression. Symptoms of CKD such as fluid retention, bone pain, peripheral neuropathy, itch or sleep disturbance as well as side effects from medication or dialysis treatments can all impact negatively on well-being and affect everyday roles and activities. Limitations on everyday activities imposed by CKD, such as fluid or dietary restrictions, and difficulty in travelling or taking holidays for those on dialysis can also affect HRQoL.

Quality of life is of direct importance to patients with CKD, and for some is a more important consideration than length of life [3]. Therefore, the need to balance the benefits and harms of CKD treatments in terms of survival and quality of life provides an important reason for clinicians to assess HRQoL when evaluating the effect of new and established treatments.

37.2 What Is Known About HRQoL in Kidney Disease?

Available literature indicates that HRQoL declines as GFR decreases, particularly in the domains of physical functioning. HRQoL is lower in incident and prevalent dialysis patients compared with the age-matched general population. Although age itself has a significant influence on physical function, older patients report less loss of HRQoL and greater satisfaction with life than do younger patients. On average, HRQoL of dialysis patients is similar to patients dealing with metastatic malignancy and is worse for renal patients with a high symptom burden (Box 37.2). Socio-demographic factors may also influence HRQoL. For patients with end-stage kidney disease (ESKD), treatment with transplantation yields higher HRQoL than dialysis. Considering dialysis modalities, home-based dialysis is associated with higher self-reported HRQoL than hospital-based dialysis [4].

HRQoL is one component of a broader suite of Patient Reported Outcomes Measurements (PROMs) and while symptoms of depression, cognitive impairment or pain are relevant to overall quality of life, HRQoL instruments are not designed to diagnose these clinical conditions. The move towards building healthcare around patient-centred outcomes, and increasing consideration of individual patient preferences, means a good understanding of HRQoL measurement and interpretation is of critical importance in modern nephrology practice.

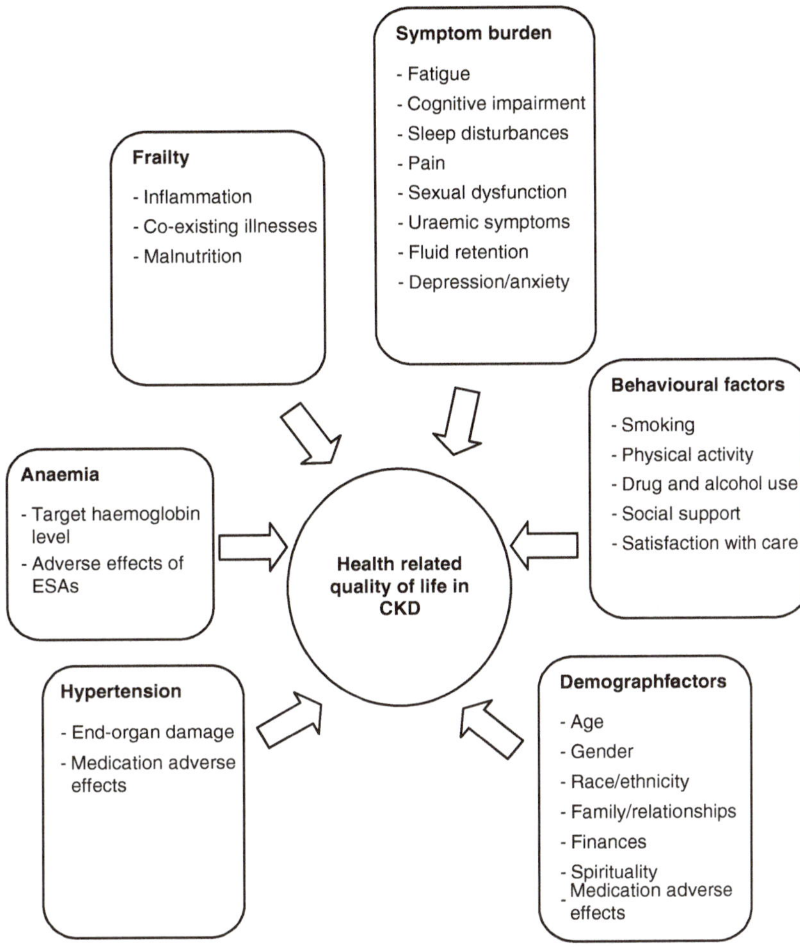

Fig. 37.1 Interaction of factors contributing to diminished HRQoL in CKD (Adapted with permission Soni et al. [2])

Box 37.2. Examples of Mean Health-Related Quality of Life Weights in CKD and in other chronic diseases

Population or health state	Quality of life weight (utility) * [0–1 scale, where 0=death and 1=full health]
CKD stage 3	0.88
Kidney transplant	0.86
CKD stage 4	0.84
CKD stage 5 (pre-dialysis)	0.79
Peritoneal dialysis	0.75
In-centre haemodialysis	0.61
Hospitalised for influenza on haemodialysis	0.50
1 year on haemodialysis	0.49
Distant metastases from breast cancer	0.76
Melanoma stage IV – stable disease	0.65
Metastatic prostate cancer	0.60
Paralysis due to spinal cord injury	0.52
Bed-ridden with pressure ulcers	0.30

Source: Data from the Cost-Effectiveness Analysis Registry – Tufts University (https://research.tufts-nemc.org/cear4/) [5].

37.3 Methods to Assess Quality of Life in CKD

While HRQoL is a subjective phenomenon in that it comprises people's perceptions, the measurement techniques used to assess, analyse and interpret HRQoL are objective. Methods to assess HRQoL include interviews, focus groups or patient diaries; however, in the vast majority of clinical applications, HRQoL is measured by questionnaire. Patients usually self-administer the questionnaire, although there may be circumstances under which a researcher-administered questionnaire is necessary. If an HRQoL questionnaire has been rigorously developed, its constituent questions should have been selected on the basis of literature review and expert or patient opinion. It will also have been subjected to testing of its reliability and validity with the populations of interest (Box 37.3).

37.3.1 Generic Versus Disease-Specific Questionnaires

Questionnaires that measure HRQoL are generally referred to as instruments. Generic instruments enable a broad evaluation of overall health across many domains and are widely used. They are designed for measuring HRQoL in the general population and in doing so allow for comparisons to be made between specific groups, e.g. patients with stage 4 CKD and the general population, or patients and their caregivers (Table 37.1). One of the downsides of generic instruments is that they may be subject to positive or negative bias for particular groups in the population. For example, an instrument with an emphasis on physical functioning may rate a lower HRQoL for a person with spinal injuries than a disease-specific instrument where there is an emphasis on mobility or independence. Similarly a generic instrument may not be sensitive enough to detect a change in HRQoL if the disease-specific symp-

Box 37.3. Reliability, Validity and Responsiveness of HRQoL Instruments

Concept	Definition
Test-retest reliability	The correlation between responses to the same questions or items administered to the same respondents at different times
Inter-rater reliability	The correlation between responses to the same items obtained by different observers, raters or interviewers (relevant for proxy-administered questionnaires)
Internal consistency reliability	The extent to which items in a commonly accepted scale measure the same concept (often measured with Cronbach's alpha)
Content validity	The extent to which an instrument includes domains relevant to the population or study
Construct validity	Involves specifying constructs that account for variance in a proposed measure and satisfy hypothesised relationships among constructs. The agreement there is between different measures meant to measure the same concept (convergent validity) and the more they differ from those intended to measure other concepts (discriminant validity)
Criterion validity	The extent to which the measurement correlates with an external assessment, such as a previously validated measure or gold standard, for example, Karnofsky Performance Status or the Beck Depression Inventory
Responsiveness	The sensitivity of the instrument to detect changes in a patient's clinical condition

Table 37.1 Summary of generic HRQoL instruments commonly used in people with CKD

Name of instrument	Developed by and for whom	Validated in	Time to complete	Domains covered	Number of questions or items	Can be converted to utility?	Where do I get it?
Short Form 36 Health Survey (SF-36)	Medical Outcomes Study for HRQoL in the general population	General population and used extensively in CKD	20 min	8 (physical functioning, role – physical, bodily pain, general health, vitality, social functioning, role –emotional, mental health)	36	Not directly – but an algorithm is available to transform SF-36 scores into utilities	www.qualitymetric.com
SF-12	Rand Corporation as a shorter version of the SF-36	General population and used in CKD	5 min	8 (physical functioning, role – physical, bodily pain, general health, vitality, social functioning, role –emotional, mental health)	12	Yes – the SF-6D provides a means for using the SF-12 data by estimating a preference-based single index measure using general population values	www.qualitymetric.com http://www.shef.ac.uk/scharr/sections/heds/mvh/sf-6d
EQ-5D	EuroQol organisation for a generic instrument that describes and values HRQoL	General population with population norms from most high income countries	5 min	5 (mobility, self-care, usual activities, pain/discomfort, anxiety/depression)	5 plus a visual analogue scale	Yes – specifically recommended for NICE submissions in the UK	www.euroquol.org
Sickness Impact Profile (SIP)	Johns Hopkins University to provide a descriptive profile of changes in a person's behaviour due to sickness	General population with any disease or illness	30 min	12 (sleep and rest, eating, work, home management, recreation and pastimes, ambulation, mobility, body care and movement, social interaction, alertness behaviour, emotional behaviour and communication)	136 – or a shorter version with 68 questions	No	http://www.mapi-trust.org/

tom or condition is not included. An example of this is the inability of an instrument with no domains for visual acuity to measure the impact of reduced vision in a population of patients with diabetic retinopathy.

The alternatives to generic instruments are disease-specific instruments. These are designed for patients with a specific disease, for patients with specific symptoms or for those undergoing a particular intervention – such as dialysis (Table 37.2). These instruments detect subtle changes in common CKD symptoms such as fatigue or pruritus if these dimensions are explicitly included. A major downside of disease-specific instruments is that they do not allow comparisons between groups, i.e. those with and those without the disease and/or between people managed with different treatment modalities, e.g. dialysis versus transplantation (Table 37.2).

Table 37.2 Summary of disease-specific HRQoL instruments commonly used in CKD

Name of instrument	Developed by and for whom	Validated in	Time to complete (min)	Domains covered	Number of questions or items	Where do I get it?
KDQ	University of Western Ontario, Canada for haemodialysis patients	Haemodialysis patients	10–15	5 (physical symptoms, fatigue, depression, relationships with others, frustration)	26	Not routinely used
Kidney Disease Quality Of Life – Long Form (KDQOL-LF)	Kidney Disease Quality of Life Working Group for patients on dialysis	Haemodialysis patients	30	Includes the SF-36 plus 8 kidney-specific domains: Symptoms and problems, effects of kidney disease, sleep quality, burden of kidney disease, cognitive function, social support, dialysis staff, encouragement and patient satisfaction	134	www.rand.org
Kidney Disease Quality Of Life – Short Form (KDQOL-SF)	A shortened version of the KDQOL-LF developed by the RAND corporation	Haemodialysis patients	20	General HRQoL including the SF-36 plus 8 kidney-specific domains: Symptoms and problems, effects of kidney disease, sleep quality, burden of kidney disease, cognitive function, social support, dialysis staff encouragement and patient satisfaction	80	www.rand.org
KDQOL™-36	RAND corporation	Haemodialysis or peritoneal dialysis patients	10–15	General HRQoL including the SF-12 instrument and 3 kidney-specific domains: burden of kidney disease, symptoms/problems, effects of kidney disease	36	www.rand.org

37.3.2 Utility-Based Quality of Life

Economic evaluations and cost-effectiveness studies of treatments in CKD often require the health outcome to be reported in quality-adjusted life years (QALYs). QALYs are a standard metric which combines the length of life with the quality of life. The quality of life is weighted in this calculation and when used in this circumstance is called a utility. Utilities are based on individuals' preferences for different health states – thereby a more desirable health state receives a greater weight. HRQoL utilities are measured on a scale ranging from 0 to 1, where 0 indicates the state 'dead' and 1 indicates 'full health'. Valuations of different health states on the 0–1 scale are available from large surveys of the general population in many countries (Table 37.3).

37.4 What Quality of Life Measure Should I Use?

The choice of HRQoL instrument will depend on your objectives (e.g. for research or for following patients), the patient population you are working with, the treatments involved and their potential side effects and the resources available. For some measurement needs, there may not be one ideal tool – you may need to use a complementary set of instruments. If feasible, pairing a generic and a disease-specific questionnaire is recommended. For any economic evaluation, a utility-based quality of life instrument should be used [4]. There are numerous HRQoL instruments available; therefore, taking the time to choose the right measure at the outset can make all the difference between negative and positive findings. It is always a good idea to get copies of the actual questionnaire so you can see exactly how the domains are covered and what you will be asking your participants to consider.

The best instruments are ones that have been validated in your population of interest and have a track record in research with objectives and treatments similar to your own study. The chosen instrument should also have face validity for the patient. Face validity means including questions that are both appropriate and meaningful for your patient context (Tables 37.1, 37.2 and 37.3; Box 37.3).

37.5 Measuring HRQoL in Special CKD Groups: End-of-Life Care for the Elderly and Caregivers

37.5.1 The Elderly and End-of-Life Care

Elderly patients often have multiple coexisting diseases such as ischaemic heart disease, diabetes, peripheral vascular disease or cancer which result in additional decrements in HRQoL. The initiation of dialysis therapies in elderly ESKD patients is often associated with decreased quality of life, increased hospitalisation and functional decline. Similarly, elderly patients managed on a conservative non-dialytic pathway may also lose HRQoL with symptoms of dyspnoea, pain and lack of energy. The goal of care at the end of life is to achieve as good a quality of life for the patient as possible, and good communication as well as proactive management of symptoms are required. There is a growing body of literature in nephrology and palliative care about practical methods to manage symptoms for ESKD patients at their end of life. Assessment of HRQoL in the elderly and palliative population requires a modified approach taking into account the illness of respondents and the particular domains of interest or importance such as spirituality and pain management. The SF-36 and the EQ-5D have been used to assess HRQoL in this population; however, newer instruments such as the ICECAP-SCM (supportive care measure) may be more sensitive to the well-being and quality-of-life needs of this population [6].

37.5.2 Caregivers

To date, the quality of life of informal caregivers of patients with CKD has rarely been targeted for intervention or measured in clinical trials. However, it is of special interest where the goal of intervention is to improve chronic care service provision such as respite for partners of home dialysis patients rather than change the severity of illness of the patient [7]. Caregivers of elderly patients on dialysis report decreased quality of life, and a substantial number also have signs of depression.

Table 37.3 Summary of utility-based instruments for use in health economic evaluations commonly used in people with CKD

Name of instrument	Instrument type	Developed by	Population valuation weights (tariffs)	Time to complete (min)	Domains covered	Number of questions or items	Where do I get it?
EQ-5D	Multi-attribute	EuroQol	UK, USA, most European countries, Australia/New Zealand	5	5 (mobility, self-care, usual activities, pain/discomfort, anxiety/depression)	5 each with 3 or 5 levels plus a visual analogue scale	www.euroquol.org
SF-6D	Multi-attribute	University of Sheffield, UK	UK	5	12 (need to complete the SF-12 questionnaire)	12	www.qualitymetric.com http://www.shef.ac.uk/scharr/sections/heds/mvh/sf-6d
Health utilities Index (HUI) version 2 or 3)	Multi-attribute	Health Utilities Index, Inc	Canada, UK	8–10	9 (vision, hearing, speech, ambulation/mobility, pain, dexterity, self-care, emotion and cognition)	15	http://www.healthutilities.com/
Assessment of Quality of Life (AQOL) version 4D, 6D, 7D or 8D	Multi-attribute	Monash University, Australia	Australia	Dependent on version: 2–6	Dependent on version (4–8 including independent living, happiness, mental health, coping, relationships, self worth, pain, senses)	Dependent on version (12–35 questions)	http://www.aqol.com.au/
Time Trade-Off (TTO)	Preference-based measure: (trading time in different health states)	Mc Master University, Canada	Not applicable	Dependent on number of time preference questions: usually 10–15	To be determined by the investigator as the time to be traded and health states are context specific	Usually 5–15 questions	Example: http://www.healthstrategy.com/tto/tto.html
Standard Gamble (SG)	Preference-based measure: (trading risk of death with time in a particular health state)	Mc Master University, Canada	Not applicable	Dependent on number of risk preference questions: usually 10–15	To be determined by the investigator as the risk of each health state is context specific	Usually 5–15 questions	Example: http://www.healthstrategy.com/sg/sg.html#anchor

More research is needed to examine potential relationships between caregivers' quality of life and how this impacts upon the quality of care they offer and the HRQoL of the people with CKD they care for. Where the quality of life of caregivers has been measured, this has generally been done using generic questionnaires designed for measuring HRQoL in the general population (e.g. the SF-36) [8]. While this approach allows results for caregivers to be compared with those for other groups, generic measures are unlikely to cover areas that are of special importance to caregivers – for example, burden of care, feelings of guilt, financial concerns and family responsibility and support. In addition, such measures may not distinguish between impacts related to the health of the person with CKD being cared for and the health of the caregiver themselves – many of whom may also be suffering from chronic illness.

37.6 Detailed Review of Most Common Instruments Used to Assess HRQoL in CKD

The Medical Outcomes Study Short Form 36 (SF-36) is the most widely used generic QOL instrument for CKD patients, their caregivers and the general population. The SF-36 v 2.0 contains 36 items and covers eight domains including physical functioning, role functioning (physical), bodily pain, general health, vitality, social functioning, role functioning (emotional) and mental health. Each domain score is transformed onto a 0–100 scale and two summary scores are calculated: the physical summary score and the mental summary score. Norms for the general population in many countries are available to enable comparisons. This instrument takes about 10 min to complete and is available in several languages and many modes of administration (e.g. paper based, online or on a tablet). Despite no specific validation of this instrument in the CKD population, numerous studies have been published using this instrument [9].

The Short Form 12 (SF-12) v2.0 is a more recent shortened version of the SF-36 instrument discussed above. It contains 12 questions to measure physical and mental health covering the eight domains in the SF-36. The instrument uses norm-based scoring that enables comparisons with the general population. One advantage of this instrument is that the responses can also be transformed into the SF-6D, a utility-based instrument for use in economic evaluations [10]. Additionally, the SF-12 is a short one-page questionnaire that takes 2–3 min to complete.

The Sickness Impact Profile measures global health status (sleep and work, eating, rest, recreation and pastimes, home management) and physical and psychosocial health domains. According to an extensive review in CKD [11], the Sickness Impact Profile shows good evidence of both reliability and validity in the ESKD population.

The EuroQol 5 dimensions (EQ-5D) is a generic instrument developed in Europe and is widely used around the world. It contains five domains: mobility, self-care, usual activities, pain/discomfort and anxiety/depression. Originally containing three response levels per domain, it has recently been updated with five response levels (no problems, slight problems, moderate problems, severe problems and extreme problems) [12]. The EQ-5D also contains a visual analogue scale (VAS). The EQ VAS records the respondent's self-rated health on a vertical, thermometer-like visual analogue scale where the endpoints are labelled 'Best imaginable health state' and 'Worst imaginable health state'. The patient's score is used as a quantitative measure of health outcome as judged by the individual respondent. Advantages of the EQ-5D are its ease of completion, availability in many languages and ability for the scores to be transformed into utilities for economic evaluation.

An example of a disease-specific HRQoL instrument is the Kidney Disease Quality of Life – short form (KDQOL-SF) instrument. It includes questions from the SF-36, plus an additional 43 items specific to kidney disease. The kidney-disease-specific questions include but are not limited to burden on the family; CKD symptoms such as cramps, pruritus, dry skin and shortness of breath; dialysis access; fluid restriction; and ability to travel. A shorter version of this instrument called the KDQOL-36 is also available, which contains the same items as in the generic SF-12 along with an additional 24 questions that are kidney-disease-specific. Many dialysis centres in the USA use the KDQOL-36 as the preferred measurement tool for its ease of administration and report relatively minimal patient and staff burden.

37.7 What Should I Do to Improve HRQoL for My Patients?

Listed below are examples of interventions to improve quality of life in patients with CKD (Table 37.4) and a summary of relevant clinical practice guidelines in nephrology (Table 37.5).

Table 37.4 Summary of suggested interventions that show improved HRQoL in CKD in research studies

Intervention	Source of evidence (ungraded)
Provide information and education to meet patient/family needs	1 Randomised controlled trial and several observational and qualitative studies
Cognitive behavioural therapy and/or group psychosocial intervention	2 Randomised controlled trials
Erythropoietin to correct anaemia	Several large randomised controlled trials and cohort studies
Structured exercise programmes	5 Randomised controlled trials
Treatment of depression – e.g. antidepressant medication	3 Cohort studies
Treatment of sleep disturbance/sleep apnoea	1 Randomised controlled trial and several observational studies
Improved pain management	1 Randomised controlled trial and 2 cohort studies
Treatment of sexual dysfunction	15 Randomised controlled trials
Improve patient satisfaction with CKD service provision	1 Cohort study
Nutritional counselling (pre-dialysis)	1 Randomised controlled trial
Financial assistance	Few observational and qualitative studies
Home dialysis modality	4 Longitudinal cohort studies, several cross-sectional studies
Frequent or extended hours haemodialysis	1 Randomised controlled trial, several observational cohort studies
Respite care	2 Cohort studies
Support for travel/vacations	Several qualitative studies
Kidney or kidney/pancreas transplantation	Several cohort studies

Table 37.5 What the guidelines say you should do: HRQoL

Guideline group[a]	Guideline	HRQoL context
Kidney Disease: Improving Global Outcomes (KDIGO)	Diagnosis, Evaluation, Prevention, and Treatment of Chronic Kidney Disease-Mineral and Bone Disorder (CKD-MBD)	The gastrointestinal side effects and high pill burden required to achieve normal serum phosphorus may lead to reduction in HRQoL. There is no good evidence that vitamin D, calcitriol, vitamin D analogues or calcimimetics improve HRQoL
Caring for Australasians with Renal Impairment (CARI)	Water and fluid in pre-dialysis patients	Sodium and water retention reduces HRQoL due to nocturnal dyspnoea and fluid overload

Table 37.5 (continued)

Guideline group[a]	Guideline	HRQoL context
	Duration and frequency of haemodialysis therapy	'…Blood pressure control and quality of life improved with more frequent, shorter dialysis. Patients acted as their own controls, and total weekly Kt/V was kept constant. Blood pressure control and quality of life both improved'.
		'In a cohort of 83 patients, patient survival was 81 % over 5 years. Compared with short thrice-weekly dialysis, nocturnal dialysis is associated with improved salt and water control, increased solute removal, improved calcium and phosphate control, and a marked improvement in quality of life'.
	Pre-dialysis education	'Multi-disciplinary clinics and [structured pre-dialysis] education programmes may facilitate the improved medical care of patients (for example, better control of anaemia and hypertension), greater patient involvement in the selection of the mode of dialysis, a reduction in the need for 'urgent start' dialysis, and improve short-term survival and quality of life after the initiation of dialysis'.
	Level of renal function at which to initiate dialysis	'Compared with patients who have timely initiation, the health-related quality of life among late starters was worse during the first 6 months after initiation, but no different at 12 months'.
	Timing of referral of chronic kidney disease patients to nephrology services (adult).	'A planned first dialysis resulted in a higher QoL in the first 6 months than a late start dialysis'.
	Acceptance onto dialysis – ethical considerations	'An expectation of survival with an acceptable quality of life is a useful starting point for recommending dialysis'.
		'The possibility that length or quality of life will not be improved by dialysis may be a relevant factor for patients and caregivers in making decisions about whether or not to start dialysis'.
	Acceptance onto dialysis – quality of life	Suggestion for clinical care (based on level III and IV evidence). A discussion of the effect of dialysis on quality of life (QOL) should be included in the decision-making process for undertaking dialysis treatment. The discussion should include effect on physical function, burden of treatment and effect on family and social life. This is best accomplished by a multidisciplinary team of appropriate health professionals
		Age alone should not be interpreted as being predictive of poorer QoL
		Poorer physical and mental health should be considered predictive of poorer QoL on dialysis
		No single QoL measure should be used to recommend acceptance or denial of dialysis
Canadian Society of Nephrology (CSN)	Use of erythropoietic stimulating agents	Anaemia is associated with reduction in QoL
European Renal Best Practice (ERBP)	Antidepressants for depression in stage 3–5 chronic kidney disease: a systematic review of pharmacokinetics, efficacy and safety	'In line with the current treatment guidelines, the high prevalence of depression in patients with CKD3-5 and its negative influence on survival and quality of life, active intervention seems justified'. Intervention – treatment with antidepressants

(continued)

Table 37.5 (continued)

Guideline group[a]	Guideline	HRQoL context
Renal Physicians Association (US)	Shared decision-making in the appropriate initiation of and withdrawal from dialysis	'Patients whose prognosis is particularly poor should be informed that dialysis may not confer a survival advantage or improve functional status over medical management without dialysis and that dialysis entails significant burdens that may detract from their quality of life'.
		Providing effective palliative care: 'To improve patient-centred outcomes, offer palliative care services and interventions to all AKI, CKD, and ESRD patients who suffer from burdens of their disease'.
Renal Association (UK)		*End-of-life care*: Conservative kidney management and withdrawal of dialysis – 'Quality of life for patients following a conservative pathway may be comparable to that in haemodialysis patients, though data are very limited'.
National Institute for Health and Care Excellence (NICE)	Assessment and optimisation of erythropoiesis	*Benefits of treatment with erythropoiesis stimulating agents (ESAs)*: 'Treatment with ESAs should be offered to people with anaemia of CKD who are likely to benefit in terms of quality of life and physical function'.
Australia and New Zealand Society of Nephrology (ANZSN)	Renal Supportive Care Guidelines 2013 – Quality of life	What constitutes a poor QOL of life varies from person to person and the potential impact of dialysis on an individual will be unique for each person
		Patients need good information in order to allow them to assess the potential impact of renal replacement therapy on their lives
		The Short Form 36 Health Survey (SF-36) QOL questionnaire is a suitable tool to be used in dialysis and non-dialysis patients to assess QOL changes

[a]*Links to guidelines*: *KDIGO*=www.kdigo.org/, *CARI*=http://www.cari.org.au/guidelines.php, *CSN*=http://csnscn.ca, *ERBP*=http://www.european-renal-best-practice.org/, *Renal Physicians Association* (*USA*)=http://www.renalmd.org/End-Stage-Renal-Disease/, *Renal Association* (*UK*)=http://www.renal.org/clinical/guidelinessection/guidelines.aspx, *ISPD*=http://ispd.org/lang-en/treatmentguidelines/guidelines, *NICE*=http://www.nice.org.uk/guidance/index.jsp?action=byType&type=2&status=3, *ANZSN*=http://onlinelibrary.wiley.com/doi/10.1111/nep.12065/pd

Before You Finish: Practice Pearls for the Clinician

- A good understanding of HRQoL measurement and interpretation is of critical importance for decision-making in modern nephrology practice. Known HRQoL estimates can be used to help patients understand the likely impact of their disease, its progression and potential treatment interventions and can help clinicians and researchers better appreciate the impact of disease and treatments in different patient groups.
- HRQoL measurement can also inform understanding of new research findings. CKD results in considerable decrement to HRQoL, which varies by stage and renal replacement therapy. Although HRQoL for different health states may be reported as an average across patient groups, it is important to understand that each patient's experience will be unique, and some side effects or interventions may impact different people to different extents.
- While several clinical practice guidelines make reference to HRQoL, there is no specific guideline focussing on HRQoL improvement. However, there is some evidence that interventions targeting specific symptoms or aimed at supporting educational or lifestyle considerations do make a positive difference to people living with CKD.

References

1. Guyatt GH, Feeny DH, Patrick DL. Measuring health-related quality of life. Ann Intern Med. 1993;118(8):622–8.
2. Soni RK, Weisbord SD, Unruh ML. Health-related quality of life outcomes in chronic kidney disease. Curr Opin Nephrol Hypertens. 2010;19(2):153–9.
3. Morton RL, Tong A, Howard K, Snelling P, Webster AC. The views of patients and carers in treatment decision making for chronic kidney disease: systematic review and thematic synthesis of qualitative studies. BMJ. 2010;340:c112.
4. Wyld M, Morton RL, Hayen A, Howard K, Webster AC. A systematic review and meta-analysis of utility-based quality of life in chronic kidney disease treatments. PLoS Med. 2012;9(9):e1001307.
5. Tufts Medical Centre. Cost-effectiveness analysis registry [internet]. c2013 [Cited 2013 July 25]. Available at: https://research.tufts-nemc.org/cear4/.
6. Sutton E CJ. ICECAP Supportive care measure EconEndLife project [internet]. Birmingham: University of Birmingham; c2013 [Cited 2013 July 25]. Available at: http://www.birmingham.ac.uk/research/activity/mds/projects/HaPS/HE/ICECAP/ICECAP-SCM/index.aspx.
7. Sulch D, Kalra L. Quality of life of caregivers. In: Carr AJ, Higginson IJ, Robinson PG, editors. Quality of life. London: BMJ Books; 2003. p. 31–9.
8. Ware Jr JE, Sherbourne CD. The MOS 36-item short-form health survey (SF-36). Conceptual framework and item selection. Med Care. 1992;30(6):473–83.
9. Liem YS, Bosch JL, Arends LR, Heijenbrok-Kal MH, Hunink MGM. Quality of life assessed with the Medical Outcomes Study Short Form 36-Item Health Survey of patients on renal replacement therapy: a systematic review and meta-analysis. Value Health. 2007;10(5):390–7.
10. Brazier J, Roberts J, Deverill M. The estimation of a preference-based measure of health from the SF-36. J Health Econ. 2002;21(2):271–92.
11. Cagney KA, Wu AW, Fink NE, Jenckes MW, Meyer KB, Bass EB, et al. Formal literature review of quality-of-life instruments used in end-stage renal disease. Am J Kidney Dis. 2000;36(2):327–36.
12. Rabin R, de Charro F. EQ-5D: a measure of health status from the EuroQol Group. Ann Med. 2001;33(5):337–43.

Index

M. Arici (ed.), *Management of Chronic Kidney Disease*,
DOI 10.1007/978-3-642-54637-2, © Springer-Verlag Berlin Heidelberg 2014

Q

R

S

FSC
www.fsc.org
MIX
Papier | Fördert gute Waldnutzung
FSC® C083411

Kolibri 360 GmbH
Ferdinand-Jühlke-Straße 7
99095 Erfurt, Deutschland
produktsicherheit@kolibri360.de